Exercise Physiology
for Health and Sports Performance

Visit the **Exercise Physiology for Health and Sports Performance** Companion Website at **www.pearsoned.co.uk/draper** to find valuable student learning material including:

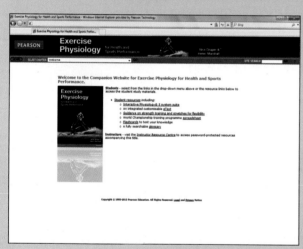

- Interactive Physiology® 5-system suite
- An integrated customisable eText
- Guidance on strength training and stretches for flexibility
- World Championship training programme spreadsheet
- Flashcards to test your knowledge
- A fully searchable glossary

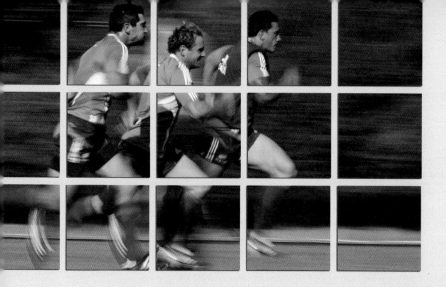

Exercise Physiology
for Health and Sports Performance

Nick Draper and
Helen Marshall

PEARSON

Harlow, England • London • New York • Boston • San Francisco • Toronto • Sydney • Auckland • Singapore • Hong Kong
Tokyo • Seoul • Taipei • New Delhi • Cape Town • São Paulo • Mexico City • Madrid • Amsterdam • Munich • Paris • Milan

PEARSON EDUCATION LIMITED
Edinburgh Gate
Harlow CM20 2JE
Tel: +44 (0)1279 623623
Fax: +44 (0)1279 431059
Website: www.pearson.com/uk

First published 2013 (print and electronic)

ISBN: 978-0-273-75562-3 (print)
      978-0-273-75564-7 (PDF)
      978-0-273-77868-4 (eText)

British Library Cataloguing-in-Publication Data
A catalogue record for this book is available from the British Library

Library of Congress Cataloguing-in-Publication Data
Draper, Nick (Nicholas)
  Exercise physiology for health and sports performance / Nick Draper and Helen Marshall.
      p. ; cm.
  Includes bibliographical references and index.
  ISBN 978-0-273-75562-3
  I. Marshall, Helen, 1976- II. Title.
  [DNLM: 1. Athletic Performance–physiology. 2. Exercise–physiology. QT 260]

  612.7'6-dc23

                                                      2012016028

10 9 8 7 6 5 4 3 2 1
16 15 14 13 12

Front cover image © Getty Images

Print edition typeset in 9.75/13 pt Minion Pro by 73
Print edition printed and bound in by Grafos SA, Barcelona, Spain

NOTE THAT ANY PAGE CROSS REFERENCES REFER TO THE PRINT EDITION

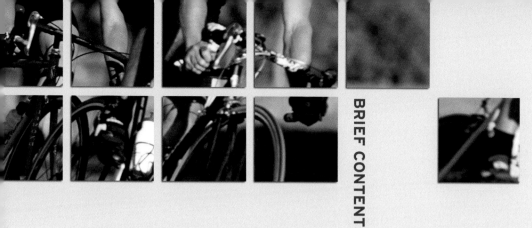

BRIEF CONTENTS

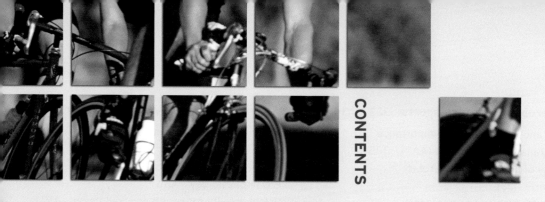

Contents

Supporting resources

Visit **www.pearsoned.co.uk/draper** to find valuable online resources

Companion Website for students

- Interactive Physiology® 5-system suite
- An integrated customisable eText
- Guidance on strength training and stretches for flexibility
- World Championship training programme spreadsheet
- Flashcards to test your knowledge
- A fully searchable glossary

For instructors

- PowerPoint slides containing all the figures from the book

Also:

The Companion Website provides the following features:

- Search tool to help locate specific items of content
- Online help and support to assist with website usage and troubleshooting

For more information, please contact your local Pearson Education sales representative or visit **www.pearsoned.co.uk/draper**

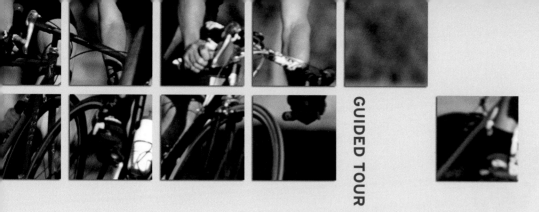

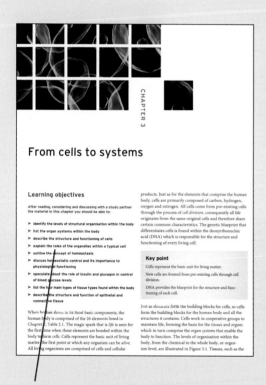

CHAPTER 3

From cells to systems

Learning objectives

After reading, considering and discussing with a study partner the material in this chapter you should be able to:

➤ identify the levels of structural organisation within the body

➤ list the organ systems within the body

➤ describe the structure and functioning of cells

➤ explain the roles of the organelles within a typical cell

➤ outline the concept of homeostasis

➤ discuss homeostatic control and its importance to physiological functioning

➤ speculate about the role of insulin and glucagon in control of blood glucose levels

➤ list the four main types of tissue types found within the body

➤ describe the structure and function of epithelial and connective tissue

When broken down to its most basic components, the human body is comprised of the 26 elements listed in Chapter 2, Table 2.1. The magic spark that is *life* is seen for the first time when these elements are bonded within the body to form *cells*. Cells represent the basic unit of living matter, the first point at which any organism can be *alive*. All living organisms are comprised of cells and cellular products. Just as for the elements that comprise the human body, cells are primarily composed of carbon, hydrogen, oxygen and nitrogen. All cells come from pre-existing cells through the process of *cell division*, consequently all life originates from the same original cells and therefore share certain common characteristics. The genetic blueprint that differentiates cells is found within the deoxyribonucleic acid (DNA) which is responsible for the structure and functioning of every living cell.

Key point

Cells represent the basic unit for living matter.

New cells are formed from pre-existing cells through cell division.

DNA provides the blueprint for the structure and functioning of each cell.

Just as elements form the building blocks for cells, so cells form the building blocks for the human body and all the structures it contains. Cells work in cooperative groups to maintain life, forming the basis for the *tissues* and *organs* which in turn comprise the *organ systems* that enable the body to function. The levels of organisation within the body, from the chemical to the whole body, or organism level, are illustrated in Figure 3.1. Tissues, such as the

---

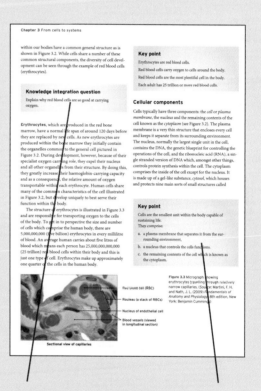

within our bodies have a common general structure as is shown in Figure 3.2. While cells share a number of these common structural components, the diversity of cell development can be seen through the example of red blood cells (erythrocytes).

Knowledge integration question

Explain why red blood cells are so good at carrying oxygen.

Erythrocytes, which are produced in the red bone marrow, have a normal life span of around 120 days before they are replaced by new cells. As new erythrocytes are produced within the bone marrow they initially contain the organelles common to the general cell pictured in Figure 3.2. During development, however, because of their specialist oxygen carrying role, they expel their nucleus and all other organelles from their structure. By doing this, they greatly increase their haemoglobin-carrying capacity and as a consequence, the relative amount of oxygen transportable within each erythrocyte. Human cells share many of the common characteristics of the cell illustrated in Figure 3.2, but develop uniquely to best serve their function within the body.

The structure of erythrocytes is illustrated in Figure 3.3 and are responsible for transporting oxygen to the cells of the body. To get in to perspective the size and number of cells which comprise the human body, there are 5,000,000,000 (five billion) erythrocytes in every millilitre of blood. An average human carries about five litres of blood which means each person has 25,000,000,000,000 (25 trillion) red blood cells within their body and this is just one type of cell. Erythrocytes make up approximately one quarter of the cells in the human body.

Key point

Erythrocytes are red blood cells.

Red blood cells carry oxygen to cells around the body.

Red blood cells are the most plentiful cell in the body.

Each adult has 25 trillion or more red blood cells.

Cellular components

Cells typically have three components: the *cell or plasma membrane*, the *nucleus* and the remaining contents of the cell known as the *cytoplasm* (see Figure 3.2). The plasma membrane is a very thin structure that encloses every cell and keeps it separate from its surrounding environment. The nucleus, normally the largest single unit in the cell, contains the DNA, the genetic blueprint for controlling the operations of the cell, and the ribonucleic acid (RNA), a single stranded version of DNA which, amongst other things, controls protein synthesis within the cell. The cytoplasm comprises the inside of the cell except for the nucleus. It is made up of a gel-like substance, *cytosol*, which houses and protects nine main sorts of small structures called

Key point

Cells are the smallest unit within the body capable of sustaining life.
They comprise:

a. a plasma membrane that separates it from the surrounding environment,

b. a nucleus that controls the cells functions,

c. the remaining contents of the cell which is known as the cytoplasm.

Red blood cell (RBC)

Rouleau (a stack of RBCs)

Nucleus of endothelial cell

Blood vessels (viewed in longitudinal section)

Sectional view of capillaries

Figure 3.3 Micrograph showing erythrocytes travelling through relatively narrow capillaries. (Source: Martini, F. H. and Nath, J. L. (2009) *Fundamentals of Anatomy and Physiology*, 8th edition, New York: Benjamin Cummings)

Learning objectives introduce topics covered and help you to focus on what you should have learnt by the end of the chapter, either individually or with a study partner.

Knowledge integration questions and **Key points** appear frequently throughout the text to develop and consolidate your learning.

Guided tour

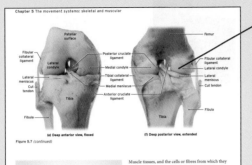

(e) Deep anterior view, flexed

(f) Deep posterior view, extended

Figure 5.7 (continued)

Numerous **full colour photos** and diagrams illustrate the text and enhance the learning experience.

Key point
The muscular system requires the skeletal system to produce the leverage necessary to bring about movement of the body.

5.2 The muscular system

The skeletal and muscular systems are interrelated and are often known together as the **musculoskeletal system**. The attachment of muscles, across joints, to the bones of the skeleton allows for the movement of body parts upon muscle contraction. In addition to the importance for sports performance, a healthy musculoskeletal system helps to maintain a high quality of life, allowing us to complete our everyday tasks. This section of the chapter covers the different types of muscle tissue before focusing on the structure and function of skeletal muscle.

 Try **Interactive Physiology:**
Muscular

Muscle tissue types and functions

Three types of muscle tissue can be found within the body: smooth, cardiac and skeletal muscle (Figure 5.8).

Muscle tissues, and the cells or fibres from which they are formed, are responsible for bringing about movement, whether it be movement of the body for playing sport, circulation of blood and nutrients around the body or the propulsion of foods through the digestive tract. The structure of each muscle tissue type differs according to its function. **Smooth muscle** is found throughout the body. It surrounds the blood vessels and airways and serves to assist with the passage of blood and air through the cardiovascular and respiratory systems. It is also part of the digestive tract walls where its contractions assist the movement of food along it. Smooth muscle, in common with cardiac muscle, is innervated by the autonomic nervous system and so we have little or no voluntary control over the contraction of these muscle groups. We cannot make the heart beat faster or push food through the digestive tract more quickly. **Cardiac muscle**, the muscle which forms the heart, is responsible for our heart beat and the subsequent pumping of blood and nutrients around the body. **Skeletal muscle** is the only muscle type that can be voluntarily contracted and is the form of tissue that enables bodily movement by contracting against the skeleton (hence the name). The human body is comprised of between 600 and 700 muscles which vary in size from 1 mm (such as those found attached to the bones of the ear) to 30 cm long in the sartorius muscle of the thigh.

120

The text links to a Premium Website which contains your annotatable eText along with Pearson's **Interactive Physiology**®5-System suite of online resources to provide interactive examples of points developed in the text.

---

aerobic capacity gains to traditional ET exercise prescription, but with a significant time saving for the SIT group. There were also significant improvements in sub-maximal exercise response (V O₂ and HR), resting blood pressure and waist circumferences, again with no statistical differences between the groups. These results indicated that (a) HIIT and SIT can provide similar reductions in health risk factors and improvements in aerobic endurance ability compared to ET in a real-world setting and (b) SIT can provide a time-efficient method of exercise for improving health and fitness. The results of the study also indicated that the increased intensity for the SIT group, along with the increased loading on the body associated with ascending and descending a slope, resulted in an increased injury incidence when compared with HIIT and ET. Consequently, researchers and health professionals involved in exercise prescription should consider the use of reduced or non-weight bearing exercise for a SIT intervention to decrease the potential risk of injury. Results from each of the studies, however, support the notion that HIIT training has the potential to provide a useful, time-saving alternative for improving health and fitness to traditional endurance training.

Knowledge integration question
What is the physiological justification of prescribing high-intensity interval training for health benefits?

Check your recall
Fill in the missing words.

➤ Delayed onset muscle soreness may occur _____ to _____ days following exercise, particularly if _____ contractions have been involved in the activity.

➤ The mechanisms responsible for DOMS are thought to be micro-trauma to the muscle fibres and _____.

➤ The most common treatments of muscular cramp are _____ and the replacement of fluid and _____.

➤ The risk of developing obesity, diabetes mellitus and cardiovascular disease can be reduced through the participation in regular _____.

➤ Many sedentary individuals cite '_____ _____' as a reason for their physical inactivity

➤ _____ (HIIT) provides a time-efficient method for improving aerobic fitness in CAD, heart failure, and metabolic syndrome patients

Review questions

1. What is DOMS? Explain why DOMS occurs and its significance for physical activity and training.
2. Discuss the possible mechanisms responsible for muscular cramps and strategies successful in its treatment.
3. What is the likely cause of the runner's stitch?
4. Through experimentation of what disease did Brooks and colleagues demonstrate that the lactate and ventilatory thresholds do not always occur at the same time point? Why was this the case in these patients?
5. What is the biggest killer worldwide and how is physical activity related to its prevention and treatment?
6. What are the health benefits of high-intensity interval training?
7. What are the likely causes and treatment for asthma?
8. Name the three groups of medication that can be prescribed in the treatment of asthma?
9. Explain the difference between overtraining and overreaching.
10. How does exercise serve to benefit people suffering from depression?

Teach it!
In groups of three, choose one topic and teach it to the rest of the study group.

1. Discuss the ways in which physical activity can benefit health.
2. Outline the key physiological changes occurring through the aging process.
3. Explain the female triad.

Check your recall, **Review questions** and **Teach it!** sections are provided for each chapter to help you revise and test your knowledge.

➤

My time at Huddersfield Town

My most memorable game, funnily enough, was not with Manchester United, but against them! I was playing my preferred midfield position for Huddersfield Town in an under-16 game. I wanted to prove myself to Manchester United in this position (they had moved me to centre half in my last year with them, but I don't like defence) and I wanted to impress. That is what I did when I scored the best goal of my career to date . . . it was 'a screamer' from 25 yards out, dropping the shoulder and cutting inside on to my right foot with rising effort. Bang! Into the top right hand corner. We won the game 2–0.
Training as an apprentice is more tactical-based than skill-based. Now

that I have moved up to training with the first team standards are higher. The other players have better ball skills and are faster on the ball. The start of training on the 1st July has been the hardest training I have ever done . . . I was exhausted. Our new fitness coach recently tested our speed over 40 yards (using timing gates). My performance (5.07 s) was close to the best (4.9 s). Some other testing involved the Yo-Yo test to assess our cardiovascular fitness and capturing video and photo data to monitor our mobility overtime as an injury prevention measure. In training, not surprisingly we do lots of running, VO₂ runs and match specific sessions, along with flexibility sessions and plyometric work with exercises such as lunges, jumps off one foot and one-foot hops.

My weekly schedule includes 2-hour intensive fast training on Monday and Tuesday, a rest day on Wednesday, a 2-hour morning session and a 1.5-hour afternoon session on Thursday, a 2-hour session on Friday, a match on Saturday and a 1-hour recovery session on Sunday. In addition to these soccer-specific sessions I do a weights session at the gym three times a week. We also have a food guideline to follow to ensure we have sufficient and appropriate nutritional intake. Since the start of the new training programme I feel fitter and faster.
The first team manager and coaching staff are developing a team that will hopefully become champions of league one this year and move into the championship next season. The future is bright!

SPORT IN ACTION

Biography: Andy Ellis
Sport: Rugby union

Born in Christchurch, New Zealand, Andy Ellis currently plays half back (scrum half) for Canterbury in provincial rugby and for the Crusaders in the Super 14 league. He was selected for the NZ under-21s side in 2005. However, due to injury in the Super 14 semi-final, was unavailable for international selection until the 2006 end of year tour when Andy made his All Blacks debut playing against England at Twickenham. Since then, Andy has been a regular selection for the All Blacks team, including selection to play in the Rugby World Cup, 2007 and 2011.

Training for rugby union at the elite level

(written with Ashley Jones, strength and conditioning coach for the Crusaders)

Strength and power conditioning

To be a successful international half back, able to withstand the physical demands of the position, and to additionally act as an extra loose forward at times (both in ball-carrying and defending around the edges of the ruck/maul and scrum), I believe my body mass must be at least 90 kg. To this end I perform a weight-training program specific to my position, to maintain upper-body

size and strength. This is either added to full body strength training or a power program, or is an

(Source: Georgie/RugbyImages)

Vibrant **Sport in action** articles written by world class elite athletes and coaches provide first-hand insight into the physiological and psychological demands of a variety of sports.

so many years of endurance training behind me and the solid base that I built at the beginning of my career, it is not necessary for me to race regularly or train over the race distance.

With all this training in place, I was finally ready to head to Australia. I flew out to Perth 14 days prior to the race, this gave me sufficient time to overcome the jet-lag, acclimatise and complete the finishing touches of the training programme. The race was on a Saturday and I completed my final training session on Tuesday evening, this left me with three full days to rest and build up my glycogen stores. I consumed a high-carbohydrate diet and plenty of fluids. Race day arrived; I was rested and ready to endure the toughest part of the race...

I raced through the pain barrier and finally I entered the home straight, there was no chance of anyone catching me now, the challenge was maintaining my focus, because all of a sudden I was distracted by the thought of another world title and that made me emotional! This was not the time to be getting emotional, I hadn't won yet! I needed to focus!

I did and finally after 2 hours 16 minutes of racing I crossed the line in first place – world title number four! I threw my arms in the air and gave a yelp of joy and relief. It was the sweetest victory yet. (If you would like to see video footage of me in action please go to my website: www.annahemmings.com.)

CLASSIC RESEARCH SUMMARY

The use of the aerobic-anaerobic transition in determining endurance training intensity by Kindermann et al. (1979)

In the 1970s, many researchers held differing views on the best criteria for the selection of the most appropriate training intensity for endurance athletes. The anaerobic threshold was suggested, in 1978, to be a suitable guideline for the determination of exercise training intensity. Kindermann and colleagues aimed to build on this suggestion by establishing an exercise intensity that could be maintained for prolonged periods of time, yet adequate for endurance training.

Kindermann and colleagues tested seven national-level cross-country skiers. Initially they completed an incremental treadmill test to volitional exhaustion. The treadmill incline was maintained at 5% throughout the test whereas velocity was increased from a starting level of 8 km·h^{-1} by 2 km·h^{-1} every three minutes. Exercise was stopped for 20 s after each three minute period to allow the testers to obtain a blood sample from the ear lobe for the analysis of arterialised blood lactate concentration. In addition, a final blood sample was taken three minutes following volitional exhaustion for the determination of maximal post-exercise lactate concentration. With the use of an Oxycon gas analysis system, $\dot{V}O_2$ and $\dot{V}_E$ were recorded and heart rate was monitored with electrocardiograms. The aerobic-anaerobic threshold was defined in this paper as a blood lactate concentration of 4 mM. Two additional treadmill tests were then completed: (1) 30 min running at the aerobic-anaerobic threshold HR (treadmill speed was continually reduced to maintain HR at this level), and (2) 30 min running at the aerobic-anaerobic threshold velocity. Heart rate was recorded every minute while $\dot{V}O_2$ was continuously monitored, and blood samples were taken from the ear lobe at rest and every 5 min during the 30-min run.

The primary finding of this paper was that running at an intensity sufficient to elevate blood lactate concentration to around 4 mM (as determined with an incremental treadmill test) can be performed by the majority for 45 – 60 min, with a few able to continue for even longer. This exercise elevated HR to an average of 170 beats·min^{-1}, although some individuals experienced HRs in excess of 180 beats·min^{-1}. Kindermann and colleagues suggested that training at an intensity around the 'aerobic-anaerobic' threshold (~4 mM blood lactate) would lead to adaptations in both the cardiovascular system and the muscle cells. It has since been determined that blood lactate measures of the aerobic-anaerobic transition are strong predictors of endurance performance in 30- >60-min races, hence its improvement with endurance training is critical for optimal performance.

Reference: Kindermann, W., Simon, G. and Keul, J. (1979). The significance of the aerobic-anaerobic transition for the determination of work load intensities during endurance training. *European Journal of Applied Physiology*, 42: 25-34.

350

Research summary boxes present key research papers relating to the topics, and highlight the importance of research within the field of exercise physiology.

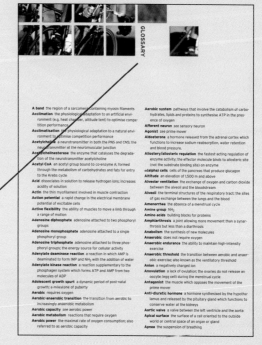

GLOSSARY

A band the region of a sarcomere containing myosin filaments
Acclimation the physiological adaptation to an artificial environment (e.g. heat chamber, altitude tent) to optimise competition performance
Acclimatisation the physiological adaptation to a natural environment to optimise competition performance
Acetylcholine a neurotransmitter in both the PNS and CNS; the neurotransmitter at the neuromuscular junction
Acetylcholinesterase the enzyme that catalyses the degradation of the neurotransmitter acetylcholine
Acetyl CoA an acetyl group bound to co-enzyme A; formed through the metabolism of carbohydrates and fats for entry to the Krebs cycle
Acid dissociates in solution to release hydrogen ions; increases acidity of solution
Actin the thin myofilament involved in muscle contraction
Action potential a rapid change in the electrical membrane potential of excitable cells
Active flexibility the ability of muscles to move a limb through a range of motion
Adenosine diphosphate adenosine attached to two phosphoryl groups
Adenosine monophosphate adenosine attached to a single phosphoryl group
Adenosine triphosphate adenosine attached to three phosphoryl groups; the energy source for cellular activity
Adenylate deaminase reaction a reaction in which AMP is deaminated to form IMP and NH_3 with the addition of water
Adenylate kinase reaction a reaction supplementary to the phosphagen system which forms ATP and AMP from two molecules of ADP
Adolescent growth spurt a dynamic period of post-natal growth; a milestone of puberty
Aerobic requires oxygen
Aerobic-anaerobic transition the transition from aerobic to increasingly anaerobic metabolism
Aerobic capacity see aerobic power
Aerobic metabolism reactions that require oxygen
Aerobic power the maximal rate of oxygen consumption; also referred to as aerobic capacity

Aerobic system pathways that involve the catabolism of carbohydrates, lipids and proteins to synthesise ATP in the presence of oxygen
Afferent neuron see sensory neuron
Agonist see prime mover
Aldosterone a hormone released from the adrenal cortex which functions to increase sodium reabsorption, water retention and blood pressure.
Allostery/allosteric regulation the fastest-acting regulation of enzyme activity; the effector molecule binds to allosteric site (not the substrate binding site) on enzyme
α(alpha) cells cells of the pancreas that produce glucagon
Altitude an elevation of 1,500 m and above
Alveolar ventilation the exchange of oxygen and carbon dioxide between the alveoli and the bloodstream
Alveoli the terminal structures of the respiratory tract; the sites of gas exchange between the lungs and the blood
Amenorrhea the absence of a menstrual cycle
Amine group NH_2
Amino acids building blocks for proteins
Amphiarthrosis a joint allowing more movement than a synarthrosis but less than a diarthrosis
Anabolism the synthesis of new molecules
Anaerobic does not require oxygen
Anaerobic endurance the ability to maintain high-intensity exercise
Anaerobic threshold the transition between aerobic and anaerobic exercise; also known as the ventilatory threshold
Anion a negatively charged ion
Anovulation a lack of ovulation; the ovaries do not release an oocyte (egg cell) during the menstrual cycle
Antagonist the muscle which opposes the movement of the prime mover
Anti-diuretic hormone a hormone synthesised by the hypothalamus and released by the pituitary gland which functions to conserve water at the kidneys
Aortic valve a valve between the left ventricle and the aorta
Apical surface the surface of a cell oriented to the outside world or central space of an organ or gland
Apnea the suspension of breathing

A comprehensive **Glossary** linked to emboldened words in the text is supplied as a reference and revision aid.

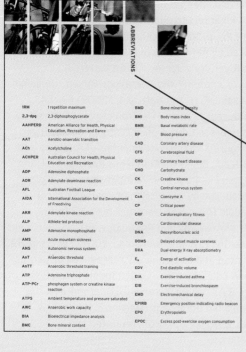

ABBREVIATIONS

1RM	1 repetition maximum	BMD	Bone mineral density
2,3-dpg	2,3-diphosphoglycerate	BMI	Body mass index
AAHPERD	American Alliance for Health, Physical Education, Recreation and Dance	BMR	Basal metabolic rate
		BP	Blood pressure
AAT	Aerobic-anaerobic transition	CAD	Coronary artery disease
ACh	Acetylcholine	CFS	Cerebrospinal fluid
ACHPER	Australian Council for Health, Physical Education and Recreation	CHD	Coronary heart disease
		CHO	Carbohydrate
ADP	Adenosine diphosphate	CK	Creatine kinase
ADR	Adenylate deaminase reaction	CNS	Central nervous system
AFL	Australian Football League	CoA	Coenzyme A
AIDA	International Association for the Development of Freediving	CP	Critical power
		CRF	Cardiorespiratory fitness
AKR	Adenylate kinase reaction	CVD	Cardiovascular disease
ALP	Athlete-led protocol	DNA	Deoxyribonucleic acid
AMP	Adenosine monophosphate	DOMS	Delayed onset muscle soreness
AMS	Acute mountain sickness	DXA	Dual-energy X-ray absorptiometry
ANS	Autonomic nervous system	E$_a$	Energy of activation
AnT	Anaerobic threshold	EDV	End diastolic volume
AnTT	Anaerobic threshold training	EIA	Exercise-induced asthma
ATP	Adenosine triphosphate	EIB	Exercise-induced bronchospasm
ATP-PCr	phosphagen system or creatine kinase reaction	EMD	Electromechanical delay
		EPIRB	Emergency position indicating radio beacon
ATPS	Ambient temperature and pressure saturated	EPO	Erythropoietin
AWC	Anaerobic work capacity	EPOC	Excess post-exercise oxygen consumption
BIA	Bioelectrical impedance analysis		
BMC	Bone mineral content		

A comprehensive list of **Abbreviations** is supplied to familiarise students with common acronyms for technical terms.

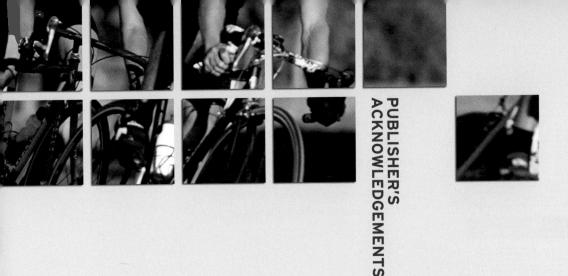

PUBLISHER'S ACKNOWLEDGEMENTS

We are grateful to the following for permission to reproduce copyright material:

Text

Article A. from *Visual Anatomy and Physiology* Benjamin Cummings (Martini, F. H., Ober, W. C. and Nath, J. L., 2011) pp. 262-5, © 2011, reprinted and electronically reproduced by permission of Pearson Education, Inc., Upper Saddle River, New Jersey; Article on page xiii from *Visual Anatomy and Physiology*, Benjamin Cummings (Martini, F. H., Ober, W. C. and Nath, J. L., 2011) p., 23, © 2011, reprinted and electronically reproduced by permission of Pearson Education, Inc., Upper Saddle River, New Jersey; Appendices on page xii from *Visual Anatomy and Physiology*, Benjamin Cummings (Martini and Ober 2011) p. 26, © 2011, reprinted and electronically reproduced by permission of Pearson Education, Inc., Upper Saddle River, New Jersey; Box on pages 260-1 from Sarissa de Vries; Box on pages 261-3 from John Hellemans; Box on pages 291-2 from Jacko Gill; Box on pages 428-9 from Karen Roberts; Case study on pages 430-1 from Ashley Jones; Box on pages 437-8 from Living with McArdle's disease – Personal Reflections on McArdle's disease, http://phosphorylase.wordpress.com/about-me/ http://phosphorylase.wordpress.com/?s=walk+over+wales by permission of Bill Corr.

Tables

Table on page 492 from *Essentials of Exercise Physiology*, 3rd ed., Williams and Wilkins (McArdle, W. D., Katch, V. L., 2006) p. 526, Table D.2 Factors to reduce moist gas to a dry gas volume at 0°C and 760 mm Hg, reproduced by permission of Fitness Techologies Press, V. L. Katch, and F. Katch.; Tables 2.7a, 2.7b from World Health Organization; Table 5.1 from *Fundamentals of Anatomy and Physiology*, 8th ed., Benjamin Cummings (Martini, F. H. and Nath, J. L., 2009) Table 6.1, p. 187, © 2009, reprinted and electronically reproduced by permission of Pearson Education, Inc., Upper Saddle River, New Jersey; Table on page 432 from Human muscle metabolism during intermittent maximal exercise, *Journal of Applied Physiology*, vol. 75(2), pp. 712-19 (Gaitanos, G. C., Williams, C., Boobis, L. H. and Brooks, S., 1993); Table 14.4 adapted from *The Practical Guide Identification, Evaluation, and Treatment of Overweight and Obesity in Adults* (NIH Publication no. 00-4084), National Institutes of Health (2000) Table 2, p. 10.

Figures

Figure 1.1b from *History of Physiology*, Krieger Pub. Co. (Rothschuh, K. E., 1973) Fig. 8, p. 51; Figure 1.2a from *History of Physiology*, Krieger Pub. Co. (Rothschuh, K. E., 1973) Figure 7, p. 50; Figure 1.12 from *Teaching Physical Education*, 5th ed., Benjamin Cummings (Mosston, M. and Ashworth, S., 2002) reproduced by permission of S. Ashworth; Figure 2.19 adapted from *Fundamentals of Anatomy and Physiology*, 8th ed., Pearson Education Ltd (Martini, F. H. and Nath, J. L., 2009) Figure 2.20, p. 55, © 2009, reprinted and electronically reproduced by permission of Pearson Education, Inc., Upper Saddle River, New Jersey; Figure 2.21 from *Fundamentals of Anatomy and Physiology* 8th ed., Benjamin Cummings (Martini, F. H. and Nath, J. L., 2009) Fig. 24.1, p. 876, © 2009, reprinted and electronically reproduced by permission of Pearson Education, Inc., Upper Saddle River, New Jersey; Figure 3.1 from *Fundamentals of Anatomy and Physiology*, 8th ed., Benjamin Cummings (Martini, F. H. and Nath, J. L., 2009) Fig. 1.1, p. 9, © 2009, reprinted and electronically reproduced by permission of Pearson Education, Inc., Upper Saddle River, New Jersey; Figure 3.2 from *Fundamentals of Anatomy and Physiology*, 8th ed., Benjamin Cummings (Martini, F. H. and Nath, J. L., 2009) Fig. 3.1, p. 69, © 2009, reprinted and electronically reproduced by permission of Pearson Education, Inc., Upper Saddle River, New Jersey; Figure 3.4 adapted from *Visual Anatomy and Physiology* Benjamin Cummings (Martini, F. H., Ober, W. C. and Nath, J. L., 2011) p. 88, © 2011, reprinted and electronically reproduced by permission of Pearson Education, Inc., Upper Saddle River, New Jersey; Figure 3.7 adapted from *Visual Anatomy and Physiology*, Benjamin Cummings (Martini, F. H., Ober, W. C. and Nath, J. L., 2011) Fig. 1, p. 19, © 2011, reprinted and electronically reproduced by permission of Pearson Education, Inc., Upper Saddle River, New Jersey; Figure 3.10 from *Visual Anatomy and Physiology*, Benjamin Cummings (Martini, F. H., Ober, W. C. and Nath, J. L., 2011) p. 125, © 2011, reprinted and electronically reproduced by permission of Pearson Education, Inc., Upper Saddle River, New Jersey; Figure 3.11 from *Visual Anatomy and Physiology*, Benjamin Cummings (Martini, F. H., Ober, W. C. and Nath, J. L., 2011) No. 3, p. 125, © 2011, reprinted and electronically reproduced by permission of Pearson Education, Inc., Upper Saddle River, New Jersey; Figure 4.3 from *Visual Anatomy and Physiology*, Benjamin Cummings (Martini, F. H., Ober, W. C. and Nath, J. L., 2011) Fig. 1,2,3. p. 30, © 2011, reprinted and electronically reproduced by permission of Pearson Education, Inc., Upper Saddle River, New Jersey; Figure 4.4 from *Visual Anatomy and Physiology*, Benjamin Cummings (Martini, F. H., Ober, W. C. and Nath, J. L., 2011) p. 369, © 2011, reprinted and electronically reproduced by permission of Pearson Education, Inc., Upper Saddle River, New Jersey; Figure 4.5 from *Visual Anatomy and Physiology*, Benjamin Cummings (Martini, F. H., Ober, W. C. and Nath, J. L., 2011) Fig. 1, p. 402, © 2011, reprinted and electronically reproduced by permission of Pearson Education, Inc., Upper Saddle River, New Jersey; Figure 4.7 adapted from *Visual Anatomy and Physiology*, Benjamin Cummings (Martini, F. H., Ober, W. C. and Nath, J. L., 2011) Figs 1-3, p. 374, © 2011, reprinted and electronically reproduced by permission of Pearson Education, Inc., Upper Saddle River, New Jersey; Figure 4.8 from *Fundamentals of Anatomy and Physiology*, 8th ed., Benjamin Cummings (Martini, F. H. and Nath, J. L., 2009) Summary Table 12.3, p. 409, © 2009, reprinted and electronically reproduced by permission of Pearson Education, Inc., Upper Saddle River, New Jersey; Figure 4.9 adapted from *Fundamentals of Anatomy and Physiology* 8th ed., Benjamin Cummings (Martini, F. H. and Nath, J. L., 2009) Fig. 12.15, 12.16, p. 410. p. 412, © 2009, reprinted and electronically reproduced by permission of Pearson Education, Inc., Upper Saddle River, New Jersey; Figure 4.10 from *Fundamentals of Anatomy and Physiology*, 8th ed., Benjamin Cummings (Martini, F. H. and Nath, J. L., 2009) Figs. 14.12(b) 4.12 © p. 481, © 2009, reprinted and electronically reproduced by permission of Pearson Education, Inc., Upper Saddle River, New Jersey; Figure 4.11 adapted from *Fundamentals of Anatomy and Physiology* 8th ed., Benjamin Cummings (Martini, F. H. and Nath, J. L., 2009) Fig. 13.3, p. 433, © 2009, reprinted and electronically reproduced by permission of Pearson Education, Inc., Upper Saddle River, New Jersey; Figure 4.13 from *Fundamentals of Anatomy and Physiology*, 8th ed., Benjamin Cummings (Martini, F. H. and Nath, J. L., 2009)

Fig. 18.1, p. 607, © 2009, reprinted and electronically reproduced by permission of Pearson Education, Inc., Upper Saddle River, New Jersey; Figure 5.2 from *Fundamentals of Anatomy and Physiology*, 8th ed., Benjamin Cummings (Martini, F. H. and Nath, J. L., 2009) Fig. 6.1, p. 186, © 2009, reprinted and electronically reproduced by permission of Pearson Education, Inc., Upper Saddle River, New Jersey; Figure 5.3b from *Fundamentals of Anatomy and Physiology*, 8th ed., Benjamin Cummings (Martini, F. H. and Nath, J. L., 2009) Figs 6.5-6.6, pp. 192-3; Figure 5.4 from *Fundamentals of Anatomy and Physiology*, 8th ed., Benjamin Cummings (Martini, F. H. and Nath, J. L., 2009) Fig. 4.14, p. 133, © 2009, reprinted and electronically reproduced by permission of Pearson Education, Inc., Upper Saddle River, New Jersey; Figure 5.5 from *Visual Anatomy and Physiology*, Benjamin Cummings (Martini, F. H., Ober, W. C. and Nath, J. L., 2011) p. 258, © 2011, reprinted and electronically reproduced by permission of Pearson Education, Inc., Upper Saddle River, New Jersey; Figure 5.6 from *Fundamentals of Anatomy and Physiology*, 8th ed., Benjamin Cummings (Martini, F. H. and Nath, J. L., 2009) p. 278, © 2009, reprinted and electronically reproduced by permission of Pearson Education, Inc., Upper Saddle River, New Jersey; Figure 5.7 adapted from *Fundamentals of Anatomy and Physiology*, 8th ed., Benjamin Cummings (Martini, F. H. and Nath, J. L., 2009) Figs 9.1b, 9.12a, 9.12b p. 270, p. 285, © 2009, reprinted and electronically reproduced by permission of Pearson Education, Inc., Upper Saddle River, New Jersey; Figure 5.8 from *Visual Anatomy and Physiology*, Benjamin Cummings (Martini, F. H. and Ober, W. C., 2011) text and figures 1-3, p. 150, © 2011, reprinted and electronically reproduced by permission of Pearson Education, Inc., Upper Saddle River, New Jersey; Figure 5.9 from *Fundamentals of Anatomy and Physiology*, 8th ed., Benjamin Cummings (Martini, F. H. and Nath, J. L., 2009) Fig. 10.1, p. 295, © 2009, reprinted and electronically reproduced by permission of Pearson Education, Inc., Upper Saddle River, New Jersey; Figure 5.10 adapted from *Fundamentals of Anatomy and Physiology*, 8th ed., Benjamin Cummings (Martini, F. H. and Nath, J. L., 2009) Fig. 10.3, 10.5a, 10.5b, p. 297 p. 300, © 2009, reprinted and electronically reproduced by permission of Pearson Education, Inc., Upper Saddle River, New Jersey; Figure 5.13 from *Fundamentals of Anatomy and Physiology*, 8th ed., Benjamin Cummings (Martini, F. H. and Nath, J. L., 2009) Fig. 10.7, p. 302, © 2009, reprinted and electronically reproduced by permission of Pearson Education, Inc., Upper Saddle River, New Jersey; Figure 5.15a after *Fundamentals of Anatomy and Physiology* 8th ed., Benjamin Cummings (Martini, F. H. and Nath, J. L., 2009) Fig. 10.4, p. 299, © 2009, reprinted and electronically reproduced by permission of Pearson Education, Inc., Upper Saddle River, New Jersey; Figure 5.16 from *Fundamentals of Anatomy and Physiology*, 8th ed., Benjamin Cummings (Martini, F. H. and Nath, J. L., 2009) Fig. 10.15, p. 313, © 2009, reprinted and electronically reproduced by permission of Pearson Education, Inc., Upper Saddle River, New Jersey; Figure 5.17 from *Fundamentals of Anatomy and Physiology*, 8th ed., Benjamin Cummings (Martini, F. H. and Nath, J. L., 2009) Fig. 10.16 (b, c, d) p. 314, © 2009, reprinted and electronically reproduced by permission of Pearson Education, Inc., Upper Saddle River, New Jersey; Figure 5.18 from *Fundamentals of Anatomy and Physiology*, 8th ed., Benjamin Cummings (Martini, F. H. and Nath, J. L., 2009) Fig. 10.17, p. 315, © 2009, reprinted and electronically reproduced by permission of Pearson Education, Inc., Upper Saddle River, New Jersey; Figure 5.21 from *Fundamentals of Anatomy and Physiology* 8th ed., Benjamin Cummings (Martini, F. H. and Nath, J. L., 2009) Fig. 11.3, Fig. 11.15a, Fig. 11.15b, pp. 343, 345, 364, © 2009, reprinted and electronically reproduced by permission of Pearson Education, Inc., Upper Saddle River, New Jersey; Figure 5.22 from *Visual Anatomy and Physiology*, Benjamin Cummings (Martini, F. H., Ober, W. C. and Nath, J. L., 2011) Fig. 10.1, p. 314, © 2011, reprinted and electronically reproduced by permission of Pearson Education, Inc., Upper Saddle River, New Jersey; Figure 6.1 from *Fundamentals of Anatomy and Physiology*, 8th ed., Benjamin Cummings (Martini, F. H. and Nath, J. L., 2009) Fig. 23.1, p. 827, © 2009, reprinted and electronically reproduced by permission of Pearson Education, Inc., Upper Saddle River, New Jersey; Figure 6.2 from *Fundamentals of Anatomy and Physiology*, 8th ed., Benjamin Cummings (Martini, F. H. and Nath, J. L., 2009) Fig. 23.9, p. 838, © 2009, reprinted and electronically reproduced by permission of Pearson Education, Inc., Upper Saddle River, New Jersey; Figure 6.3 adapted from *Visual Anatomy and Physiology*, Benjamin Cummings (Martini, F. H., Ober, W. C. and Nath, J. L., 2011) Figures and captions p. 738, © 2011, reprinted and electronically reproduced by permission of Pearson Education, Inc., Upper Saddle River, New Jersey; Figure 6.4 from *Fundamentals of Anatomy and Physiology*, 8th ed., Benjamin Cummings (Martini, F. H. and Nath, J. L., 2009) Fig. 23.11, p. 840, © 2009, reprinted and electronically reproduced by permission of Pearson Education, Inc., Upper Saddle River, New Jersey; Figure 6.5 from *Fundamentals of Anatomy and Physiology*, 8th ed., Benjamin Cummings (Martini, F. H. and Nath, J. L., 2009) Fig. 23.19, p. 854, 2009, reprinted and electronically reproduced by permission of Pearson Education, Inc., Upper Saddle River, New Jersey; Figure 6.10 adapted from *Visual Anatomy and Physiology*, Benjamin Cummings (Martini, F. H., Ober, W. C. and Nath, J. L., 2011) Figs1-6, p. 578, © 2011, reprinted and electronically reproduced by permission of Pearson Education, Inc., Upper Saddle River, New Jersey; Figure 6.14 from *Visual Anatomy and Physiology*, Benjamin Cummings (Martini, F. H., Ober, W. C. and Nath, J. L., 2011) Module 20.11, diag. 2 and text, p. 744, © 2011, reprinted and electronically reproduced by permission of Pearson Education, Inc., Upper Saddle River, New Jersey; Figure 6.15 from *Fundamentals of Anatomy and Physiology*, 8th ed.,

Benjamin Cummings (Martini, F. H. and Nath, J. L., 2009) Fig. 20.3, Fig. 20.6(a), p. 685, p. 688; Figure 6.16 from *Fundamentals of Anatomy and Physiology*, 8th ed., Benjamin Cummings (Martini, F. H. and Nath, J. L., 2009) Fig. 20.7, p. 690, © 2009, reprinted and electronically reproduced by permission of Pearson Education, Inc., Upper Saddle River, New Jersey; Figure 6.17 from *Fundamentals of Anatomy and Physiology*, 8th ed., Benjamin Cummings (Martini, F. H. and Nath, J. L., 2009) Fig. 21.18, p. 748, © 2009, reprinted and electronically reproduced by permission of Pearson Education, Inc., Upper Saddle River, New Jersey; Figure 6.18 from *Fundamentals of Anatomy and Physiology*, 8th ed., Benjamin Cummings (Martini, F. H. and Nath, J. L., 2009) Fig. 20.12a, Fig. 20.12, p. 696, p. 697, © 2009, reprinted and electronically reproduced by permission of Pearson Education, Inc., Upper Saddle River, New Jersey; Figure 6.21 from *Fundamentals of Anatomy and Physiology*, 8th ed., Benjamin Cummings (Martini, F. H. and Nath, J. L., 2009) Fig. 21.20, Fig. 21.27, p. 751, p. 760, © 2009, reprinted and electronically reproduced by permission of Pearson Education, Inc., Upper Saddle River, New Jersey; Figure 6.22 from *Fundamentals of Anatomy and Physiology*, 8th ed., Benjamin Cummings (Martini, F. H. and Nath, J. L., 2009) Fig. 21.2, Fig. 21.1, p. 723. p. 721, © 2009, reprinted and electronically reproduced by permission of Pearson Education, Inc., Upper Saddle River, New Jersey; Figure 6.23 from *Fundamentals of Anatomy and Physiology*, 8th ed., Benjamin Cummings (Martini, F. H. and Nath, J. L., 2009) Fig. 21.6, p. 728, © 2009, reprinted and electronically reproduced by permission of Pearson Education, Inc., Upper Saddle River, New Jersey; Figure 7.7 from *Paediatric Osteology: New Developments in Diagnostics and Therapy*, Elsevier (Schoenau, E. (ed.) 1996) Fig. 2, p. 138, Copyright Elsevier 1996; Figure 7.8 from Volumetric bone mineral density in normal subjects, aged 5-27 years., *Journal of Clinical Endocrinology and Metabolism*, vol. 81(4) (Lu, PW 1996); Figure 7.9 adapted from Influence of puberty on muscle area and cortical bone area of the forearm in boys and girls (Fig. 1), *Journal of Clinical Endocrinology and Metabolism*, Vol.85(3), p.1096 (Schoenau, E. et al., 2000); Figure 7.11 adapted from Grip strength performances by 5-19 year olds, *Perceptual and Motor Skills*, 109, pp. 362-70 (Butterfield, S. A., Lehnhard, R. A., Loovis, E. M., Coladarcie, T., and Saucier, D., 2009), reproduced with permission of authors and publisher; Figure 7.22 adapted from Longitudinal Changes of Maximal Short-Term Peak Power in Girls and Boys during Growth, *Medicine and Science in Sports and Exercise*, 36 (3), pp. 498-503 (Martin, et al., 2004); Figure 7.23 from Assessment arid interpretation of aerobic fitness in children and adolescents, *Exercise Sports Science Review*, vol. 22, pp. 435-76 (Armstrong, N., and Welsman, J. R., 2011); Figure 7.24 from Aerobic fitness: what are we measuring? (Fig. 2), *Medicine and Sport Science*, vol. 50(R), p. 18 (Armstrong, N., and Welsman, J., 2007), reproduced by permission of S. Karger AG, Basel; Figure 7.25 from *Pediatric Anaerobic Performance*, Human Kinetics (van Praagh, E.) Fig. 9.14, p. 213; Figure 7.26 from *Paediatric Exercise Science and Medicine*, 2nd ed., Oxford University Press (Armstrong, N., and van Mechelem, W., 2008) Fig. 8.1, p. 102; Figure 10.12 adapted from Basketball Bioenergetics: Practical applications, *National Strength and Conditioning Association Journal*, December, vol. 6(6), pp. 45 (Semenick, D., 1984); Figure 13.2c from VX Sport location report, reproduced by permission of Visuallex Sport International Ltd; Figure 13.3 adapted from The assessment of an intermittent high intensity running test, *Journal of Sports Medicine and Physical Fitness*, 45(3), pp. 248–56 (Psotta, R. et al., 2005), reprinted by permission of Edizioni Minerva Medica; Figure 13.8 adapted from The reliability and validity of a field hockey skill test, *International Journal of Sports Medicine*, vol. 27(5), pp. 395–400 (Sunderland, C., Cooke, K., Milne, H., and Nevill, M. E., 2006), Adapted and reprinted by permission; Figure 13.9 after The development of a test of reactive agility for netball: a new methodology, *Journal of Science and Medicine in Sport*, vol. 8(1), pp. 52–60 (Farrow, D., Young, W., and Bruce, L., 2005), copyright 2005, with permission from Elsevier; Figure 13.10 adapted from Physiological characteristics of elite and sub-elite badminton players, *Journal of Sports Sciences*, vol. 27(14), pp. 1,591–9 (Ooi, C. H., et al., 2009); Figure 13.11 adapted from Game analysis and energy requirements of elite squash, *Journal of Strength and Conditioning Research*, vol. 21(3), pp. 909–14 (Girard, O., et al., 2007); Figure 13.12 adapted from Physiological aspects of surfboard riding performance, *Sports Medicine*, vol. 35(1), pp. 55–70 (Mendez-Villanueva, A., and Bishop, D., 2005); Figure 15.1 adapted from The pathophysiology of hypothermia, *International Reviews of Ergonomics*, pp. 201–18 (Mekjavic, I. and Bligh, J., 1987), reproduced by permission of the publisher and the author.

Picture credits

The publisher would like to thank the following for their kind permission to reproduce their photographs:

(Key: b – bottom; c– centre; l – left; r –right; t – top)

British Judo/Bob Willingham: p. 387, p. 482; **Corbis:** Glow Images p. 323, Nice One Production p. 264; **David Sykes:** p. 429; **Didier Poppe:** p. 204 (b), p. 291; **Digital Vision:** p. 229; **Dr Susan Dewhurst:** p. 205; **Georgie/RubyImages:** p. iii; p. 279, p. 282, p. 430, **Getty Images:** p. 204 (t); **GNU Free Documentation License: Wikipedia:** p. 11, p. 121; **Illustrated London News Picture Library:** Ingram Publishing Alamy p. 3; **iStockphoto:** Mads Abildgaard p. 1, p. 109, Martin McCarthy p. 27, Monika Wisniewska p. 82, Paul Vasarhelyi p. 189, Sebastian Kaulitzki p. 66, p. 150; **John Foxx Images:** p. 351, p. 433; **Mark Lloyd:** p. 349, p. 384; **Nicky Norris:** p. 177, p. 247, p. 305 (c), p. 450; **PhotoDisc:** p. 225, Sean Thompson p. 294; **Science Photo Library Ltd:** p. 7 (r), 12 (r), p. 15l, ABECASIS p. 8, Bill Longcore p. 71, Christopher Vander Eecken/Reporters p. 195 (tr), Doncaster & Basset Law Hospitals p. 195 (bl), National Library of Medicine p. 7l, US National Library of Medicine p. 13, p. 14; **Smithsonian Institute:** p. 15 ®; **The Benjamin Cummings Publishing Company:** p. 59, p. 70, p. 100, p. 114, p. 116, p. 135, p. 157, p. 169, p. 172; **Trevor Chapman:** p. 347.

All other images © Pearson Education

In some instances we have been unable to trace the owners of copyright material, and we would appreciate any information that would enable us to do so.

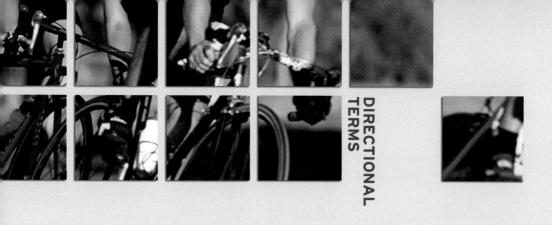

Term	Region or reference	Example
Anterior	The front surface	The navel is on the *anterior* surface of the trunk.
Ventral	The belly side (equivalent to anterior when referring to the human body)	The navel is on the *ventral* surface of the trunk.
Posterior or **dorsal**	The back surface	The shoulder blade is located *posterior* to the rib cage.
Cranial or **cephalic**	The head	The *cranial*, or *cephalic*, border of the pelvis is on the side toward the head rather than toward the thigh.
Superior	Above; at a higher level (in the human body, toward the head)	In humans, the cranial border of the pelvis is *superior* to the thigh.
Caudal	The tail (coccyx in humans)	The hips are *caudal* to the waist.
Inferior	Below; at a lower level	The knees are *inferior* to the hips.
Medial	Toward the body's longitudinal axis; toward the midsagittal plane	The *medial* surfaces of the thighs may be in contact; moving medially from the arm across the chest surface brings you to the sternum.
Lateral	Away from the body's longitudinal axis; away from the midsagittal plane	The thigh articulates with the *lateral* surface of the pelvis; moving laterally from the nose brings you to the cheeks.
Proximal	Toward an attached base	The thigh is *proximal* to the foot; moving proximally from the wrist brings you to the elbow.
Distal	Away from an attached base	The fingers are *distal* to the wrist; moving distally from the elbow brings you to the wrist.
Superficial	At, near, or relatively close to the body surface	The skin is *superficial* to underlying structures.
Deep	Further from the body surface	The bone of the thigh is *deep* to the surrounding skeletal muscles.

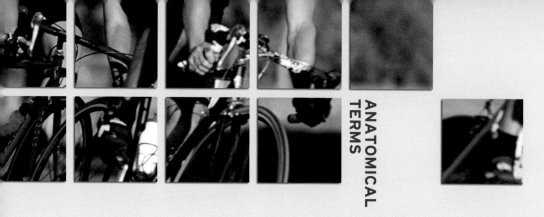

Important word roots, prefixes, suffixes, and combining forms in anatomy

a-, *a-*, without: avascular

aer-, *aeros*, air: aerobic metabolism

-algia, *algos*, pain: neuralgia

arter-, *arteria*, artery: arterial

arthro-, *arthros*, joint: arthroscopy

auto-, *auto*, self: autonomic

bio-, *bios*, life: biology

-blast, *blastos*, germ: osteoblast

bronch-, *bronchus*, windpipe, airway: bronchial

cardi-, cardio-, -cardia, *kardia*, heart: cardiac, cardiopulmonary

cerebr-, *cerebrum*, brain: cerebral hemispheres

cervic-, *cervicis*, neck: cervical vertebrae

chondro-, *chondros*, cartilage: chondrocyte

cranio-, *cranium*, skull: craniosacral

cyt-, cyto-, *kytos*, a hollow cell: cytology, cytokine

derm-, *derma*, skin: dermatome

-ectomy, *ektome*, excision: appendectomy

end-, endo-, *endon*, within: endergonic, endometrium

epi-, *epi*, on: epimysium

ex-, *ex*, out of, away from: exocytosis

hemo-, *haima*, blood: hemopoiesis

hemi-, *hemi*, one-half: hemisphere

histo-, *histos*, tissue: histology

homo-, *homos*, same: homozygous

hyper-, *hyper*, above: hyperpolarization

hypo-, *hypo*, under: hypothyroid

inter-, *inter*, between: interventricular

iso-, *isos*, equal: isotonic

leuk-, leuko-, *leukos*, white: leukaemia, leukocyte

lyso-, -lysis, -lyze, *lysis*, a loosening: hydrolysis

meso-, *mesos*, middle: mesoderm

micr-, *mikros*, small: microscope

morph-, morpho-, *morphe*, form: morphology, morphotype

myo-, *mys*, muscle: myofilament

nephr-, *nephros*, kidney: nephron

neur-, neuri-, neuro-, *neuron*, nerve: neural, neurilemma, neuromuscular

-ology, *logos*, the study of: physiology

-osis, *osis*, state, condition: neurosis

ost-, oste-, osteo-, *osteon*, bone: osteal, ostealgia, osteocyte

oto-, *otikos*, ear: otolith

path-, -pathy, patho-, *pathos*, disease: pathergy, idiopathy, pathogenesis

peri-, *peri*, around: perineurium

phago-, *phago*, to eat: phagocyte

-phil, -philia, *philo*, love: neutrophil, hemophilia

-phot, -photo, *phos*, light: photalgia, photoreceptor

physio-, *physis*, nature: physiology

pre-, *prae*, before: precapillary sphincter

pulmo-, *pulmo*, lung: pulmonary

retro-, *retro*, backward: retroperitoneal

sarco-, *sarkos*, flesh: sarcomere

sclera-, sclero-, *skleros*, hard: sclera, sclerosis

-scope, *skopeo*, to view: colonoscope

sub-, *sub*, below: subcutaneous

super-, *super*, above or beyond: superficial

-trophy, *trophe*, nourishment: atrophy

vas-, *vas*, vessel: vascular

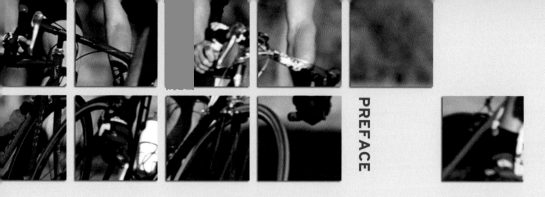

It is highly dishonourable for a reasonable soul to live in so divinely built a mansion as the body she resides in, altogether unacquainted with the exquisite structure of it.

(Robert Boyle, 1664)

Robert Boyle (1627–91), in one aspect of his research, determined through experimentation that there was a substance within air that was vital for sustaining life. While our understanding of oxygen, and indeed of physiology, has developed enormously since Boyle's time, his quotation is as true today as it was then. The human body is an incredibly complex structure and the mechanisms through which life is sustained are both amazing and fascinating. Within exercise physiology, the subject of this textbook, the wonders of the molecular structure of cells, the mechanisms through which human movement is brought about and the processes through which energy is generated for all cellular activity provide captivating illustrations of the exquisite structure and function of the human body.

Exercise Physiology for Health and Sports Performance has been written for physical education, sports coaching and exercise science students and professionals with an interest in, and passion for, the health and performance aspects of exercise physiology. *Exercise physiology*, a branch of physiology devoted to the study of the functioning of the body during physical activity (exercise), is founded from the disciplines of anatomy, physiology and biochemistry. *Anatomy* concerns the structure of the body, its parts and their inter-relationship, while (human) *physiology* concerns the functioning of the structures – cells, tissues, organs and organ systems. *Biochemistry* concerns the functioning of structures within the body on a chemical and molecular level. An understanding of foundations in each of these disciplines is essential to developing knowledge in exercise physiology.

Part I of this textbook is devoted to the foundations of exercise physiology and provides important information regarding the anatomy, physiology and biochemistry of the body that underlie the exercise physiology of health and sports performance. With knowledge of the foundations of exercise physiology it is possible to gain a far deeper understanding of the applied aspects of exercise physiology as they relate to health and sports performance.

Part II of this textbook, building on the foundations of exercise physiology, examines sports and health from an applied perspective. The physiological demands of a sport such as weight-lifting are fundamentally different from those for marathon running or game-related sports such as football (American, soccer, Aussie rules, rugby union or league), netball, basketball or hockey. The key differences relate to the energy demands of the sport, and as such, Part II of *Exercise Physiology for Health and Sports Performance* is divided into chapters based around these varied demands.

The energy demands of any sport are based on its intensity and duration. The human body has a number of mechanisms for generating the energy necessary to meet demands during sports as diverse as shot putt and multi-day cycling events such as the Tour de France. In evolutionary terms these mechanisms were developed to enable our ancestors to outrun predators (speed and power) and for their own hunting and gathering (endurance) purposes. Sports test these mechanisms in a modern context. Part II of this textbook comprises chapters based around the mechanisms underlying the energy delivery for sports with differing relative intensities and durations. While the physiological aspects of every sport could not hope to be covered individually within this textbook, with an understanding of applied exercise physiology it is possible to devise a programme to monitor and improve performance for any sport. The more knowledge a person has regarding the nature of a sport, its intensity and duration, the more precise and applied such a programme could become.

Exercise physiologists, as well as studying exercise in a performance context, are also interested in health-related aspects of exercise. The link between exercise and health is not new, however, and early records of the relationship between them date back to the times of the Greek and Roman Empires. The common saying of 'healthy body, healthy mind' comes from a Latin phrase *mens sana in corpore sano* (a sound mind in a sound body) which was taken from a poem by the Roman poet Juvenal (55–127 CE). Later

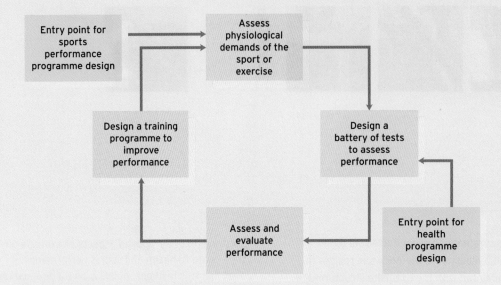

Figure 1 The cycle of exercise physiology assessment and programme design for sports performance and health.

Galen (129-200 or 217 CE), physician to Emperor Marcus Aurelius, wrote treaties (articles) describing the importance of exercise, amongst other considerations, for health. Sport and exercise, as well as being pursued for recreational and performance reasons, can be undertaken to improve health and well-being.

Exercise physiologists seek to better understand the what, where, when, how and why of sports for health and performance reasons. Regardless of whether an individual takes part in sport or exercise for performance or health reasons or both, exercise physiologists can monitor fitness levels and design programmes to improve both exercise goals. The role of an exercise physiologist involves a number of stages that can be seen as part of a cycle. The starting point might be different for an individual starting exercise for health or performance reasons; the pattern, though, would be common to both, as illustrated in Figure 1. Exercise physiologists design a battery of tests to assess fitness and then devise a training intervention which is monitored throughout to assess achievement towards a goal, whether that be for an improvement in sports performance or in health status.

General structure of the book

Exercise Physiology for Health and Sports Performance is divided into two parts. The first provides foundations in exercise physiology; the second examines applied exercise physiology as related to specific sports performance or health aspects. At the end of each chapter a summary is presented and questions are provided for you to assess your understanding of the material covered. All references have been included at the end of the book to make for ease of reading but are presented by chapter as sources of further reading. Each of the chapters in Part II include an example of research paper that relates to either a sport or classic exercise physiology study. These examples are provided in 'Classic research summary' textboxes which have been included as examples of important studies in the field of exercise physiology. The chapters within Part II also have 'Sport in action' sections which were written by elite athletes and coaches from a number of sports and provide interesting insights into the physiological demands of their sport.

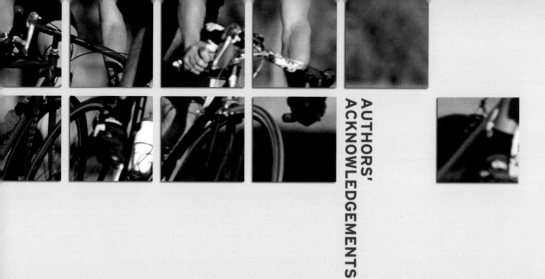

AUTHORS'
ACKNOWLEDGEMENTS

The publication of any textbook requires the help of a team to see it to fruition. There are many people who helped with the development of our idea and the completion of this work - thank you to each of them.

Firstly, to the team at Pearson who supported and guided the project and provided important deadlines and feedback throughout the process to improve the final result - to Rufus Curnow, Pat Bond, Helen Leech, Carole Drummond and Elizabeth Harrison - thank you.

To David and Kirsty Milne - thank you for your impeccable grammatical editing and being a fresh set of eyes, which have greatly improved the final version of this book. We are indebted to Ian Culpan for his help in the writing of Chapter 1 and to Gail Gillon, PVC of the College of Education at the University of Canterbury, for providing the time to complete this project. Thank you to Gavin Blackwell for his technical support - finding copies of articles and helping to construct the reference list for the completed book. To David Winter, Ashley Garrill and Andy Pratt at the University of Canterbury - thank you for your knowledge and great technical assistance around biochemical and chemical aspects of the book, your help was invaluable and the discussions invigorating!

Thank you to Simon Fryer who was the photographer for many figures within this book and to Cirrus Tan for agreeing to be a subject in the photographs included in our book. We owe a large debt of gratitude to the athletes and coaches who wrote the Sport in Action pieces for the book: thank you very much to Sarissa de Vries, John Hellemans, Jacko Gill, Katherine Schirrmacher, Anna Hemmings, Tim Brabant, Ben Ainslie, Karen Roberts, Andy Ellis and Matt Crooks.

Then perhaps most importantly, there are our family members who supported us every step of the way during the completion of *Exercise Physiology for Health and Sports Performance*. To Jeanne and Lester Marshall - for coming to the rescue and looking after Helen's children (on several occasions) when time was running out and we were behind schedule. To Johnny, thank you for giving me the time and strength to complete the book, and for your continued patience and support throughout, and to Katie and Sophie for keeping me smiling! To Lara, Sam, Matt and Joe - thank you for everything!

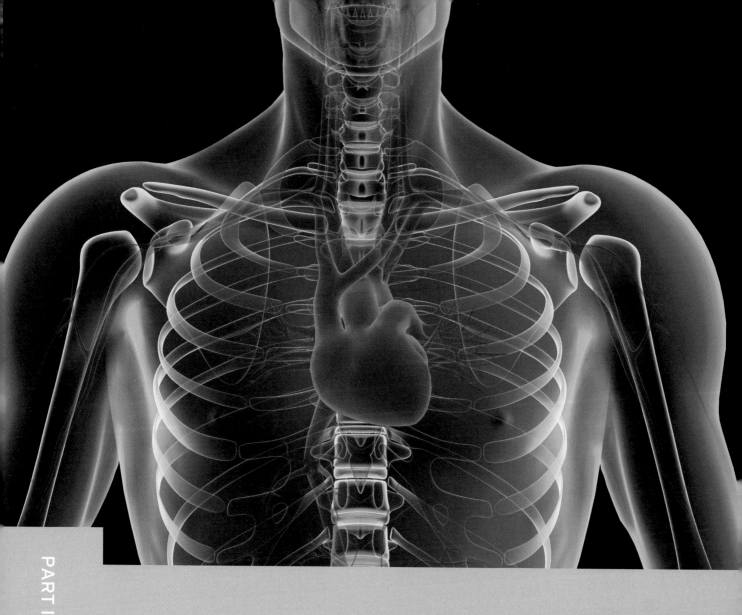

PART I

Foundations of exercise physiology

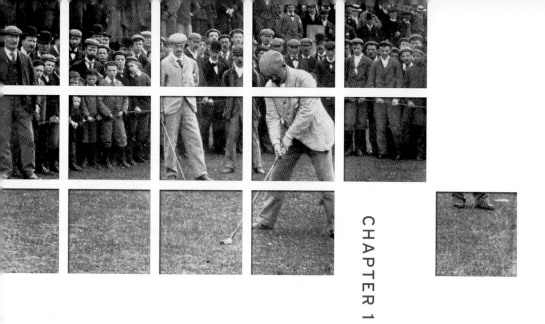

CHAPTER 1

Exercise physiology, sport and pedagogy:
an historical perspective

Learning objectives

After reading, considering and discussing with a study partner the material in this chapter you should be able to:

➤ describe a range of developments regarding our knowledge in the fields of anatomy, physiology and exercise physiology

➤ identify researchers who have made significant contributions to our understanding of contemporary exercise physiology

➤ outline how sport and physical education have changed over the centuries and how this might affect the role of exercise physiologists

➤ be challenged to use a range of teaching pedagogies in your teaching or coaching of exercise physiology

1.1 An historical perspective: the context of contemporary exercise physiology

This section is designed to highlight some of the interesting and significant developments in knowledge that led to our current understanding in the field of exercise physiology. For future physical education teachers, especially those who after graduation might well teach exercise physiology, this section can provide useful examples and contexts through which to bring your teaching sessions alive. For example, until the work of William Harvey (1578–1657), physiologists thought the blood within our bodies ebbed and flowed like the sea, rather than circulated, as he demonstrated through his research. Examples such as these highlight how our knowledge of human functioning has changed over time.

The early physiologists

Perhaps not surprisingly, much of the early work regarding human physiology related to describing the structures within the body (the anatomy) rather than the functioning (the physiology). The Greeks, during the times of the Greek Empire, were responsible for a great number of advances in our early understanding of anatomy and physiology. Greek scholars were very good at assimilating knowledge from other cultures as their empire expanded and they learned from the observations made by scholars in Mesopotamia, Egypt and India. From around 600 BCE to the fall of the Greek Empire to Rome in 201 BCE, Greek scholars, often philosophers at that time, such as Empedocles (495–435 BCE), Hippocrates (460–377 BCE), Plato (427–347 BCE) and Aristotle (384–322 BCE) developed existing physiological knowledge, much of which remained unchallenged for over 1,000 years.

As happens now in the development of our modern physiological knowledge, each generation built upon, or challenged, the accepted theories of the time. Empedocles, in developing his theories of physiological knowledge, viewed the world as comprising various elements that required a balance to be maintained between them. To Empedocles, humans were comprised of four elements: earth, fire, air and water. To maintain health, it was essential to maintain a balance between the four human components. Ill-health was the result of an imbalance between the four elements. The soul, Empedocles maintained, was located in the blood. Hippocrates and his disciples, based on the Island of Cos, wrote many medical papers or 'treaties'. Hippocrates, through his work in the field of medicine, has become known as the founder of western medicine. Indeed, doctors today still undertake to follow the Hippocratic Oath. Hippocrates and his son-in-law Polybos developed Empedocles' theories concerning the four components that comprised the human body and referred to them as four antagonist humours (from Greek, *chymos* meaning juice or fluid). These humours were black bile (earth), yellow bile (fire), blood (air) and phlegm (water), a balance between each being required to maintain health. Figure 1.1 provides an illustration of the relationship between the elements and the humours.

Galen, whose contribution to physiology is discussed in more detail in the next section, went on to link the bodily aspects of the humours to a person's bodily temperament, which was associated with their personality type and susceptibility to disease. He described these temperaments as warm, cold, moist and dry, such that the humour of blood, as can be seen in Figure 1.1, was associated with warm and moist temperament qualities. Indeed, the personality traits associated with being phlegmatic, sanguine or melancholic originate from Galen's temperaments.

Maintaining a balance between the humours was important for good health and reflected a balanced temperament. In contrast, imbalances between the humours were detrimental to health. It was the influence of humourism that led to the introduction of bloodletting, often using leeches, which remained a common practice amongst physicians for over 1,000 years. It was thought that by releasing fluid from the body the balance between the humours, and therefore good health, could be restored. Interestingly, blood was considered a special element, as it was thought to contain all four humours; blood, black bile, yellow bile and phlegm. In the 1920s a Swedish physiologist Fåhræus, when considering why such a theory might have arisen, examined blood after it was left in an open tray for one hour and found evidence of components within the sample that might have led the early physiologists to such a conclusion. After being left the blood began to separate into layers and to clot. As a result there were red (red blood cells), black (blood clots), yellow (plasma) and white (buffy coat or white blood cells) layers which the early physiologists might have interpreted as evidence of the four humours, blood, black bile, yellow bile and phlegm, respectively.

Hippocrates and his followers believed that the balance between the humours was assisted by the heat provided through an internal fire, that was maintained in the bloodless left ventricle of the heart. To maintain the internal fire, life-giving air or *pneuma*, along with food and drink for nourishment, was required. All food and drink was made up of blood, bile (black and yellow) and phlegm. It was at this time that the theory of blood ebbing and flowing was developed by the followers of Hippocrates. Through simple dissections, largely of animals, the early physiologists determined, mistakenly, that blood ebbed and flowed rather than circulated and only entered the right side of the heart. The left side of the heart was associated with the internal fire of life. The left auricle of the heart received pneuma on each inspiration, which was supplied to the left ventricle to help nourish the internal fire. The heat created by the internal fire was believed to be responsible for the beating of the heart.

Plato's view of physiology differed little from those of Hippocrates and Aristotle, although he saw the soul as being made up of three parts, the sensual soul located in the liver, the emotional part in the chest and the eternal, rational soul contained in the brain. As part of his philosophy of humans, Aristotle saw all organisms as comprising two elements, matter and spirit, the combination of which brought about life. Aristotle believed the soul

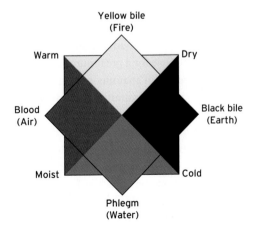

Figure 1.1 The elements, qualities and humours of the human body according to Hippocratic medicine.

lay within the heart and was the central human organ. In contrast, Aristotle believed the brain to be an insensitive organ, a fact supported by the lack of blood found there. Furthermore, he believed the cerebrum was responsible for cooling the heat of the body resulting in the secretion of mucus products that were eliminated from the body through the nose.

Although by modern-day standards there were many flaws in the thinking of the early physiologists, they did identify some of the anatomical structures of the body such as the ventricles of the heart, the auditory canal, middle and inner ear, and various organs such as the liver, brain and blood vessels. Their work paved the way for Galen who was one of the first experimental physiologists.

Galen (129-200 or 217 CE)

If Hippocrates can be seen as the founder of western medicine, then Galen must be viewed as the most influential physician of all time. He took and developed the Greek theories of physiology and medicine and created a body of medical knowledge that was largely unchallenged for over a thousand years. By the time of Galen's birth the Greek empire had fallen to Rome, where he spent much of his career working on physiological research and as physician to emperors such as Marcus Aurelius.

Born in Pergamos, now part of modern-day Turkey, Galen began learning about medicine when he was 16 years old and by the time of his death had produced between 400–500 treaties on medicine, physiology and health. His work has been criticised in the past for the mistakes in some of his findings and his beliefs as they predominated for such a long period of history. This, however, was perhaps due more to the control the church had over the development of knowledge until the beginning of the Renaissance period and the lack of printing presses, rather than anything to do with the nature of the ideas proposed by Galen.

Galen was responsible for the identification of a wide range of organs and tissues within the body as well as, in some cases, correctly identifying their functioning. He carried out many experiments, occasionally on humans, but mainly on animals such as pigs, cows, goats and horses, designed to identify anatomical parts and establish their function. In addition to being physician to emperors, he also treated gladiators after they had been in the arena, devising new treatments for injuries and using his observations to further his anatomical knowledge. In one of his treaties he described the functioning of muscles, correctly identifying the existence and role of muscles, tendons, ligaments, bone and nerve. He explained the functioning

of muscles in antagonistic pairs and that the contraction of a muscle was innervated from the brain or spinal cord. He identified previously unidentified muscles such as the popliteus and plantaris of the lower leg. Contrary to previous physicians and philosophers he demonstrated through experiment the existence of blood in the left ventricle, which had previously been thought to contain the heat of life but no blood. Through ligation of the ureters Galen demonstrated the role of the kidneys in the excretion of waste products and water. With regard to pulmonary gas exchange he deduced correctly that blood was enriched by a vital element in the air that was subsequently delivered to the tissues around the body. He wrote many essays on health and the recommendations he made then have value today. In his laws of health he advised people to take regular fresh air, eat proper foods, exercise regularly (he developed training programmes for this purpose), and ensure adequate periods of sleep along with praising the virtues of a daily bowel movement.

These discoveries represented a major step forward in physiological knowledge However, there were areas where he mistakenly continued, or further developed, flawed thinking from previous physiologists. When Galen was unable to demonstrate the existence of a particular finding he would change the language of his papers to include phrases such as 'no sane person can doubt . . .' to implore the reader to accept his assertions. Galen continued to mistakenly refer to the four humours and the necessity to maintain a balance between them to maintain health. He believed that matter was brought to life through the existence of 'spirits' existing within the brain, heart and liver. He mistakenly believed blood was formed in the liver and that the cardiac septum (the wall between the left and right side of the heart) had pores in it to allow blood to flow from the left to the right side.

Despite the errors in some of Galen's findings and reports, he moved physiological understanding forward from the work of previous physiologists. He made some original discoveries about human and animal physiology. Although it took nearly 1,400 years before his work was seriously followed up (and refuted where necessary) he demonstrated, as perhaps the first experimental physiologist, the need to base findings on research observations.

Andreas Vesalius (1514-64)

When in 1543 the Belgian physician Andreas Vesalius brought out a new text *De Humani Corporis Fabrica* (The Structure of the Human Body) a new epoch in anatomy and physiological discovery began. The origins of the discoveries Vesalius made can perhaps be traced to the start of the separation of scholastic endeavour from religious control. The twelfth and thirteenth centuries saw some of the great universities for the first time make a separation between theological and philosophical faculties (Bologna in about 1119, Paris in 1200, Padua in 1222, Oxford in 1249 and Cambridge in 1284) which allowed for a gradual, but sometimes painful, separation of science and religion. An example of this was the death of Michael Sevetus (1511–53), burned at the stake for heresy, after suggesting the true nature of pulmonary circulation which was in disagreement with the Galenist views of medicine as supported by the church.

The development of the printing press by Bi Sheng in China in 1041 and by Johann Gutenberg in Europe in the 1450s brought about a fundamental shift in the transfer of knowledge. One hundred years later Vesalius benefited greatly from the use of the printing press for the dissemination of his new textbook on human anatomy and physiology. With the advent of the printing press Vesalius' work created a watershed in medical thinking.

Andreas Vesalius, born in 1514 in Brussels, had a fascination with medicine and anatomy from an early age and was said to have conducted dissections of animals as a boy, a practice that might cause consternation for parents and teachers nowadays. For Vesalius it led to a career in the medical profession and he started medical school in Paris at the age of 17. He studied under Jacobus Sylvius, a follower of Galen, who continued the practice of having servants carry out dissections for students to observe. Sadly this meant the dissections were of a very poor quality, as the servants were untrained in such practices. At one such dissection Vesalius, annoyed by the poor techniques being used, took over and completed the dissection in a more exact and scientific manner. During his time in Paris he had to acquire bodies from various sources for dissection. Through this work he began to gain a better understanding of human anatomy. His research led him to question the findings of both Sylvius and Galen and also the accepted anatomical and physiological knowledge. Early in 1537 he moved to Venice to continue his work. Later that same year, at the age of 22, Vesalius was made Doctor of Medicine and put in charge of anatomy and surgery at the University of Padua. Here he continued his research in a city and atmosphere where he was allowed access to human bodies to conduct dissections. He worked under the protection of the rulers of Venice who had noticed his brilliance and appointed him to this role. His continued work led to the discoveries he published in his *De Humani Corporis Fabrica*.

Praise for Vesalius' work comes not only for the hundreds of anatomical differences he observed from Galen's work, but from the brilliant illustrations provided for the text by the Belgian artist Jan Stephan (1499–1546). The developments brought about through Vesalius' work on human anatomy, and made available for the medical profession by the invention of the printing press, can be seen in the skeletons depicted in Figure 1.2. The skeleton on the left shows the extent of knowledge and accuracy in the 14th century. The depiction by Stephan shows the extent of Versalius' work and knowledge of human anatomy.

There were mistakes in Versalius' work. He did not refute the pores Galen described in the septum wall and he added an extra muscle for controlling the eye, but his work overthrew the dogma of a thousand years and paved the way for later physiologists following his methods of experimentation and observation.

William Harvey (1578-1657)

Born in Folkestone, William Harvey studied medicine first at Cambridge and then at the University of Padua (which had continued its support for the development of anatomy and physiology after earlier guidance by Vesalius) before moving to London to begin his medical career. During his medical work he was physician to Francis Bacon and Charles I. He had a great fascination with the circulation of the blood and in 1616 he began lecturing on the subject. It was not until 1628, however, that he set down his ideas in text when he wrote *Exercitatio Anatomica de Motu Cordis et Sanguinis* (an Anatomical Treatise on the Movement of the Heart and Blood). In this work Harvey explained correctly for the first time how the blood circulated around the body. Through experimentation and observation with animals and humans, Harvey was able to determine that blood was forced into the aorta and pulmonary artery with each contraction of the heart, returning to the heart from the lungs via the pulmonary veins and from the body via the other veins of the body. He concluded that circulation of the blood was a one-way journey in a closed system. In addition, he was the first to denounce the notion of pores in the septum between the left and right side of the heart stating:

> . . . if the pulmonary vein were destined for the conveyance of air, it has the structure of a blood vessel here . . . Still less is that opinion to be tolerated which . . . supposes the blood to ooze through the septum of the heart from the right side to the left ventricle by certain secret pores . . .

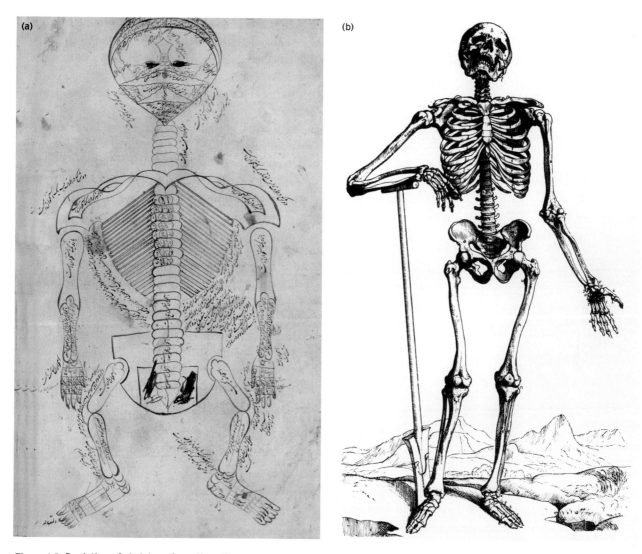

Figure 1.2 Depiction of skeletons from the 14th century (a) and by Jan Stephan, artist for Versalius' *De Humani Corporis Fabrica* (b). (*Source*: Science Photo Library Ltd (*right*))

> But, in faith, no such pores can be demonstrated, neither in fact, do any such exist.
>
> (William Harvey, 1628).

With this statement he correctly rejected over 1,500 years of medical thinking. Despite the moves forward since the times of Vesalius there were still those who clung to the old beliefs. Jean Riolan, Chair of Anatomy at the University of Paris in the 1640s claimed that Galen's interpretation of blood circulation was still correct and if Harvey had found differently then his subjects must have been abnormal.

Robert Boyle (1627–91)

During his career, Irish natural philospher Robert Boyle (Figure 1.3) devised a number of ingenious experiments based in his laboratories in Oxford and London and was a founding member of the Royal Society.

He was the first to analyse the components of blood, also describing its properties including taste, colour, weight and temperature. Working with Robert Hooke (1635–1703) he constructed an air pump which they used to examine the nature of air for combustion and living creatures. During different experiments using the pump, Boyle and Hooke extracted air from a jar containing mice, birds or candles. With the reduction of air the animals became unconscious and the flame on the candle died. When they reintroduced air the animals often recovered. Boyle and Hooke concluded that air contained was a substance that maintained both life and combustion.

7

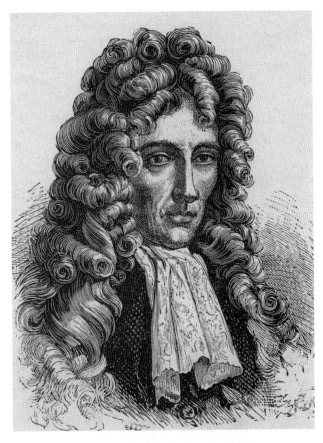

Figure 1.3 Robert Boyle. (*Source*: Science Photo Library Ltd (SPL))

In other research, Boyle (1660) designed and employed a mercury-filled column to determine atmospheric pressure. With this knowledge he went on to devise an experiment in 1662 to examine the effects of pressure on the volume of a gas. The apparatus, was a J-shaped glass tube sealed at one end with air trapped between mercury and the end of the tube. Boyle found that the volume of the gas varied proportionally with the pressure of mercury on the gas. It was from this work that Boyle's law was created. Later (in 1676) this was amended slightly by a French scientist Edme Mariotte (1620–84), who noted that Boyle's finding held true when the temperature of the gas remained constant.

Marcello Malpighi (1628–94) and Anton van Leeuwenhoek (1632–1723)

Further development of physiology was greatly helped during this time by the development of microscopes and magnifying glasses. Malpighi, born and educated in Bologna, became a celebrated microscopist working with two-lens microscopes, while van Leeuwenhoek, a tradesman born

in Delft, was famous for the observations he made using his own hand-crafted (single-lens) magnifying glasses. Malpighi, following up Harvey's work, was able to demonstrate under the microscope the direct link between the arteries and the veins in the lungs of a frog. He also identified erythrocytes (red blood cells) for the first time, although he thought they were globules of fat. Later van Leeuwenhoek identified them correctly; he was also the first to notice the striated nature of muscle fibres and the rods and cones in the retina. The advent of microscopes revealed a new world to the scientists of the day.

Sir James Lind (1716–94)

Born and trained in Edinburgh, James Lind was a naval physician who carried out a number of experiments whilst working on the many journeys he undertook with the Navy. Lind recognised the effects of cold water immersion and also recognised the need to re-warm victims of body temperature cooling. In 1747 he ran what was probably the first crossover design study to examine the effects of adding citrus to the diet of sailors on board HMS Salisbury, where he was serving as physician. Scurvy was responsible for the death of many sailors and Lind found that by adding lemons and oranges to their diet sailors could avoid this terrible disease. Although his results were ignored for almost 40 years his ideas were eventually taken on by the Navy and Army.

Joseph Black (1728–99)

Born in Bordeaux, but of Scottish descent, Joseph Black was taught to read and write by his mother before studying medicine at Glasgow University and then taking a lecturing post at the University of Edinburgh. Through his research into gases and their properties he made a number of discoveries that helped future researchers including Antoine Lavoisier. He proved to be a very popular lecturer with hundreds of students often attending his sessions where he frequently carried out practical experiments for those present. Prior to Black's work, air had been generally considered an element. Through his research, however, Black demonstrated that air was made up of a number of different parts. By heating calcium carbonate (limestone) in separate experiments he found it lost weight. He concluded that limestone lost part of its volume to air, which he termed 'fixed air' and we now call carbon dioxide. In another experiment he collected a sample of fixed air and bubbled the gas through a solution of lime to produce calcium carbonate. In doing this he not only discovered carbon dioxide, but also demonstrated that a gas could combine with a solid, which had previously been believed to be impossible.

Joseph Priestley (1733-1804) and Carl Scheele (1742-86)

Between 1772 and 1774, without knowing the exact nature of it, both Joseph Priestley and Carl Scheele discovered what Scheele termed 'fire air' and we know as oxygen. Clinging to old theories of the past, Priestley, a Yorkshireman born near Leeds, and Scheele, from Köping in Sweden, discovered oxygen when they burned red oxide of mercury. In a further experiment Priestley added plants to a room filled with fixed air (carbon dioxide), and demonstrated that a lighted flame was extinguished due to the lack of oxygen. He left the room for ten days and then tried to light a flame again. This time the flame continued to burn, from which Priestley concluded plants had the ability to clean air.

William Hewson (1739-74)

A British physician, William Hewson, continued the work of previous physiologists on blood, and during his research he correctly identified the coagulation during blood clotting. As part of this research he also identified leukocytes – white blood cells – and fibrinogen which he called 'coagulable lymph'.

Antoine Lavoisier (1743-94)

Working as a tax collector provided Antoine Lavoisier, who was born and educated in Paris, with sufficient time to work on the physics and chemistry experiments he loved. He conducted many experiments into the properties of gases and specifically air. After removing fixed air (carbon dioxide) from air he determined that there still existed a gas that was not used as part of respiration or combustion. This gas, nitrogen, which had also been identified by Daniel Rutherford, he termed 'azot' (meaning no life). From this work and the work of Priestley and Scheele, who both communicated their results to Lavoisier, he determined that 'fire air' or 'burnable air' was necessary for combustion and respiration. He called this component of air 'oxygène'. In further research he recognised that oxygen was converted into carbon dioxide in the body as part of respiration and that heat was generated by this process. He also measured the amount of oxygen used and the carbon dioxide produced in respiration and determined that the

amount of carbon dioxide produced was smaller than the oxygen utilised. From this he deduced that some of the oxygen taken into the body combined with hydrogen within the body to produce water. His work moved respiratory and metabolic physiology forward into a new age. Indeed, it could perhaps be argued that he was the father of exercise physiology, for in his respiratory experiments he also measured oxygen consumption at rest, after food and during exercise. Despite the value of his work he was guillotined during the French Revolution in 1794.

Per Henrik Ling (1776-1839) and Hjalmar Ling (1820-86)

Originally studying divinity, Per Henrik Ling, who was born in Ljunga, Sweden, became fascinated with exercise as a medium for improving health after he improved his own health while teaching fencing at Lund University and taking regular exercise. As a result of this experience he continued his studies, completing a medical degree and then developing his own system of gymnastics. In 1813, with the support of the Swedish Government, he opened the Royal Gymnastics Central Institute in Stockholm and began to teach his method of using exercise to promote health. Later his son Hjalmar, who studied medicine under Claude Bernard (see section below), returned to Stockholm and introduced courses in the biological sciences to complement the teaching of his father's gymnastic methods. This represented perhaps the first university programme course in exercise physiology.

William Prout (1785-1850)

Born in Horton, Gloucestershire, William Prout was not from a rich family and left school aged 13 to work on his father's farm. Realising this was not where his interests lay, he joined a private academy to further his education, working to pay his way, and eventually undertook medicine at the University of Edinburgh. During his career he worked as a urinary specialist at both St. Thomas' Hospital and Guy's Hospital in London, where he conducted numerous experiments during his non-contact hours. He was the first person to advocate following a balanced diet including four essential components: 'hydrates of carbon', fat, protein and water. In this same paper he advocated milk as the 'great alimentary prototype'. In 1823 he demonstrated that gastric juice was in fact hydrochloric acid and in other work helped to improve the barometer. Building upon Lavoisier's research, he also measured carbon dioxide production at rest, after food and during exercise. He demonstrated that while we are walking, carbon dioxide production reaches a plateau. This finding formed the basis for the later concept of 'steady-state' exercise at sub-maximal levels.

Heinrich Magnus (1802-70)

Born in Berlin, Heinrich Magnus studied in Berlin, Stockholm and Paris before returning to teach at the University of Berlin where he was an excellent and popular teacher. He carried out research across a number of aspects of physiology, but his most significant findings for the future of exercise physiology related to the concentrations of oxygen and carbon dioxide in the blood. In 1837 he demonstrated that oxygen and carbon dioxide were carried in arterial and venous blood. Further to this his research was able to show that higher concentrations of oxygen were present in arterial blood, with higher carbon dioxide concentrations being present in venous blood.

Claude Bernard (1813-78)

Hailed as one of the greatest physiologists of all time, Frenchman Claude Bernard who was born in Villefranche, near Lyon, often worked in very difficult conditions. France was not blessed with the number of medical and physiological laboratories that existed in countries like Britain and Germany at this time, nor did it have the same resources to fund equipment. In fact, the rooms within which Bernard worked at the Collège de France in Paris were cold, damp and dark. Despite these difficulties, and the reluctance of the French to use microscopes, he produced over 300 scientific writings and was responsible for a large number of significant research findings in his 35-year career. Through experimentation he was able to reveal that plasma glucose levels varied in healthy individuals. This research, in turn, led to the discovery of the glycogenic (glycogen-forming) function of the liver, and helped to increase general knowledge about diabetes. He investigated and identified the nerves responsible for vasodilation and vasoconstriction and discovered the deleterious effect of carbon monoxide on arterial and venous oxygenation. In the 1860s, when he was spending less time in his laboratory for health reasons, Bernard began to consider the internal environments of living things. He described how cells on the inside of any living matter could not survive if revealed to the outside, external environment. The internal environment was essential for life and components within this environment had to work to maintain these stable conditions. These thoughts were taken forward by Cannon (1871–1945) who, based on Bernard's work, introduced the term **homeostasis**.

Edward Smith (1819-74)

A physician working in London, Edward Smith was interested in improving health and conditions for the poorer in society including prisoners. During the 1820s treadwheels (forerunners to the treadmills we know now) had been introduced to prisons such as Brixton as a further corrective measure for inmates. Interested in their effects on the inmates, Smith designed and built a closed-circuit breathing apparatus to measure carbon dioxide production during treadwheel climbing. Through this research, during the 1850s, Smith was able to demonstrate that CO_2 production increased during exercise and to estimate energy expenditure during climbing. Smith also examined the diets of prisoners and observed that diets were inadequate for the exercise demands of treadwheel climbing. He concluded that the combined effect of poor diet and treadwheel exercise regimes left prisoners too sick to perform manual labour, and therefore to gain work, when leaving prison. He concluded that the exercise regime, combined with the poor diet in prisons, rather than helping reform the inmates was probably more likely to result in reoffending due to prisoners being unable to work upon release from prison.

In other research Smith measured heart rate, respiration rate and inspiratory air volumes during a variety of forms of exercise including swimming, rowing and walking. In addition, he led the first survey of the nutrition of the poor in London, the results of which indicated that diets were inadequate for healthy living.

Adolf Fick (1829-1901)

Born in Kassell in Germany, Adolf Fick (Figure 1.4) became a renowned physicist, mathematician and physiologist. He graduated from the University of Marburg as a Doctor of Medicine in 1851 and one year later took the Chair of Anatomy and Physiology at the University of Zurich, later returning to Germany to a similar position at the University of Würzburg, where he remained for the rest of his career.

During a distinguished career Fick carried out numerous experiments, wrote textbooks on physics and physiology, as well as explaining the intensity of diffusion rates in liquids and the distribution patterns of compounds in solvents. With regard to physiology, he is perhaps best known for creating a way of measuring cardiac output which became known as the Fick principle or equation. This theory, which could not be measured at the time of its development as the technology did not exist, was published in 1870, and was much ahead of its time. It was not

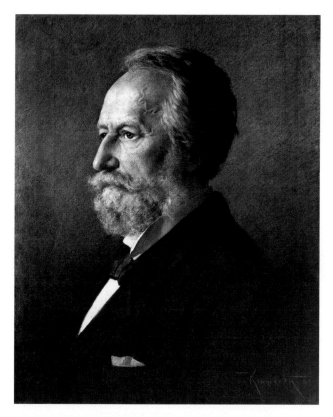

Figure 1.4 Adolf Fick in the early Zurich years. (*Source*: Reproduced with permission from the Photographic Collection of the Boston Medical Library in the Francis A. Countway Library of Medicine, Boston, MA.)

until 1930 that it was verified by André Cournand, Werner Forssmann and Dickinson Richards who later (in 1956) received the Nobel Prize in Physiology or Medicine for their demonstration of the Fick principle.

Christian Bohr (1855–1911) and August Krogh (1874–1949)

Christian Bohr, born in Copenhagen, became Professor of Physiology when he was just 30 years old and produced much of his research in the area of muscular contractions and blood gases. Part of his research legacy was the Bohr effect through which the impact of temperature and relative acidity on the oxyhaemoglobin dissociation curve was described. Danish physiologist August Krogh was born in Jutland, Denmark and studied medicine and then zoology at the University of Copenhagen. After graduation he worked, initially, as assistant to Christian Bohr at the laboratory of medical physiology at the University of Copenhagen. Inspired by Bohr's work August Krogh went on to conduct research in a wide range of areas including disproving the findings of one of his mentor's theories relating to the transport of gas into the blood. Bohr, and

indeed J. S. Haldane, whose contribution to physiology is discussed below, maintained that gases entered the blood via secretion. Through his research Krogh was able to demonstrate that gas exchange took place via diffusion rather than secretion. In later research he went on to conduct studies that led to the identification of the methods by which gases were transported by the blood and demonstrated that there was an increase in muscle capillary opening in response to exercise. In 1912, with his colleague Johannes Lindhard (1870–1947), he went on to describe the cardiovascular response to exercise, and the relative contributions of fat and carbohydrate to exercise metabolism.

Nathan Zuntz (1847–1920)

A German physiologist born in Bonn, Nathan Zuntz was an important scientist in the area of exercise and environmental physiology. He studied medicine at the University of Bonn and then worked briefly in Berlin and Bonn before becoming established for 37 years as the Head of Animal Physiology at the Agricultural University in Berlin. In his career Zuntz carried out numerous experiments and produced over 430 articles in areas such as blood, gas kinetics, respiration and energy metabolism, as well as the effects of altitude. He led expeditions to Monta Rosa and Tenerife to study altitude physiology and, with his colleague August Julius Geppert (1856–1937), developed an apparatus to analyse expired air gases in the laboratory and even a portable system (carried on the back) which he used to assess energy metabolism. In the laboratory he used his gas analysis equipment in conjunction with several treadmills that were developed specifically for the purpose, including one for cows. As part of his study of expired air, working again with Geppert, he developed the equations necessary to make the Haldane transformation some years before John Haldane (after whom the equation was named) developed his version.

John Scott Haldane (1860–1936)

The Scottish physiologist John Haldane (Figure 1.5) was born in Edinburgh where he later went to university to study medicine. Two years after graduating he moved to the Department of Physiology at Oxford University. After the disappointment of not receiving a promotion he left the university and opened his own laboratory, the Cherwell Laboratory, in his own back garden. One of his early research projects, in a career where his main focus was on human respiration and the practical application of physiology, was conducted on the London Underground where he set about testing carbon monoxide levels on and around underground trains. The results of his study led directly to the electrification of trains due to the poor air quality. In other work underground he carried out many studies of mines and was responsible for advocating the use of canaries in mines to detect carbon monoxide, due to their being more susceptible to the effects of the gas and thus presenting an early-warning system for miners.

Although he mistakenly continued in his belief about gas secretion in the lungs he made several very important findings with regard to gas kinetics. In 1905, working with his colleague John Gillies Priestley (1880–1941), Haldane identified the role of the partial pressure of carbon dioxide in the regulation of ventilation. In order to study carbon dioxide and oxygen concentrations in expired gases he developed an instrument to carry out such analyses. He also conducted research in the area of diving and, using goats as subjects (as they were the cheapest and most readily available animal akin to the size of humans), investigated the causes of the bends. He subsequently developed tables for decompression that were adopted by the British and American navies and are still in use today. He also designed decompression chambers for deep-sea divers. He carried out many simulated altitude studies and went on expeditions to examine the effects of altitude on respiration.

His son, J. B. S. Haldane (1892–1964) (Figure 1.6), was a brilliant and colourful British scientist. He received a very early taste of the world of science, being involved in a number of his father's studies including testing an experimental submarine when he was 16 years old; he went on to attend Oxford University. Being a subject for his own research was an experience that stayed with JBS (as he preferred to be called) throughout his career and included testing his wife in a variety of pressure studies and research to examine the effects of nitrogen narcosis. He was very casual about the side effects of involvement in his research, once commenting on the incidence of burst eardrums in his decompression studies that 'the drum generally heals up; and if a hole remains in it, although one is somewhat deaf, one can blow tobacco smoke out of the ear in question, which is a social accomplishment'. His accomplishments included popularising science through essays he wrote, investigating the effects of breathing pure oxygen when diving (from which research guidelines were established for safe diving depths using oxygen) and studying the effects of elevated carbon dioxide levels on manual dexterity and functioning.

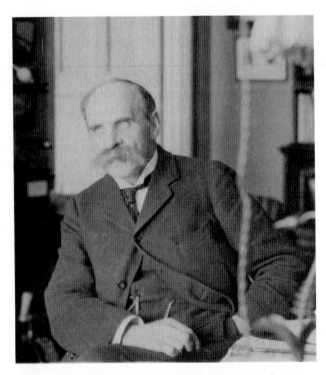

Figure 1.5 J. S. Haldane. (*Source*: GNU Free Documentation License: Wikipedia)

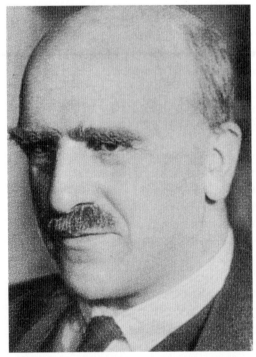

Figure 1.6 J. B. S. Haldane. (*Source*: Science Photo Library Ltd)

Ernest Starling (1866-1927)

A London-born physiologist who studied across a range of research areas, Ernest Starling is perhaps best known for his part in the development of the Frank–Starling Law, along with the German physiologist Otto Frank (1865–1944), which describes the effects of ventricular filling on contraction force. In the description of his research it was stated that:

> Experiments carried out in this laboratory have shown that in an isolated heart . . . within physiological limits . . . the larger the diastolic volume . . . the greater is the energy of the contraction.
>
> (Starling and Visscher, 1926)

Within his career Starling did much more than this; he was instrumental in the commencement of research into hormone function and was the person who coined the term 'hormone' to describe the chemical messengers at the heart of the endocrine system.

Sir Frederick Gowland Hopkins (1861-1947)

Sir Frederick Gowland Hopkins, born in Eastbourne, studied medicine at Guy's Hospital in London and then went on to work at Cambridge University. During his career, most of which he spent at Cambridge University, he made many discoveries including vitamins, or as he termed them 'accessory food factors', for which he and Christiaan Eijkman (1858–1930) won the Nobel Prize in Physiology for Medicine in 1929 (although these discoveries were made well before this, between the 1890s and 1906). In 1907, working with Sir Walter Morley Fletcher (1873-1933), Hopkins made an important discovery in the biochemistry of muscle contraction. In this research conducted with isolated muscle tissue, Hopkins and Fletcher demonstrated that a working muscle produces lactic acid. Hopkins went on to identify the subsequent creation of glycogen from lactic acid and was also one of the first to see cells as independent machines within the body.

Archibald Vivian Hill (1886-1977)

Educated in Devon and then at Trinity College, Cambridge (where he studied mathematics), Archibald Hill (Figure 1.7) who was born in Bristol, made a significant contribution to exercise physiology across a long career at Cambridge and Manchester Universities and University College, London. Hill's mentor at Cambridge was John Langley (1852–1925) who, as Head of Physiology, drew his attention to the work of Hopkins and Fletcher on lactic acid and the links to oxygen for recovery. This work formed the basis for much of his future study and he completed his doctorate under the supervision of Fletcher. Working with his colleague Hartley Lupton in 1923 they proposed and demonstrated for the first time a theory of maximum oxygen intake which has now become known as $\dot{V}O_{2\,max}$ or maximal oxygen uptake. The researchers stated 'there is clearly some critical speed for each individual . . . above which . . . the maximum oxygen intake is inadequate'. Hill and Lupton went on to describe for the first time the term oxygen debt and the maximal anaerobic level which they termed maximal oxygen debt. In addition, Hill developed a method for predicting running performance from knowledge of maximal oxygen intake and the

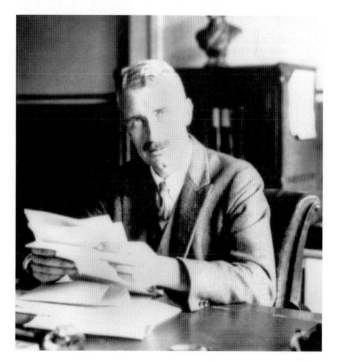

Figure 1.7 Archibald Hill. (*Source*: US National Library of Medicine)

running speed at which this was attained. In other research Hill described the phases in muscular heat production that occur in response to exercise. He also identified for the first time that heat was produced during the transmission of a nerve impulse.

Andrew Huxley (1917–)

Discoverer of two major aspects of physiology, Andrew Huxley (Figure 1.8) was born in London and spent much of his career at Trinity College, Cambridge. His half-brother was the famous writer Aldous Huxley who wrote *Brave New World*.

Working with Sir Alan Hodgkin (1914–98) he identified the roles of potassium and sodium ions in the transmission of nerve impulses or action potentials for which they received the Nobel Prize in Physiology for Medicine in 1963. Interestingly, Huxley and Hodgkin used the axon from a giant squid to measure the ionic current, as human axons were too small to be measured using the equipment they had available at the time. During the 1950s Andrew and Hugh Huxley (1924–) (no relation) from Birkenhead, Liverpool and also educated at Cambridge, working

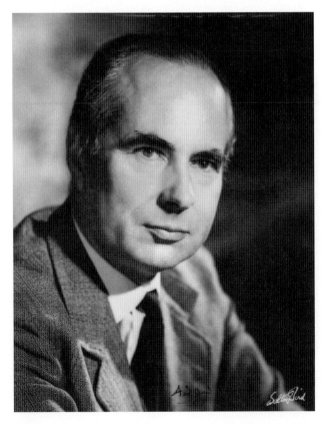

Figure 1.8 Andrew Huxley. (*Source*: US National Library of Medicine)

independently, described the nature of muscular contraction in the Sliding Filament Theory. The two met in 1953, shared their ideas and, soon after, these were published in side-by-side articles in the journal *Nature* in 1954.

Sir Joseph Barcroft (1872–1947)

Born in Northern Ireland, Joseph Barcroft moved to England to study Natural Sciences at Cambridge in 1893. After graduating he continued at Cambridge within the Physiology department for virtually his entire career. He carried out further research in the area of gas diffusion with his findings later supported through Krogh's work regarding the concept of gas diffusion rather than secretion. He carried out many experiments with himself as the subject, including spending six days in a chamber with low oxygen concentration. He also demonstrated the differing effects of gases on animals in an experiment where he, and a dog, were exposed to the gas from hydrocyanic acid – the dog being much the worse for the experiment, while he (Barcroft) recovered. He also took part in many high-altitude studies including directing a study on Cerro de Pasco in Peru. As part of this aspect of his research he successfully examined the effects of decreased oxygen on the dissociation curve for haemoglobin.

Otto Meyerhof (1884–1951)

After graduating as a doctor of medicine from the University of Heidelberg, Otto Meyerhof, who was born in Hannover, initially began a career in psychology before moving on to work in the area of physiological chemistry. With the collaboration of a variety of workers such as Jacob Parnas, Carl Neuberg, Otto Warburg, Carl Cori (1896–1984) and Gerty Cori (1896–1957), Meyerhof was able to demonstrate the pathway suggested in 1933 by Gustav Embden that detailed glycolysis – the complete breakdown of glucose to pyruvate or lactic acid. Carl and Gerty Cori, born in Prague and graduates from the German University of Prague later emigrated and continued their careers in the USA. In other studies the Coris went on to identify the pathway for the regeneration of muscle glycogen stores in the liver from lactic acid, in what has become known as the Cori cycle.

Hans Krebs (1900–81) and Fritz Hipmann (1899–1986)

Born in Hildesheim, Germany, Hans Krebs (Figure 1.9) spent the early part of his career working there, before moving to Britain in 1933.

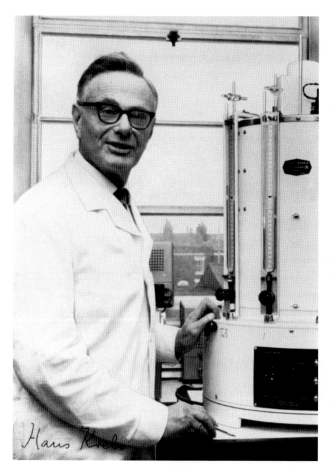

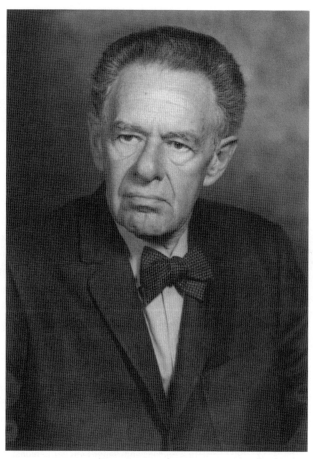

Figure 1.9 Hans Krebs. (*Source*: Science Photo Library Ltd (SPL))

Figure 1.10 Fritz Albert Lipmann. (*Source*: Smithsonian Institute)

During a distinguished career he worked at Oxford, Cambridge and Sheffield universities on a variety of research projects based around the area of intermediary metabolism. He is perhaps most renowned for his proposal, in collaboration with William Johnston in 1937, of the citric acid cycle or, as it is otherwise known, the tricarboxylic acid cycle or Krebs cycle. There were some gaps in the pathway at that time; however, further research by Fritz Lipmann (1899–86) and Nathan Kaplan (1917–86) published in 1945, identified co-enzyme A and completed the cycle as it is known today. Fritz Lipmann (Figure 1.10) was born in Koenigsberg, Germany and educated there before taking positions in the Netherlands, Germany, Denmark, and the USA. He was also responsible in 1941 for identifying the high-energy bond in adenosine triphosphate (ATP) and the phosphagen system.

A useful way to summarise the developments that have taken place in exercise physiology since early times is to present them as a timeline of discovery. Figure 1.11 (see overleaf) provides such a summary and it is interesting, as

well as noting the achievements that have been made, to also recognise the gaps in development that occurred during times such as the Dark Ages. This age is described in further detail in the next section which describes the developments in contemporary sport and physical education as we know them now.

1.2 An historical perspective: the context of contemporary sport, exercise and physical education[1]

Since recorded history, sport, exercise and physical education have played important but diverse roles in the development and functioning of individuals and society. Depending on social conditions and needs at any given time, sport, exercise and physical education have been often critically important factors in personal survival, the

[1]By Ian Culpan.

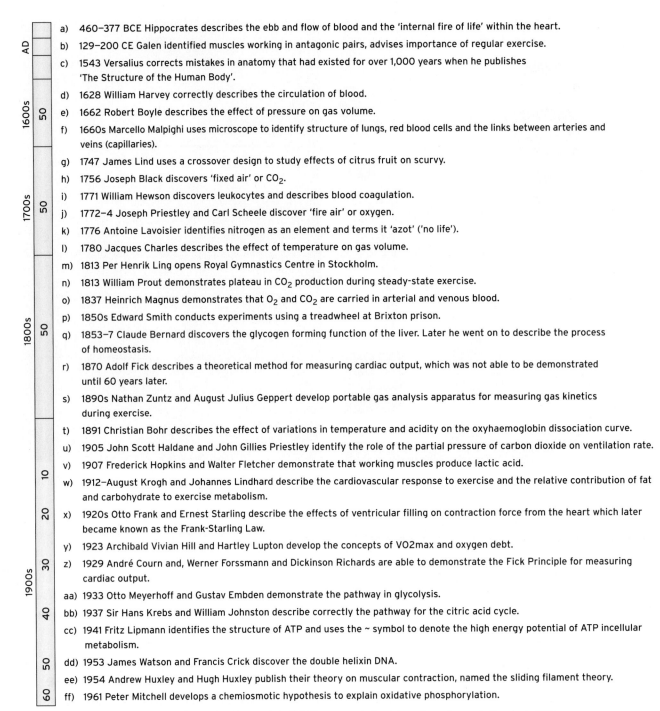

a) 460–377 BCE Hippocrates describes the ebb and flow of blood and the 'internal fire of life' within the heart.

b) 129–200 CE Galen identified muscles working in antagonic pairs, advises importance of regular exercise.

c) 1543 Versalius corrects mistakes in anatomy that had existed for over 1,000 years when he publishes 'The Structure of the Human Body'.

d) 1628 William Harvey correctly describes the circulation of blood.

e) 1662 Robert Boyle describes the effect of pressure on gas volume.

f) 1660s Marcello Malpighi uses microscope to identify structure of lungs, red blood cells and the links between arteries and veins (capillaries).

g) 1747 James Lind uses a crossover design to study effects of citrus fruit on scurvy.

h) 1756 Joseph Black discovers 'fixed air' or CO_2.

i) 1771 William Hewson discovers leukocytes and describes blood coagulation.

j) 1772–4 Joseph Priestley and Carl Scheele discover 'fire air' or oxygen.

k) 1776 Antoine Lavoisier identifies nitrogen as an element and terms it 'azot' ('no life').

l) 1780 Jacques Charles describes the effect of temperature on gas volume.

m) 1813 Per Henrik Ling opens Royal Gymnastics Centre in Stockholm.

n) 1813 William Prout demonstrates plateau in CO_2 production during steady-state exercise.

o) 1837 Heinrich Magnus demonstrates that O_2 and CO_2 are carried in arterial and venous blood.

p) 1850s Edward Smith conducts experiments using a treadwheel at Brixton prison.

q) 1853–7 Claude Bernard discovers the glycogen forming function of the liver. Later he went on to describe the process of homeostasis.

r) 1870 Adolf Fick describes a theoretical method for measuring cardiac output, which was not able to be demonstrated until 60 years later.

s) 1890s Nathan Zuntz and August Julius Geppert develop portable gas analysis apparatus for measuring gas kinetics during exercise.

t) 1891 Christian Bohr describes the effect of variations in temperature and acidity on the oxyhaemoglobin dissociation curve.

u) 1905 John Scott Haldane and John Gillies Priestley identify the role of the partial pressure of carbon dioxide on ventilation rate.

v) 1907 Frederick Hopkins and Walter Fletcher demonstrate that working muscles produce lactic acid.

w) 1912–August Krogh and Johannes Lindhard describe the cardiovascular response to exercise and the relative contribution of fat and carbohydrate to exercise metabolism.

x) 1920s Otto Frank and Ernest Starling describe the effects of ventricular filling on contraction force from the heart which later became known as the Frank-Starling Law.

y) 1923 Archibald Vivian Hill and Hartley Lupton develop the concepts of VO2max and oxygen debt.

z) 1929 André Courn and, Werner Forssmann and Dickinson Richards are able to demonstrate the Fick Principle for measuring cardiac output.

aa) 1933 Otto Meyerhoff and Gustav Embden demonstrate the pathway in glycolysis.

bb) 1937 Sir Hans Krebs and William Johnston describe correctly the pathway for the citric acid cycle.

cc) 1941 Fritz Lipmann identifies the structure of ATP and uses the ~ symbol to denote the high energy potential of ATP incellular metabolism.

dd) 1953 James Watson and Francis Crick discover the double helixin DNA.

ee) 1954 Andrew Huxley and Hugh Huxley publish their theory on muscular contraction, named the sliding filament theory.

ff) 1961 Peter Mitchell develops a chemiosmotic hypothesis to explain oxidative phosphorylation.

Figure 1.11 A timeline of some significant developments in thinking around physiology from the early Greeks to 1961.

military protection of citizens, thanksgiving to the god(s), the social control and discipline of individuals and groups, demonstration of political superiority, the development of healthy bodies and moral character, the celebration of special events, competitive contests, entertainment, the productive use of leisure time and of course part of the holistic education of citizens. What has become clear is that over time, as civilisations have developed, prospered and waned, sport and physical education have had many and varied goals and purposes. What is also equally clear is the fact that for some, sport and physical education were hard and dangerous work, e.g. military soldiering, but for others they were a sombre and spiritually reflective practice, e.g. ritualistic and religious ceremonies. For some they were glorifying an imperfect body which was considered by some as a pagan and sinful activity, while for others they were a joyous leisurely and playful time, for example, amusement for the wealthy and privileged classes.

Early historical societies

It would appear that very early societies such as those in Egypt, Mesopotamia and China did not necessarily focus on formal education. Instead, the emphasis in these early societies was essentially using physical activity as a basis for survival, the propagation of human life and to ward off possible raiders. This was manifested through the inculcation of skills and attributes necessary to hunt and gather food in order to survive, and the development of combative skills to protect their possessions and communities. It could be argued, of course, that sport and physical education practices were restricted to the learning of skills associated with how to throw, run, fight and dance in order to secure enough food for their collective living and to pay homage to the gods for the provision of such. The limited education that did exist was for the collective good of community living as opposed to any desire for individual development. In essence education was for ensuring that a particular society survived and that the young understood its importance in adult life. As a consequence, some physical training activities included young men in the ancient world learning to throw spears, wrestle and box, shoot bow and arrow and ride horses. Young men participated in these activities as soon as they were physically capable. Prior to that, just like in contemporary society today, the young played games to learn cultural traditions, values and practices and of course simply to have fun. Many of these sorts of activities exist today in the contemporary world and are legacies of this time, but in many cases the reasons for doing such are quite different from ancient times.

Greek society (1600 BCE-150 CE)

The achievements of ancient Greece have had a major impact on the way we think about sport, exercise and physical education today. At an obvious level are the legacies associated with gymnasiums, stadiums, contests and competitions, the Olympic Games, body care and perfection, athletic performance, and of course the rituals and ceremonies associated with sporting festivals and the worshipping of their gods. However, from a philosophical perspective, the Greeks left us with the dilemma that has stretched and exercised the minds of great philosophers over time. The debate about education dualism was central

to Greek education. Greek educational philosophers, at the time, argued two quite distinct positions. One particular educational view argued that the human body needed to be developed, cultivated and educated in order for the mind to function efficiently and creatively. This view believed that ultimately the mind, because of its ability to think logically and rationally, was superior to the body. As a consequence, this view promoted that the role of sport and physical education was simply to enhance the mind, and that the body was a servant to that process. Even today we often hear coaches, physical educators and sports people justifying their practices by stating 'a healthy body means a healthy mind'. The other quite opposite view in Greek society argued that every person had a duality about them. That duality was their mind and their body and each was as important as the other. As a consequence, sport, exercise and physical education needed to develop both the mind and body in a harmonious and balanced manner so that each could reach its potential. Today this argument of harmonious balanced development of the mind, body and spirit is a worthy educational justification for sport and physical education in schools. Despite these two differing philosophical positions, the importance of physical education, sport and athletic movements was recognised. The Greeks perceived their gods to be both physically beautiful and perfect with outstanding physical and intellectual skills and abilities. As a result it was the responsibility of every young male citizen to try and emulate the gods. Sport and physical education were the means by which they could attempt to achieve this physical and intellectual excellence. Even today similar arguments are used to justify the combined quest for physical and intellectual excellence. While contemporary society has moved away from trying to emulate the gods the presence of sport and physical education in schools is an attempt to develop this all-round excellence.

While two philosophical positions dominated Greek thinking about the educational worth of sport, exercise and physical education they did have a marked effect on how they were practised. In Sparta, for instance, the education of young men used the training of the body, that is, *education of the physical*, to achieve superb physical specimens for combative and military purposes. The Spartans did not place importance on the development of cultural and aesthetic understanding. However, in Athens, sport, exercise and physical education were used as *education through the physical*. For the Athenians these were not only for military purposes but also for the all-round holistic development of the person. This was aimed at producing moral citizens who had good values and attitudes to community life and who had an appreciation of the arts and cultural aspects of Greek society. Despite the different purposes, it was considered irresponsible in both Sparta and Athens for a young man to be physically unfit and unskilled. If a young man was flabby, out of shape and unfit, his fellow citizens considered it a disgrace and a sign of poor education. Interestingly enough, both Spartan and Athenian sport, exercise and physical education practices included similar content and activities. These included ball games, boxing, gymnastics, running, throwing the javelin, and wrestling.

In examining Greek sport, exercise and physical education it is very clear that the Greeks, perhaps more than any other society in human history, valued this aspect of their culture, placing high importance on it. Such has been the impact of the Greek sporting legacy that many contemporary sporting practices and events show evidence of its influence. While many of these practices still exist, it is the philosophical thinking about sport and physical education that is perhaps the Greeks' greatest legacy. Given this importance it is not surprising that Greek society placed high importance on athletic contests and festivals which were essentially spectacular religious tributes to the many Greek gods. The most important, of course, was the Olympic festival held at Olympia in honour of the most powerful Greek god Zeus. Originally (376 BCE) athletes from all over the Greek empire would come to pay homage to Zeus and compete in sporting events that put high emphasis on the ideals of honesty, courage, respect, justice and excellence. However, over time, just like today, these athletic ideals became secondary to the quest for individual fame and fortune, and the need for the many Greek states to demonstrate their political superiority. Over the centuries the religious purpose and spirit of the Olympic Games deteriorated and in 394 CE the Roman emperor declared that the once-magnificent spectacle paying homage to the Greek god Zeus, through the demonstration of certain human excellences, was no longer appropriate. It wasn't until 1894, many centuries later, that the French educator/philosopher Pierre de Coubertin re-established the Olympic Movement and the first Olympic Games of the modern era were held in Athens in 1896.

The demise of the Olympic Games in Greece was symbolic of the fact that the Greeks, over time, had gradually moved away from the emphasis on physical development (physical education and sport) as an essential part of individual holistic education. However, while this golden period of sport, exercise and physical education in society ended, the inspirational legacy that Greece has left contemporary society should be of interest to all those involved in sport.

The Romans (100 BCE–500 CE)

Sport, exercise and physical education during the Roman Empire were important for reasons significantly different from those of the Greeks. Whereas the Greeks had a sophisticated philosophical positioning for sport and physical education which emphasised individual development combined with military purposes and paying homage to the gods, the Romans were far more pragmatic. In Rome the initial focus was on order, obedience, and respect for the rule of law. Essentially Romans were educated (trained) to become soldiers and useful citizens. The ability to fight to protect and expand the empire and to obey authority was an important initial priority. The pragmatic nature of the Romans saw their young trained to fight and to live healthy efficient lives. Compared with the Greeks there was a distinct lack of education for body perfection, aesthetics, intellectual and cultural development. Instead the Roman societal machine was more interested in promoting physical development for team unity (military legions) and health. It is true that the Romans did acknowledge their gods on sporting occasions but certainly not to the same extent as the Greeks. In Rome the key promoters of the aims and purposes of sport and physical education were Roman fathers who took their sons to training temples to teach them physical skills associated with archery, boxing, chariot driving, fencing, horse-riding, jumping, running, swimming, and wrestling. While unity and healthy adherence to exercise were important, the education of the young (boys) through these physical pursuits also served as an entry into Roman manhood. Putting all this into context, the pursuit of war in an efficient and brutal manner was a very prestigious profession for the Romans.

The emphasis on efficient brutal military combat and healthy lifestyles gave rise to two key developments during the rise of the Roman Empire. Firstly, as Rome became more and more successful, its wealth increased markedly. As the wealth increased the need for the 'efficient societal machine' began to diminish and citizens of Rome became more hedonistic. There developed a need for festivities associated with large spectator appeal. This took the form of brutal physical contests involving professional soldiers (athletes) or prisoner slaves and/or animals (apes, boars, bulls, elephants, lions, tigers). Spectacular gladiatorial fights resulted, and the once active disciplined citizen became a blood-hungry participant observer who rejoiced in the brutality of the contest and the slaughter and carnage of the vanquished. This was Roman entertainment designed either to make political points between rival noblemen or for the leaders of Rome to entertain the masses.

The second key development was in the pursuit of healthy active lifestyles. Here the citizens of Rome shed the need for efficient team unity and the pursuit of vigorous exercise. Instead, sport, exercise and physical education became more individual leisure pursuits, often involving ball games followed by visits to the Roman baths. These events, the brutal spectacle and the pursuit of more sedate exercise diminished the need for physical education. As a result the aims of sport, exercise and physical education in Roman society became somewhat less important in the development of the *efficient citizen*. This dwindling of importance continued until the eventual demise of the Empire.

Given the characteristics of Roman sport and physical education it is not surprising that a number of citizens of Rome became interested in the exercise/sport health link. Claudius Galen (129–200 or 217 CE), whose contribution to physiology was described in detail in section 1.1 (above), through his interest in sport, can also perhaps be credited as being the first sports medicine practitioner. He became famous for his treatment of gladiators, the use of drugs for medicinal purposes and the science of exercise. He developed considerable practical knowledge in nutrition/diet, exercise and the social and physical benefits these can have. Galen particularly favoured the Greek notion of exercise for balanced development and was opposed to the use of sport as a brutal entertainment. Furthermore he expressed views and concerns that are still evident today, particularly among teachers, coaches and parents. Galen's concern was focused on young people being 'talent-spotted' in order for them to become professional athletes and being directed away from a holistic education, which he believed was an important developmental need of the young. Many of Galen's beliefs originated with his experimental physiological dissections of animals and of course his treatment of injured gladiators. Galen's knowledge of physiology, sports medicine and anatomy lasted throughout the Middle Ages when his works were held in the very highest esteem.

The Dark (500–900 CE) and Middle Ages (900–1400 CE)

Once the Roman Empire had fragmented into smaller pockets of social control and existence, right across Europe the only unifying aspect of life seemed to be the power and influence of the Christian Church – in particular the Roman Catholic Church. Much of this time was characterised by a feudal and agricultural economy dominated politically and academically by the Church. Many of the advanced sport and physical education philosophies and practices of the Greeks, and the applied pragmatic knowledge of the Romans, seemed to have been lost. For sport and physical education, the Dark and Middle Ages were a very bleak time indeed. During the Middle Ages, the philosophical understanding of the body and its relation to religious interpretations was a central tenet in understanding sport and physical education. As described above, the Greeks glorified the human body and sought to perfect it through sport and physical education practices. This glorification occurred as a celebration of the pagan god Zeus, and the Olympic Games in Olympia were a testament to this practice. However, given the power of the Church during the Middle Ages, a common belief propagated by it was that the body was an instrument of sin and to participate in such dedicated physical pursuits to glorify the body was indeed sinful and actually contaminated it. The contamination of the body meant that *man's* spiritual essence, housed within the body, was also corrupted. Essentially the Greek focus was about living in the world. Instead, dominant thinking by the Church was about living in the 'hereafter' and it encouraged the nourishment of the soul through obedience to the Church's laws and dogma. Being controlled by the Church was the only way to true and infinite glory and salvation. As a result, for many centuries, practices associated with sport and physical education in the Middle Ages were practically nonexistent.

While the Church's dominant thinking argued that the body and pursuits associated with its development were evil, not all Christian followers accepted this. For instance some Christian scholars at this time argued that God would not purposely create something that was inherently harmful and evil. They concluded that God was in all things and as a result, the body was filled with godliness. One such scholar was Thomas Aquinas who argued that individuals, to achieve true happiness and perfection, needed to nourish both the body and soul. He argued that for people to become knowledgeable they needed to learn through their bodies and their minds. As a result he, and other like-minded scholars at this time, believed that physical exercise was beneficial to the physical, mental, social, and moral well-being of Christians. This was an important breakthrough, for essentially this was the first time, in western thinking at least, that caring for the body through physical exercise was justified from a philosophical and religious point of view. Interestingly enough this was not unlike the Athenian Greek philosophy or the argument physical educators promote today.

Given this development, the Church, reluctantly at first, began to tolerate fun, games and recreational past times. Pragmatically they could not stop them anyway, but the Church did interfere when the behaviour of the peasants became unruly and drunken. It was not really until the 11th and 12th centuries that the real changes started to gather a little momentum. Ball games that were popular in Roman times started to reappear in modified forms. These modifications were essentially early forms of football, handball, hockey, and tennis. In addition to these, the rich nobleman and landowners hunted and held tournaments in the form of jousting and hand-to-hand fighting, both sports associated with warrior knight activities.

With the change in the Church's acceptance of sport and recreation came the corresponding interest in the body as an object of medical research. As indicated earlier, Galen's work, done many centuries previously, served as the source of medical development. During this medieval period many medical practices involved the administration of herbal, mineral and animal materials in the form of poultices, prescriptions and liquid intakes. This was combined with the therapeutic beliefs associated with superstition, magic and astrology. While this was an important development, medical science during the Dark Ages was dominated by the Church and its saints, often resulting in the necessary therapy. The treatment of disease was multi-therapeutic but essentially such was the dominance of the Church in people's psyche, that sickness was considered a mortal sin punishable by God and recovery was simply a heavenly intervention. On analysis, this belief demonstrated that while the Church had gone some way to accepting the need for care of the body through exercise, the deeply held belief that the body was an imperfect structure and an instrument of sin and corruption still prevailed. However, the domination of the Church was about to change along with an intellectual re-awakening that spread right across Europe towards the end of the Middle Ages. There appeared to be no single cause. However, a range of factors such as dissatisfaction with the power and influence of the Church resulting from intellectual curiosity, the invention of the printing press, the Black Death, the shortage of food and other resources were highly influential. Together they resulted in the re-awakening of society that occurred during the Reformation and Renaissance.

The Reformation and Renaissance (13th–16th century)

For centuries the Roman Catholic Church had a huge influence on the cultural and spiritual beliefs of the population and in so doing had a significant influence on all aspects of human existence. Sport, exercise and physical education were not to escape this influence. Throughout the Dark and Middle Ages, the Church's position on the imperfect and sinful body negated any significant advancement on Greek and Roman philosophies associated with the importance of sport and physical education and its contribution to human development and education. However the period of history following the Dark and Middle Ages was to prove significant in terms of the Church's influence and the intellectual and cultural development particularly of the noble and land-owning classes. This phase in history incorporated the Reformation and the Renaissance. The Reformation, as the name implies, was related to efforts to change or reform the Church. This resulted in the Christian church splitting into two faiths; the Roman Catholic church and the Protestant form of Christianity. The Renaissance was a time for a significant re-awakening of cultural and intellectual curiosity. The Renaissance period drew heavily on Greek and Roman philosophy and resulted in the development of freedom of thought, that is, the open debate of competing philosophies about the nature and purpose of human existence, and the establishment of robust nations and economies characterised by trade and commerce. This period in history saw the emergence of the 'Renaissance man', a person who valued all-round development that used, amongst other pursuits, sport and physical education to develop intellectual, social, spiritual and moral character. This philosophy has become known as 'humanism'. Furthermore the Renaissance man viewed the body as central to achieving this holistic development. In effect Renaissance philosophy, as with Greek philosophy before it, provided a strong foundation for the justification of sport and physical education in western civilisations. Indeed humanism has come to have a profound effect on the educative and social value of sport, exercise and physical education in contemporary society and many school curricula reveal links to humanist principles.

The transformation from the Middle Ages to the philosophies and beliefs of the Reformation and Renaissance periods was not without tension. While many scholars promoted the balanced development of body and mind in education and advocated for sport, exercise and physical education (Petrus Vergerius, Vittorino de Feltre, Thomas Elyot and Aeneas Piccolonini), others did not (Desiderius

Erasmus, John Calvin). Those who were not in favour of sport and physical education as part of education argued that the body should be used for God's work. Calvin argued that goodness was measured by one's work ethic and that if you were playing you were baring your soul as a sinner. Those who advocated for sport, exercise and physical education as important in a holistic education promoted activities such as ball games, dancing, fencing, horse-riding, leaping (jumping), outdoor activities, running, swimming, vaulting, and weapons. Perhaps a key consideration in the promotion of sport, exercise and physical education during this period was that such activities had to be purposeful, as opposed to fun. Fun and enjoyment was considered to lead to sexual pleasures and idleness, which were considered to be ungodly. What was important at this time was that education had to demonstrate tangible benefits. One Renaissance scholar in particular, Thomas Elyot, tried to improve the practices of physical education by relating sport and physical education to medical science. By drawing on his knowledge of anatomy and physiology he argued that a number of benefits could be derived from exercise – it aided digestion and excretion, body temperature regulation, and improved appetite and longevity. He believed that sport, exercise and physical education led to enhanced health which in turn led to a greater capacity to work, and consequently, God's time was put to good use.

Science and the Enlightenment (16th-19th century)

The freedoms sought and gained during the Reformation and Renaissance periods gave rise to the next important period of history, namely the Enlightenment, dominated initially by scientific discovery, but also involving shifts in political governance. It was during this period that scientific thought and the development of technologies such as the barometer and telescope allowed humanity to explore the universe better and to explain it through scientific laws and theorems. Many ideas from the past were now enlightened by new ways of thinking that insisted on careful and more analytical processes as opposed to non-evidence-based dogma. For sport, exercise and physical education this became a critical development, as medical science involving anatomy and physiology focused on elementary investigations of how the body worked and how it responded to exercise. Perhaps one of the best examples of how the age of science and enlightenment affected sport and physical education is through the work of Isaac Newton whose three laws of motion are central to most contemporary biomechanical programmes of study.

While this time was dominated by scientific evidence, philosophers still provided intellectual enlightenment as well. The mind/body debate has raged for centuries and was particularly prominent during this period However, it is important to highlight that during the age of Enlightenment some profound support for sport, exercise and physical education was forthcoming. The philosopher John Locke argued the body was far more important than was recognised by other philosophers. He believed that the body became the instrument by which the mind was developed. He was a strong supporter of sport, exercise and physical education. While Locke believed in the mind and body as two separate entities, he saw practical (bodily) activities as a source of pleasure, refreshment and reinvigoration for the mind. He believed in the need to develop the body in order to enhance personal health, particularly through good diet, adequate sleep and regular and vigorous exercise. In agreement, Jean Rousseau, a follower of Locke, argued for the need for harmony between the mind and the body. Rousseau argued that intellectual development could only follow after strong foundations had been laid in exercise and physical activity. The health of the body was crucial for intellectual development. He therefore highlighted the need for play, adventure, freedom of physical expression and for children to roam in the outdoors in order to gain a plethora of sensory body and motor experiences. This, he argued, was the true basis for physical, intellectual and moral development. Other writers who supported the importance of exercise and physical activity for healthy development included Johann GutsMuths, Johann Basedow and Richard Mulcaster. GutsMuths stressed the importance of a vigorous regime of physical exercise that included balance activities, fencing, flexibility activities, gymnastics, lifting and carrying, running, strength exercises, walking and wrestling. Like Rousseau he argued that the development of the body should precede any other form of education.

Europe in the 19th century

In Europe during the 19th century, the philosophy of idealism became very influential in education with particular relevance to sport, exercise and physical education. The philosophy of idealism had its roots in many of the beliefs and arguments emanating from Greek times, particularly from Plato and Socrates. Essentially idealism was concerned with how people treat each other, how we behave and conduct ourselves and the morality and ethics associated with both these concerns. When we define idealism as simply as this we can see immediately how it is manifested in sport through fair play and sportsmanship. The philosophers who promoted idealism were concerned with three major components: the existence of God, the development of self and the development of knowledge.

Given that idealism places importance on the mind, the implication for sport and physical education becomes very important. It is through the body experiencing physical sensory stimuli that the mind can process these experiences to develop awareness. Idealism strongly supports the inclusion of sport and physical education in the educative process for this very reason. This is commonly known today as *learning through movement*. In effect, therefore, physical educators drawing on the philosophy of idealism would start with the belief that education is about ideals, and therefore construct their teaching curriculum around the development of moral and ethical behaviours that can be learned through movement. They *would not* look upon students as simply bodies to be developed, shaped, moulded, and trained so as to perform physical feats of performance. Instead they would look upon sport and physical education as a means of educating their students *through movement* for them to learn and practise virtuous behaviours in order for them to lead good lives. By focusing on idealism the role and purpose of sport and physical education then becomes very clear. It becomes a form of character education that focuses on the holistic development of the person particularly in the physical, social, moral, ethical, spiritual and intellectual sense, and this development starts with bodily sensory-motor experiences.

With this philosophy in mind sport and physical education became very important in the education systems of Europe. Put simply, educators saw the excellent contributions that physical education could contribute to the physical, social, moral and intellectual development of the young person and their society. For instance, German physical educators seized upon this opportunity and developed very rigorous programmes that included the importance of play as a spiritual activity which could cultivate the inner life of the person particularly in regards to joy, freedom and self-sacrifice. Furthermore the Germans believed that play for the young paved the way for learning about humanity through interactive activity, and the need for rules and traditions to create order. Friedrich Jahn for instance, the famous German educator, believed passionately in sport and physical education for older youth. In particular he based his work on GutsMuths and promoted vigorous physical exercise to

promote unity between the body and mind. Jahn developed a system of gymnastics which involved the training of the bodily senses in order to train the mind. He believed that vigorous exercise was a precondition for physical and moral health. For Jahn his system of structured and systematised sport and physical education – predominately gymnastics – was essential for discipline and order. The quest for this discipline would ultimately turn to a very strong belief in creating national unity for the German people. This quest for national unity was essentially aimed at liberating the German people from Prussian and French rule.

It was during Jahn's development of a staunch gymnastic discipline to create national German unity that the Turnverein Movement (Turners) developed. Their goal was to educate through gymnastics. This education was essentially to produce true Germans who were vigorous, virtuous, courageous, pure and manful. The ultimate aim of the Turners was to bring national unity to Germany and liberate it from external controls.

While the German system focused on developing national unity through sport and physical education, other educators drew on the philosophy of idealism to develop different forms of sport and physical education in order to develop the all-round citizen. The Swede Per Henrik Ling, whose work was described in more detail in section 1.1 (above), used gymnastics and other forms of exercise for health-related purposes. Ling based his exercise system on science and perhaps his greatest contribution was relating physical education to the medical profession. For years Ling experimented with exercise as a form of medical therapy. Here, anatomy and physiology became very important not only in therapeutic exercise but also in general game-playing and sports. Ling did not subscribe to the overly vigorous German form of exercise. His Swedish exercise programme has left us with a legacy particularly around the invention of certain equipment, e.g. Swedish beams, benches and bars. Of course his intellectual understanding of exercise and science has left a lasting legacy and paved the way for exercise science today.

Much later in the 19th century the French educator philosopher Pierre de Coubertin drew heavily on the philosophy of Humanism from the Renaissance period, and idealism from the 19th century, to articulate the importance of physical education and sport. De Coubertin's lasting legacy for sport has been through the establishment of the modern Olympic Games. However, de Coubertin's thinking around sport and physical education was quite profound and has influenced contemporary thinking. For de Coubertin, sport and physical education were critical in the all-round development of the individual. He believed that through carefully structured sport and physical education programmes, the individual could be educated in order to shape character and moral behaviour. For de Coubertin education through sport was essentially a philosophy of life or a way of being. Drawing heavily on the ancient Greek philosophy and the British system of schooling, where he observed that sport and physical education provided a form of moral training through game-playing, de Coubertin developed the concept of the Olympic ideal. This philosophy of life was an educative system that took into account the method and ethic of learning through sport. De Coubertin saw the Olympic ideal, on a global scale, as a framework for thinking and living and a major factor in drawing people together to understand better each other's cultures and achieving peaceful existence. To achieve this internationally de Coubertin argued that sport and physical education programmes in schools needed to focus on the all-round development of the person. He did not give priority to the mind or the body but instead, argued for a balanced development between the mind, body and spirit. Within this balanced context de Coubertin argued that learning through sport should also incorporate the practice of universal ethics such as tolerance, generosity, unity, respect for others, friendship and non-discrimination.

American sport and physical education (19th century onwards)

As in Europe, America focused on how sport and physical education contributed to health. During the latter half of the 19th century and early 20th century the whole area of health became very important, and was characterised by the publication of books and the establishment of education programmes in schools and universities. Perhaps one of the most significant developments during the late 19th century was the establishment of the professional preparation of teachers. With the move to specialisation and professional status, physical educators were considered to be in the best position to deliver health-related courses which focused on health promotion through active lifestyles. In 1892 through to 1911, courses for the preparation of physical education teachers were established at California, Harvard, Ohio, and Stanford. This training was a significant development which was adopted by many other American universities. The content of the training bore a close relationship to that used today, and included anatomy, first aid, health and hygiene, motor control, physiology and psychology.

While sport and physical education during the 19th and 20th centuries was largely influenced by a developing scientific approach, social development objectives also became stronger. Many of these social development objectives were evident in the increasing importance given to physical play for younger children. The previous centuries had focused on sport and physical education for health, and had strong associations with the medical professions. The emerging philosophy in America towards the end of the 19th century and the early 20th century was now focusing on a much broader view of physical education and sport. This view not only encapsulated the health and lifestyle orientation, but also began to focus on a strong competitive sports emphasis and the development of social skills for character development. At this time physical educators began to promote the importance of sport and, as a consequence, the teaching of sports skills became a major thrust in school and university curricula. Later the philosophy of 'sport for all' became very popular and as a result, sport and athletic competition had significant influences on school curricula. The philosophical justification centred around the notion that involvement in sport led to the development of good moral, healthy and socially adjusted citizens, who sharpened their minds through competitive sport and active lifestyles.

The development of sport within schools and society led to an increasing concentration on high-performance or elite sport. As a consequence, sports coaching became an important professional addition to the world of physical education and as a result, university programmes began to employ sports coaches to develop their talented athletes and indeed market their programmes.

These changes paved the way for the development of modern approaches to sport. During the early 20th century, sport became highly organised on a regional, national and international basis. It developed formal standardised rules, introduced professional codes, recorded statistics of performance and informed the public of events and happenings. Of course, the modernisation of sport did not occur in a vacuum. There were huge changes within society that have also directly affected and influenced the direction of modern sport. Industry and commerce grew, improved travel and communication technologies became available, many people had increased leisure time, education was more accessible and sport was recognised as a legitimate education and career pathway. All of these facts contributed to this modern concept of sport. The developing interest in high-performance sport towards the end of the 19th century, its popular explosion in the 20th century and into the 21st century along with the health and movement aspects of physical education courses, led to an increasing focus on the science associated with sport and exercise physiology as a discipline.

Concluding remarks

This brief overview has highlighted a number of the significant influences that have moulded modern-day sport, exercise and physical education, and their place in society. From early Greek times where the relationship between the mind and the body influenced the manner in which they lived; to the Middle Ages where the Church considered the physical body as sinful; to the age of Science and the Enlightenment which offered an alternative view to the Church; to the ethical idealism of Kant and the resultant vigorous nationalism of the Germans, and to the American influence dominated initially by health and social objectives, and eventually to competitive sport. Each of these phases in history has had its influence, and brought us to where we are today, with regard to each country's unique conceptualisation of sport, exercise and physical education. Exercise physiology has a major role to play within sports science, indeed many of its findings have stemmed from testing sports men and women. The development of physiology for health and sports performance has its origin in times when physicians, philosophers and educators began to consider the notion of a healthy body and mind.

1.3 Pedagogy for contemporary exercise physiology[2]

> I keep six honest serving-men
> (They taught me all I knew);
> Their names are What and Why and When
> And How and Where and Who.
>
> Rudyard Kipling (1902)

The term pedagogy originates from a Greek word παιδαγωγέω (paidagōgeō) which means 'leading a child', and at that time referred to the role played by a slave who was responsible for guiding the master's son through his education. In a modern context, in keeping with the Latin-derived meaning, pedagogy refers to the education of children and more specifically to the teaching and learning of children and the study of theories of learning associated with education.

We have included this section on pedagogy, which is often not a theme covered in exercise physiology textbooks, to highlight a number of aspects of teaching and learning that could be considered by those reading this textbook who will go on to, or who already do, teach exercise physiology

and indeed exercise science in school, sporting or university contexts. Given the nature of the subject area, it is possible for exercise physiologists to play less attention to the pedagogy associated with the delivery of courses than to the content to be covered. The range of pedagogies available for teachers, coaches and lecturers makes it pertinent for exercise physiologists to consider whether a change in teaching style, or developing sessions using a range of pedagogies, might be beneficial to student enjoyment and enhance engagement and learning. As a consequence, the main focus of this section will be to highlight a number of pedagogical approaches that might be considered by interested teachers, coaches and lecturers as providing alternative methodologies for facilitating learning in exercise science courses, and, specifically in the context of this textbook, exercise physiology classes.

If, as exercise physiologists, we take time to consider the pedagogies associated with our classes it is also useful to consider other aspects at the same time. Not only *how* we teach, but also, as with the poem by Rudyard Kipling the *what*, *why*, *when*, *where* and *who* we teach. The *what* refers to the course content, the *why* should lead us to question what has been included and the *when* the timing for introducing key topics or concepts. The *where* should require us to consider a range of teaching facilities, the use of which should help us to bring our subject to life, while the *who* should perhaps be the most important of all, with the learner being at the heart of what we do as teachers, coaches and lecturers. We should perhaps teach students rather than a subject.

With regard to the *what*, in a school context, the past two decades have seen firstly the commencement, and subsequently the expansion, of exam-based physical education courses within the curricula of many countries. For the most part such courses have been heavily influenced by the content of degree courses in exercise science and physical education. As a more widely accepted exam subject it is perhaps pertinent for those involved in curriculum development for physical education, and specifically exercise physiology, to consider the syllabus content. Discussion between teachers and lecturers may provide an opportunity to develop complementary, rather than repetitious, syllabi such that programmes in schools lead into and complement those offered at university level.

On a similar note, physical education teachers might usefully pursue close professional relationships with staff in other subject areas to help students make links in their learning. The importance of such links can be highlighted when talking with students who have taken chemistry and physical education as exam subjects in their final years of school (years 12 and 13). If you ask such a student what

---

[2]By Ian Culpan and Nick Draper.

they learned about breaking chemical bonds, a good chemistry student will be able to explain that breaking a bond between chemicals requires energy, it is an endothermic process. But ask the same student, using knowledge from exercise physiology covered within physical education lessons, how energy is derived from ATP and the most likely reply is that the energy is released by breaking the bond with the final phosphate group, which by implication infers that bond breaking is an exothermic process. These answers are contradictory and highlight two key issues that should be considered by exercise physiology teachers. Firstly, during the translation of some aspects of science to a sporting context, knowledge has strayed from the first principles of science, in this case the fundamentals of thermodynamics. Secondly, by fostering closer links with colleagues in chemistry and biology, not only can we avoid contradictions in teaching for students but we can actually enhance the learning of students by enabling them to make cross-curricular links – something that primary school teachers have been doing for many years.

A further content-related aspect for exercise physiologists to consider is the currency of their knowledge and the curriculum of students. Our understanding of human functioning, particularly in an exercise or sporting context, is constantly evolving, and as a consequence it is vital for exercise physiologists to continue their professional development throughout their careers. More recent findings relating to the mechanisms behind fatigue and the operation of the electron transport chain highlight two key areas where accepted theories have been challenged by research developments. It is therefore essential for exercise physiologists to retain currency in their thinking and teaching.

While sport and physical education have been an educational concern for many centuries, a focus on how to teach, in order to maximise the learning process, has been a relatively recent phenomenon. Behaviourism and the principles associated with this form of learning theory provide a number of useful attributes that have often been adopted by teachers and lecturers, and these include:

- the principle of small steps (progressions)
- the principle of self-pacing – the learner learns at their own speed
- the principle of the learner actively responding
- the principle of reduction of errors – keeping mistakes to a minimum
- the principle of providing immediate feedback on performance
- the principle of repetition
- the principle of learner testing.

Within sport and physical education, including exercise physiology, behavioural pedagogy has had a huge influence on the way teachers, coaches and lecturers teach motor skills, games, and the exercise sciences. For instance, in the teaching of motor skills and games the most common method of teaching has been to break skills down into small steps, while encouraging the learner to practise and giving feedback to correct errors. In a similar manner exercise physiologists have broken down course content into small progressions to assist learning. Recent developments with software products to support learning for subjects such as anatomy and physiology follow such principles and break content into smaller steps and allow students to work at their own pace.

This approach, however, is very much teacher (or software) dependent and can present fewer opportunities for active student involvement in the learning process. This style of teaching has been referred to by Mosston and Ashworth (2002) as the command style, as the teacher makes all the decisions about the learning experience. If as teachers we rely predominantly on such a teacher-led approach, this could be detrimental to learning and limit the opportunities for students to become independent and creative learners. As a consequence, Mosston and Ashworth (2002) suggested that a number of alternative teaching styles might be considered by teachers (in our case, exercise physiologists) to improve student learning. Research indicates that the use of a range of teaching styles can promote increased student involvement in the learning process, thereby enhancing student success.

Mosston and Ashworth (2002) developed a continuum or spectrum of 12 teaching styles which are illustrated in Figure 1.12 and, moving from A–K, present a range of teaching methodologies. For example, in the command style (style A), as mentioned, the teacher makes all the decisions regarding the learning episode whereas, in the self-teaching style (style K), which would not be possible in a school environment, there is no teacher, the 'student' being responsible for all decisions in the learning process. Mosston and Ashworth do not advocate the predominance of one style over another, but have suggested that using a range of teaching styles can improve learning.

For teachers, coaches and lecturers of exercise physiology, Mosston and Ashworth's (2002) spectrum of teaching styles would provide an excellent starting point for developing teaching methodologies that move beyond the command style. Further pedagogical approaches that could be considered by exercise physiology teachers include Bruner's 'Concept Learning', Bruner's 'Discovery Learning', Gagne's 'Instructional Processes',

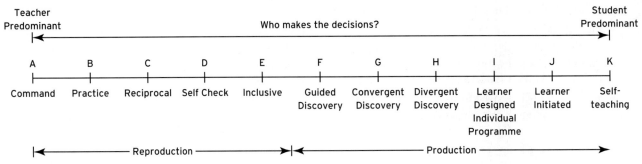

Figure 1.12 Mosston and Ashworth's spectrum of teaching styles.

Bandura's 'Social Learning' or 'Imitation Learning' model, Ausubel's 'Advanced Organisers' model, Gardner's 'Multi Intelligences', Vygotsky's 'Socio-cultural Learning' and Johnson and Johnson's 'Cooperative Learning'.

An example

If a topic to be studied was 'alterations in blood pressure during exercise' a teacher or lecturer could draw on Bruner's 'Discovery Learning' model to promote inquiry and discovery learning, then the following might be a useful approach to this topic.

1. Pose the question for investigation
   What happens to blood pressure during exercise of differing intensities?

2. Prior knowledge
   Learners would have a basic knowledge of the anatomy of the heart, how the heart responds to exercise and the meaning of blood pressure. They would also know how to take heart rates, use a stethoscope and a sphygmomanometer.

3. Sequence of lesson

   - *Collection of data: Learners would, in threes, record each other's blood pressure while at rest. They would then be expected to record blood pressure immediately after different forms of exercise moving from light exercise intensity to heavy exercise intensity.*
   - *Investigative questions: learners would develop a series of sub-questions which would attempt to answer the main question of investigation.*
   - *Provide a tentative answer based on their findings*
   - *Confirm their answer by consulting literature*
   - *Formulate explanations*
   - *Test their explanation against the explanations in the literature*

   - *Finalise their explanation*
   - *Draw some principles from their work.*
   - *Write a concluding statement about what happens to blood pressure during different exercise intensities.*

This example is intended to outline briefly how a research and discovery approach might be used in an exercise physiology context. Further information about possible pedagogical approaches for teaching exercise physiology along with generic examples can be found in the excellent textbook by Joyce, Weil and Calhoun (2000) entitled *Models of Teaching*.

Readers of this section are encouraged and challenged to experiment with their teaching, the what, when, where, who, why and how, to develop a range of methods to suit their learners. In experimenting with these models it is useful to keep in mind that what we are doing in exercise physiology is trying to get students to:

- better understand moving bodies by developing knowledge to solve problems
- justify solutions to these problems
- listen to alternative possibilities
- agree or disagree with alternative views
- ask questions to clarify thinking and meaning
- apply this new knowledge to authentic sport, physical education and coaching situations.

Perhaps the most important thing that research teaches us, irrespective of being a teacher or a student, is that we need constantly to reflect on our own teaching and learning. We need to reflect on the content of exercise physiology and determine its relevance, importance, meaning and usefulness. We need to understand and reflect on how best to maximise the learning process for students.

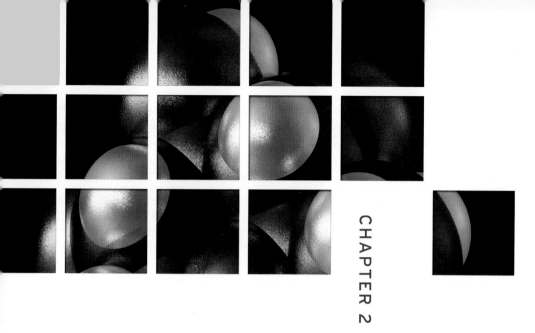

CHAPTER 2

Nutrition for health and sports performance

Learning objectives

After reading, considering and discussing with a study partner the material in this chapter you should be able to:

➤ identify the most abundant chemicals that comprise the human body

➤ outline how and why chemical bonding occurs between atoms

➤ describe briefly the role of enzymes in chemical reactions within the body

➤ explain the different types of chemical reactions that can occur within the body

➤ distinguish between the different types of macronutrient within our diet

➤ teach others about the structural differences between saturated and unsaturated fats

➤ describe the structure and functions of carbohydrates

➤ explain the role of proteins within our diet

➤ teach others about the calorific content of food and explain how food labels express the calorific content of food

➤ summarise the micronutrients necessary within our diet

➤ highlight the role of some key minerals within the body and their sources from foods in our diet

➤ discuss the importance of water for physiological functioning

➤ highlight the key aspects of digestion

➤ list the components of a healthy balanced diet

2.1 Introduction to nutrition

Humans, as omnivores, have the capacity to provide the nutrients to sustain life from a wide variety of plant and animal sources. The ability of humans to thrive in their natural environment has largely been due to their adaptability, and this includes diet. Throughout history and around the world humans have been able to adapt from vegetarian to extreme meat diets. Inuits have traditionally followed an almost exclusively animal-based diet over the centuries. Even with this diet and in extreme environmental conditions they have continued to thrive, although they now often have sucrose and lactose intolerances. The Hindu religion, on the other hand, has had a long traditional link with vegetarianism since around the 4th century BCE. The *Bhagavada Gita* – Hindu scriptures, literally the 'song of god' – first proposed the principle of *ahimsa* which advocated non-violence to all forms of life. Mahatma Gandhi (1869–1948) who led the campaign for independence for India was one of the most famous vegetarians with the *ahimsa* as a central tenant of his philosophy of life. India has the highest number of vegetarians in the world with around 399 million representing 40% of the population. Typically around 2–6% of the population in developed countries are estimated to be vegetarian (USA 7.3 million [3.2%]; Australia 1.1 million [5%]; New Zealand 75,000 [2%]; and in the UK 4 million [6.5%]). These figures include vegan, lacto and lacto-ovo vegetarians. Many cultures now exist on a mixed diet of plant and animal foods; however, it is possible for humans to thrive on a wide variety of diets.

The food we, our students or our athletes take into our bodies is important, not only for its impact on our performance for that day or the next, but also for long-term health. The importance of nutrition for health was recognised over two thousand years ago by some of the earliest researchers interested in health and the human body. Since this early identification many discoveries about the nature of the foods we take into our bodies have been made. As far as this research has taken us it still remains apparent that the basis for sound nutrition lies in the adoption of a *well-balanced diet*.

Key point

It is possible, through careful selection of foods, for a vegetarian diet to provide all the nutrients necessary for successful sports performance.

Traditionally, from a physiological perspective, six food components are required to satisfy and support optimal human functioning. Carbohydrates, proteins, fats, vitamins, minerals and water have been identified as essentials for healthy living. These macro-nutrients (carbohydrates, fats and proteins) and micro-nutrients (vitamins and minerals), along with water (the second most important substance, after oxygen, needed to maintain life), serve two main functions in humans: to provide the *fuel* for living and to maintain the *structure and functioning* of the body. This chapter examines the nature of these nutrient groups and their role in maintaining health and performance for all athletes.

The foods that form the basis of our diet are made up from chemical elements. Over 112 elements have been identified or produced artificially, the main ones of which are shown on the inside cover of this textbook within the periodic table. Ninety-two of these elements are found naturally, and of these, 26 are commonly found in humans. Table 2.1 provides details of the elements identified in the body. As can be seen from this table, oxygen,

carbon, hydrogen and nitrogen represent 96% of each person's chemical composition. In addition, they form the basis for the three macronutrients and the vitamins necessary for a well-balanced diet. Carbohydrates, fats and some vitamins (A, C, D, E, and K) all include carbon, hydrogen and oxygen within their chemical structure. Proteins and the vitamin B complex, as well as comprising carbon, hydrogen and oxygen, also contain nitrogen and a number of additional elements in their structures. These 26 elements form the structure of our bodies and are essential to our healthy functioning. They are the building blocks for the cells, tissues and systems that make up our bodies and are found in the food that we eat. To better understand human structure (anatomy) and functioning (physiology) in a sporting context it is essential to have an understanding of the principal aspects of chemistry that govern these building blocks and their interactions within our bodies.

Key point

The six main nutrients for healthy living are:

➤ carbohydrates
➤ fats
➤ proteins
➤ vitamins
➤ minerals
➤ water

Additionally, fibre facilitates digestion (described in section 2.7).

Nutrients serve to:

➤ maintain the structure and functioning of the body
➤ provide the energy necessary for sports performance.

2.2 Essential elements of chemistry

The human body and everything around us, all known as **matter**, are comprised of elements in their pure form, or combined with other elements. The simplest form of any element is the atom. Until the 20th century, an atom, meaning 'not cut' or 'indivisible', was thought to be the smallest unit of matter. First proposed as a planetary model by Niels Bohr in 1913 after earlier work by Ernest Rutherford, it has subsequently been confirmed that atoms, the building blocks for us as humans and the food we eat, are actually composed of subatomic particles of which protons, neutrons and electrons are vitally important to chemistry.

Table 2.1 The 26 elements found within the human body.

Chemical element	Percentage	Symbol	Atomic number	Atomic mass
Oxygen	65.0%	O	8	15.9994
Carbon	18.5%	C	6	12.0107
Hydrogen	9.5%	H	1	1.0079
Nitrogen	3.2%	N	7	14.0067
Calcium	1.8%	Ca	20	40.078
Phosphorus	1.0%	P	15	30.9738
Potassium	0.4%	K	19	39.0983
Sulphur	0.3%	S	16	32.066
Sodium	0.2%	Na	11	22.9898
Chlorine	0.2%	Cl	17	35.4527
Magnesium	0.1%	Mg	12	24.3050
Iron	0.007%	Fe	26	55.845
Zinc	0.002%	Zn	30	65.39
Selenium	0.0003%	Se	34	78.96
Manganese	0.0003%	Mn	25	54.9380
Copper	0.0002%	Cu	29	63.546
Molybdenum	Trace	Mo	42	95.94
Chromium	Trace	Cr	24	51.9961
Fluorine	Trace	F	9	18.9984
Iodine	Trace	I	53	126.9045
Silicon	Trace	Si	14	28.0855
Boron	Trace	B	5	10.811
Cobalt	Trace	Co	27	58.9332
Aluminium	Trace	Al	13	26.9815
Tin	Trace	Sn	50	118.710
Vanadium	Trace	V	23	50.9415

Some elements' symbols are derived from their Latin, Greek or Arabic names. Potassium (K) from the Latin *kalium*, sodium (Na) from the Latin *natrium*, iron (Fe) is from the Latin *ferrum*, copper (Cu) from the Latin *cuprum* and tin (Sn) from the Latin *stannum*. The percentages refer to the proportion of the body's total 'wet' mass. The elements in red represent the 'big four' by weight within the body, those in blue the major minerals, green the minor minerals and those in orange the lesser known minerals.

Atomic structure

Each atom has a nucleus comprised of positively charged protons and neutrons (no charge). Orbiting around the nucleus, in a planetary fashion as proposed by Bohr, are one or more negatively charged electrons (Figure 2.1). The movement of electrons around the nucleus, however, is now thought to be more complex than Bohr's original model. It is now believed that, rather than tracking around the nucleus in a regular pattern, electrons move randomly in cloud layers that surround the nucleus. The two-dimensional image of Figure 2.1 shows electrons to conform to a pattern of shells around the nucleus. The inner shell of an atom can contain a maximum of two

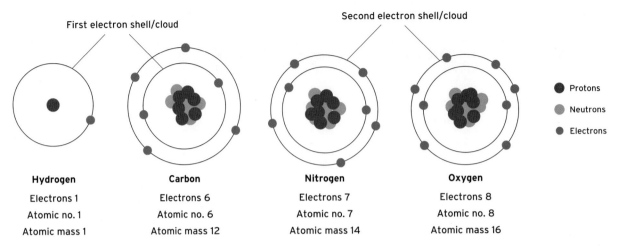

Figure 2.1 Structural models for the most common elements in the human body. The *atomic number* represents the number of protons (positively charged) in the nucleus (which is equal to the number of negatively charged electrons). The *atomic mass number* (u) represents the mass of the atom and is the sum of the number of protons and neutrons within the nucleus.

electrons. The second shell, which actually has two sub-shells, can hold up to 8 electrons (2 in the first and 6 in the second). The third shell can hold a maximum of 18 electrons arranged in three sub-shells each holding 2, 6 and up to 10 electrons respectively. In reality the electrons in each shell are actually thought to move randomly within a cloud, such that the first two electrons would orbit or move within the first cloud layer.

The positive and negative charges associated with protons and electrons are fundamental to the chemical reactions that take place within the body. The existence of these charges means that particles will attract or repel each other depending on their charge. When two objects carry opposite electrical charges they will attract each other; when of the same charge, such as is the case with two protons, they will repel each other. The electrons associated with an atom move around the nucleus and are held within their shells due to the forces of attraction between the electrons and the protons found in the nucleus. Although protons are positively and electrons are negatively charged, an undisturbed atom will always remain neutral as there are an equal number of protons and electrons. The **atomic number** for an atom refers to the number of protons; for example the number of protons in an atom of oxygen is 8 and so the atomic number is 8, and this will be matched by the number of electrons so that an oxygen atom is neutral. The number of protons in an atom determines its size and the type of element that it forms. Figure 2.1 shows the structure of the four most common elements found in our food and bodies; oxygen, carbon, hydrogen and nitrogen.

Protons and neutrons are very small. However, electrons are 1836 times smaller and therefore the mass of an atom is determined by the number of protons and neutrons in the nucleus. Ernest Rutherford received the Nobel prize in 1908 for the discovery that atoms are mostly empty space, with the mass being concentrated in the nucleus. Such is the difference in weight between the particles of the nucleus and electrons, that for a 70 kg person the total mass of electrons in their body would amount to little over 38 g. As a result, the **atomic mass** of an atom, expressed in atomic mass units (u), refers to the total number of protons and neutrons and hence, as can be seen in Figure 2.1, hydrogen is the smallest element with an atomic mass of 1 u.

Many elements naturally exist in slightly different versions of the same substance, for example chlorine has two types or **isotopes**. Approximately three quarters of chlorine atoms exist with 18 neutrons whereas almost a quarter have 20 neutrons. Both isotopes possess 17 protons with the result that the atomic masses are 35 u and 37 u for the two chlorine isotopes, respectively. The averaged atomic mass for chlorine can be calculated as shown on the next page.

This atomic mass of chlorine is therefore often written as 35.5 u. As can be seen from Table 2.1, or the periodic table on the inside cover of this book, chlorine is more correctly shown to have an atomic mass of 35.4527 u. This is because the ratio of ^{35}Cl and ^{37}Cl is only approximately 3:1. However, it is important to know that different isotopes of the same element do exist, differentiated by the number of neutrons present in each form.

Key point

Atomic number refers to the number of protons an element contains.

Atomic mass refers to the number of protons and neutrons.

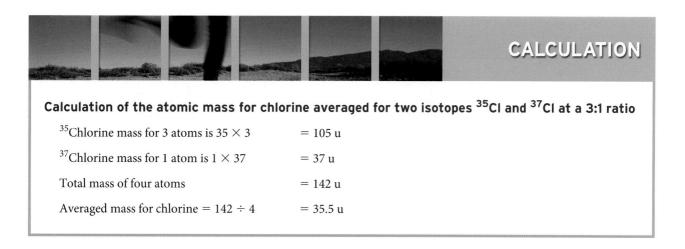

CALCULATION

Calculation of the atomic mass for chlorine averaged for two isotopes ^{35}Cl and ^{37}Cl at a 3:1 ratio

^{35}Chlorine mass for 3 atoms is 35×3 = 105 u

^{37}Chlorine mass for 1 atom is 1×37 = 37 u

Total mass of four atoms   = 142 u

Averaged mass for chlorine = $142 \div 4$ = 35.5 u

Chemical bonding

As can be seen from Figure 2.2, atoms, which comprise the smallest units of our foods, come together in groups to form matter. The force that holds atoms together is called chemical bonding. Chemical reactions occur to form these bonds and, through this bonding force, atoms join to form our foods and our bodies. It is the positive and negative charges of atoms that provide the basis for chemical bonding. There are two main forms of chemical bonding and both involve the use of electrons to create the bond. **Ionic bonds** involve the donation of one or more electrons from one atom to another and **covalent bonds** involve atoms sharing electrons.

The atoms in Figure 2.1 have one or two shells of electrons. Each of the electrons in these shells has energy stored within it, and the greater the distance electrons are from the nucleus, the more energy they possess. The electrons furthest from the nucleus are the most likely to interact with other atoms. Each shell of electrons has a maximum number of electrons and atoms will try to undergo processes to fill their outer shell. This is due to the fact that when a shell is filled the atom is more stable. The number of electrons in the outer shell of an atom and its need to donate, accept or share electrons with other atoms

is known as its **valency** and relates to the combining power of an atom to bond with other atoms.

An ionic bond is formed between two atoms when one of the atoms donates an electron to another, thus completing the outer shell of electrons for each and creating a stable chemical product. An example of this can be found in Figure 2.3 where chlorine (Cl) accepts one electron from sodium (Na). By doing this Cl becomes a negatively charged chloride ion (Cl^-) as it has more electrons than protons and Na becomes a positively charged sodium ion (Na^+) because it has one electron fewer. Atoms that lose electrons and become positively charged are called **cations** (to remember this think of the t as + and positive) and those that accept electrons and become negatively charged ions are called **anions** (think of the n as **n**egative). The resultant compound for this example is sodium chloride (NaCl) or table salt. It is this compound in our sweat that gives sweat a salty taste.

Key point

Cations are positive ions – they have donated electrons

Anions are negative ions – they have accepted electrons

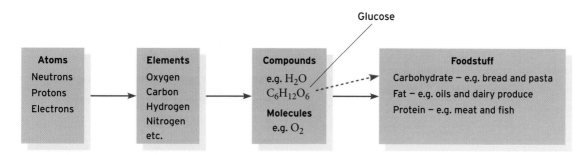

Figure 2.2 The chemical components of our food.

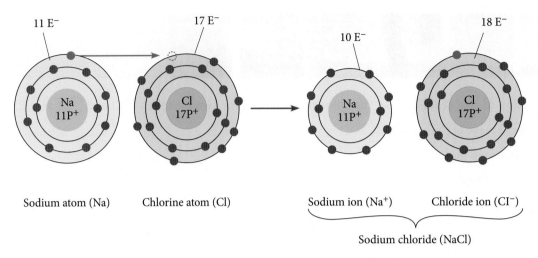

Figure 2.3 The formation of sodium chloride (table salt) from the donation of electrons by sodium to chlorine as an example of ionic bonding.

The creation of ions through electron donation and acceptance, such as that for the formation of NaCl, are crucial for human structure, functioning and sporting performance. Ions such as calcium (Ca^{2+}) which donates two electrons (hence the $^{2+}$) are vital components in the structure of bones and teeth. Hydrogen ions (H^+) are important in the acid-base balance of the body which, as we will discuss in Chapter 9 (lactate tolerance and management sports), is a key determinant of fatigue during high-intensity sporting activities. In addition, when dissolved within bodily fluids the anions and cations of compounds such as NaCl are able to conduct an electrical current. Such soluble compounds, that can conduct an electrical current, are called **electrolytes**. Electrolytes within the human body enable the electrical conduction necessary for nerve impulse transmission and muscle contraction. Ions are therefore vital for physiological functioning. Table 2.2 provides an overview of key ions, their function within the body and common electrolytes associated with specific ions.

 Try **Interactive Physiology:**
Fluids, electrolytes and acid-base balance: Electrolyte homeostasis

Key point

Substances that contain ions are called electrolytes.

Key electrolytes within the body include:

Ca^{2+}, Mg^{2+}, Na^+, K^+, and Cl^-

A covalent bond is formed when two or more atoms share a pair of electrons and form a compound or molecule.

Figure 2.4 provides examples of covalent bonds where the atoms involved share one pair (a single covalent bond), two pairs (a double covalent bond), or three pairs (a triple covalent bond) of electrons. A simple way to remember the specific bonding of the common elements for human nutrition is the acronym **HONC**. HONC stands for **H**ydrogen (one bond), **O**xygen (two bonds), **N**itrogen (three bonds) and **C**arbon (four bonds). Each of the gases in Figure 2.4 exists in this structure to share electrons. The sharing of electrons enables each atom to complete its outer shell without losing or gaining electrons.

Knowledge integration question

Explain how the term HONC helps with explaining chemical bonding.

An example of covalent bonding of atoms from two different elements is the formation of water from two hydrogen and a single oxygen atom ($2H + O = H_2O$). This can be seen diagrammatically in Figure 2.5.

Key point

Matter comprises bonded atoms.

Two important types of chemical bonds are:

➤ ionic – atoms donate or accept electrons
➤ covalent – atoms share electrons

Bonding enables atoms to complete the outer electron shell, making them chemically more stable (less reactive).

Table 2.2 Important ions and associated electrolytes for human structure and functioning.

Ion	Symbol	Function within the body	Example of associated electrolytes	Formula
Cations				
Calcium	Ca^{2+}	Muscle contraction, bone and tooth structure	Calcium phosphate	$CaPO_4$
Potassium	K^+	Nerve impulse conduction, muscle contraction	Potassium chloride	KCl
Hydrogen	H^+	Acid-base balance		
Magnesium	Mg^{2+}	Component for enzymes	Magnesium chloride	$MgCl_2$
Ammonium	NH_4^+	Acid-base balance		
Sodium	Na^+	Nerve impulse conduction, muscle contraction	Sodium chloride	$NaCl$
		Hydration level regulation		
Anions				
Chloride	Cl^-	Hydration level regulation		
Hydroxide	OH^-	Acid-base balance		
Bicarbonate	HCO_3^-	Acid-base balance	Sodium bicarbonate	$NaHCO_3$
Phosphate	PO_4^{3-}	Bone and tooth structure, energy storage and release, acid-base balance		

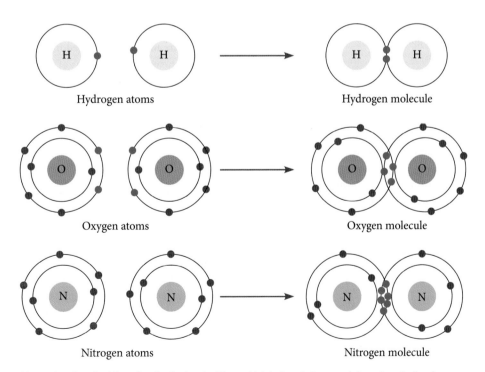

Hydrogen atoms   Hydrogen molecule

Oxygen atoms   Oxygen molecule

Nitrogen atoms   Nitrogen molecule

Figure 2.4 Covalent bonding in single, double and triple bonds to complete outer shells of electrons for hydrogen, oxygen and nitrogen respectively.

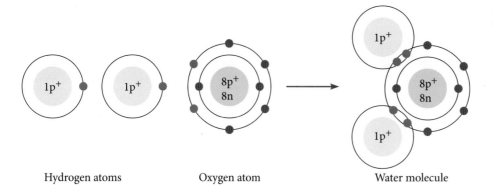

Hydrogen atoms   Oxygen atom   Water molecule

Figure 2.5 Covalent bonding: the formation of water.

Chemical reactions

A **chemical reaction** is a process in which a chemical change occurs, where the starting materials (reactants) differ from the end products. Chemical bonds are broken, rearranged or formed during chemical reactions, generally due to the motion of electrons.

Chemical notation

Chemical reactions can be written in a shorthand symbolic form, as **chemical equations**, to simplify the description of chemical structures and reactions. There are a number of rules that apply to chemical notation that will help you understand chemical equations. A simple chemical equation indicating the joining of two hydrogen atoms to form a hydrogen molecule (see Figure 2.4) is written as:

$$H + H \longrightarrow H_2 \text{ (hydrogen gas)}$$

Reactants   Products

Notice from this chemical equation that the symbol of an element indicates one atom of that element. When two atoms of the same element chemically bond, as in the production of hydrogen gas above, the product is called a **molecule**. A number written as a *subscript* (as seen in the product in this example, H_2) indicates that that number of atoms are joined by chemical bonds to form a molecule. The arrow indicates the direction of the equation from reactants to products.

When the bonding of different elements occurs, the product is termed a **compound**, such as the formation of water (see Figure 2.5) in the following chemical equation:

$$2H + O \longrightarrow H_2O \text{ (water)}$$

It must be noted, however, that sometimes the bonding of different elements can also be referred to as a molecule, as is the case with a molecule of CO_2. In contrast to a *subscript* number which indicates bonded atoms, a number written as a *prefix* denotes the number of molecules. For example,

in the above chemical equation, 2H signifies two unbonded hydrogen atoms, whereas H_2O indicates that two hydrogen atoms are bonded with oxygen to form a molecule of water. *Note that the term molecule is often used interchangeably to refer to a compound or a molecule.*

Key point

Molecules are formed when two of the same elements bond in a reaction and sometimes, as with CO_2, when different elements bond.

Compounds are formed when different reactants bond.

Often the term molecule is used interchangeably to describe both products.

Atoms are not created or destroyed in chemical reactions, they are merely rearranged into new combinations. Therefore, the number of atoms of each element must be balanced on each side of the equation (i.e. reactants versus products). The following chemical equations demonstrate an unbalanced and a balanced equation:

$$H_2 + O_2 \longrightarrow H_2O \text{ Unbalanced}$$
$$2H_2 + O_2 \longrightarrow 2H_2O \text{ Balanced}$$

Talking about atoms and molecules in chemical equations is not, however, very practical as it is impossible to measure one atom or one molecule. It may be more practical to read the equation in terms of **moles**, e.g. 2 moles of hydrogen plus one mole of oxygen yields 2 moles of water. One mole is a quantity of an element or compound having a mass in grams equal to the element's atomic weight or to the compound's molecular weight. One mole of a given element contains the same number of atoms as one mole of another element.

In theory, chemical reactions are reversible. This reversibility is indicated by a double arrow:

$$A + B \rightleftharpoons AB$$

This equation indicates the consecutive occurrence of a synthesis (from left to right) and a decomposition (from right to left) reaction (discussed further in the following section). When the rates of the two reactions are equal a state of **equilibrium** is reached, that is, there is no net change in the amount of reactants or products. The addition of reactants, or removal of products, will increase the rate of one of the reactions above that of the other and hence disturb the state of equilibrium. An example of this would be when the carbon dioxide formed from the breakdown of glucose (see example of an exchange reaction, p. 36) enters the bloodstream and is ultimately exhaled by the lungs. The continual removal of the product, carbon dioxide, means that the reverse reaction cannot occur.

Types of chemical reaction

Three of the most important are: *synthesis, decomposition* or *exchange* reactions.

Synthesis reaction

As suggested by its name, a *synthesis* (or combination) *reaction* involves bond formation between atoms and/or molecules to form larger, more complex molecules. The formation of water from hydrogen and oxygen molecules is an example of a synthesis reaction. A simple synthesis reaction can be represented as:

$$A + B \longrightarrow AB$$

The synthesis of new molecules within the body's cells and tissues is collectively known as **anabolism**. All anabolic activities in our bodies' cells involve synthesis reactions. These reactions are obviously common in the growing child, as body tissues grow in size. A more specific role of synthesis reactions in the human body is the formation of peptide bonds as amino acids are joined together to form a protein molecule (discussed in the section on Proteins; see Figure 2.18).

Dehydration, or condensation, is a chemical reaction that involves the loss of water from the reactants. The two monosaccharides glucose and fructose can combine to form the disaccharide sucrose by dehydration synthesis (discussed in the section on Disaccharides; see Figure 2.9).

Decomposition reaction

A **decomposition reaction** involves the breaking down of molecules into smaller molecules or its constituent atoms, and can be simply represented as:

$$AB \longrightarrow A + B$$

Decomposition reactions are the opposite of synthesis reactions and underlie **catabolism**, the degradative processes within our cells. In addition, decomposition reactions also occur outside the body's cells (within the digestive tract) during the digestion of our food. The carbohydrates, proteins and fats that we consume are too large to be absorbed straight into our bloodstream or lymphatic system, hence decomposition reactions occur along the digestive tract to break these large molecules down into their simplest forms of glucose, amino acids and free fatty acids, respectively. These small molecules are then able to be absorbed into the blood or lymph.

The breakdown of complex molecules in the body into two parts by the addition of water is known as **hydrolysis**. One of the bonds in a complex molecule is broken, and one part of the parent molecule gains a hydrogen ion (H^+) from the water molecule (H_2O) while the other part gains the remaining hydroxyl ion (OH^-) as shown below:

$$A\text{-}B + H_2O \longrightarrow A\text{-}H + B\text{-}OH \quad \text{Hydrolysis}$$

Many reactions in the human body involve hydrolysis. The most significant example is the hydrolysis of **adenosine triphosphate** (ATP) and subsequent release of energy to maintain the function of the cell, for example muscle cells rely on increased ATP hydrolysis to allow our muscles to contract faster and more powerfully during sport. Another example would be the hydrolysis of sucrose to form glucose and fructose, the opposite to the dehydration synthesis described above.

Exchange reaction

Exchange reactions (also called displacement reactions) involve both decomposition and synthesis reactions as bonds are initially broken, then new bonds are formed. The components of the reactants are broken down and then reformed to produce new products. Examples of exchange reactions are shown below:

$$AB + C \longrightarrow A + CB \quad and \quad AB + CD \longrightarrow AD + CB$$

An important exchange reaction occurs in the body when glucose enters a cell and reacts with ATP to form glucose phosphate and **adenosine diphosphate** (ADP), ensuring the glucose fuel molecule remains within the cell. Oxidation-reduction reactions, called **redox reactions** for short, are sometimes exchange reactions, and are vital for the survival of living systems. Redox reactions involve the exchange of electrons between reactants – the reactant losing electrons is the electron donor and is said to be **oxidised**, whereas the reactant gaining electrons is called the electron acceptor and is said to become **reduced**. An important example of a redox reaction involves the major pathway by which glucose is broken down to form cellular energy:

$$C_6H_{12}O_6 + 6O_2 \longrightarrow 6CO_2 + 6H_2O + ATP$$

glucose   oxygen   carbon   water   energy
                                        dioxide

In this reaction, it can be seen that glucose is oxidised to carbon dioxide as it loses its hydrogen atoms, and oxygen is reduced to water by the acceptance of the hydrogen atoms. This reaction is discussed in more detail in Chapter 9.

Energy transfer in chemical reactions

Chemical bonds are a source of chemical energy, hence reactions ultimately result in the net release or absorption of energy. Reactions that occur spontaneously and release energy are called **exergonic** reactions. As a general rule, catabolic and oxidative reactions are exergonic with **cellular respiration** being an important example. **Endergonic** reactions, in contrast, are those in which energy is absorbed including all anabolic reactions.

The food we eat contains energy and our bodies break the food down and reassemble it in order to harness this energy. The energy stores we create are through endergonic reactions storing energy that we can release later through exergonic reactions.

Catalysts and chemical reactions

Catalysts are substances that speed up chemical reactions but themselves remain unchanged following the reaction, ready to catalyse another reaction. In the human body, **enzymes** act as catalysts. Chemical reactions are necessary throughout the body to provide the body's cells with energy required to fuel cellular work. Without the presence of enzymes, however, chemical reactions in our body would proceed at an extremely slow rate and life would not be maintained. Enzymes, created within our body, speed up chemical reactions to enable us to function more efficiently.

Knowledge integration question

Explain why enzymes are essential for the functioning of humans, given that we are homeotherms (animals that maintain a constant temperature).

Forms and sources of energy

Chemical bonds are essential to the structure of all matter, whether it be our bodies or the food we eat. The food we take into our bodies to maintain health and for sports performance is broken down and used for growth and repair of the cells within our bodies, stored for later use or used directly to provide the energy we need for living. The chemical bonds made between atoms store energy that can be liberated by breaking these bonds (as discussed in the section on Chemical reactions).

Energy is the capacity to do work and exists as two types; *potential* energy (stored energy) and *kinetic* energy (motion energy). Energy cannot be destroyed, but can be changed from one form to another, always remaining as either potential or kinetic energy. This represents the *first law of thermodynamics* – the conservation of energy. In accordance with this principle the human body does not create or destroy energy, merely transforms it from one form to another. There are six forms in which energy can be stored or used: chemical, nuclear, mechanical, heat, light and electrical (Table 2.3).

Table 2.3 The forms of energy.

Form of energy	Examples
Chemical	The bonds within our food or made by our bodies in chemical reactions store and release energy. Fossil fuels also represent a store of chemical energy.
Nuclear	The splitting of atoms through nuclear fission releases energy that can be harnessed to drive turbines for the creation of electricity such as that carried out at nuclear power stations.
Mechanical	Physical work or movement in humans and animals. Wind turbines carry out physical work to harness electrical energy for our homes and industry.
Heat	Electricity and fossil fuels can be used to release heat energy. In our bodies, the reactions that take place to enable us to swim, bike or play rugby, release heat energy as a by-product. In cold climates this can be a useful by-product, in hot environments this can be detrimental to performance.
Light	The sun during the day, a gas lantern, torch, fire or electric power in our homes can provide light energy.
Electric	Created from many sources, electric energy can be used to power domestic and industrial machinery.

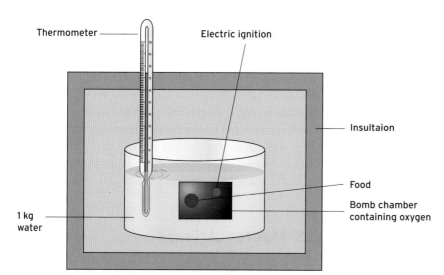

Thermometer

Electric ignition

Insultaion

Food

Bomb chamber
containing oxygen

1 kg
water

Figure 2.6 Bomb calorimeter.

When taking part in physical activity or sport our movements are brought about through the transformation of chemical energy to mechanical energy with heat being released as a by-product.

It is possible to measure the stored energy in food using a bomb calorimeter; an example of this is shown in Figure 2.6. In a bomb calorimeter the food to be tested is burned completely within a chamber containing oxygen and started by an electrical ignition. The burning of the foodstuff will result in the release of heat energy.

The heat energy released by a particular foodstuff is measured by recording the rise in temperature of the water surrounding the bomb chamber. The rise in water temperature brought about through the burning of food has traditionally been measured in **calories**. A calorie represents the amount of heat required to raise the temperature of 1 g of water by 1°C. As a gram of water is very small, the term

kilocalorie is most commonly used when referring to the energy contained within our foods. A kilocalorie (kcal) represents the amount of heat required to raise the temperature of 1 kg of water by 1°C. Sometimes you may see 'calorie' written with a small 'c' – *calorie*, and 'kilocalorie' written with a capital 'C' – *Calorie*. When looking at the label on the side of a food product the energy value of the food is presented in kilocalories. In recent years there has been a move to adopt the joule or kilojoule as the unit of energy value for food. The energy expended in applying a force of 1 newton through a distance of 1 meter is equal to 1 joule. The système international (SI) unit for the measurement of work is the joule, so as a consequence food labels in a number of countries now also show the energy value in kilojoules (kJ) as well as kcal. It is easy, however, to convert from one to the other. To convert from kcal to kJ simply multiply by 4.184, or to move from kJ to kcal divide by 4.184.

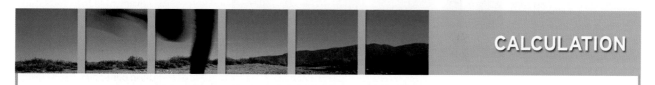

CALCULATION

Calculation of kcal and kJ using the 4.18 conversion

The energy value of a typical can of baked beans is listed as 301 kJ or 72 kcal per 100 grams.

To convert from kcal to kJ multiply by 4.184

$72 \times 4.184 = 301.2$ kJ

To convert from kJ to kcal divide by 4.184

$301 \div 4.184 = 71.94$ kcal

Table 2.4 Net calorific values for the macronutrients.

Macronutrient	Calorific value from 1 gram
Carbohydrate	4 kcal
Fat	9 kcal
Protein	4 kcal

It is possible through the use of a bomb calorimeter to identify the energy value of the main macronutrients. When 1 g of an average fat is combusted it liberates between 9.2 and 9.5 kcal of energy. Carbohydrates and proteins completely burned in the same way yield 3.7–4.2 kcal and 5.65 kcal respectively. It is clear, therefore, that a much greater amount of energy can be obtained through the **metabolism** of the same mass of fat compared to carbohydrate or protein.

Knowledge integration question

Explain why the inefficiency in chemical reactions (much of the energy for work is lost during a reaction) is helpful for humans.

The human body, however, is not as efficient at digesting and processing the foodstuffs taken into the body as a bomb calorimeter. As a consequence, research has identified the values in Table 2.4 as appropriate for the energy value of food when combusted within the body. An example of the energy value of carbohydrates, fats and protein can be illustrated again by the contents within a typical can of baked beans.

As part of this introduction to nutrition the range of diets that humans can survive and indeed thrive on has been discussed. This was followed by a review of the need for food, what food is made of, how the energy in food is stored and how the energy value of food can be measured. The following sections in this chapter will go on to look at each of the macronutrients and micronutrients necessary for healthy living, how our food is digested and absorbed into our bodies, the necessary components for a healthy diet and general dietary recommendations.

2.3 Macronutrients

There are three primary **macronutrients** in the human diet: carbohydrate, fat and protein. These are the compounds which we consume in the largest quantities and which are potential sources of energy for the human body.

Carbohydrates

Carbohydrates are compounds formed from carbon, hydrogen and oxygen. The main purpose of carbohydrate in the diet is as an energy source for the chemical reactions that take place in the body. The basic currency for carbohydrate-based energy production is the simple sugar **glucose**. When exercising, particularly during high-intensity short- to medium-duration exercise, carbohydrates provide the main fuel supply. Some cells/tissues of the body, for example red blood cells and the nervous system, rely entirely on carbohydrate energy supply. Carbohydrates can be classified as simple sugars, sugars or complex carbohydrates. *Monosaccharides* are classified as simple sugars and *disaccharides* as sugars, while

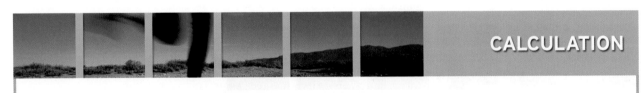

CALCULATION

Calculation of energy value of carbohydrates, fats and protein in baked beans

A typical can of baked beans contain protein (4.6 g), carbohydrates (12.9 g) and small amounts of fat (0.2 g). The energy value listed is 301 kJ or 72 kcal per 100 g.

The energy provided by carbohydrates is	12.9 g × 4 kcal = 51.6 kcal
The energy provided by fats is	0.2 g × 9 kcal = 1.8 kcal
The energy provided by protein is	4.6 g × 4 kcal = 18.4 kcal
Total energy value of baked beans	**= 71.8 kcal**

Figure 2.7 The chemical composition of three hexose monosaccharides. All three can be represented by the chemical formula $C_6H_{12}O_6$. However, the structure of each is different, making three distinct substances.

```
        H                      H                       H
        |                      |                       |
   H —C—OH                  C = O                   C = O
        |                      |                       |
     C = O                 H—C—OH                  H—C—OH
        |                      |                       |
  HO—C—H                  HO—C—H                  HO—C—H
        |                      |                       |
   H—C—OH                  H—C—OH                  HO—C—H
        |                      |                       |
   H—C—OH                  H—C—OH                  H—C—OH
        |                      |                       |
   H—C—OH                  H—C—OH                  H—C—OH
        |                      |                       |
        H                      H                       H

    Fructose                Glucose                 Galactose
```

complex carbohydrates are formed from chains of simple sugars and are called *polysaccharides*.

Fruits, grains and vegetables all contain carbohydrates. Plants create glucose during photosynthesis, when carbon dioxide (CO_2) and water (H_2O) are combined in the presence of chlorophyll and sunlight (light or solar energy). Chlorophyll absorbs sunlight and with the help of a variety of enzymes enables glucose to be produced. A vitally important by-product of this process is the production of oxygen which sustains all animal life.

Monosaccharides

As with all carbohydrates, monosaccharides contain carbon, hydrogen and oxygen atoms, hence the short form CHO is often used for the carbohydrate group. Monosaccharides are the most simple carbohydrates, consisting of a single basic sugar unit with the general formula $C_xH_{2x}O_x$. They primarily range from three to seven carbon atoms. However, the most important monosaccharides for humans have five (pentoses, $C_5H_{10}O_5$) or six (hexoses, $C_6H_{12}O_6$) carbon atoms.

Figure 2.7 illustrates the bonding for the three nutritionally important hexoses: fructose, glucose and galactose. Often monosaccharides bond in a three dimensional structure and so can be represented more correctly using a ring notation (Figure 2.8) rather than as shown in Figure 2.7 as this is closer to their structure in reality. The differences between the simple sugars in this group come from the distribution of the hydrogen and oxygen atoms. Glucose

Figure 2.8 Three-dimensional and ring representations of the chemical structure of glucose.

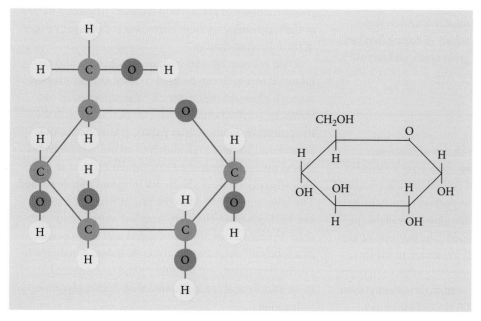

Monosaccharide	+	Monosaccharide	$\rightleftharpoons$	Disaccharide

$C_6H_{12}O_6$ (Glucose) + $C_6H_{12}O_6$ (Fructose) $\rightleftharpoons$ $C_{12}H_{22}O_{11}$ **Sucrose** (table sugar) + H_2O

$C_6H_{12}O_6$ (Glucose) + $C_6H_{12}O_6$ (Fructose) $\rightleftharpoons$ $C_{12}H_{22}O_{11}$ **Maltose** (malt sugar) + H_2O

$C_6H_{12}O_6$ (Glucose) + $C_6H_{12}O_6$ (Fructose) $\rightleftharpoons$ $C_{12}H_{22}O_{11}$ **Lactose** (milk sugar) + H_2O

Figure 2.9 The structure of disaccharides. (*Source*: Martini, F. H. and Nath, J. L. (2009) *Fundamentals of Anatomy and Physiology*, 8th edition, New York: Benjamin Cummings)

(sometimes referred to as dextrose) is a building block for more complex sugars such as cellulose (found in plants) and is perhaps the most plentiful organic substance on earth. Glucose forms naturally in plants and animals break down (catabolise) carbohydrates to glucose through digestion. Fructose, another common simple sugar is found in fruits and honey. Galactose is most commonly found as a building block for the milk sugar lactose but is also present in peas. Ribose and deoxyribose are important pentoses for humans as they form part of the structure for DNA (deoxyribonucleic acid) and RNA (ribonucleic acid), the blueprint and genetic coding for the development of each cell in our bodies.

Disaccharides

As the name suggests, disaccharides are formed when two monosaccharides are combined. In terms of nutrition, sucrose, maltose and lactose are the most important disaccharides. As can be seen from Figure 2.9, each of these two sugar units is formed when two hexoses are combined. Sucrose (table sugar) is most commonly found in sugar beet or cane, maltose occurs less widely in nature, but can be found present in germinating grain seeds, and lactose is produced in the milk of mammals.

Polysaccharides

Polysaccharides are formed from chains of monosaccharides ranging in size from three up to several hundred thousand. There are two forms of polysaccharide, plant and animal. In animals only a small proportion (approximately 10–20 g for a sedentary adult) of the glucose available to produce energy is stored in the blood. The majority of glucose supplies held within the body are stored in the form of glycogen (around 400 g for a sedentary adult). Glycogen is the storage form of glucose for mammals with anywhere from several hundred to 25–30,000 glucose molecules

linked to form chains. Glycogen is stored in the liver, where it is able to increase levels of blood glucose when required and in the muscles where it is used directly for energy production. Most of the body's glycogen stores are held in the muscles (about 350 g) with the remaining 50 g stored in the liver.

Key point

Carbohydrate 4 kcal of energy per g

Around 400 g glycogen stored in the muscles and liver

Energy store of ~1,600 kcal

Glycogen stores insufficient to complete a marathon

This is the reason why energy drinks can be helpful during a race (see Chapters 12 and 13)

Glycogen is stored in long highly branched chains of glucose molecules, as can be seen in Figure 2.10. The hormones glucagon and insulin control the rate of **glycogenesis** (glycogen formation) and **glycogenolysis** (the breakdown of glycogen to glucose). The exact nature of the functioning of these hormones is discussed further in the following chapter.

Plant polysaccharides include starch, fibre and cellulose all of which can be used to store glucose created through photosynthesis. Starch, is synthesised in two forms, as *amylose* and *amylopectin* chains, as to carbohydrate store. Food such as pastas, grains, beans and potatoes all contain high starch contents. Amylopectin chains are highly branched in a similar fashion as glycogen, whereas amylose chains are long and non-branched. The branching is linked to the rate at which the starch can be digested when eaten. Amylose starch chains (non-branched) are slower to digest and when present in a foodstuff decrease the glycemic index. Amylopectin chains (branched), on the other hand, are digested more readily and are associated with higher glycemic index foods.

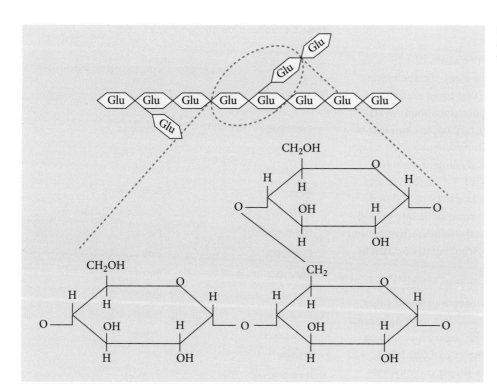

Key point

Carbohydrate can be classified as:

➤ **Monosaccharides** – single sugars. Examples: glucose and fructose.

➤ **Disaccharides** – two sugar molecules. Examples: sucrose (table sugar) and maltose (malt sugar).

➤ **Polysaccharides** – chains of sugar molecules (simple sugar stores). Examples include starch and glycogen.

Fibre, not traditionally included as one of the six necessary nutrients for healthy living, has been recognised as an important omission from many western diets. There is a variety of forms fibre can take within plants and these include cellulose and pectin. Within plants, fibre is used to give the plant its structure and is found within the stems, roots, leaves and fruit. The fibrous (hence the name), nature of this polysaccharide means that it is resistive to digestive processes. This resistance means dietary fibre increases bulk in human waste products (fibre contains a relatively high water content) and decreases the time taken for food to exit the body. Western diets, often including highly processed foods, have lower fibre content which has been linked with poor digestive tract health and increased incidence of cancers and haemorrhoids. Increasing the fibre in your diet, by changing to whole wheat grains, pastas, cereals and breads has been shown to improve digestive function.

Foods containing carbohydrate

There is a wide variety of foods that have a high proportion of carbohydrate within them. Examples of these foods are listed in Table 2.5. When making decisions about which of these foods to include within a healthy diet it is appropriate to identify the nature of the carbohydrate – its relative complexity and glycemic index – which is discussed in the next section.

Table 2.5 Foods with high carbohydrate content.

Simple or processed carbohydrates	More complex carbohydrates
Table sugar	Bananas
Honey	Apples
Gatorade	Kidney beans
Powerade	Lentils
Power bars	Chick peas
White bread	Whole wheat or multigrain bread
Quick-cook and white rice	Whole grain brown rice
Pasta	Whole wheat pasta
Oven-cook chips	Potatoes

Glycaemic index

It is recommended for healthy active adults that 55–60% of our food intake should be in the form of carbohydrate. There is another factor, however, that could usefully be taken into account when making decisions about which carbohydrates should form the dietary staples, and that is the type of carbohydrate. In its simplest context this relates to the interplay between simple and complex carbohydrates that form the basis of our diet. Research indicates the glycaemic index of foods should also be considered when making decisions about the range of dietary carbohydrates. Simple carbohydrates include monosaccharides and disaccharides, whereas complex carbohydrates pertain to polysaccharides such as starch.

Complex carbohydrates generally take longer to digest, result in a lower postprandial (after eating) blood sugar peak and consequently would be available for longer as an energy source when compared with sugary foods. Pasta and potatoes are examples of complex carbohydrates and table sugar is an example of a simple carbohydrate. The division between simple and complex carbohydrates works as a general rule; however, the reality is more complex. Potatoes, for example, are more quickly absorbed than pasta. In addition, the more processing a food rich in starch undergoes during manufacture, the less complex its resultant chemical structure. As a consequence, the use of the food glycaemic index has become popular when describing the complexity of a carbohydrate. The glycemic index for a food is based on its rate of digestion and absorption and the spike in blood sugar levels it creates. A rating regarding the glycaemic index of a range of food items can be seen in Table 2.6. A score of 100 represents the glycaemic index for white bread and glucose and is used to inform decisions around low (<80) and high (>80) index foods.

Table 2.6 High and low glycaemic index foods.

High glycaemic index (>80)	Low glycaemic index (<80)
Table sugar	Kidney beans
Honey	Chick peas
Doughnuts	Lentils
Bagels	Baked beans
White rice	Whole grain brown rice
Watermelon	Pasta
Pineapple	Figs
Raisins	Dates
Carrots	Peaches
Potatoes	Sweet potatoes
Rice cakes	Plums
Waffles	Milk
Rice Crispies	Yoghurt
Corn flakes	All Bran
Shredded Wheat	Apples
Corn tortilla chips	Peanuts
White bread	Bananas

Note: The glycaemic index scale is based on 100 representing the score for glucose and white bread.

Key point

Choice of carbohydrate (CHO) should take into account:

➤ Complexity of the CHO

➤ Glycaemic index

➤ Rate at which it is required

Simple sugars are absorbed rapidly:

➤ Ideal for maintaining and restoring levels

Complex CHO takes much longer to digest and be absorbed:

➤ Ideal for restoring levels and increasing stores

Fats

Fats or lipids (from the Greek word for fat – *lipos*), as they are also known, are our most dense form of energy store, able to provide on average 9 kcal of energy per gram compared with 4 kcal for carbohydrates and proteins. Fats, like carbohydrates are comprised of carbon, hydrogen and oxygen. The nature of their structure and bonding, however, differs from carbohydrates. This results in fats being more energy-dense compounds that have limited water solubility. As well as an energy source, fats provide protection and support for vital organs, are essential parts of each cell's membrane, help increase the speed of nerve impulse transmission, assist in the preservation of body heat and are the storage and transport system for fat-soluble vitamins. Lipids can be classified as fatty acids, triglycerides (sometimes referred to as triacylglycerols), sterols (which include cholesterol), phospholipids, glycolipids and lipoproteins.

Common foods containing fats include meat, dairy products and plant-based oils. Fats represent the energy store for the body and excess carbohydrate and protein intake are converted to fat and stored within specialist adipocytes (fat cells) that form the adipose tissue. Available fat within the muscle, the blood and stored in the adipocytes can provide 90,000–100,000 kcal of energy. This represents a plentiful energy supply, especially when compared with the 1,500–2,000 kcal of stored carbohydrate.

Dietary fat is an essential macronutrient. However, in recent years excess fat intake has been associated with increased obesity rates and incidence of cardiovascular disease in many western societies (Table 2.7).

In the UK a great emphasis has been placed upon the need to decrease dietary fat consumption as a percentage of total caloric intake. In 1986–7 fat consumption represented 40% of the average British citizen's food consumption. With an emphasis on decreasing fat intake, the Department of Health targeted a reduction in total fat intake to <35% in their 2004 Choosing Health campaign. This target has recently been reported to have been reached (35.1%).

Table 2.7a The top twenty countries, as reported by WHO, for incidence of obesity (%) in males (15+ year olds) in 2002 and those countries' rankings and incidence in 2010.

Country	2002 ranking	2002 percentage	2010 ranking	2010 percentage
Nauru	1st	82.3	1st	84.6
Cook Islands	2nd	67.9	2nd	72.1
Federated States of Micronesia	3rd	64.3	3rd	69.1
Tonga	4th	58.7	4th	64.0
Samoa	5th	36.2	6th	42.2
Nuie	6th	34.4	7th	40.7
USA	7th	32.0	5th	44.2
Kuwait	8th	29.6	13th	29.6
Palau	9th	29.0	9th	35.0
Argentina	10th	28.0	8th	37.4
Kiribati	11th	27.6	10th	33.6
Greece	12th	26.2	11th	30.3
Malta	13th	24.6	17th	28.1
United Arab Emirates	14th	24.5	21st	24.5
Canada	15th	23.1	20th	25.5
Saudi Arabia	16th	22.3	25th	23.0
Egypt	17th	22.0	27th	22.0
Bahrain	18th	21.2	30th	21.2
Australia	19th	21.2	16th	28.4
Mexico	20th	20.3	12th	30.1

Note: Obesity rates are defined as the percentage of the population with a Body Mass Index (BMI) ≥30 kg·m^{-2}. WHO is the World Health Organisation.

Table 2.7b The top twenty countries, as reported by WHO, for incidence of obesity (%) in females (15+ year olds) in 2002 and those countries' rankings and incidence in 2010.

Country	2002 ranking	2002 percentage	2010 ranking	2010 percentage
Nauru	1st	77.7	1st	80.5
Tonga	2nd	74.8	2nd	78.1
Federated States of Micronesia	3rd	71.3	3rd	75.3
Cook Islands	4th	69.0	4th	73.4
Nuie	5th	58.6	5th	64.7
Samoa	6th	55.0	6th	60.9
Palau	7th	52.2	7th	69.4
Kuwait	8th	49.2	9th	55.2
Barbados	9th	46.7	8th	57.2
Trinidad and Tobago	10th	41.9	10th	52.7
Dominica	11th	41.8	11th	52.6
Jordan	12th	40.2		
Egypt	13th	39.3	14th	48.0
Kiribati	14th	37.9	15th	46.1
United Arab Emirates	15th	37.9	17th	42.0
United States	16th	37.8	13th	48.3
Jamaica	17th	36.4	12th	48.3
Seychelles	18th	35.8	16th	43.2
South Africa	19th	34.3		
Malta	20th	33.8		

Note: Obesity rates are defined as the percentage of the population with a Body Mass Index (BMI) ≥30 kg·m^{-2}. WHO is the World Health Organisation.

However, saturated fat intake was reported to be 12.8% of energy intake, greater than the recommended level of 11% (National Diet Nutrition Survey 2008/2009). In Australasia, the percentage energy from total fat was similarly advised by the New Zealand Nutrition Taskforce (1991) to be ≤ 33% and the 'Nutrient Reference Values for Australia and New Zealand' (2006) recommend an upper limit of 35%. The contribution of fat to energy intake in New Zealand adults has fallen from 37% in 1989–90 to 35% in 1997 (NZ National Nutrition Survey, 1997). Saturated fat, however, was still the predominant source of fat (15%) which has more recently been recommended to have a limit of 8–10% of energy from saturated and trans-fats combined (Nutrient Reference Values for Australia and New Zealand, 2006). A Norwegian policy 'Recipe for a Healthier Diet' is an action plan on nutrition (2007–2011). With a reduction in total fat consumption of Norwegians from 40% of total calorie intake in 1977–1979 to 34% in 2002–2004, their current nutritional action plan recommends an intake of ~30% total fat. Similarly, the consumption of saturated fats and trans-fats have decreased from 17% to 14%, and 4% to < 1%, respectively, with the current recommended level standing at ≤ 10% intake of saturated fat and < 1% intake of trans fats (as suggested by WHO European Action Plan for Food and Nutrition Policy 2007–2012). It is interesting to note that the American Heart Association have moved further, recommending a maximum of 30% total fat in the diet with 6–9% comprising saturated fats. Excess lipid levels have been associated with an increase risk of colon, rectum and prostate cancer, hence the American Cancer Society has moved further to suggest a total fat intake of 20% to reduce these risks. For an active sports performer, maintaining fat intake at a level below 30% of total caloric intake is believed to be beneficial for health. In addition to this, reducing cholesterol and saturated fat intake as a part of this 30% would appear to be beneficial.

Key point

Fats or lipids are the body's major energy store

Lipid stores (90% as triglyceride) are held within the adipocytes

Fats are energy dense ~9 kcal of energy per g

Fats are an essential dietary component:

➤ but excess intake associated with increased coronary heart disease and diabetes risk

➤ ideally fat intake up to 30% of caloric intake

➤ saturated fat recommended < 10% of total caloric intake

Fatty acids, glycerol and triglycerides

The lipid equivalent to glucose for energy production from fats is the fatty acid. Free fatty acids are long carbon chains with hydrogen atoms attached. As can be seen from Figure 2.11 one end of a fatty acid contains a COOH (*carboxylic acid*) unit and this is known as the head. The head will form bonds when in water because it is **hydrophilic** (water-friendly). However, the tail of a fatty acid is **hydrophobic** (water-fearing). While glucose is stored as glycogen in the muscles and liver, free fatty acids are stored as triglycerides within the adipocytes. Triglycerides are composed of a glycerol molecule attached to three fatty acids. Unlike the fatty acids, glycerol is a carbohydrate-based molecule that can be converted to glucose when a triglyceride is broken down. When fatty acids are required as an energy source the triglyceride can be catabolised (broken down) again to release the fatty acids. The process by which fats are released from their glycerol backbone is called *lipolysis* and during low-intensity exercise, when fat becomes the predominant fuel source for aerobic metabolism, the rate of lipolysis will increase. Fatty acids are released into the blood and attach to albumin, a blood protein, and travel to the exercising muscles as *free fatty acids*.

Fatty acids exist in saturated and unsaturated forms. Figure 2.11 shows the chemical structure of the saturated fat palmitic acid and the unsaturated fat linolenic acid. Palmitic acid, as the name suggests, is a major component of palm oil and coconut oil. It is one of the most common saturated fats found in plants and animals. Linolenic acid, or more correctly α-linolenic acid, is found in seed oils such as rapeseed, soybeans, flaxseed and kiwifruit seeds. Research indicates that consumption of α-linolenic acid is associated with decreased risk of cardiovascular disease. The saturation of a fatty acid refers to the number of hydrogen atoms attached to the carbon chain. Carbon makes four covalent bonds to share electrons. In a saturated fat the carbon atoms are saturated with hydrogen atoms, such that each carbon atom is attached to its neighbouring carbon atoms and two hydrogen atoms. It cannot hold any more hydrogen atoms and remain attached to the fatty acid chain, and is therefore a saturated fatty acid. In an unsaturated fatty acid one or more of the carbon atoms makes a double bond with a neighbouring carbon atom. This means that while the double carbon-bonded atoms maintain four covalent bonds for chemical stability it remains unsaturated with hydrogen atoms. In the example shown, α-linolenic acid has three unsaturated carbon atoms.

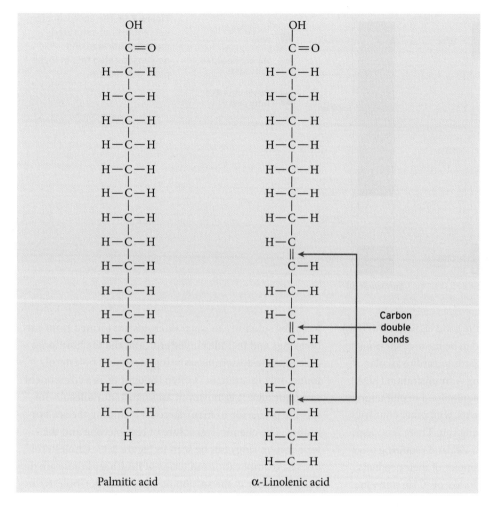

Figure 2.11 Chemical structure of palmitic acid ($C_{16}H_{32}O_2$ – a saturated fatty acid) and α-linolenic acid ($C_{18}H_{30}O_2$ – an unsaturated fatty acid). The palmitic acid molecule has no carbon double bonds and is therefore *saturated* with hydrogen atoms whereas α-linolenic acid has 3 carbon double bonds and is consequently not saturated (or *unsaturated*) with hydrogen atoms.

The ratio of hydrogen atoms to oxygen atoms reveals part of the structural differences between carbohydrates and fats. Fats have a higher density of hydrogen atoms to oxygen atoms than carbohydrates. For example glucose, with a chemical formula of $C_6H_{12}O_6$, has an H:O ratio of 2:1 whereas the fatty acids in Figure 2.11, palmitic acid ($C_{16}H_{32}O_2$) and α-linolenic acid ($C_{18}H_{30}O_2$), have ratios of 16:1 and 15:1 respectively.

Unsaturated fatty acids can be **monounsaturated**, where they have one carbon double bond or **polyunsaturated** with more than one carbon double bond. α-linolenic acid, with its three unsaturated carbon atoms, is an example of a polyunsaturated fatty acid. Olive oil contains largely monounsaturated fat, while sunflower oil and corn oils are predominantly polyunsaturated fats (Figure 2.12). Common sources of saturated fats include cheese, whole milk, beef and pork. Oils from plants, such as coconut oil, sunflower oil and olive oil, contain all three forms of fatty acid, but vary in the amount they contain of each type. Figure 2.12 shows the percentages of each fatty acid in these three plant-derived oils

and, as can be seen from this figure, one of the three types of fatty acids is predominant for each of the oils.

In terms of health, dieticians recommend that saturated fats are best kept as a small percentage (6–9 %) of total food and lipid intake. Research strongly indicates that individuals with diets rich in saturated fats, found in items such as red meats and many processed foods, are linked with an increased risk of cardiovascular disease.

It is interesting to note that in order to create solid fats (at room temperature) for margarine, hydrogen is forced through a vegetable oil to create a higher level of hydrogen saturation and enable it to solidify. This is known as **hydrogenation** and leads to the fatty acid becoming saturated and being referred to as a trans-fatty acid. These trans-fatty acids are not essential and have no apparent benefit to health. The British Heart Foundation (BHF) has highlighted research suggesting that such trans-fatty acids have a negative effect on cholesterol levels, another factor linked with the development of cardiovascular disease. In addition, it has been reported that trans-fats not only increase the bad

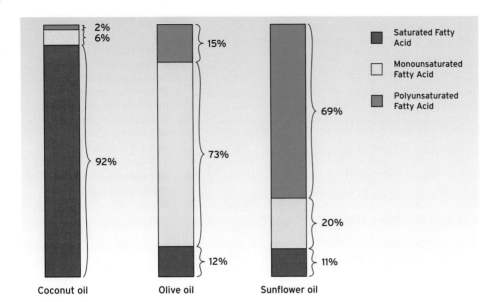

Saturated Fatty Acid

Monounsaturated Fatty Acid

Polyunsaturated Fatty Acid

Coconut oil: 2%, 6%, 92%
Olive oil: 15%, 73%, 12%
Sunflower oil: 69%, 20%, 11%

Figure 2.12 The approximate percentages of saturated, monounsaturated and polyunsaturated fats in these plant-derived oils.

cholesterol (LDL) but also lower the good cholesterol (HDL) and have therefore been suggested to be more deleterious than saturated fatty acids with regards to cardiovascular disease. In 2003 the Food and Drug Administration (FDA) in the US implemented a law to require food manufacturers to label trans-fats within the contents, with other countries, such as Brazil and Canada, following suit. There is no legislation in the UK, Australia or New Zealand requiring food manufacturers to label trans-fat content of their products. The WHO recommend a dietary intake of < 1% trans-fat, and advocates phasing out the use of trans-fats as has been accomplished in Denmark, Switzerland and parts of the US and Canada. The BHF suggests consumers look at the labels of food for hydrogenated fat or hydrogenated oils. The lower they come down the list, the smaller the percentage of the ingredients they represent. We do, however, require lipids as part of our diet, so as a consequence of the health implications of some fatty acids, it is perhaps beneficial to maintain a diet where the majority of fats are from mono- or polyunsaturated sources.

Key point

Excess saturated fat intakes can be harmful to health.

Monounsaturated or polyunsaturated fats provide healthier choices.

Sterols

Sterols or steroids are lipid derivatives and have a different chemical structure from other lipids, although they still have low solubility in water. Steroids are formed from carbon rings and include cholesterol, and the sex hormones oestrogen, testosterone and progesterone. Cholesterol, found only in animals, is often thought of as a component of a poor diet. It is, however, an important molecule, for it is the precursor to many steroids including the sex hormones. The chemical structure of testosterone and the four carbon rings can be seen in Figure 2.13. Cholesterol does have implications in terms of health and these are discussed further in the section on lipoproteins. Cholesterol represents one of the lipoprotein group and it is in this role that its presence can be harmful to health.

Phospholipids and glycolipids

Phospholipids and glycolipids are involved in a variety of functions within the body including providing the insulating (myelin) sheath around nerve fibres, assisting in blood clotting and maintenance of each cell's membrane and structure. Phospholipids and glycolipids, as their names suggest, are comprised of a lipid and a phosphate or glucose component respectively. Their structure is similar

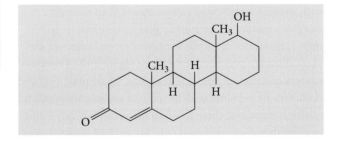

Figure 2.13 The chemical structure of testosterone $C_{19}H_{28}O_2$.

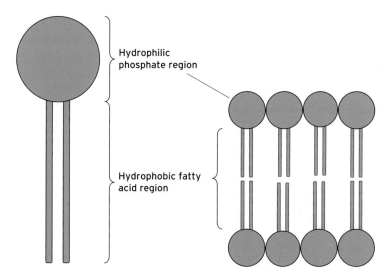

Figure 2.14 The structure of a phospholipid (*left*) and an illustration of phospholipid bonding to establish the bilipid layer that forms the protective cell membrane for animal cells.

Hydrophilic phosphate region

Hydrophobic fatty acid region

to that of a triglyceride with the exception that one of the fatty acids is replaced with a phosphate group and usually a nitrogen group in the case of a phospholipid, and a carbohydrate group in the case of glycolipids. A phospholipid bilayer, along with small amounts of glycolipids and cholesterol, forms the basic structure of the plasma membrane of cells. The phospholipid molecules have hydrophilic phosphate heads and hydrophobic fatty acid tails. The glycolipid structure is similar, with a glucose-based hydrophilic head. The structure of the plasma membrane is depicted in Figure 2.14. These unique properties enable phospholipids and glycolipids to create a sealed membrane that separates cells from their outside environment. The forces of attraction are strong enough that no covalent bond is needed between adjacent molecules to maintain the structural integrity of the cell membrane.

Knowledge integration question

What is special about the structure of phospholipids that makes them ideal to form a cell's plasma membrane?

Lipoproteins

Lipoproteins, usually metabolised in the liver, are formed when phospholipids or triglycerides are joined with a protein, with cholesterol being an important one. The major function of lipoproteins is to enable blood transport of fats. Lipoproteins, unlike lipids, are water soluble and as such can be carried within the plasma of the blood. There are a number of lipoproteins including chylomicrons, low-density lipoproteins (LDL) and high-density lipoproteins (HDL). Chylomicrons are formed in the small intestine and

are the blood lipid carriers for fats that have been digested from our food. After entry to the bloodstream from the intestines, chylomicrons carry fat to muscle and adipose cells. The muscle cells and adipocytes adjacent to blood vessels release the enzyme lipoprotein lipase and this enables chylomicrons to release fatty acids and monoglycerides (a fatty acid attached to a glycerol molecule) for use or storage in those tissues. The remnants of the chylomicrons, which include cholesterol, are then returned via the bloodstream to the liver for reuse or excretion from the body as necessary.

Within the liver low-density lipoproteins (LDLs), often referred to as 'bad cholesterol', are synthesised from chylomicrons as they arrive in the hepatocytes. As they are formed, LDLs diffuse from the liver into the bloodstream. Cells throughout the body absorb LDL and extract the cholesterol for uses such as the synthesis of the membrane and the formation of hormones. Cholesterol not used by a cell diffuses back into the bloodstream where it is absorbed by high-density lipoproteins (HDLs), which are also released from the liver, but serve to transport unused cholesterol to the liver where it is either repackaged or excreted from the body. Low-density lipoproteins are seen as the 'bad' cholesterol because LDLs have been found to be strongly attracted to the tissues of the arterial wall where they damage the lining and create plaques (made up of cholesterol-based deposits) that eventually narrow the artery in which they are formed. High-density lipoproteins, on the other hand, appear to reverse this process by clearing cholesterol from the arterial walls and blocking the entrance of LDL to the arterial cells, and are hence referred to as 'good cholesterol'. Increasing the monounsaturated and polyunsaturated fats in your diet, as well as not smoking and taking regular exercise, appears to decrease LDL and increase

HDL levels. Having low total cholesterol levels and a high proportion of that cholesterol as HDLs appears to lower the risk of cardiovascular disease (CVD).

> **Key point**
>
> Cholesterol is an essential part of our diet.
>
> Lipoproteins contain cholesterol.
>
> Low-density lipoproteins (LDL) are associated with plaque formation and CVD.
>
> High-density lipoproteins (HDL) appear to be more beneficial in the body:
>
> ➤ attack plaque deposits
>
> ➤ block LDL attachment to arterial walls
>
> The HDL:LDL ratio can be improved by:
>
> ➤ avoiding smoking
>
> ➤ increasing the proportion of mono- and polyunsaturated in diet
>
> ➤ regular exercise

Proteins

Proteins, from the Greek word *proteios* meaning of first or prime importance, are an essential component of a balanced diet and can be found from plant and animal sources. Proteins are broken down to amino acids in the small intestine and transported via the bloodstream to be used throughout the body for a myriad of functions. Proteins are involved in nearly every reaction that takes place within the body. They play a major role in the structure of all body tissues being the building blocks for synthesising hair, skin, bones, tendons and muscles. Proteins form the basis for all enzymes and many hormones,

provide the necessary amino acids to enable blood clotting, muscular contraction, growth and repair, regulation of metabolism and immune function. In addition, proteins provide an alternative to carbohydrates and fats for energy production and play a major role in oxygen and carbon dioxide transport in the body.

> **Key point**
>
> Proteins play a crucial role in nearly all physiological processes.
>
> Amino acids are the building blocks for proteins.

Amino acids

The building blocks for proteins are **amino acids**. Figure 2.15 shows the general chemical structure common to amino acids. Similar to carbohydrates and fats, amino acids contain carbon, hydrogen and oxygen. However, the nitrogen atom within the **amine group** of the molecule distinguishes them from carbohydrates and fats. The acid section of the amino acid is the **carboxyl group**, which, as for the head of fatty acids, contains one carbon, two oxygen and one hydrogen atom (COOH).

Each amino acid also contains a unique *R group* that distinguishes it from other amino acids. In the simplest amino acid, glycine, the R group contains a hydrogen atom which is covalently bonded to a carbon atom (Figure 2.16). The R group for alanine, a structurally more complex amino acid, comprises a carbon atom bonded to three hydrogen atoms. This R group is covalently bonded to a carbon atom (Figure 2.17).

The R group differs for all amino acids and can include sulphur, hydrogen, carbon or iron in their structure.

The amine group – which contains nitrogen.

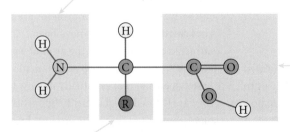

The carboxyl group – the acid part of the amino acid, similar in structure to carbohydrates and fats.

The R group – which contains a variety of components for each amino acid. This component differentiates one amino acid from another.

Figure 2.15 The general structure of an amino acid.

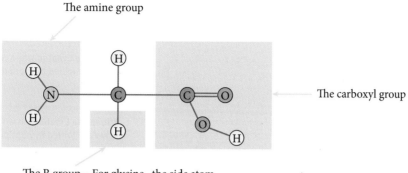

The amine group

The carboxyl group

The R group – For glycine, the side atom is hydrogen.

Figure 2.16 The chemical structure of glycine ($C_2H_5NO_2$) - the simplest amino acid.

Amino acids form proteins when they are covalently bonded by peptide bonds. The formation of a peptide bond between the amino acids glycine and alanine, to form the dipeptide glycylalanine, is shown in Figure 2.17. The bond is made between the carboxyl group of one amino acid (in this example glycine) and the amine group of the other (alanine). The synthesis of all dipeptides causes the liberation of one molecule of water.

When three amino acids bond to form a tripeptide molecule through the creation of two peptide bonds, two molecules of water are liberated. This continues for each amino acid that joins the chain to form polypeptides

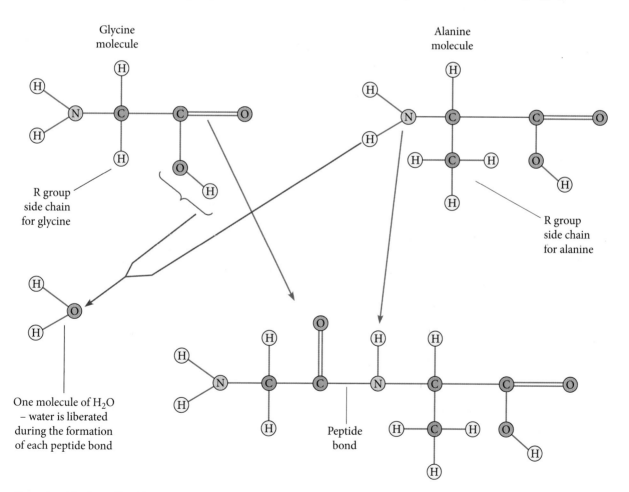

Glycine molecule

Alanine molecule

R group side chain for glycine

R group side chain for alanine

One molecule of H_2O – water is liberated during the formation of each peptide bond

Peptide bond

Figure 2.17 The formation of the dipeptide glycylalanine through the creation of a peptide bond between glycine ($C_2H_5NO_2$) and alanine ($C_3H_7NO_2$).

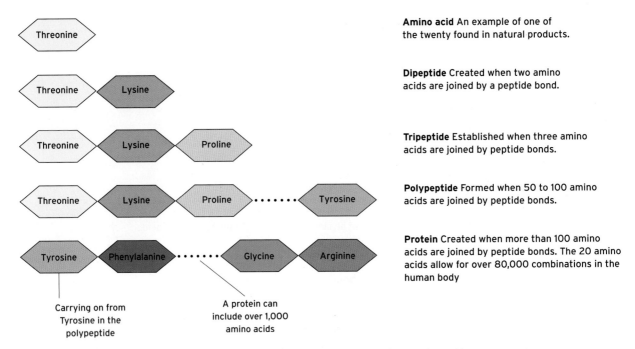

Amino acid An example of one of the twenty found in natural products.

Dipeptide Created when two amino acids are joined by a peptide bond.

Tripeptide Established when three amino acids are joined by peptide bonds.

Polypeptide Formed when 50 to 100 amino acids are joined by peptide bonds.

Protein Created when more than 100 amino acids are joined by peptide bonds. The 20 amino acids allow for over 80,000 combinations in the human body

Carrying on from Tyrosine in the polypeptide

A protein can include over 1,000 amino acids

Figure 2.18 The formation of dipeptides, tripeptides, polypeptides and proteins from amino acids.

and eventually proteins. An illustration of the formation of protein from amino acids is provided in Figure 2.18. The named amino acids in the figure are a sample of the 20 amino acids found within the body. Amino acids can be bonded in a diverse range of combinations as dictated by the type of protein to be synthesised. This versatility is essential because of the myriad of functions performed by proteins within our bodies.

In comparison to carbohydrates and fats, proteins are very large molecules. While the chemical composition of glucose is $C_6H_{12}O_6$ and palmitic acid is $C_{16}H_{32}O_2$ haemoglobin, a fairly small protein, comprises $C_{2952}H_{4664}O_{832}N_{812}S_8Fe_4$. Proteins have a complicated four-level structure to provide the structural integrity necessary for these long chain molecules and to enable their formation in a relatively confined space. Figure 2.19 illustrates the four structural levels amino acids conform to in the creation of a protein. The example provided is similar to the structure for the protein-based molecule, haemoglobin.

The 20 amino acids necessary for human growth and health are shown in Table 2.8. Amino acids are, by convention, usually classified as essential and non-essential. All 20 amino acids are essential for a healthy diet but this classification refers to the fact that the non-essential amino acids can be synthesised within the body and consequently we can survive without including them in our diet. The essential amino acids, however, must be included within our diet

because they cannot be synthesised within the body. To maintain a well-balanced dietary food intake it is beneficial to consume a full range of amino acids on a regular basis.

Many sports people, particularly those involved in power and strength events, believe, mistakenly, that protein supplements are necessary for muscle growth and function.

Table 2.8 The essential and non-essential amino acids.

Essential amino acids	Non-essential amino acids
Isoleucine	Alanine
Leucine	Arginine
Lysine	Asparagine
Methionine	Aspartic acid
Phenylalanine	Cysteine
Threonine	Glutamic acid
Tryptophan	Glutamine
Valine	Glycine
Histidine	Proline
	Serine
	Tyrosine

Note: Histidine is an essential amino acid for children. However, adults have the ability to synthesise it within the body. For adults histidine is a non-essential amino acid.

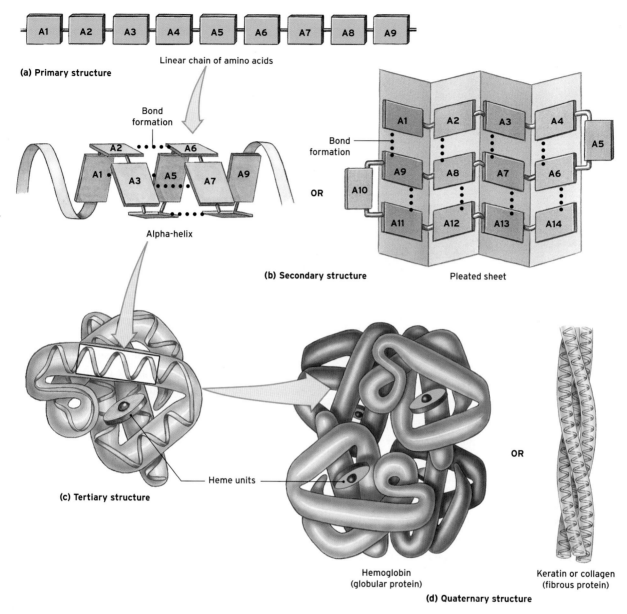

Figure 2.19 The four structural levels of a protein. (*Source*: Martini, F. H. and Nath, J. L. (2009) *Fundamentals of Anatomy and Physiology*, 8th edition, New York: Benjamin Cummings)

Research indicates that this is not the case and normally all the necessary amino acids can be found within a healthy balanced diet. It is also a misconception that vegetarians cannot obtain all the amino acids from their diet. An increasing number of sports participants, including elite athletes like Dave Scott (World Champion Ironman triathlete) have adopted vegetarian or nearly vegetarian diets and it is perfectly possible for them to provide all 20 amino acids within their normal food.

Proteins can be sourced from a variety of plant and animal-based foods. The difference between the two sources is that plant-based foodstuffs, with the possible exception of soybeans, are less protein-dense than animal-based sources of protein. In addition, they often contain an incomplete amino acid range, whereas animal-based protein sources such as milk, eggs, chicken and fish are complete proteins and contain all 20 amino acids. A vegetarian will have to eat a higher volume of food, from a range of sources, to consume the same amount of protein as could be found from animal sources. With a well-balanced diet, however, vegetarians can obtain all the amino acids necessary for health and performance. For instance, rice and beans as a meal choice can provide all twenty amino acids and are common staples in South American countries such as Bolivia.

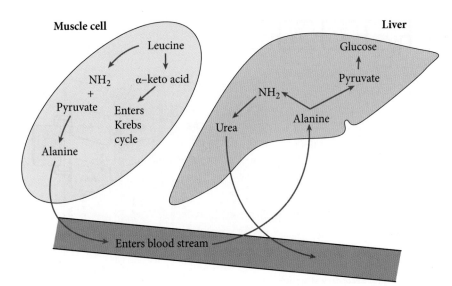

Figure 2.20 The glucose-alanine cycle – an example of how amino acids can be utilised as an energy source.

Key point

There are 20 amino acids required for human functioning.

8 are essential and 12 are nonessential.

Non-essential amino acids can be synthesised within the body.

A well-balanced diet should provide all necessary amino acids.

Protein supplements are not normally necessary.

Protein metabolism

As building blocks, amino acids undergo frequent change and renewal within the body. There is a variety of processes that take place to **anabolise** and **catabolise** amino acids, polypeptides and proteins. Dietary proteins, broken down to their constituent parts in the small intestine, are absorbed into the bloodstream and taken up by cells that require them to anabolise cellular proteins.

Within a cell, amino acids can be further catabolised through a process called **deamination** which, as the name suggests, involves the removal of the amine group with an α-keto acid remaining. The nitrogen element (the amine), once detached from the α-keto acid, can be removed from the body as urea or, in a process called **transamination,** can be attached to another α-keto acid to create a new amino acid. The remains of the deaminated molecule, the α-keto acid, can then be catabolised to provide energy.

Depending on the duration of the exercise an athlete is engaged in, and their diet before and during the activity, proteins are thought to provide up to 10% of the required energy. The **glucose-alanine cycle**, illustrated in Figure 2.20, provides an example of a mechanism through which amino acids can become a source of energy, particularly during prolonged exercise or when an athlete is in a fasted state. It has been suggested that during such conditions the amino acid leucine is deaminated to release the amine group. The released amine group then bonds with an intramuscular pyruvate molecule to synthesise the amino acid alanine. Once formed, alanine is transported to the liver via the bloodsteam, where it in turn is deaminated. The pyruvate component is converted to glucose for use as a carbohydrate energy source, and the amine unit is removed as urea and excreted from the body. Interestingly, it is thought that the remaining α-keto acid from the deaminated leucine molecule is also used for energy production within the muscle by entering the Krebs cycle, as discussed further in Chapters 8 and 12.

2.4 Micronutrients

Vitamins

Vitamins are a significant group of **micronutrients** and in small amounts are vital to optimal physiological functioning. While not formally discovered until the 20th Century, it was understood as long ago as during the Greek Empire that there were substances in foods that could prevent diseases.

An interesting example regarding the discovery of the disease-preventative effects of vitamins can be seen from the work of James Lind. In 1747 Lind conducted an excellent experiment on HMS Salisbury to test the use of citrus fruit as a protection against the effects of scurvy. Before Lind's experiment, and indeed for some time afterwards (until his results were accepted), scurvy was rife in the

British Navy. As we now know, scurvy was caused in sailors by a lack of Vitamin C in the diet during the long sea voyages. The symptoms of scurvy were bleeding and spongy gums, bleeding from almost every mucous membrane, depression, and then physical incapacitation. In his experiment, which included a control group who did not receive the treatment, sailors were given daily rations of citrus fruits to test if they would ward off the effects of scurvy. The study proved successful and, after the results were accepted, the British Navy were supplied with rations of citrus fruits, particularly limes, to protect against the disease. It was for this reason that the British gained the name 'Limeys'. The actual discovery of the chemical structure of vitamin C was not made until 1928.

The term 'vitamin' was originally proposed by a Polish biochemist, Casimir Funk, who discovered the vitamin thiamine in 1912. Seven years prior to Funk's discovery, Frederick Hopkins (who was also involved with the discovery and isolation of lactic acid – see Chapter 1) found that keeping the husks on rice prevented the development of beriberi, a disease which can affect the gastrointestinal, nervous, cardiovascular and musculoskeletal systems. Moving on from this discovery, Funk was able to isolate thiamine (later called vitamin B and now known as vitamin B1) as the substance responsible for preventing the development of the disease. Funk recognised the importance of this discovery and as a consequence coined the term 'vitamine' from the words *vita* meaning 'life-giving' and *amine* because the chemical structure included an amine (nitrogen group). This term was later changed to vitamin (dropping the 'e') because as further vitamins were discovered, it was found that some (e.g. vitamin C) had no amine group as part of their chemical structure. The vitamins were discovered between 1912 and 1941, with the year of discovery of each vitamin presented in Table 2.9.

Vitamins were given alphabetical names according to the date of their discovery and isolation, although for some it is difficult to pin-down the exact date. Some vitamins continue to be referred to by the alphabetical name, whereas others such as Niacin, which was originally named Vitamin B$_3$, are known by the substance name. There are 13 essential vitamins, although there were more in the past when vitamins B$_4$, B$_8$, B$_{10}$, B$_{11}$, were included. These substances were later found not to be essential to our diet and were consequently removed from the list.

Vitamins are organic compounds that, in common with carbohydrates, fats and proteins, include carbon, hydrogen and oxygen atoms in their structure. The 13 essential vitamins are shown in Table 2.9: of these, nine are water soluble and four are fat soluble. Vitamins, while not providing an energy source for metabolism, have a wide number of crucial functions within the body. The major roles of vitamins include ensuring appropriate growth and development of cells such as epithelial cells (associated with the skin) and red blood cells (RBC), the eyes, nerves, muscles, teeth, bones and digestive tract, enabling efficient energy metabolism, assisting in the formation of enzymes and hormones, along with acting as antioxidants. Foods that contain the essential vitamins, the main function of each vitamin and their associated recommended daily allowances (RDA) can be seen in Table 2.9.

Although essential to our diet they are needed in tiny amounts relative to the volume of food we consume each day. With a few exceptions, such as the need for pregnant women to supplement their diet with folic acid (which has been shown to decrease the chances of a child developing a neural tube defect) a healthy balanced diet should provide all our vitamin requirements. The vitamin and dietary supplements industry is worth millions of dollars around the world and yet with a balanced diet we should be able to meet all our vitamin needs from our diet. We need to be particularly careful about the levels of fat soluble vitamins (A, D, E and K) we consume. By taking a vitamin supplement we may consume more water-soluble vitamins than our bodies need, but we can excrete them from our bodies in our urine. This is not possible with vitamins A, D, E and K. There is a danger of us encountering a toxic reaction (vitamin toxicosis) if we include too many of these vitamins in our diet through supplementation.

Key point

There are 13 essential vitamins:

➤ 9 water soluble – B vitamins and vitamin C

➤ 4 fat soluble – vitamins A, E, D and K

Vitamins are organic compounds:

➤ They serve a wide number of vital functions

Supplementation should not be necessary

➤ Healthy diet should provide all required vitamins

➤ Exceptions include during pregnancy

➤ Excess can cause vitamin toxicosis

Vitamins as enzymes

The water-soluble vitamins play a key role in the structure of enzymes. Vitamins form co-enzymes that combine with protein compounds to form enzymes that are particularly vital in energy metabolism. Riboflavin forms part of the

Table 2.9 Vitamins, their functions and recommended daily allowance (RDA).

Vitamin	Discovered	Food sources	Function within the body	EU RDA
Vitamin A (Retinol)	1917	Preformed Vitamin A: milk, butter, egg yolk, liver. Proformed Vitamin A (beta carotene) green leafy vegetables, orange fruit and vegetables, e.g. carrots	Repair and growth of body tissues (especially epithelial), maintains night vision, peripheral vision and an antioxidant. **Deficiencies:** Night blindness	0.7-0.9 mg
Vitamin B1 (Thiamine)	1912	Yeast, wholemeal grains, oranges, wholegrain rice, sunflower seeds, nuts, liver and pork	Coenzyme for metabolism, normal function of nervous system, digestion and muscles. **Deficiencies:** Beriberi, profound fatigue	1.4 mg
Vitamin B2 (Riboflavin)	1933	Milk and dairy products, eggs, green beans, bananas, popcorn	Component of co-enzymes for metabolism (e.g. FAD), protects vision and skin. **Deficiencies:** cracks on corners of mouth, blurred vision	1.1-1.3 mg
Vitamin B3 (Niacin)	1937	Meat, fish, eggs, nuts, sunflower seeds, whole grains, vegemite/ marmite	Component of co-enzyme for metabolism (NAD), protects nervous function and skin. **Deficiencies:** Skin lesions, nervous disorders, pellagra	14-16 mg
Vitamin B5 (Pantothenic acid)	1933	Fish, liver, chicken, eggs, nuts, milk, broccoli, avocados, whole grains and whole grain rice, yeast	Part of co-enzyme A for metabolism. **Deficiencies:** Very rare, fatigue and nausea	5.0 mg
Vitamin B6 (pyridoxine)	1938	Fish, chicken, bananas, nuts, beans and whole grains	Coenzyme for amino acid metabolism, normal function of nervous system. **Deficiencies:** Irritability, confusion	1.3-1.7 mg
Vitamin B7 (Biotin)	1940	Nuts, peas (black eye), egg yolks and green leafy vegetables	Co-enzyme in synthesis of fat, glycogen and amino acids. **Deficiencies:** Very rare, fatigue, hairloss, dermatitis	none set
Vitamin B9 **(Folate, folic acid)**	1941	Name from fact green leafy vegetables (foliage) are rich in folate, also liver, beans and eggs.	Co-enzyme for metabolism and DNA, RBC production, protects baby during pregnancy. **Deficiencies:** Anaemia, spina bifida risk in newborns, neural deficits.	0.2-0.4 mg
Vitamin B12 (Cobalamin)	1918	Richest sources are from animals, meat, dairy foods, eggs, but also from enriched breakfast cereals	Co-enzyme for DNA, RBC and nerve production. **Deficiencies:** nervous system damage, nervous disorders	0.0025 mg
Vitamin C (Ascorbic acid)	1912/1928	Best sources are from plants, citrus fruits, strawberries, tomatoes, broccoli, green leafy vegetables and peppers	Collagen formation, an antioxidant, promotes immune function and cell structure. **Deficiencies:** Scurvy, impaired immunity	75-90 mg
Vitamin D (D_1 – D_5 exist)	1922	Exposure to sunlight 10-20 minutes, 2–3 per week. Fish oils, milk and eggs	Helps with absorption of calcium – promotes bone growth. **Deficiencies:** Rickets and osteomalacia	0.01 mg
Vitamin E (Tochopherol)	1922	Most widely available in food, found in polyunsaturated oils, nuts, eggs, green leafy vegetables	Promotes growth and development and works as an antioxidant. **Deficiencies:** Very rare, possibly anaemia	15 mg
Vitamin K (K_1 – K_5 exist)	1929	Green leafy vegetables, broccoli, eggs, cheese, tea	Promotes correct blood coagulation (clotting). **Deficiencies:** Defective blood clotting, bruising.	0.1 mg

Note: Water-soluble vitamins are shaded in blue, fat soluble vitamins are shaded in yellow. The name in bold is the most common name by which the vitamin is generally referred. Vitamin C was identified as a vitamin in 1912; however, it was not isolated as a substance until 1928.

structure of flavin adenine dinucleotide (FAD), niacin is part of the nicotinamide adenine dinucleotide (NAD) structure and pantothenic acid is part of co-enzyme A. These, together with vitamins B6 and B12, are involved in catalysing the breakdown of protein. Thiamine is involved in the breakdown of pyruvate to acetyl coenzyme A (acetyl CoA) and vitamin C forms part of enzymes involved in protein synthesis. Each of these enzymatic functions of vitamins is discussed in more detail in subsequent chapters of the book.

Vitamins as antioxidants

One of the functions performed by vitamins A, C, and E is to serve as antioxidants. They perform this antioxidant role against **free radicals**. Free radicals are destructive molecules that develop naturally as part of metabolism or enter the body through cigarette smoking, and air pollutants. In section 2.2, the nature of electrons and the need to complete the outer shell of electrons in order for the atom to become more stable was discussed. Free radicals act in the same way seeking out additional electrons. Free radicals are highly reactive molecules (or parts of molecules) that contain missing electrons from their outer shells. They seek out other compounds with which to bond and can be very destructive to other cellular components as they search for additional electrons. Vitamins A, C, and E react with, and then remove, free radicals from cells. If left unchecked in the body free radicals can prevent the body from removing carcinogens and also promote increases in LDL levels which are associated with the development of atherosclerosis and cardiovascular disease.

Minerals

The 26 elements that comprise the human body were presented in Table 2.1. The elements oxygen, carbon, hydrogen and nitrogen represent 96% of the structure of the human body. The remaining 4% is formed from varying amounts of the other 22 elements found within the human body. These 22 elements, which largely comprise metallic substances, are collectively known as the **minerals**. As a group they can be subdivided into the *major minerals* and the *minor* or *trace minerals*. The major and minor minerals are presented in Table 2.10 along with food sources and the functions of most of the elements. While research has revealed significant details about the function of most minerals (19 of the 22 known to be found within humans), the function of some minerals within the body remains unclear. These minerals, aluminium, tin and vanadium are listed at the bottom of Table 2.10. The RDA for each of the minerals (where known)

is also provided in Table 2.10. Research indicates, as with vitamins, that there are no apparent health benefits to consuming minerals in excess of these allowances.

> ### Key point
>
> There are 22 major and minor minerals found in the body
>
> They comprise about 4% of our body mass
>
> Minerals originate from within the soils, rivers, lakes and seas around us
>
> Minerals form inorganic micronutrients (do not contain carbon)
>
> Minerals serve many vital functions within our bodies

Vitamins and minerals can be distinguished by the fact that minerals do not contain carbon, thus minerals are the inorganic micronutrients and vitamins the organic micronutrients. The minerals necessary for healthy physiological functioning originate in the soils and water of the earth's crust. By consuming mineralised water and foods from plant or animal sources humans can obtain all the minerals essential to life.

While not providing a source of calorific energy, minerals serve three important functions within the body. They combine with other chemicals to synthesise the building blocks for tissues, are integral to the structure of enzymes and assist in the regulation of many physiological functions within the body. As can be seen from Table 2.10, calcium is the most abundant mineral and its role includes structural, metabolic, regulatory and enzymatic functions. Calcium is an essential element for healthy bones and teeth and a lack of calcium within the diet has been linked to osteoporosis which is a bone mineral deficiency. Weight-bearing exercise and a diet with the RDA for calcium can help to prevent the development of osteoporosis. Phosphorus, the second most plentiful mineral in the body, is also an essential structural component for healthy bones and teeth. Calcium, sodium and potassium, as will be discussed in the next chapter, have a particularly important role in nerve impulse transmission and muscle contraction.

Sodium, which often enters our bodies as sodium chloride, has important functions within the body, but excess levels have also been associated with the development of hypertension and cardiovascular disease. Sodium occurs widely and naturally within our foods so adding extra salt to foods is not normally necessary. About a third of the people with high blood pressure (hypertension) find that its induction was by excess salt intake in the diet. Sodium within the diet assists with regulation of osmosis (the

Table 2.10 Major, minor and lesser known minerals and their functions within the body.

Mineral	Food sources	Function within the body	EU RDA
Calcium	Dairy products, green vegetables, beans	Bone and tooth growth, nerve transmission, muscle contraction. **Deficiencies:** Osteoporosis, stunted growth	1300 mg
Phosphorus	Dairy products, chicken, whole grains, nuts	Energy metabolism, bone and tooth growth, acid-base balance. **Deficiencies:** Weakness	700 mg
Potassium	Dairy products, meat, potatoes, bananas	Nerve conduction, fluid and acid-base balance, muscle contraction. **Deficiencies:** Muscular weakness, paralysis	4700 mg
Sulphur	Contained within dietary proteins	Liver function, component of certain amino acids. **Deficiencies:** Very rare, symptoms of protein deficiency.	Unknown
Sodium	Contained within salt	Nerve transmission, fluid and acid-base balance. **Deficiencies:** Muscle cramps, reduced appetite	1500 mg
Chlorine	Part of salt (NaCl as chloride)	Fluid balance. **Deficiencies:** Very rare, muscle cramps, reduced appetite	2300 mg
Magnesium	Whole grains, green leafy vegetables	Enzyme formation, **Deficiencies:** Nervous system disturbances, tremors, muscle weakness, hypertension	300–400 mg
Iron	Red meats, liver, chicken, eggs, whole grains, legumes, nuts	RBC production, enzyme formation. **Deficiencies:** Anaemia, weakness, impaired immunity.	Males 8 mg; females 16–18 mg
Zinc	Meat, beans	Part of digestive and metabolic enzymes. **Deficiencies:** Growth problems, loss of taste and smell, impaired immunity.	Males 11 mg; females 8 mg
Selenium	Sea food, freshwater fish, meats, sunflower seeds	Component of enzymes, antioxidant, links with iodine function. **Deficiencies:** Very rare, anaemia	0.05–0.07 mg
Manganese	Nuts, wholewheat pasta and rice, vegetables, fruits	Metabolism, skeletal development. **Deficiencies:** Very rare, abnormal bone and cartilage	2.5 mg
Copper	Eggs, wholewheat grains, beans, liver, nuts, seafood	Iron metabolism, enzyme component. **Deficiencies:** Very rare, anaemia	0.9–1.5 mg
Molybdenum	Dairy products, eggs, liver, beans, sunflower seeds, some vegetables	Enzyme function, DNA/RNA synthesis. **Deficiencies:** Very rare, disorder in excretion of nitrogen-containing compounds	0.045 mg
Chromium	Beans, liver, yeast, meat, whole grains, seafood, some vegetables, wine	Insulin function and glucose metabolism. **Deficiencies:** Very rare, impaired glucose metabolism, diabetes mellitus	0.035 mg
Fluorine	Fluoridated tap water, seafood, tea	Skeletal and teeth strength and structure. **Deficiencies:** Very rare, higher frequency of tooth decay	3–4 mg
Iodine	Sea food, dairy products	Promotes thyroid function, linked with metabolism. **Deficiencies:** Goitre	0.15 mg
Silicon	Whole grains, whole grain rice	May help lower **Al** levels and assist with calcium function. **Deficiencies:** Problems with bone growth	No RDA

Table 2.10 (*continued*)

Mineral	Food sources	Function within the body	EU RDA
Boron	Dried fruits, vegetables, fruits, nuts	Assists calcium in bone structure. **Deficiencies:** Excess calcium loss	No RDA
Cobalt	Animal food sources, dairy products, eggs, enriched breakfast cereals	An element within vitamin B_{12}, RBC production	No RDA
Aluminium	Processed foods, medicines	Not required for health, may be detrimental to bone growth/brain	No RDA
Tin	Tinning for foods, low levels in foods	Not known in new born children, may be toxic	No RDA
Vanadium	Widely distributed in foods	Not known	No RDA

Note: Major minerals shaded in blue, minor minerals are shaded in green and the lesser known minerals in orange. Mineral abundancy decreases from top to bottom.

movement of water between the cells in the body and their outside environment) and, combined with bicarbonate (also referred to as hydrogen carbonate), is involved in helping to lower levels of acidity in cells (buffering), a function to which phosphorus also contributes. To facilitate nerve impulse conduction and muscle contraction, the body takes advantage of the potential for sodium chloride and potassium chloride to dissociate in water to their ionic forms. Within the body's aqueous internal environment, these three ions serve as electrolytes and enable an electrical potential to be created which is essential to the conduction of a nerve impulse or muscle contraction.

As well as having roles in buffering and bone structure, phosphorus has a major role in metabolism (all the reactions that take place within the body). When combined with hydrogen and/or oxygen it forms a phosphate ion, a key component of the high-energy fuel **adenosine triphosphate** (ATP). ATP is the petrol for our bodies, providing the fuel for most of the reactions that take place. Just as crude oil is refined to produce petrol, carbohydrates, fats and proteins are broken down through digestion and metabolism to form ATP.

Iron, one of the best understood minor minerals, plays a vital role in the formation of haemoglobin and myoglobin (a related substance to haemoglobin found within the muscles) which facilitate oxygen transport within the blood and muscle tissue respectively. In addition, iron is involved in the chemical structure of a number of enzymes and tissues within the body. Females generally, and female athletes in particular, need to ensure that their diet includes sufficient iron content. Where an individual's diet is iron-deficient this can result in the development of anaemia. Iron-deficiency-induced anaemia results in a decrease in the haemoglobin content of blood which reduces the body's oxygen-carrying capacity and leads to lack of energy, headaches and loss of appetite.

2.5 Water

Water is not one of the macronutrients or micronutrients, yet it is vital to life. Water is second only to oxygen in its importance to the human body. As such, water balance is a vital aspect when considering nutrition for health and sports performance. Water is a major body component, representing around 60% of total body mass depending upon age, gender and body composition. It is not by accident that around two-thirds of the human body is comprised of water. Not only does it provide the internal environment necessary for metabolism, but water also has a number of special properties that make it a unique substance vital to sustaining life. Water has a high solubility factor, meaning that many organic and inorganic molecules will dissolve in water. This means that water can host and enable the great number of chemical reactions necessary to sustain life. For instance, sodium chloride in aqueous solution (water) will dissociate to its component sodium and chloride ions. Water is able to disrupt the ionic bonds of substances such as sodium chloride because of its polar nature. The oxygen atom in water has a strong attraction for the electrons in the O-H bonds which leave a slight positive charge on the hydrogen atoms. This enables the hydrogen atoms to attract electrons from other atoms. It is through the attraction to neighbouring atoms that water can disrupt the bonds of inorganic compounds like sodium chloride and cause them to dissociate into their component ions. As described in the section on chemical reactions, not only can water play host to chemical reactions, it also participates in dehydration and hydrolysis reactions.

Water balance is regulated by the amount of water consumed each day and the water lost through evaporation and excretion. We obtain most of the water we consume, about 60%, through drinking, a further 30% from our food and the remaining 10% is produced via metabolic pathways such as the water liberated when two amino acids join (see Figure 2.17). Regular exercise and sports participation creates greater loss of water through evaporation than for sedentary individuals. This is likely to be due to an increase in the sweat output per gland. Those taking part in physically active sports must therefore ensure they replenish the additional water loss to maintain their water balance.

Water plays a number of key roles within the body, each of which serves to sustain life. Water is a significant component of synovial fluid (the fluid that fills synovial joint cavities, such as the shoulder) and its ability to serve as a lubricant is essential to smooth and low-friction movement. It is a major component of blood plasma and as such is the solution in which red blood cells and the other components of blood are carried. Water loss through evaporation plays a major role in cooling the body during exercise and in hot environments. It is vital that the body maintains its core temperature within a narrow band to maintain optimal functioning and ultimately life itself. During exercise, core temperature gradually rises due to the metabolic production of heat, stimulating the secretion of sweat onto the skin surface. It is the evaporation of the sweat, and loss of body water, that results in the release of heat energy from the body, ultimately blunting the increase in, maintaining or lowering the core temperature (dependent on factors such as exercise intensity and environmental conditions). Water is also vitally important in maintaining the concentration of ions and nutrients on the inside and outside of a cell. The fluid inside a cell is the **intracellular fluid,** that outside the cell is the **extracellular fluid.** The extracellular fluid is made up of **interstitial fluid,** that which bathes and surrounds cells, and **plasma,** the fluid component of blood. Our body fluid is made up largely of water, with about two-thirds of the water being contained within cells and the rest, interstitial fluid and blood plasma, surrounding the cells.

Key point

Intracellular fluid refers to the fluid within a cell.

Extracellular fluid, the fluid outside the cell, is composed of interstitial fluid and plasma:

➤ *interstitial fluid* is the fluid that surrounds the cell.

➤ *plasma* comprises the fluid component of blood.

In terms of performance during regular and prolonged exercise a key concern for athletes is water loss and a consequence of this is **dehydration.** Dehydration has a negative effect on performance and as a consequence a status of **euhydration** (normal hydration) should be maintained prior to, during and after exercise. Euhydration involves maintaining a balance between water intake and water loss. Research has indicated that a loss of only 2% in body weight through sweating during exercise will have a negative impact on performance. Loss of fluid from the body results in a decrease in the blood plasma volume which decreases the volume of blood reaching the working muscles. As a consequence, heart rate has to increase to meet demand (a phenomenon known as **cardiac drift**), placing a greater strain on the cardiovascular system. An additional consequence of the decrease in plasma volume is that less blood reaches the skin for cooling purposes, so the body does not lose heat as effectively, and core temperature rises to greater levels.

Knowledge integration question

A middle-distance athlete wants to know why they should rehydrate during training. Explain the physiological benefits of drinking during training and advise whether the fluid should be in the form of water or a sports drink.

Weight loss during exercise, and when in hot environments, is a simple method to monitor fluid loss. Fluid lost must be replaced to maintain performance, and this must be initiated rapidly, not waiting for the sensation of thirst. The thirst mechanism is sluggish and responds after dehydration and its negative effects on performance have occurred. As a consequence, in normal conditions, fluid should be replaced by athletes during exercise to minimise water loss through sweating and its detrimental effect on the body. The thirst mechanism is triggered by the build-up of sodium and chloride ions in the kidneys in response to the hormone aldosterone which is released due to the effects of dehydration. Dehydration also results in an increase in the concentration of both sodium and chloride ions in the blood. This increase is detected by special sensory receptors called **chemoreceptors** which send a message to the brain and trigger the thirst response.

 Try **Interactive Physiology:**
Fluids, electrolytes and acid-base balance: Water homeostasis

2.6 Digestion

Once food enters our mouths and we start to chew, the process of **digestion**, the breakdown of our macronutrients and micronutrients, begins. Digestion represents the initial processing of our food. Once absorbed into our bodies from the digestive tract, the extracted nutrients are either further broken down for immediate use for energy production or structural purposes, or they are synthesised into storage forms (glucose to glycogen, fatty acids to triglycerides). This section describes the structure of the digestive system and the processes that take place to break down the food we eat.

The digestive system and accessory digestive organs

The digestive system is comprised of the gastro-intestinal (GI) tract, also referred to as the alimentary canal, and a number of digestive organs that assist the GI tract with the digestive process. The GI tract consists of a canal or tube which extends from the mouth to the anus and is up to five to six metres in length. From the mouth the GI tract continues to the oesophagus, stomach, small intestine (duodenum, jejunum, ileum), large intestine (colon), rectum and finally ends at the anus, from which waste products are expelled. The organs that assist in the digestive process are the liver, gall-bladder and pancreas. The structures within the digestive system can be seen in Figure 2.21.

The digestive process involves five actions that help to bring about the breakdown of food for absorption to the bloodstream and the expulsion of waste products. These actions are: *peristalsis, secretion, digestion, absorption,* and *excretion.* **Peristalsis**, the movement of food by muscular contraction of the smooth muscle within the GI tract, results in the propulsion of the food along the GI tract and the mixing of the food to enable maximal contact with

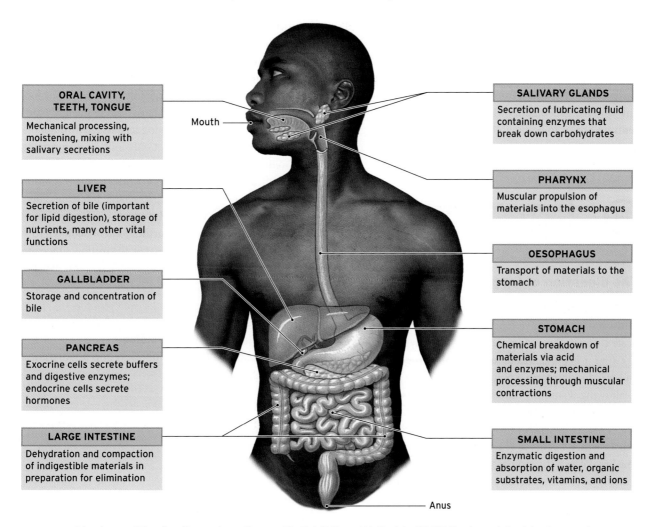

Figure 2.21 Structures of the digestive system. (*Source*: Martini, F. H. and Nath, J. L. (2009) *Fundamentals of Anatomy and Physiology*, 8th edition, New York: Benjamin Cummings)

digestive juices and walls of the tract for absorption. As food is moved through the digestive tract, starting with saliva in the mouth, juices are *secreted* into the canal to enable *digestion* – the breakdown of macronutrients and micronutrients. Once food has been broken down into its component parts it is made available for *absorption* into the blood and lymph via the walls of the digestive tract. Indigestible foods, such as fibre and other waste products, are then *excreted* from the anus.

The organs that assist with digestion, the pancreas, liver and gall-bladder, produce digestive juices which are utilised within the duodenum. The pancreas has two main functions, one exocrine – the production of pancreatic juice to assist with digestion, and the other endocrine – the production of the hormones insulin, glucagon and somatostatin which are transported via the blood for use elsewhere in the body. Pancreatic juice neutralises the acids of digestion in the stomach and further digests carbohydrate, fat and protein ready for absorption. The liver produces bile, a yellowy-brown or dark green liquid, which is involved in the facilitation of lipid breakdown by helping to emulsify the fats in food, that is, the production of small lipid droplets (micelles) ready for absorption to the blood. The ducts from the liver that carry bile also link with the gall-bladder where bile is stored and concentrated prior to being used in the duodenum. The gall-bladder, a 7–10 cm pear-shaped chamber, is situated just below the liver.

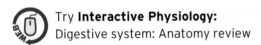 Try **Interactive Physiology:**
Digestive system: Anatomy review

The digestion of food

The initial digestion of food begins in the mouth where saliva starts to dissolve food and breakdown carbohydrate through the action of the enzyme amylase. The chewing process serves to mechanically process, moisten and mix food to form a bolus (lump of food) prior to swallowing. From the mouth each food bolus passes via the oesophagus to the stomach by peristalsis. The stomach contains hydrochloric acid, which kills bacteria, and pepsin which begins the breakdown of protein. During this breakdown the stomach will absorb some nutrients, water ions and fatty acids. Food within the stomach is dissolved and along with the digestive enzymes forms a soupy substance called **chyme**. The chyme passes from the stomach to the small intestine where most of the

digestion and absorption of food takes place. To allow time for these processes the small intestine is up to three metres in length, which increases the absorptive area and the transit time for digestion. Within the small intestine, carbohydrate in the form of the disaccharides sucrose, lactose and maltose are broken down to monosaccharides by the enzymes, sucrase, lactase and maltase, respectively, ready for absorption. Fat molecules are broken down to smaller units by the action of bile salts (contained within bile) and subsequently acted upon by pancreatic lipase to produce fatty acids and monoglycerides for absorption. Protein which began initial breakdown in the stomach is broken down to peptides in the small intestine by trypsin and similar enzymes. Once in the form of peptides the enzymes aminopeptidase and dipeptidase break protein down to its component amino acids for absorption.

The majority of the absorptive process takes place within the small intestine, with the macronutrients absorbed during the transit of chyme through the small intestine. In addition, 90% of water absorption, along with the major part of micronutrient uptake, takes place within the small intestine, leaving very few nutrient components in the chyme as it enters the large intestine. When the food enters the large intestine it will have been in the body for between 3–10 hours and following its passage through the small intestine will have lost not only most of its nutrients, but also most of its water and as such is known as the solid substances faeces by this time. Very little further digestion and absorption take place within the large intestine. The exceptions are some continued absorption of water (about 10% of total absorption) and further food breakdown to release some additional vitamins for absorption. Once this process is complete the remaining faecal matter is expelled from the body.

 Try **Interactive Physiology:**
Digestive system: Digestion and absorption

Key point

Nutrient digestion largely takes place in the mouth, stomach and small intestine.

Nutrient absorption mainly takes place from the small intestine.

Fibre assists the passage of food through the large intestine.

2.7 Components of a healthy balanced diet

A healthy diet is the basis for sound nutrition and the need for supplements and dietary manipulation is seldom necessary if a sports performer has a well-balanced diet. A healthy balanced diet should include the macronutrients (including fibre as part of carbohydrate intake), micronutrients and water as previously described within this chapter. The RDA for micronutrients – vitamins and minerals – are provided in Tables 2.9 and 2.10 respectively. For a sedentary person the Department of Health guidelines for the UK recommend an average intake of 1,940 kcal (nearly 2,000 kcal) for females and 2,500 kcal for males per day. For people involved in sports this amount would obviously need to be increased to account for energy expended during training and performance. Elite performers, particularly those participating in endurance events, may conduct high-volume training sessions as often as six days per week and hence their calorie intake requirements could be 2–3 times greater than the guidelines. In contrast, the energy requirement for adolescents tends to increase with age, and during peak growth may exceed that recommended for adults. Dietary recommendations for adolescents must allow for growth and development to progress at the same time as normal metabolism for sustaining life. Table 2.11 presents the recommended energy intake (kcal) for adolescents in the US, the UK, and Australia and New Zealand.

Knowledge integration question

Explain why the phrase 'you are what you eat' makes perfect chemical sense.

Calorie intake to maintain a balance between input and expenditure is highly individual and is dependent on factors such as age, gender, body size and composition, frequency, intensity and duration of training, and individual metabolic differences. Calorie intake should be matched to energy requirements to maintain a healthy body composition. Maintaining fluid balance, as well as nutritional balance, is vital for health and sports performance. For general health, water should ideally be consumed in small quantities at regular intervals throughout the day, such as continuous sipping from a water bottle. Similarly, during sporting activities, it is recommended that fluid should be drunk regularly (every 15–20 minutes) in small volumes (around 200 ml). This is feasible in some activities, such as cycling and running; however, other sports are limited to drinking during breaks in play (e.g. soccer, rugby, netball, field hockey). Water is generally the best form of fluid to maintain euhydration during the day. Sports drinks, containing carbohydrates and electrolytes, may be beneficial during and post exercise as not only do they provide a rapid energy supply, but the presence of electrolytes and glucose increases the speed at which fluid enters the blood. Fluid replacement, however, can be achieved almost as quickly by drinking plain water, and at a fraction of the cost.

In terms of calorie intake from the macronutrients that make up the bulk of our diet, it is recommended that we consume 55–60% of our calories from carbohydrates, up to 30% from fats (but ideally less than this, with under 10% through saturated and trans fats) and 10–15% from proteins. The above recommendation for fat consumption is lower than some governmental recommendations (35% of total energy intake), as research suggests that maintaining a total fat intake below 30% (and below 10% for saturated fats) is more beneficial to health.

Table 2.11 Recommended daily energy intakes (kcal) for adolescents in the US, the UK, and Australia and New Zealand.

	Males			Females		
Age (years)	11-14	15-18		11-14	15-18	
US	2510	2988		2199	2199	
Age (years)	11-14	15-18		11-14	15-18	
UK	2216	2751		1893	2110	
Age (years)	8-11	12-15	16-18	8-11	12-15	16-18
Aus/NZ	2079-2175	2199-2820	2796-3227	1840-1960	1936-2342	2103-2390

Note: US data, National Research Council 1989; UK data, Department of Health 1991; Australia/New Zealand data, Truswell et al. 1990. Converted to kcal from MJ. http://www.moh.govt.nz/moh.nsf/0/0697F789B648D3304C25666F0039933A/$File/foodnutritionguidelines-adolescents.pdf

Key point

A healthy diet should include:

➤ 55–60% carbohydrate (including fibre)

➤ ≤ 30% fat

➤ 10–15% protein

➤ vitamins

➤ minerals

➤ water

Recommended caloric intake:

➤ sedentary: 2,000 kcal for females and 2,500 kcal for males

➤ total caloric intake for a sports person is dependent upon:

  • age

  • volume and intensity of training

➤ for sports people, caloric intake could be more than double that of a sedentary person

An alternative way of viewing the macronutrient recommendations is provided in Figure 2.22. The food pyramid provides a guide to the distribution of food groups that should form the basis of a healthy diet. Consuming foods from these groups can, in a natural way without the need for supplements, provide all the nutrients necessary for a healthy athletic life.

The recommended daily servings for each of the food groups within the pyramid are shown in Figure 2.22. For the bread etc. group an example of a serving size for bread would be one slice, or a half-cup (cooked) of pasta or rice. For the fruit and vegetable groups, examples of a serving would be an apple, a small banana, a medium tomato, or a small stalk of broccoli. For the meat etc. group, example serving sizes would be one egg, 1/3 of a can (small) of tuna or 3 oz (75 grams) chicken breast (about the size of a pack of cards).

In Britain people are encouraged to eat five portions of fruit and vegetables a day. Similarly, the New Zealand Ministry of Health (2003) recommends that adults eat at least three servings of vegetables and two servings of fruit per day. The Center for Disease Control (CDC) in the US has updated its recommendations for the consumption of fruits and vegetables from the '5-A-Day' programme to the 'Fruits and Veggies – More Matters' campaign, re-emphasising the importance of fruit and vegetables in the diet. The food pyramid includes both fruit and vegetables as selecting both in your diet helps to achieve a greater variety. It is better to eat a mixture of fruits and vegetables rather than eating five apples a day. Including fibre in your diet will aid digestion and can be found in vegetables, fruits, whole wheat grains, some cereals, beans and peas.

With regard to carbohydrate it is beneficial to consume a mixture of forms at different times of the day. During training, and immediately after, it is perhaps most useful to consume carbohydrate in the form of simple sugars.

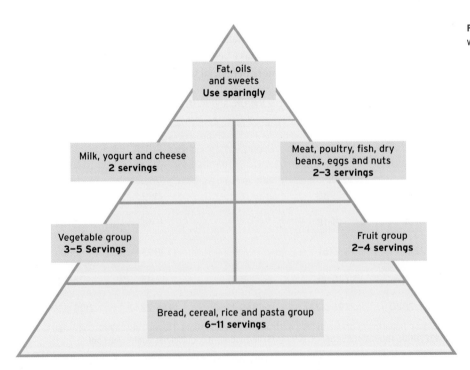

Figure 2.22 Food guide pyramid with suggested daily servings.

Fat, oils and sweets
Use sparingly

Milk, yogurt and cheese
2 servings

Meat, poultry, fish, dry beans, eggs and nuts
2–3 servings

Vegetable group
3–5 Servings

Fruit group
2–4 servings

Bread, cereal, rice and pasta group
6–11 servings

Simple sugars provide a rapid source of energy which can be utilised during training or, following training, they can replenish blood glucose levels. Complex carbohydrates should form the basis for recovery meals, main meals during each day, and as part of the food during longer activities such as triathlon (greater than sprint distance), multisport racing or simply when out for a day walking or tramping or hiking. In addition, it is beneficial to pay attention to the glycaemic index of the foods to include lower as well as higher glycaemic index carbohydrates. Lower glycaemic index foods will last longer as a fuel source for training or performance.

Protein requirements are generally not as high as athletes often presume, with a balanced diet generally supplying the body's requirements. Normally there would be no need for expensive (or inexpensive) protein supplements. For sedentary people, the protein requirement per day is about 0.8 g per kg of body mass, such that a 70 kg person would require 56 (0.8 g × 70 kg) grams of protein a day. A 227 g (8 oz) tin of tuna fish or 200 g (7 oz) chicken breast, for example, contains 67 g and 61 g of protein respectively. One of these servings would more than satisfy the daily protein requirement. For those involved in power sports the requirement might rise to 1.0–2.0 g per kg of body mass, dependent upon the type of activity and the athlete. However, these requirements can still be easily supplied by dietary means.

It is essential to maintain some fat within your food to maintain a healthy diet. Fat is a necessary component of our diets. When choosing foods it is beneficial, however, to examine the types of fats they contain. Where possible choose foods with a high proportion of the fat in the form of monounsaturated and polyunsaturated fats. Look at food labels, and where possible, try to avoid hydrogenated (trans) fats which are very common in processed, super-market-prepared foods. It is also useful to check the fat content or percentage relative to carbohydrate and protein. The percentage of fat though, is presented in a number of different ways, such as by the weight of the food. It is the percentage of total calories that are supplied by fat that is important, not simply the percentage of total fat within the food. A simple way to check the total calorific value of the fat content is to use the total calorific value of the food and the grams of fats. Remembering that one gram of an average fat contains 9 kcal it is possible to calculate the percentage of calories from fat and importantly saturated fat.

In addition to the basic diet there are some useful considerations you can make to improve upon these basic guidelines. Variety, moderation and naturalness will add to a healthy diet. There is no one food that can provide all the nutrients we need, having *variety* with meals helps us to gain all the nutrients we need. There is nothing wrong with having occasional treats as these add variety to the diet and increase enjoyment of your food. The secret to this is *moderation* and cutting back in other areas. The more *natural* your food is, that is, the less it has been processed by manufacturers before you consume it, the better. Processed food tends to have fewer nutrients than natural foods. Choosing wholemeal bread over white bread, whole grain rice over quick cook rice, along with cooking foods yourself rather than buying processed meals can make a difference. The choice of

CALCULATION

Calculation of fat percentage in a breakfast cereal

One healthy breakfast cereal on the market contains 12 g fat and 4.5 g saturated fat per 100 g. The energy value listed is 1690 kJ or 404 kcal per 100 g.

The energy provided by fat is 12 g × 9 kcal		= 108 kcal
The energy provided by saturated fat is 4.5 g × 9 kcal		= 40.5 kcal
The percentage of total fat is	108/404 × 100	= **26.7%**
The percentage of saturated fat is	40.5/404 × 100	= **10%**

This breakfast cereal satisfies the recommended daily fat intake percentages (less than 30% total fat and less than 10% saturated fat).

CALCULATION

Simplified calculation of fat percentage in a breakfast cereal

To simplify the above calculation make an allowance of **3 g of fat per 100 kcal** of total energy in any food (3 g = 9 kcal × 3 = 27 kcal of energy from fat (27/100 kcal from fat), i.e. less than 30% from fat).

The rule of thumb *allowance* = **3 g fat per 100 kcal** to stay below 30% fat.

In the breakfast cereal example:

404 kcal = approximately 400 kcal per 100 g of which 12 g = fat

12 g fat per 400 kcal total energy means = **3 g (12/4) in 100 kcal is fat** (about 27% from fat).

---

whole grains and home food preparation add to and help to retain the nutrients in the food you consume. It is interesting when looking at Tables 2.9 and 2.10, to see how many useful dietary micronutrients are to be found in whole grains.

Chapters 8 to 12 include further information about specific dietary adaptations that can be made for specific types of intensity and duration sports. For example there are a number of dietary manipulations that can be made for power or endurance athletes.

Key point

A balanced diet becomes a healthy balanced diet when we pay attention to:

➤ consuming a *variety* of foods

➤ maintaining as far as possible the *naturalness* of our food

➤ *moderating* our intake of certain food groups

What we eat does count for maintaining and improving health and performance.

Check your recall
Fill in the missing words.

➤ Human beings use food for two distinct purposes: to provide _____ and as building blocks for the maintenance of the body's structure.

➤ There are six food groups consisting of:

• Carbohydrates

• _____

• Fats

• Vitamins

• _____

• Water

➤ _____ elements make up the human body.

➤ Carbohydrates and fats are made of carbon, hydrogen and oxygen. Proteins contain _____ in addition to these three elements.

➤ Carbon, hydrogen, oxygen and nitrogen make up _____ % of our bodies.

➤ The number of protons in an element can be found from its atomic _____.

➤ Elements can bond by accepting or donating electrons (ionic bonding) or by sharing electrons (_____ bonding).

➤ Anabolic reactions synthesise new molecules, whereas _____ reactions result in the decomposition of a molecule.

➤ Enzymes catalyse reactions but remain _____ after the process.

➤ The three forms of carbohydrate are monosaccharides, _____ and polysaccharides.

➤ Two examples of a polysaccharide are _____ and _____.

➤ The glycaemic index for white bread is _____.

➤ Fats are primarily stored in the adipocytes as _____.

➤ A healthy percentage intake of fat with a normal diet should be around _____ of which ≤ 10% should be in the form of saturated fats.

➤ Protein in our diet is broken down in to one of 20 _____ of which _____ are essential and _____ are non-essential, as they can be synthesised within the body.

➤ The chemical structure of glucose is $C_6H_{12}O_6$, while the structure of palmitic acid a typical fat is _____ and that for haemoglobin, a relatively small protein is _____.

➤ Vitamins are known as the organic micronutrients because they contain _____.

➤ Around _____ of our total body mass is comprised of water.

➤ We obtain water from three sources, through drinking, our food and from _____.

➤ Normal hydration is known as _____ .

➤ The sensory mechanisms through which we detect dehydration are called _____.

➤ The five actions within the process of digestion are peristalsis, secretion, digestion, _____ and excretion.

➤ The recommended caloric intake for males is _____ kcal and for females is _____ kcal. Athletes in full-time training can often require two or three times these amounts.

➤ In normal circumstances the maximum required amount of protein for a power athlete would be around _____ g per kg.

➤ In addition to a balanced diet, adding variety, _____ and moderation to your food intake can be beneficial to short-term and long-term health.

Review questions

1. What are the three macronutrients that humans require and what is the basic role of each of these?

2. What elements make up the chemical composition of the macronutrients? How does this relate to the composition of the human body?

3. Explain the difference between an exergonic chemical reaction and an endergonic chemical reaction. Why is it important that both occur within the human body?

4. Give the scientific definition of the calorie. What is a kilocalorie and why is food normally labelled in kilocalories (kcal or Calorie)?

5. What is the glycaemic index and why is it important in food choices for sports performers? What would be a good choice of carbohydrates for a mountain biker in a 24-hour endurance race?

6. What chemical differences are there between saturated fats, monounsaturated fats and polyunsaturated fats? What is the advice for long-term health in relation to these?

7. How does a protein molecule like haemoglobin differ from a carbohydrate molecule like glucose? What do the terms anabolise and catabolise mean in relation to protein structures within the body?

8. What are the two kinds of micronutrient? How is their function in the body different from the macronutrients?

9. Why can dehydration impact on cardiovascular performance during endurance events? What are the three ways our body gets the water it requires to function effectively?

10. What are the average daily calorific needs of a sedentary individual? How might these be different for an endurance-based sports performer involved in marathon running or cycle road racing?

Teach it!

In groups of three, choose one topic and teach it to the rest of the study group.

1. Explain, using diagrams, the structural differences between saturated, unsaturated and monosaturated fats and how/why unsaturated fats can be converted into transfats.

2. Outline how and why chemical bonding occurs between atoms

3. Explain how we work out the caloric content of a food item. Use a food label from home as the basis for explaining the ingredients and how they contribute to total caloric intake.

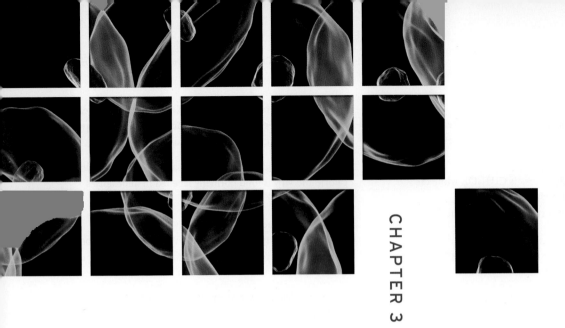

CHAPTER 3

From cells to systems

Learning objectives

After reading, considering and discussing with a study partner the material in this chapter you should be able to:

➤ identify the levels of structural organisation within the body

➤ list the organ systems within the body

➤ describe the structure and functioning of cells

➤ explain the roles of the organelles within a typical cell

➤ outline the concept of homeostasis

➤ discuss homeostatic control and its importance to physiological functioning

➤ speculate about the role of insulin and glucagon in control of blood glucose levels

➤ list the four main types of tissue types found within the body

➤ describe the structure and function of epithelial and connective tissue

When broken down to its most basic components, the human body is comprised of the 26 elements listed in Chapter 2, Table 2.1. The magic spark that is *life* is seen for the first time when these elements are bonded within the body to form *cells*. Cells represent the basic unit of living matter, the first point at which any organism can be *alive*. All living organisms are comprised of cells and cellular

products. Just as for the elements that comprise the human body, cells are primarily composed of carbon, hydrogen, oxygen and nitrogen. All cells come from pre-existing cells through the process of *cell division*, consequently all life originates from the same original cells and therefore share certain common characteristics. The genetic blueprint that differentiates cells is found within the deoxyribonucleic acid (DNA) which is responsible for the structure and functioning of every living cell.

Key point

Cells represent the basic unit for living matter.

New cells are formed from pre-existing cells through cell division.

DNA provides the blueprint for the structure and functioning of each cell.

Just as elements form the building blocks for cells, so cells form the building blocks for the human body and all the structures it contains. Cells work in cooperative groups to maintain life, forming the basis for the *tissues* and *organs* which in turn comprise the *organ systems* that enable the body to function. The levels of organisation within the body, from the chemical to the whole body, or organism level, are illustrated in Figure 3.1. Tissues, such as the

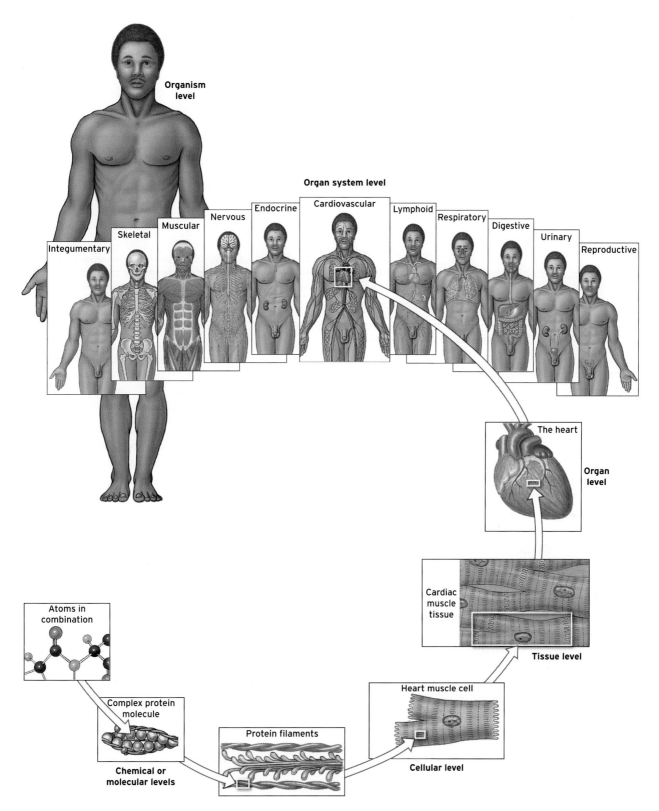

Figure 3.1 Levels of structural organisation. (*Source*: Martini, F. H. and Nath, J. L. (2009) *Fundamentals of Anatomy and Physiology*, 8th edition, New York: Benjamin Cummings)

cardiac muscle illustrated in Figure 3.1, are comprised of specialised cells and their products that perform a specific function within an organ and within the body. This can be demonstrated by the heart which represents a structure composed of cardiac muscle tissue along with connective and epithelial tissues (Figure 3.1).

Knowledge integration question

Think of an example to describe how organ systems can work together during exercise to maintain performance.

There are 11 organ systems commonly described within the body and these, along with their functions, are shown in Table 3.1. The primary role of cells and the organ systems they comprise is to maintain **homeostasis**. The following sections of this chapter describe the structure and function of cells and the importance of homeostasis to human functioning. Within this textbook seven of the eleven organ systems in Table 3.1 are covered in detail due to their importance for sport performance. The digestive system, because of its role in catabolising the food we eat, was covered in Chapter 2, followed by presentation of the control systems (nervous and endocrine) in Chapter 4. Then in Chapter 5, where the focus is upon the fundamental systems for human movement, the structure and functioning of the skeletal and muscular systems is covered. The final two organ systems covered in this book, the cardiovascular and respiratory systems, which play roles in transport and exchange, are covered in Chapter 6. Students and readers interested in finding out more about the integumentary, lymphatic, reproductive and urinary systems could consult a textbook such as Martini and Ober (2011) which covers these systems thoroughly and very clearly. These systems are not covered in our textbook because the primary focus is on the key physiological systems that impact upon sports performance. To better understand the nature of sports performance it is essential to have knowledge of the key systems that enable movement and ultimately exercise and sport. Human performance in any sport, however, is reliant on the cells within the body and so the first main focus of this chapter is upon the structure and function of cells – the building blocks for the body and its energy systems.

Key point

Cells provide the building blocks for tissues and organs.

Tissues and organs make up the 11 organ systems within the body.

Table 3.1 The eleven organ systems that comprise the human body.

System	Function within the body
Digestive system	Responsible for the breakdown and absorption of macronutrients, micronutrients and water into the body, along with the excretion of waste products.
Skeletal system	Supports and protects body parts and along with the muscular system is responsible for bringing about movement. Site of red blood cell production and storage of minerals and lipids.
Nervous system	Divided into the central nervous system and the peripheral nervous system it is responsible for receiving, processing and effecting a response to sensory input. Along with the endocrine system it is responsible for control and regulation within the body.
Endocrine system	The longer term control system. Responsible for the production of hormones that regulate the control of function throughout the body.
Muscular system	Along with the skeletal system is responsible for bringing about human movement, as well as producing heat through the reactions that bring about movement.
Respiratory system	Responsible for exchange of O_2 and CO_2 with the outside environment.
Cardiovascular system	Includes the heart, blood vessels and blood and is responsible for transport of nutrients and waste products including O_2 and CO_2, hormones and ions. Also involved in temperature regulation and defence against infection.
Integumentary system	Comprises the skin, hair and nails and provides a barrier between the body and the outside environment as well as being involved in temperature regulation.
Lymphatic system	Includes the lymph and white blood cells and is involved in defence against disease. Lymph controls the level of interstitial fluid within the body and it absorbs and transports fatty acids and fats from the blood.
Reproductive system	The reproductive systems are different for males and females and are chiefly responsible for perpetuation of the species and determining individual sex characteristics, but also have an endocrine function.
Urinary system	Responsible for the excretion of waste products and maintaining fluid balance within the body.

3.1 The cellular basis for life

The foundation of all living things is the cell – the smallest unit capable of carrying out all the processes associated with life. Each human being starts from one cell and, through the process of cell division, is able to grow to adult size. Nevertheless, cells are tiny, with five or more typical cells fitting into the dot above the letter 'i' printed here. Due to their size, a light or electron microscope is needed to study cells and reveal the structure of these tiny building blocks. Through a light microscope it is possible to see structures such as mitochondria; however, an electron microscope would be required to view much smaller organelles such as ribosomes. These organelles are illustrated in Figure 3.2.

Humans are made up of around 200 different types of cell that work in coordinated groups to accomplish functions within the body. The organ systems such as the skeletal, muscular, respiratory and nervous systems are comprised of cells working in cooperative units. All cells have specialised functions that contribute to the overall functioning of the body and are dependent on other groups of cells carrying out their functions for survival of the organism. For example, muscle cells use energy to bring about movement, but are dependent on the cardiovascular system (heart, blood vessels and blood) for supplying oxygen and nutrients and for removing the waste products that result from energy production. Cells within the body have to work cooperatively in this integrated fashion to sustain life. Although serving different functions, the various cells

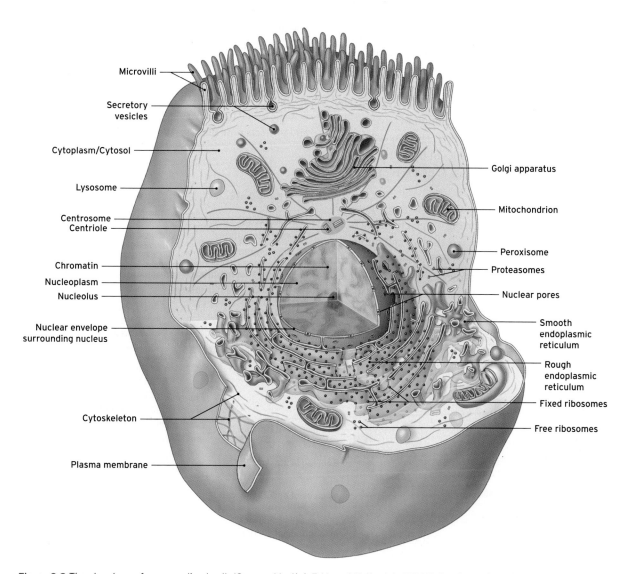

Figure 3.2 The structure of a generalised cell. (*Source*: Martini, F. H. and Nath, J. L. (2009) *Fundamentals of Anatomy and Physiology*, 8th edition, New York: Benjamin Cummings)

within our bodies have a common general structure as is shown in Figure 3.2. While cells share a number of these common structural components, the diversity of cell development can be seen through the example of red blood cells (erythrocytes).

Knowledge integration question

Explain why red blood cells are so good at carrying oxygen.

Erythrocytes, which are produced in the red bone marrow, have a normal life span of around 120 days before they are replaced by new cells. As new erythrocytes are produced within the bone marrow they initially contain the organelles common to the general cell pictured in Figure 3.2. During development, however, because of their specialist oxygen carrying role, they expel their nucleus and all other organelles from their structure. By doing this, they greatly increase their haemoglobin-carrying capacity and as a consequence, the relative amount of oxygen transportable within each erythrocyte. Human cells share many of the common characteristics of the cell illustrated in Figure 3.2, but develop uniquely to best serve their function within the body.

The structure of erythrocytes is illustrated in Figure 3.3 and are responsible for transporting oxygen to the cells of the body. To get in to perspective the size and number of cells which comprise the human body, there are 5,000,000,000 (five billion) erythrocytes in every millilitre of blood. An average human carries about five litres of blood which means each person has 25,000,000,000,000 (25 trillion) red blood cells within their body and this is just one type of cell. Erythrocytes make up approximately one quarter of the cells in the human body.

Key point

Erythrocytes are red blood cells.

Red blood cells carry oxygen to cells around the body.

Red blood cells are the most plentiful cell in the body.

Each adult has 25 trillion or more red blood cells.

Cellular components

Cells typically have three components: the *cell* or *plasma membrane*, the *nucleus* and the remaining contents of the cell known as the *cytoplasm* (see Figure 3.2). The plasma membrane is a very thin structure that encloses every cell and keeps it separate from its surrounding environment. The nucleus, normally the largest single unit in the cell, contains the DNA, the genetic blueprint for controlling the operations of the cell, and the ribonucleic acid (RNA), a single stranded version of DNA which, amongst other things, controls protein synthesis within the cell. The cytoplasm comprises the inside of the cell except for the nucleus. It is made up of a gel-like substance, *cytosol*, which houses and protects nine main sorts of small structures called

Key point

Cells are the smallest unit within the body capable of sustaining life.
They comprise:

a. a plasma membrane that separates it from the surrounding environment,

b. a nucleus that controls the cells functions.

c. the remaining contents of the cell which is known as the cytoplasm.

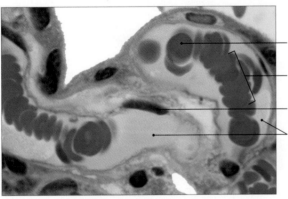

Sectional view of capillaries

Red blood cell (RBC)

Rouleau (a stack of RBCs)

Nucleus of endothelial cell

Blood vessels (viewed in longitudinal section)

Figure 3.3 Micrograph showing erythrocytes travelling through relatively narrow capillaries. (*Source*: Martini, F. H. and Nath, J. L. (2009) *Fundamentals of Anatomy and Physiology*, 8th edition, New York: Benjamin Cummings)

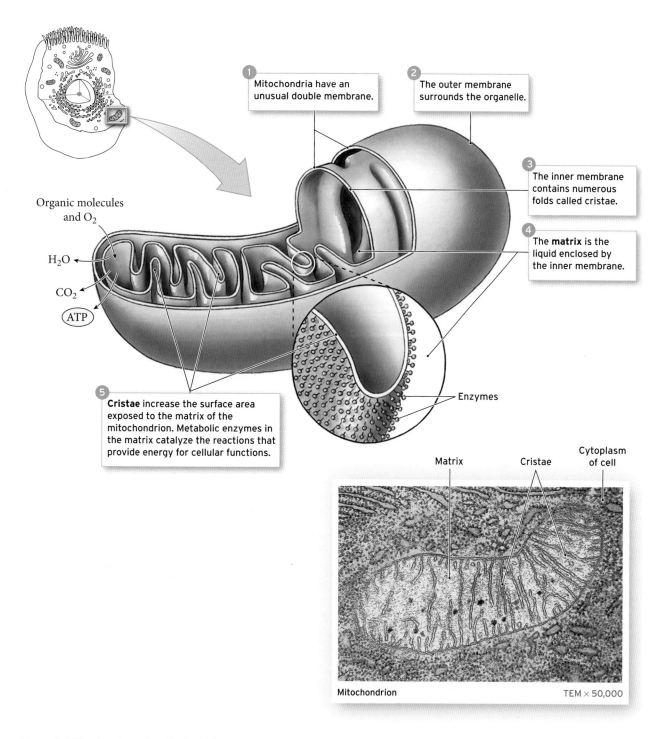

1 Mitochondria have an unusual double membrane.

2 The outer membrane surrounds the organelle.

3 The inner membrane contains numerous folds called cristae.

4 The **matrix** is the liquid enclosed by the inner membrane.

Organic molecules and O_2

H_2O

CO_2

ATP

5 **Cristae** increase the surface area exposed to the matrix of the mitochondrion. Metabolic enzymes in the matrix catalyze the reactions that provide energy for cellular functions.

Enzymes

Matrix

Cristae

Cytoplasm of cell

Mitochondrion

TEM × 50,000

Figure 3.4 The structure of a mitochondrion.

organelles. These organelles serve a variety of roles for the cell. An illustration of one such organelle, a *mitochondrion*, is provided in Figure 3.4. Mitochondria are the power plants of many cells and are responsible for producing about 90% of human energy.

Plasma membrane

The plasma membrane maintains a barrier between the cell's internal contents and the external environment, as shown in Figure 3.5. It is a *phospholipid bilayer* composed, as the

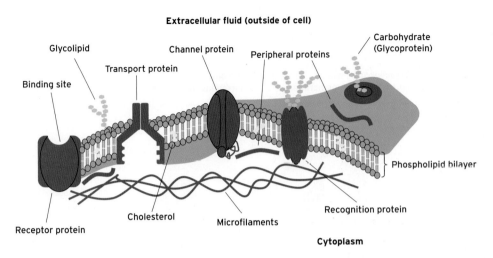

Extracellular fluid (outside of cell)

Glycolipid

Channel protein

Peripheral proteins

Carbohydrate
(Glycoprotein)

Transport protein

Binding site

Phospholipid bilayer

Receptor protein

Cholesterol

Microfilaments

Recognition protein

Cytoplasm

Figure 3.5 The structure of the cell membrane.

name suggests, of two layers of phospholipid molecules that are dually hydrophilic and hydrophobic in nature (as was described in Chapter 2). As a result of the forces of attraction between the heads of the phospholipid molecules in each layer, and between the tails of the adjacent layers, no covalent bonds are required to maintain the integrity of the plasma membrane. The avoidance of chemical bonding between molecules means that individual phospholipids are free to move in a fluid fashion on their side of the plasma membrane and this means the membrane is very flexible. Despite the movement possible within each layer, the forces of attraction between the hydrophobic and hydrophilic components of each phospholipid molecule mean it is not possible for molecules to move between the two layers (pass from the inside of the cell to the outside or vice versa).

Knowledge integration question

Explain the structure of the plasma membrane and what is special about it.

If each cell was a self-contained living organism, not requiring any substances to be moved into or out of the cell, the plasma membrane might only consist of the phospholipid bilayer. However, the need to move molecules, such as nutrients and waste products into and out of the cell, means the plasma membrane has to be more complex in structure. As can be seen in Figure 3.5, each cell's plasma membrane has a large number of *transmembrane proteins* and carbohydrate-based molecules that facilitate transport and communication between the inside and outside of each cell. In addition, peripheral proteins, cholesterol and glycolipids, along with microfilaments within the cell, help to maintain the complex

structure of the plasma membrane. Chemical analysis shows that the protein and lipid components of the plasma membrane are approximately equal amounts by weight.

There are four main types of transmembrane protein: recognition proteins, receptor proteins, channel proteins and transport proteins. *Recognition proteins* are glycoproteins, meaning that they have carbohydrate (glucose) and protein components. Their role is to set an identity for each cell type so that it can be recognised as normal by the immune system. *Receptor proteins* have a binding site, specific to a particular signal molecule, on the outside of the plasma membrane which, when receiving the appropriate signal, will trigger a change in the cell's functioning. An example of this that can be seen as movement at the whole-body level is muscle contraction which is triggered by specific chemicals binding to receptor proteins within *muscle fibre* (*muscle cell*) plasma membranes. This process will be covered in more detail in Chapter 5. *Channel proteins* enable specific ions to diffuse into the cell. Channel proteins are often gated (see Figure 3.5) to enable diffusion of a specific ion only when the gate is open. There are usually many channel proteins for potassium and chloride ions, but fewer for calcium and sodium ions. Whereas ions pass through channel proteins into the cell by diffusion (from higher to lower concentration), sometimes the same ions and larger molecules must be actively transported into the cell against the concentration gradient. This process is mediated by *transport proteins* which use adenosine triphosphate (ATP), the energy currency for all cells, to bring ions or molecules into the cytosol. An example of active transport, as carried out through the sodium-potassium pump, is depicted in Figure 3.6. The breakdown of ATP is necessary to provide the energy to enable the transport of sodium out of the

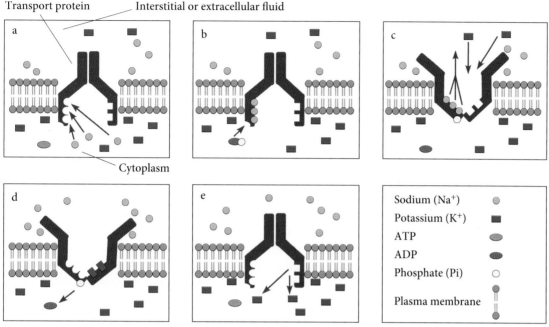

The sodium-potassium pump is an example of active transport across the plasma membrane. The sodium-potassium pump works continuously moving sodium ions (Na^+) to the outside of the cell and potassium ions (K^+) into the cell. (a) Three sodium ions bind with the transport protein, which triggers (b) the hydrolysis of ATP to ADP and releases a phosphate ion to bind the protein. (c) The binding of the phosphate ion (Pi) alters the shape of the protein, opening it to the extracellular fluid. This change in shape causes a release of the $3Na^+$ as the protein then favours binding with K^+. (d) Two K^+ attach to the protein which triggers the release of the Pi and (e) the protein returns to its original shape and releases the K^+ into the cytoplasm. The released phosphate is then free to bind with ADP within the cytoplasm to form another ATP molecule.

Figure 3.6 The sodium-potassium pump.

cell and potassium into the cell. By doing this it is possible for nerve and muscle cells to establish an electrical charge differential between the inside and outside of the cell. This electrical differential is know as an *action potential* and will be discussed further in the section on the nervous system (Chapter 4).

 Try **Interactive Physiology:**
Fluids and electrolytes: Electrolyte homeostasis

Key point

The cell or plasma membrane is a phospholipid bilayer that encloses the cell.

The bilayer is composed of phospholipids and cholesterol.

Trans-membrane proteins (TMP) transect the lipid bilayer.

TMP controlling the flow of ions and molecules into and out of the cell.

The carbohydrate components of the plasma membrane serve three main purposes: cell recognition, binding of cells to one another and lubrication of the cell surface. *Glycoproteins* are involved in cell–cell interactions as they serve as part of the identity structure of recognition proteins, for example, they are important in white blood cell and antibody recognition. *Glycolipids* extend into the extracellular environment where they also act as recognition sites for specific chemicals, in addition to helping cells to attach to one another to form tissues and to decrease friction on the outer surface of the plasma membrane. For cells such as erythrocytes, low friction levels are essential to assist their passage through the narrow constrictions within capillaries.

Nucleus

The nucleus, usually found at the core of each cell, is the control centre. It is encapsulated within a double-layered membrane that separates it from the rest of the cytoplasm but contains nuclear pores that enable substances to pass between the nucleus and the cytoplasm. Most cells have one nucleus, although as already mentioned red blood cells expel their nucleus during development to increase oxygen-carrying capacity and muscle cells and some bone cells are multinucleated. The nucleus represents the single largest component within the cell and contains DNA which enables the nucleus to govern the cell's functions.

Deoxyribonucleic acid contains the blueprint or genetic code for the cell and therefore controls replication of the cell and directs protein and enzyme synthesis. Deoxyribonucleic acid does not, however, leave the nucleus to control the cells function, therefore RNA, of which there are three types, is employed for this purpose. The genetic code for a particular protein is passed from DNA to messenger RNA (mRNA). Messenger RNA leaves the nucleus via the nuclear pores and enters the cytoplasm where it delivers the genetic transcript to ribosomal RNA (rRNA) where it is interpreted and translated into amino acid sequences for a particular protein synthesis. Transfer RNA (tRNA) is then used to move the necessary amino acids within the cytoplasm for the synthesis of the protein.

Knowledge integration question

Explain the role of deoxyribonucleic acid.

Cytoplasm

The cytoplasm, meaning cell-forming matter, comprises cytosol, a cytoskeleton and organelles which carry out a wide range of functions within the cell. *Cytosol* or *intracellular fluid* is a gel-like substance, largely composed of water that contains suspended and dissolved particles such as ATP, glucose, lipids, amino acids and a variety of different ions. Many metabolic reactions take place within the cytosol including glycolysis, one of the major pathways for synthesising ATP. The *cytoskeleton* is literally that, a cellular 'skeleton' within the cytoplasm which is made out of protein (see Figure 3.2). It includes three main types of protein filament that, among other roles, maintain cell structure and hold in place many of the cell's organelles. The *microtubules* are responsible for support and structure within the cell giving the cytoskeleton strength and rigidity. The *intermediate filaments* give the cell strength, help to maintain the structure and stabilise the position of the cells organelles, while *microfilaments* (which are illustrated in Figure 3.5) help to give the cell shape by anchoring the

cytoskeleton to the plasma membrane. The microfilaments (which are comprised of the protein actin) are also one of the filaments responsible for muscular contraction (see Chapter 5).

The organelles located within each cell serve a variety of purposes to assist with cell functioning, under direction from the nucleus. Situated near the nucleus, each cell has a *centrosome*, which contains two *centrioles* that play an important role in cell division during the creation of new cells. The central location of the centrosome is linked to its function within the cell. As the name indicates, it serves as a central hub for the cytoskeleton and many of the microtubules radiate out from the centrosome (see Figure 3.2). There are two types of *endoplasmic reticulum* which are associated with the synthesis, storage and transport of a variety of molecules required to maintain cell functioning. Endoplasmic reticulum is a system of membranes which are continuous with the nuclear membrane and extend throughout the cytoplasm. The *rough endoplasmic reticulum* is a membrane network of *cisternae* (sac-like structures) and is named as such because its outer membrane is littered with ribosomes. *Ribosomes* are responsible for protein synthesis and are linked with RNA which determines the composition of each protein. Ribosomes are found throughout the cytoplasm, but attach to the rough endoplasmic reticulum when they start to synthesise proteins intended for the secretory pathway. Within the rough endoplasmic reticulum ribosomal proteins are modified, some to form enzymes or other proteins, while others are combined with glucose to form glycoproteins. Most of these modified proteins are subsequently transported in *transport vesicles* (membrane-bound containers) to the *Golgi apparatus*. The *smooth endoplasmic reticulum* is a tube-like network continuous with the rough endoplasmic reticulum. The smooth endoplasmic reticulum can be differentiated from the rough endoplasmic reticulum by its shape and the fact that it does not have ribosomes attached. These differences are clearly illustrated in Figure 3.2. The key roles of the smooth endoplasmic reticulum relate to the synthesis and storage of a range of lipids and carbohydrates including phospholipids, cholesterol, steroid hormones, glycerides such as triglyceride, and glycogen.

The *Golgi apparatus,* a continuous series of flattened discs, is the packaging and shipping centre for a cell. Proteins formed in the rough endoplasmic reticulum are collected in the Golgi apparatus for further modification, sorting and packaging. Within the Golgi apparatus lipids and glucose are added to proteins to form lipoproteins and glycoproteins. These and other proteins are transferred to transport vesicles which are used to ship the contents to either the cell's plasma membrane or other organelles within the cell while keeping them separate from the rest of the cytoplasm during transport. A further function of the Golgi apparatus is the creation of lysosomes. *Lysosomes* are a form of vesicle responsible for carrying over fifty different enzymes involved in a range of processes. One of their primary functions is the destruction of bacteria and damaged organelles. This clean-up process is completed with the use of digestive enzymes contained within the vesicle that would otherwise be toxic to the cell. *Peroxisomes* are smaller than lysosomes, but play a similar role, transporting enzymes within the cell and catabolising unwanted molecules. In the case of peroxisomes, the enzymes they carry are linked with the breakdown of fatty acids and amino acids. *Mitochondria*, illustrated in Figure 3.4, play a vital role in energy production within the cell. Some cells have several hundred, while muscle fibres, which require large volumes of ATP for contraction, contain thousands of mitochondria.

Key point

The cytoplasm comprises all parts of the cell within the plasma membrane, with the exception of the nucleus.

The cytoplasm consists of cytosol, a water-based gel-like mass that surrounds the organelles (tiny cellular organs).

A cytoskeleton provides a structure to support a cell's organelles.

Organelles provide a wide range of functions to support the cell's activities.

3.2 Homeostasis

French physiologist Claude Bernard was one of the first to confirm the importance of maintaining a stable environment within the body. Later, based on his work and that of others working at the time, American physiologist Walter Canon coined the term *homeostasis* to describe the need to maintain a stable internal environment. Homeostasis is vital to all living organisms, from unicellular amoeba to the most complex multicellular animals including humans. Homeostasis comes from the Greek words 'homoios' meaning 'similar' and 'stasis' meaning 'standing', and refers to the need of an organism to provide constancy in its internal environment. For an amoeba, as a single cell

organism, this is a more simple process because the cell is in contact with its external environment to exchange nutrients and waste products. For humans, not all cells are immediately in contact with the external environment and as a consequence must work in cooperative units to maintain a stable internal environment. For example, muscle fibres do not have contact with the environment outside the body and so must rely on other cells to provide the nutrients and remove the waste products necessary to maintain a stable environment within each fibre. Cells within the human body are *mutually dependent* and work together to sustain life.

Knowledge integration question

Explain why homeostasis is important to multicellular organisms.

Homeostatic control refers to alterations in physiological functioning to maintain the internal environment of the body within a narrow range tolerable for the cells of the body. For example, the pH (acid-base balance), temperature and electrolyte balance all need to be maintained within a narrow band to protect against damage to the cells and the structures within them. The tolerance ranges can appear quite narrow; however, the systems within the body are excellently adapted to maintain homeostasis. The normal pH range for the blood is between 7.35 and 7.45. Outside of this range the body will alter physiological functioning to return the pH to normal levels. If homeostatic control mechanisms were unable to respond to changes in pH within the blood and the pH rose to above 7.8 or fell below 7.0, death would follow. Fortunately, the body has a number of mechanisms, such as pH buffering which will be covered in detail in Chapter 10, to protect against threats to homeostasis. Homeostatic control is about maintaining the internal environment within these narrow tolerance bands in order to allow the cells of the body to continue their work and sustain life. Homeostatic control is brought about through three mechanisms. Information about the physiological functioning of the body is picked up by *receptors* that are spread throughout the body and these relay environmental changes to the brain which serves as the *control centre* within the body. The brain interprets the incoming message and, when necessary, when there is a threat to homeostasis, a response through an *effector* organ is initiated. The heating in your home can serve as an excellent example of how homeostatic control

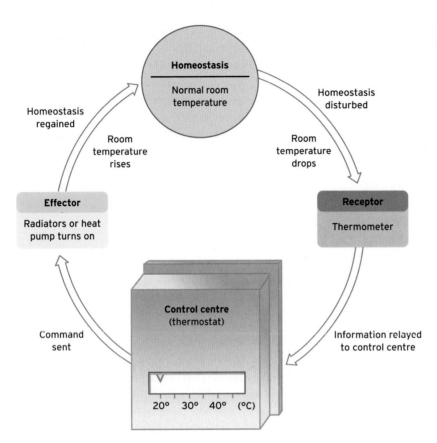

Figure 3.7 Illustration of homeostatic control.

functions (Figure 3.7). In this example a thermometer detects the temperature in the room and sends a signal to the control centre, in this case the thermostat, if the temperature falls below a set point (e.g. 20°C). When this happens the thermostat triggers the radiator or heat pump to turn on, increasing the temperature back to the set point. Importantly, once the temperature has returned to the set point the heating will be switched off to keep the room temperature at the set point.

The nervous and endocrine systems, which will be described in more detail in Chapter 4, play a vital role in the regulation of homeostasis. They are the *control mechanisms* that regulate the functioning of other systems to maintain the body's internal environment. The *nervous system* is the body's fast-response mechanism and the *endocrine system* the slower, sustained regulation process. Throughout the body there is a variety of *receptor* or *sensory mechanisms* that pick up and relay homeostatic status reports to the brain. The brain processes the sensory information and provides either a nervous or endocrine response. For example, if receptors detect a lack of glucose in the blood (a necessary energy supply for all cells) the brain interprets this information and stimulates an

endocrine response in the form of a release of *glucagon*, a hormone that stimulates the breakdown of glycogen to release glucose into the circulating blood. Alternatively, where a more immediate response is required, nervous control can be altered. When you start to run there is an immediate increase in the demand for oxygen for the working muscles. Receptors detect this (and a rise in carbon dioxide concentrations in the blood) and send sensory information to the brain where it is processed and a nervous response effected. In this case it would include a rise in respiration (breathing rate) and heart rate to match demand. The most common control mechanism for ceasing a nervous or endocrine response is through a *negative feedback* loop. For example, when running at a steady pace there is, as already mentioned, a rise in heart rate in response to the increased energy and oxygen demands of the working muscles. The rise in heart rate would continue until the receptors detected that oxygen and carbon dioxide concentrations had returned to their normal range. At this point the demand for oxygen and the clearance of carbon dioxide would have matched supply. In exercise physiology, when heart rate plateaus in response to exercise this condition is termed *steady-state exercise*.

Homeostatic balance can be threatened by a wide range of *threats* or, as Hans Selye (who will be discussed further in Chapter 8 in the section concerning periodisation of training) refers to them, *stresses*. These stresses can include environmental, exercise, circadian, nutritional threats and illness or disease, and can provide significant challenges to human homeostasis, particularly when operating as multiple stressors. Desert marathon runners, such as those taking part in the Marathon des Sables in the Sahara, place exercise, nutritional (water and energy) and environmental (heat) demands upon their bodies. Perhaps though the ultimate number of challenges to homeostasis comes from alpine ascents of mountain peaks, where the participant can face exercise, environmental (cold, altitude), circadian (alpine ascents often start at 1:00 or 2:00 am when you would normally be asleep) and, due to the length of the day, nutritional (water and energy) threats. To survive, the body must maintain homeostasis. As educators, coaches or sports people it is vital to understand this delicate balance and the threats that taking part in any activity present.

Try **Interactive Physiology**:
Fluids and electrolytes: Acid/base homeostasis; Water homeostasis; Electrolyte homeostasis

Key point

Homeostasis is vital for sustaining life for a biological organism.

Homeostasis refers to maintaining constancy within the internal environment.

Cells within the body work cooperatively in systems to maintain homeostasis. To maintain homeostasis these organ systems control the:

➤ supply of nutrients
➤ removal of waste products
➤ temperature
➤ pH balance
➤ electrolyte balance

3.3 Tissues

Atoms combine to form the particles necessary for the formation of cells, the smallest units of living matter. Within the human body, cells work in specialised groups, and together with the materials and fluids in their immediate extracellular environment, form the tissues of the body. The body is comprised of four main tissue types – *epithelial, nervous, muscle, connective* – that are interwoven to form all structures within the human body. An overview of these tissue types, including examples, is presented in Figure 3.8 with more detail about the cell types and materials that comprise each of the four tissue types provided in Figure 3.9. A description of the structure and functioning of epithelial and connective tissues follows, with detailed information on the nervous and muscle tissues found in Chapters 4 and 5, respectively.

Key point

There are four main tissue types:

➤ Epithelial tissue provides protective layers.
➤ Nervous tissue provides a network for communication and control.
➤ Muscle tissue enables movement.
➤ Connective tissue provides a framework, connections and protection.

Epithelial tissue

A layer of cells that separates the body's internal environment from the outside world (the skin) or lines the hollow organs of the body (e.g. gut, lungs, urinary tract) is known as *epithelia*. Epithelia form a barrier to protect surfaces that would otherwise be exposed, with skin being an epithelial tissue we see every day. There are two main classes of epithelia, covering epithelia and glandular epithelia.

Epithelia can be classified based on either the number of cell layers (simple: single layer; stratified: more than one layer) or the shape of the cell (squamous, cuboidal, columnar). These different classifications of epithelial are illustrated in Figure 3.10. Squamous (flattened) epithelia are found lining blood vessels and the alveoli of the lungs, while the small intestine is lined with columnar epithelia. An illustration of a typical epithelial cell is shown in Figure 3.11. They have many of the organelles found within the general cell (as depicted in Figure 3.2), but are also specialised to carry out their specific functions within the body. One of the prime functions of the epithelia is to provide physical protection for the underlying layers. The *apical surface* of an epithelial layer is oriented to the outside world or central space (of an organ or gland) and

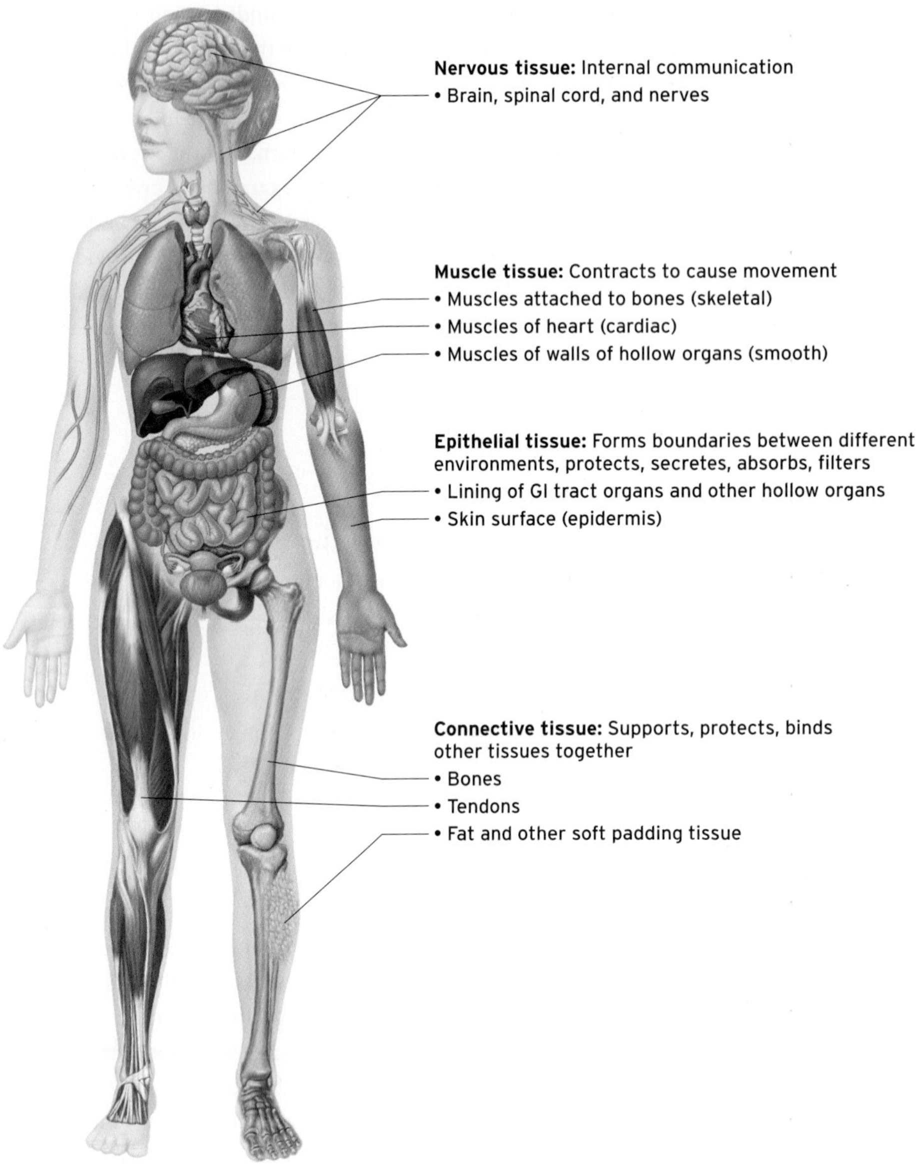

Figure 3.8 Types of tissue found within the human body.

Nervous tissue: Internal communication
• Brain, spinal cord, and nerves

Muscle tissue: Contracts to cause movement
• Muscles attached to bones (skeletal)
• Muscles of heart (cardiac)
• Muscles of walls of hollow organs (smooth)

Epithelial tissue: Forms boundaries between different environments, protects, secretes, absorbs, filters
• Lining of GI tract organs and other hollow organs
• Skin surface (epidermis)

Connective tissue: Supports, protects, binds other tissues together
• Bones
• Tendons
• Fat and other soft padding tissue

provides the barrier between the body's internal and external environments. Within internal passageways microvilli or cilia are often present on the apical surface to increase the surface area of the cell (enhancing functions such as absorption and secretion) or facilitate movement through the tract, respectively. For example, microvilli are found on the epithelia of the small intestine aiding the absorption of nutrients, and cilia found on the lining of the trachea (windpipe) help to sweep dirt and mucus from the lungs. Epithelia are also selectively permeable depending on their location and function, but can control the passage of any substance into or out of the body or a tissue. The epithelia share a close link with nervous tissue, for contained within

the tissue are specialist epithelial cells that function as receptors that detect changes in their environment for relay via neurons to the brain.

Glandular epithelial tissue produces specialised secretions from exocrine and endocrine glands. Exocrine glands release their secretions into ducts that open on to the epithelial surface in which they are situated. There is a variety of exocrine glands (e.g. the pancreas, salivary glands and sweat glands) and their structure is determined by their role. Mucus, sweat, salivary, breast milk, gastric and sebaceous oil secretions are all produced by exocrine glands. In contrast, endocrine glands lack a duct and secrete material directly into the blood. Endocrine glands

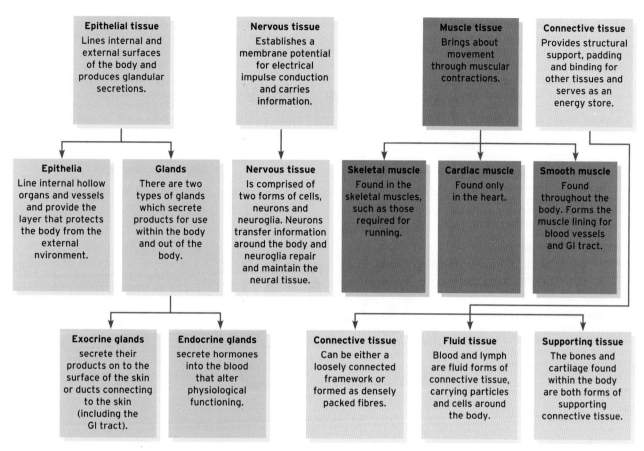

Figure 3.9 Cell types and materials that comprise each of the four tissue types.

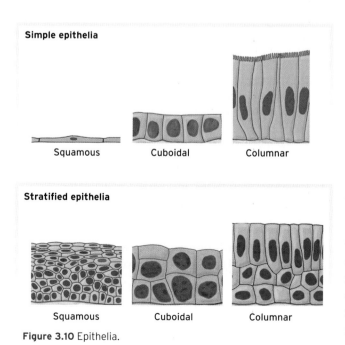

Figure 3.10 Epithelia.

and the hormones they produce are described later in Chapter 4.

Connective tissue

Connective tissue is found throughout the body, has a wide variety of functions, and as a consequence, the structure differs for each type. This tissue type not only provides a framework for the body and connects the parts of the body, but it also functions as an energy store, provides protection and insulation as well as facilitating transport of substances round the body. Connective tissue includes bone, cartilage, blood, lymph and adipocytes, as well as providing a loose and dense network that provides the framework and support for other cells and tissues. The following chapters provide further information about many of these forms of connective tissue.

The cells of any epithelium share a number of basic features. An epithelium has an **apical** (Ā-pi-kal) **surface**, which faces the exterior of the body or some internal space, and a **base**, which is attached to adjacent tissues. The term polarity refers to the presence of structural and functional differences between the exposed and attached surfaces

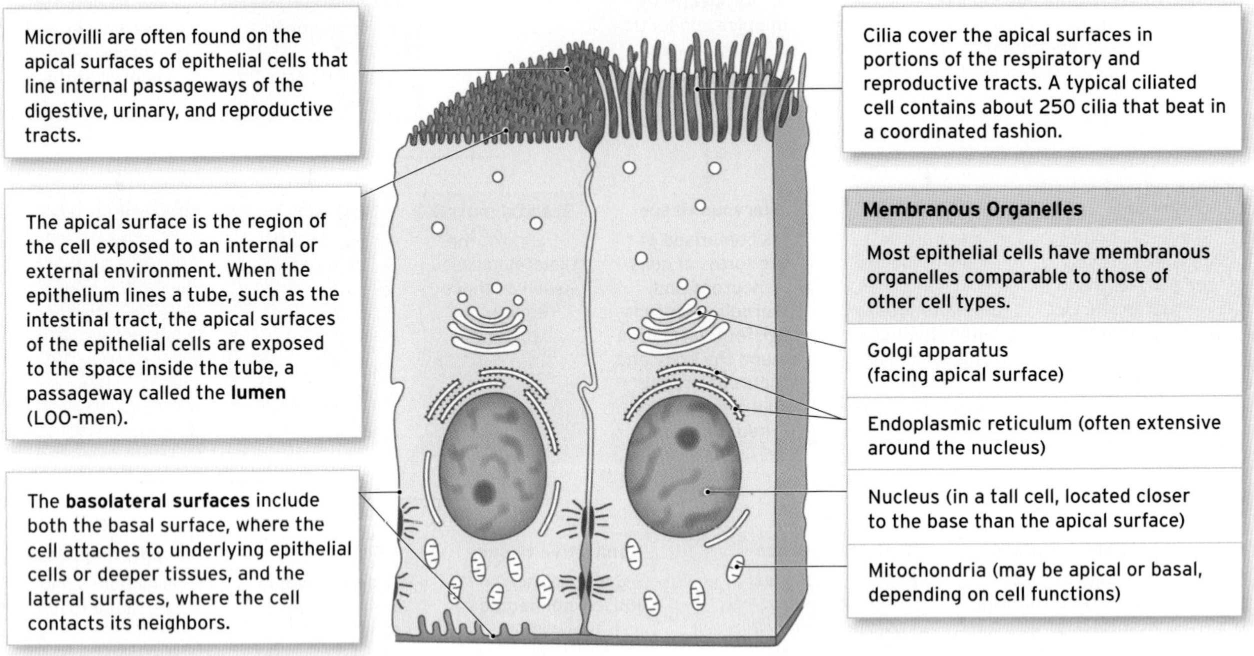

Microvilli are often found on the apical surfaces of epithelial cells that line internal passageways of the digestive, urinary, and reproductive tracts.

Cilia cover the apical surfaces in portions of the respiratory and reproductive tracts. A typical ciliated cell contains about 250 cilia that beat in a coordinated fashion.

The apical surface is the region of the cell exposed to an internal or external environment. When the epithelium lines a tube, such as the intestinal tract, the apical surfaces of the epithelial cells are exposed to the space inside the tube, a passageway called the **lumen** (LOO-men).

Membranous Organelles

Most epithelial cells have membranous organelles comparable to those of other cell types.

Golgi apparatus (facing apical surface)

Endoplasmic reticulum (often extensive around the nucleus)

Nucleus (in a tall cell, located closer to the base than the apical surface)

The **basolateral surfaces** include both the basal surface, where the cell attaches to underlying epithelial cells or deeper tissues, and the lateral surfaces, where the cell contacts its neighbors.

Mitochondria (may be apical or basal, depending on cell functions)

Figure 3.11 Structure of a typical epithelial cell.

Check your recall
Fill in the missing words.

➤ Cells are the basic _____ of living things.

➤ Within the body, cells are organised into a hierarchy of tissues, organs and _____ systems.

➤ In human beings around 200 different types of cell make up the _____ different organ systems.

➤ Cells are composed of three major parts:

  • a plasma membrane that surrounds the cell,

  • a _____ responsible for controlling its functions, and

  • cytoplasm that contains _____ that carry out the other work of the cell.

➤ The plasma membrane is responsible for maintaining a _____ between the cell's internal environment and the external environment.

➤ The plasma membrane also contains _____ proteins that enable communication and the transportation of selected ions or molecules in and out of the cell.

➤ There are four main kinds of _____ proteins: recognition proteins, receptor proteins, _____ _____ and transport proteins.

➤ The nucleus is the control centre of the cell. Most cells have one nucleus. However, red blood cells expel their nucleus during development and muscle cells are _____, containing many nuclei.

➤ The key component of the nucleus is the _____ which contains the genetic code, or blueprint, for the cell and directs its structure and functioning.

➤ The cytoplasm consists of cytosol (intracellular fluid) and _____.

➤ The cytosol provides the structure and rigidity of the cell through its network of protein filaments referred to as the _____.

➤ Cells actively work to maintain a constant internal environment and this process is referred to as _____.

➤ Cells within the human body work _____ in order to achieve _____.

➤ The four types of tissue are:

• _____

• Muscle

• Nervous

• _____

Review questions

1. Describe the relationship between cells, tissues, organs and systems within the human body. How does the differentiation of cells allow the body to function?

2. What are the three main parts of the cell? What are the basic functions of each of these?

3. What is meant by the term homeostasis? Why is homeostasis important within the human body?

4. Why do erythrocytes contain no nucleus?

5. What is the structure of the plasma membrane?

6. What are the functions of glycolipids and where are they found?

7. What role does the nucleus play in cell functioning? How does RNA assist the nucleus in the functioning of the cell?

8. Which organelles are involved in the synthesis, modification, packaging and transport of proteins?

9. What function does epithelial tissue play within the body? How can epithelia be classified?

10. What are the functions of connective tissue?

Teach it!
In groups of three, choose one topic and teach it to the rest of the study group.

1. Explain, using a diagram, how temperature is regulated as a part of homeostasis.

2. Given that insulin stimulates cells to take up glucose and glucagon stimulates the breakdown of glycogen, explain the homeostatic processes that might be undergone to maintain normal blood glucose levels (a) after a meal and (b) during exercise.

3. Describe the structure and function of each of the organelles within a cell.

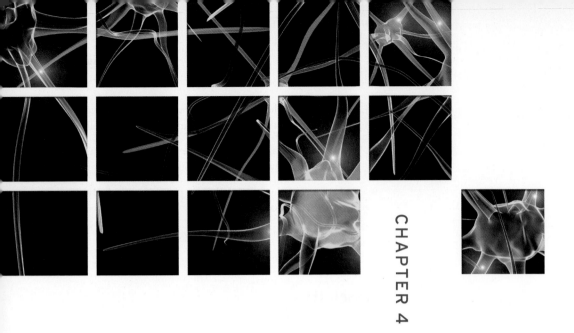

CHAPTER 4

The control systems:
nervous and endocrine

Learning objectives

After reading, considering and discussing with a study partner the material in this chapter you should be able to:

➤ describe the structure and function of nervous tissue

➤ distinguish between the divisions within the nervous system

➤ explain the sodium-potassium pump and its role in nerve impulse conduction

➤ teach others about how a nerve impulse or action potential is conducted along a neuron

➤ identify the differences between the central and peripheral nervous systems

➤ list the key endocrine organs, highlighting those that have another role within the body in addition to their endocrine function

➤ explain the essential components of endocrine messaging

➤ summarise the function of a number of key hormones

➤ describe the relationship and interaction between the nervous and endocrine systems

Human cells are the smallest living units within the body and work in specialised groups to form our tissues and organs. Under the control of the nervous and endocrine systems, the body's other organ systems carry out specialised functions to maintain homeostasis, that is, to provide a stable internal environment for optimal physiological functioning. The nervous system is the main controller of the body. Through electrical and chemical signals, the nervous system is the immediate response mechanism of the body. It collects and interprets information from the senses and effects the appropriate response within milliseconds. Through interaction with the nervous system, the endocrine system plays a role in the control of metabolic activity through the release of hormones (chemical messengers) into the blood and lymph. Compared to the nervous system, the endocrine system is slower to initiate a response. However, the response is sustained longer than those initiated by the nervous system. The combined work of the nervous and endocrine systems allows the internal environment of the body to remain within a narrow range required for cell and organism survival.

The first section of this chapter includes an overview of the organisation, structure and functioning of the nervous system, with the endocrine organs and hormonal functions discussed in section two. The responses of these two control systems to acute exercise are considered in the final section.

4.1 The nervous system

The nervous system is comprised of the brain, spinal cord, ganglia, nerves and sensory receptors. Despite its importance to the body, the nervous system comprises less than 5% of total body mass, with a mass of around 2 kg. The nervous system plays multiple roles during sports performance, including the initiation of muscular contractions that bring about movement. It is through the nervous system that we are able to respond to the ever-changing environment of the sports field, for example, a defender coming in to make a tackle, a tennis ball lobbed over your head, maintaining balance on a gymnastics beam. In a movement response, such as the start of a 100 m sprint race, nerve impulses from the brain or spinal cord link with the effector organ (muscle fibres) at neuromuscular junctions where the nervous stimulation is passed to the muscle fibre to initiate contraction of that fibre. This movement response is the result of three overlapping functions of the nervous system:

1. *Sensory input* – the information collected via sensory receptors which allows the nervous system to monitor changes both within, and outside, the body (e.g. the BANG of the starter's gun).
2. *Integration* – the method of processing and interpreting the sensory input and deciding on the appropriate course of action.
3. *Motor output* – the response initiated by the nervous system by activation of the effector organs (muscles and glands) (e.g. the sudden, explosive push off the starter blocks).

In addition to their roles in sports performance, these three overlapping functions of the nervous system enable the maintenance of homeostasis, and hence, survival.

Divisions of the nervous system

The nervous system is divided into two main divisions, the **central nervous system** (CNS) and the **peripheral nervous system** (PNS). The CNS includes the brain and spinal cord and is responsible for interpreting the sensory input and dictating the motor response. The PNS is the part of the nervous system outside the CNS and consists of peripheral nerves (12 pairs of cranial nerves, 31 pairs of spinal nerves), sensory receptors and ganglia. These nerves serve as the communication network between all parts of the body and the CNS. The PNS is further subdivided into the afferent (sensory) and efferent (motor) divisions. All divisions of the nervous system are illustrated in Figure 4.1.

The **sensory** or **afferent division** of the PNS comprises sensory (afferent) neurones which, as the name suggests, detect internal and external (to the body) signals and relay them to the central nervous system. There are five main types of sensory receptors within the body:

- **Mechanoreceptors** are responsive to stretching and pressure and are associated with the senses of touch, pressure, sound and balance. **Proprioception**, the awareness of where the body is in space, is a vital sense for many sports and is brought about through specific mechanoreceptors that are also referred to as proprioceptors.
- **Photoreceptors** are sensitive to light and are the basis for the sense of vision.
- **Chemoreceptors** detect chemicals that bind with their cell membranes and are responsible for the senses of smell and taste as well as detecting chemical changes within the body. The detection of increased CO_2 in the blood vessels, which is a trigger for an increase in heart and respiration rates, is brought about by chemoreceptors.

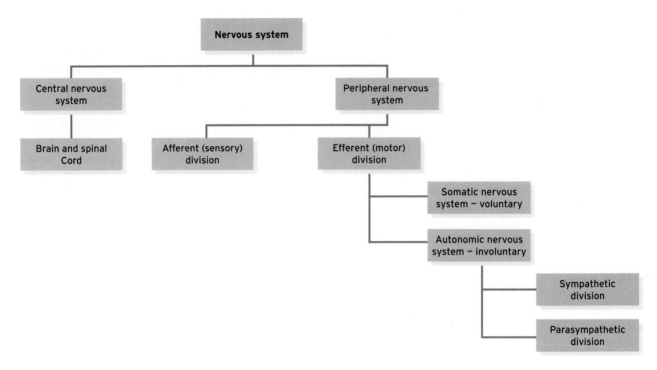

Figure 4.1 Divisions within the nervous system.

- **Thermoreceptors** detect changes in temperature and relay this information to the brain and spinal cord.
- **Nociceptors** detect pain and respond to mechanical, thermal and chemical sources which can be from internal or external sources.

Once sensory information has been relayed to and processed by the CNS, the nerves of the **motor** or **efferent division** transmit a response to the relevant tissues, organs or systems. We have conscious control over some motor responses, such as the movement of our limbs. However, others, such as the change in heart rate that occurs when playing sport, we have little or no control over. The **somatic nervous system** describes the parts of the nervous system which give us control of our skeletal muscles. The **autonomic nervous system** (ANS) refers to those parts over which the brain and spinal cord have control without us consciously having to think, such as breathing and the movement of food along the GI tract. The final division of the nervous system is within the autonomic nervous system which can be further separated into the **sympathetic** and **parasympathetic** divisions. The *sympathetic division* is responsible for speeding up the body systems in what is sometimes called the 'fight or flight' response. In contrast, the *parasympathetic division* is responsible for returning the body to normal functioning and can be thought of as the 'rest and digest' response.

Knowledge integration question

Explain the fight or flight response.

Nervous tissue

At a cellular level the nervous tissue is made up of two principal types of cell, **neurons** and **neuroglia** (or **glial cells**). Neurons (nerve cells) are excitable cells that process and transmit information by electrical and chemical signalling. In contrast, the much smaller neuroglia, are non-excitable cells that provide the neurons with structural and metabolic support. Neurons and neuroglia are formed during development from neuroblasts, the nervous system equivalent of the osteoblasts found in the skeletal system.

Neurons

Neurons and the nerves they comprise, in common with muscle tissue, are **excitable**, meaning that they can conduct an electrical impulse. This **nerve impulse**, or **action potential**, is the signal that passes along a neuron. **Sensory neurons** conduct information from the tissues and organs of the body to the brain and spinal cord and **motor neurons** relay messages from the CNS to the response organs. Some specialised neurons pass information from one neuron to another and as a result are called **interneurons** or **association neurons**.

Neuron structure

Neurons are normally made up of three main components, **dendrites**, a **cell body** and a single **axon**. Dendrites receive information (sensory or neurotransmitter stimuli) which is conveyed toward the cell body for processing. The axon then generates nerve impulses and conducts them away from the cell body, along the **axolemma** (axon plasma membrane), to the secretory axon terminals. The axon is a specialised cellular filament that arises from the cell body at a site known as the **axon hillock**. There are three main structural classifications of neurons related to the number of processes extending from the cell body. These are shown in Figure 4.2 with the direction of impulse travel indicated by an arrow. Although all neurons have only one axon leaving the cell body, **multipolar neurons** have many dendrites connecting to the cell body, **bipolar neurons** have a single dendrite coming to the cell body, and **unipolar neurons** have a joint dendrite axon process connecting with the cell body. Generally, motor neurons are multipolar in structure and sensory neurons are mainly unipolar although some specialist neurons, such as those of the rods and cones of the eye, are bipolar. Figure 4.3 shows a multipolar neuron in more detail.

Neurons vary greatly in both length and diameter depending on their function within the body. Some

nerve cells, such as those responsible for bringing about muscular contraction of the lower leg and feet, are over one metre in length. Like other cells within the body, the cell body (**soma** or **perikaryon**) comprises of a cell membrane, a nucleus and cytoplasm. The plasma membrane of the cell body and dendrites is called the **neurilemma**. However, the cell membrane of the axon is usually referred to as the **axolemma** because the function of axons necessitates differences in structure when compared with the rest of the cell. In a similar way the cytoplasm of the cell body is known as **neuroplasm** whereas that in the axon is called **axoplasm**. The cytoplasm of neurons contains many organelles common to other cells, such as lysosomes, ribosomes, mitochondria and a Golgi apparatus. In addition to generalised organelles, they contain some neuron-specific components, such as *neurofibrils*, neuron-specific *microtubules* and *Nissl bodies*. **Neurofibrils** are comprised of protein filaments and are designed to maintain the structure of the cell body. The neuron-specific **microtubules** provide a transport structure through which substances pass between the cell body and the axon. **Nissl bodies** are small rough endoplasmic reticulum structures that are responsible for synthesising proteins to be used for growth and repair.

Axons propagate action potentials to the receiving neuron or organ. Due to their often great length and lack of Nissl bodies, axons have two specialist transport systems (slow and fast axonal transport) that enable essential substances to be moved between the axon and the cell body. *Slow axonal transport* (transports at a speed of about 0.1 mm per hour) is responsible for the movement of axoplasm and *fast axonal transport* (around 12 mm per hour – ten times quicker than its slow counterpart) is responsible for moving

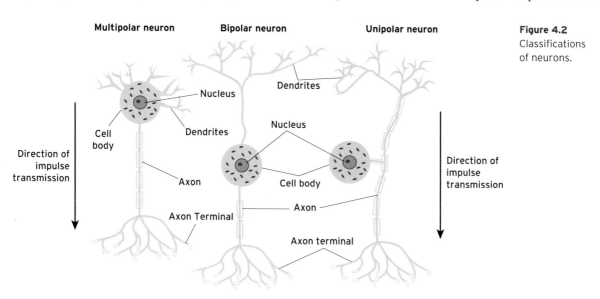

Figure 4.2
Classifications
of neurons.

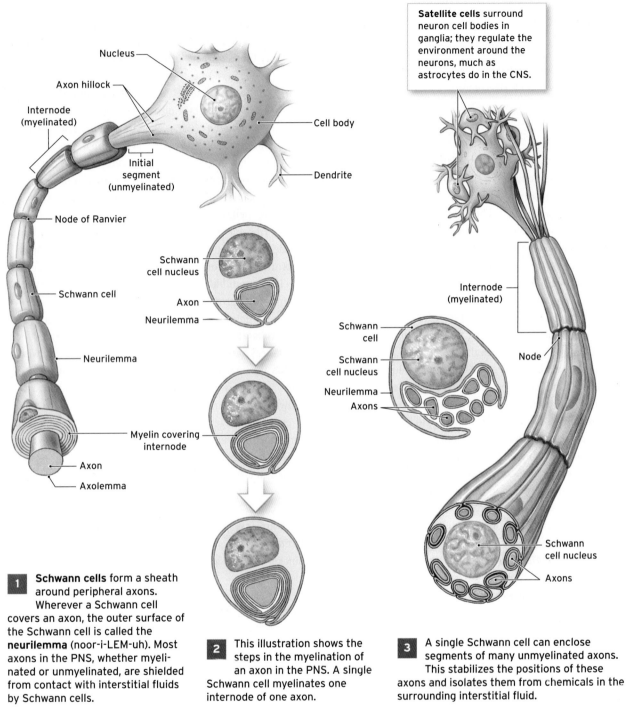

Nucleus

Axon hillock

Internode (myelinated)

Cell body

Initial segment (unmyelinated)

Dendrite

Node of Ranvier

Schwann cell nucleus

Axon

Neurilemma

Schwann cell

Neurilemma

Myelin covering internode

Axon

Axolemma

Satellite cells surround neuron cell bodies in ganglia; they regulate the environment around the neurons, much as astrocytes do in the CNS.

Internode (myelinated)

Schwann cell

Schwann cell nucleus

Neurilemma

Axons

Node

Schwann cell nucleus

Axons

1   **Schwann cells** form a sheath around peripheral axons. Wherever a Schwann cell covers an axon, the outer surface of the Schwann cell is called the **neurilemma** (noor-i-LEM-uh). Most axons in the PNS, whether myelinated or unmyelinated, are shielded from contact with interstitial fluids by Schwann cells.

2   This illustration shows the steps in the myelination of an axon in the PNS. A single Schwann cell myelinates one internode of one axon.

3   A single Schwann cell can enclose segments of many unmyelinated axons. This stabilizes the positions of these axons and isolates them from chemicals in the surrounding interstitial fluid.

Figure 4.3 The structure of a multipolar neuron.

organelles (such as mitochondria) and proteins between the cell body and axon terminals. After information from the dendrites is received and processed by the nucleus the nerve impulse is propagated from a trigger zone which is situated just below the axon hillock. Although each neuron has only one axon leaving the cell body, axons occasionally have branches from them called **axon collaterals** which lead to another set of axon terminals. Whether an axon is undivided or has collaterals, it usually has profuse branching at the end, enabling communication with many target cells (see Figure 4.2). The **axon terminals** form the link with other tissues or neurons. When the axon terminals of a motor neuron meet a muscle fibre the junction is called a **neuromuscular junction**, whereas the junction between two neurons is called a **synapse**.

The axons of many neurons are myelinated, meaning they are covered by a **myelin sheath**. This is a protective layer of segmented, electrically insulating, fatty material and is found particularly on neurons that are long or large in diameter. The principle function of the myelin sheath is to greatly increase the speed of transmission of nerve impulses. Type A axons, which comprise all efferent neurons and many afferent neurons (e.g. proprioceptors) within the peripheral nervous system, are the largest diameter fibres (between 4–20 μm) and are myelinated. The larger surface area and myelinated nature of the axons means that nerve impulses travel at the highest speeds in these fibres which can be as fast as 140 m·sec^{-1} or over 300 mph. Type B axons are smaller (between 2–4 μm), but still myelinated and as a consequence impulses still travel at relatively fast speeds, up to 18 m·sec^{-1} or around 36 mph. Type B axons form the majority of pre-ganglionic autonomic nervous system neurons (described in the section on the PNS). Type C, the smallest axons, are up to 2 μm in diameter and are unmyelinated, consequently, nerve impulses travel at slower speeds of 1–2 m·sec^{-1} or up to 4 mph. Post-ganglionic neurons within the autonomic nervous system predominantly comprise Type C axons.

Key point

There are three types of neuron: multipolar, bipolar and unipolar.

Multipolar neurons are mainly motor neurons (carry a response from the brain).

Unipolar and bipolar neurons are usually sensory neurons (carry information to the brain).

There are four types of neuroglia in the CNS: astrocytes, ependymal cells, microglia and oligodendroctyes.

There are two types of neuroglia in the PNS: Schwann cells and satellite cells.

Neuroglia

Neuroglia are much smaller cells than neurons and are the most common type of nerve tissue cell found in the body, comprising over half of the nervous system. They provide structural and metabolic support for the nervous system and are found in both the central nervous system and the peripheral nervous system. There are four types of neuroglia found in the CNS; astrocytes, ependymal cells,

microglia and oligodendroctyes, which can be seen in Figure 4.4, and two types found in the PNS, Schwann cells and satellite cells (see Figure 4.3).

Astrocytes are the most abundant CNS neuroglia and have several functions which include providing support for neurons, maintaining chemical balance and regulating nervous tissue growth. **Ependymal cells** line the central cavities of the brain and spinal cord and have hair-like structures protruding from them called *microvilli* and *cilia* which help with the flow of cerebrospinal fluid (CSF). **Microglia** are involved in repair of neurological tissue and help by removing debris from the interstitial environment. **Oligodendrocytes** are responsible for creating a myelin sheath around neurons of the CNS and to create a structural framework for the CNS. **Schwann cells** are the equivalent of oligodendrocytes in the PNS and, as can be seen in Figure 4.3, each Schwann cell is responsible for myelination of one section of a neuronal axon. Schwann cells also have a role in providing a coordinated structure and protection for unmyelinated neurons and can enclose up to 10 or 20 of these neurons. **Satellite cells** (Figure 4.3), the second form of neuroglia found in the PNS, help to supply nutrients to the surrounding neurons.

Knowledge integration question

Explain the differences between neurons and neuroglia.

Nerves

Neurons are found collected in groups or bundles, with unmyelinated neurons forming the grey matter of nervous tissue and myelinated neurons forming the white matter (myelin is whitish in colour and formed from lipid and protein). The structure of a nerve, which can be seen in Figure 4.5, has some similarities with muscle in that individual fibres or neurons are grouped together into fascicles and are surrounded by three protective sheaths. The protective sheaths for nerve fibres are the **epineurium**, the **perineurium** and the **endoneurium**.

The structure of an unmyelinated nerve also includes Schwann cells that wrap around the fibres, but unlike myelinated nerves, many fibres are encapsulated by one Schwann cell, but are not individually myelinated (see Figure 4.3). The majority of nerves, however, are myelinated which increases the speed of nervous transmission. Within the PNS, the presence of Schwann cells, and the neurilemma surrounding each axon, provide a protective tube in the event of injury (providing the nerve fibres remain aligned). In this situation, the protective tube created by the Schwann

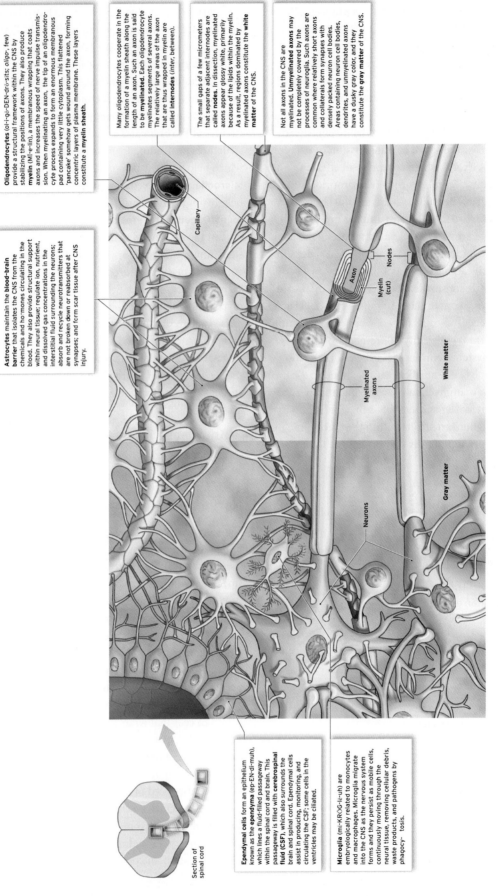

Oligodendrocytes (ol-i-go-DEN-dro-sits; *oligo-*, few) provide a structural framework within the CNS by stabilizing the positions of axons. They also produce **myelin** (MĪ-e-lin), a membranous wrapping that coats axons and increases the speed of nerve impulse transmission. When myelinating an axon, the tip of an oligodendrocyte process expands to form an enormous membranous pad containing very little cytoplasm. This flattened 'pancake' somehow gets wound around the axon, forming concentric layers of plasma membrane. These layers constitute a **myelin sheath**.

Many oligodendrocytes cooperate in the formation of a myelin sheath along the length of an axon. Such an axon is said to be **myelinated**. Each oligodendrocyte myelinates segments of several axons. The relatively large areas of the axon that are thus wrapped in myelin are called **internodes** (*inter*, between).

The small gaps of a few micrometers that separate adjacent internodes are called **nodes**. In dissection, myelinated axons appear glossy white, primarily because of the lipids within the myelin. As a result, regions dominated by myelinated axons constitute the **white matter** of the CNS.

Not all axons in the CNS are myelinated. **Unmyelinated axons** may not be completely covered by the processes of neuroglia. Such axons are common where relatively short axons and collaterals form synapses with densely packed neuron cell bodies. Areas containing neuron cell bodies, dendrites, and unmyelinated axons have a dusky gray color, and they constitute the **gray matter** of the CNS.

Astrocytes maintain the **blood-brain barrier** that isolates the CNS from the chemicals and hormones circulating in the blood. They also provide structural support within neural tissue; regulate ion, nutrient, and dissolved gas concentrations in the interstitial fluid surrounding the neurons; absorb and recycle neurotransmitters that are not broken down or reabsorbed at synapses; and form scar tissue after CNS injury.

Ependymal cells form an epithelium known as the **ependyma** (ep-EN-di-muh), which lines a fluid-filled passageway within the spinal cord and brain. This passageway is filled with **cerebrospinal fluid (CSF)**, which also surrounds the brain and spinal cord. Ependymal cells assist in producing, monitoring, and circulating the CSF; some cells in the ventricles may be ciliated.

Microglia (mī-KROG-lē-uh) are embryologically related to monocytes and macrophages. Microglia migrate into the CNS as the nervous system forms and they persist as mobile cells, continuously moving through the neural tissue, removing cellular debris, waste products, and pathogens by phagocy‐ tosis.

Section of spinal cord

Capillary

Nodes

Axon

Myelin (cut)

Neurons

Myelinated axons

White matter

Gray matter

Figure 4.4 The structure of neuroglia.

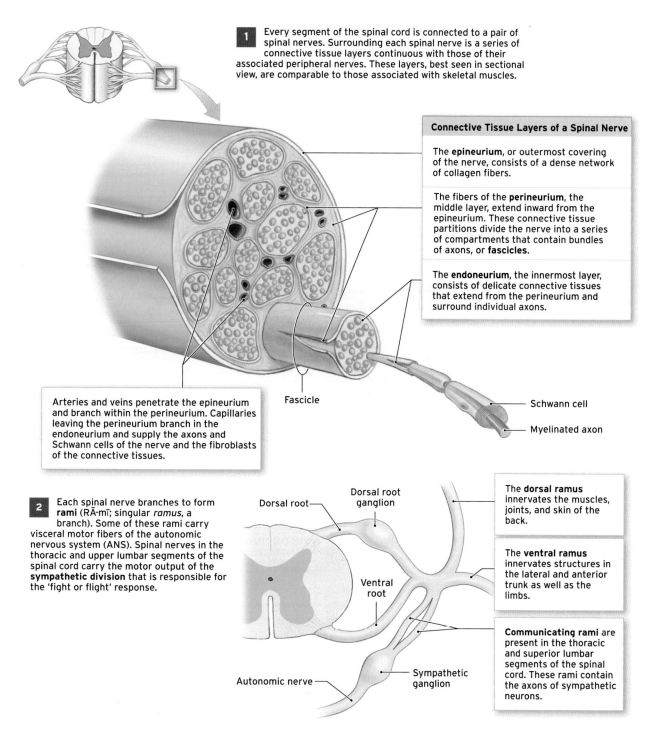

1 Every segment of the spinal cord is connected to a pair of spinal nerves. Surrounding each spinal nerve is a series of connective tissue layers continuous with those of their associated peripheral nerves. These layers, best seen in sectional view, are comparable to those associated with skeletal muscles.

Connective Tissue Layers of a Spinal Nerve

The **epineurium**, or outermost covering of the nerve, consists of a dense network of collagen fibers.

The fibers of the **perineurium**, the middle layer, extend inward from the epineurium. These connective tissue partitions divide the nerve into a series of compartments that contain bundles of axons, or **fascicles**.

The **endoneurium**, the innermost layer, consists of delicate connective tissues that extend from the perineurium and surround individual axons.

Arteries and veins penetrate the epineurium and branch within the perineurium. Capillaries leaving the perineurium branch in the endoneurium and supply the axons and Schwann cells of the nerve and the fibroblasts of the connective tissues.

Fascicle

Schwann cell

Myelinated axon

2 Each spinal nerve branches to form **rami** (RĀ-mī; singular *ramus*, a branch). Some of these rami carry visceral motor fibers of the autonomic nervous system (ANS). Spinal nerves in the thoracic and upper lumbar segments of the spinal cord carry the motor output of the **sympathetic division** that is responsible for the 'fight or flight' response.

Dorsal root

Dorsal root ganglion

Ventral root

Autonomic nerve

Sympathetic ganglion

The **dorsal ramus** innervates the muscles, joints, and skin of the back.

The **ventral ramus** innervates structures in the lateral and anterior trunk as well as the limbs.

Communicating rami are present in the thoracic and superior lumbar segments of the spinal cord. These rami contain the axons of sympathetic neurons.

Figure 4.5 The structure of a nerve.

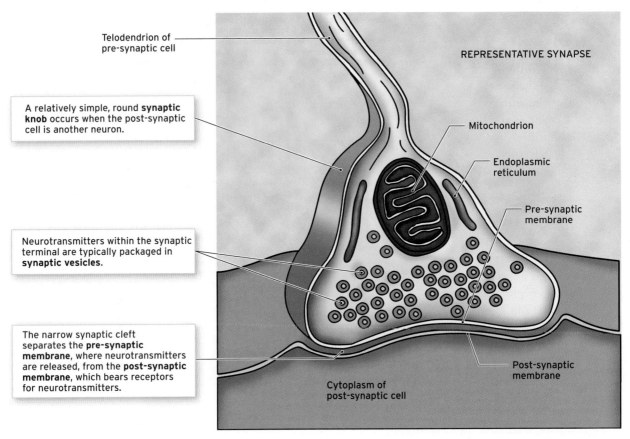

Telodendrion of pre-synaptic cell

REPRESENTATIVE SYNAPSE

A relatively simple, round **synaptic knob** occurs when the post-synaptic cell is another neuron.

Mitochondrion

Endoplasmic reticulum

Neurotransmitters within the synaptic terminal are typically packaged in **synaptic vesicles.**

Pre-synaptic membrane

The narrow synaptic cleft separates the **pre-synaptic membrane**, where neurotransmitters are released, from the **post-synaptic membrane**, which bears receptors for neurotransmitters.

Post-synaptic membrane

Cytoplasm of post-synaptic cell

Figure 4.6 The structure of a synapse.

cell and neurilemma enables **neurogenesis** (new tissue growth). However, if the damaged neuron is misaligned during injury the tissue may not be able to repair itself. In the CNS there is currently little or no chance of nervous tissue regeneration, although research into medical stimuli for neurogenesis is progressing.

The brain has 12 pairs of cranial nerves that emerge from and return to the CNS and serve sensory and motor roles in and around the head for both the somatic (muscular system) and autonomic nervous systems. The spinal cord has 31 pairs of nerves that serve somatic and autonomic function roles for the rest of the body. The cell bodies of the neurons that form these 43 pairs of nerves are normally located within **ganglia**, small masses of nerve tissue that exist on the outside of the CNS. As a consequence, it is the axons of each neuron that form the nerves that extend from the CNS.

Neuron junctions

A **synapse** is formed at the junction between two neurons or a neuron and its effector cell, as shown in Figure 4.6. Synapses enable an action potential to pass from one neuron to another. The neuron carrying the action potential (already stimulated and conducting a nerve impulse) is called the **pre-synaptic neuron**, and the one to which it will pass is the **post-synaptic neuron**. The sequence of events for the transfer of the action potential from one neuron to the next is very similar to that at a neuromuscular junction which will be described in the next chapter. As can be seen from Figure 4.6, the arrival of the nerve impulse at the axon terminal of the pre-synaptic neuron causes voltage-gated transmembrane protein channels to open. These channels allow Ca^{2+} to enter the axon terminal. The presence of calcium within the pre-synaptic neuron causes vesicles containing a neurotransmitter (chemical message) to fuse with the plasma membrane and open the vesicle to the synaptic cleft.

The neurotransmitter is able to diffuse across the extracellular fluid within the synaptic cleft and bind with ligand-gated channels to enable sodium to pass into the post-synaptic neuron and initiate a nerve impulse. Ligand-gated channels are trans-membrane proteins which have special receptor cells on their outside (open to the synaptic cleft) that will only enable a particular neurotransmitter to bind with them and open the channel. The neurotransmitter for many neurons in the PNS and neuromuscular junctions is **acetylcholine**. Within the CNS, along with acetylcholine, there are several proteins that are involved in synaptic neurotransmittion. Aspartic acid, glutamic acid, and glycine work directly as neurotransmitters, and the catecholamines adrenalin (also known as epinephrine), noradrenalin (also known as norepinephrine) and dopamine are neurotransmitters within the brain.

Knowledge integration question

Describe how an action potential crosses from one neuron to another.

Key point

Neuron cell bodies are located in ganglia (knots of nervous tissue located outside the brain and spinal cord).

Axons form the structures for nerves.

Neurons are generally:

➤ sensory (afferent) – relaying information to the CNS, or

➤ motor (efferent) – transmitting responses from the brain.

The 43 pairs of nerves are composed of sensory and motor axons.

Nerve impulse conduction

Stimulation of a neuron results in the generation of an electrical current, known as an *action potential* or *nerve impulse*, which is propagated along the length of the axon. The ability of a neuron to generate an *action potential* is dependent on the movement of electrolyte ions, primarily sodium and potassium, across the axolemma via the *sodium-potassium pump*. To fully appreciate how an action potential is generated, we must first understand the basic principles of electricity.

Principles of electricity

The same number of positive and negative charges exist within the body. A simple rule of electricity is that 'like charges repel', whereas 'opposite charges attract' each other. Due to this attraction, the separation of oppositely charged molecules, for example by a plasma membrane, requires work and so creates **potential energy**. This energy is termed the **potential difference**, also called **voltage**, and is measured in volts, a measure of the energy of electricity between two points, e.g. intracellular compared to extracellular. When the potential difference results in the movement of charged particles (ions within the body) this is called a **current** which is responsible for the propagation of an action potential.

Key point

The Na^+-K^+ pump establishes a potential difference across a neuron membrane.

The potential difference enables the propagation of an action potential.

Establishment of resting membrane potential

The electrical potential across the axolemma is created by the *sodium-potassium pump* (Na^+-K^+ pump) which was described earlier in Chapter 2 and illustrated in Figure 3.6. It is well worth reading this section again before reading about nerve impulse conduction. The Na^+-K^+ pump creates a differential in the concentration of Na^+ and K^+ on either side of the plasma membrane, by expelling three Na^+ from, and importing two K^+ into, the cytoplasm. It is this (resting) **membrane potential** or **potential difference** that enables nerve impulse conduction. The selectively permeable nature of the cell's plasma membrane, along with the actions of the sodium-potassium pump, enable the resting membrane potential to be established (Figure 4.7).

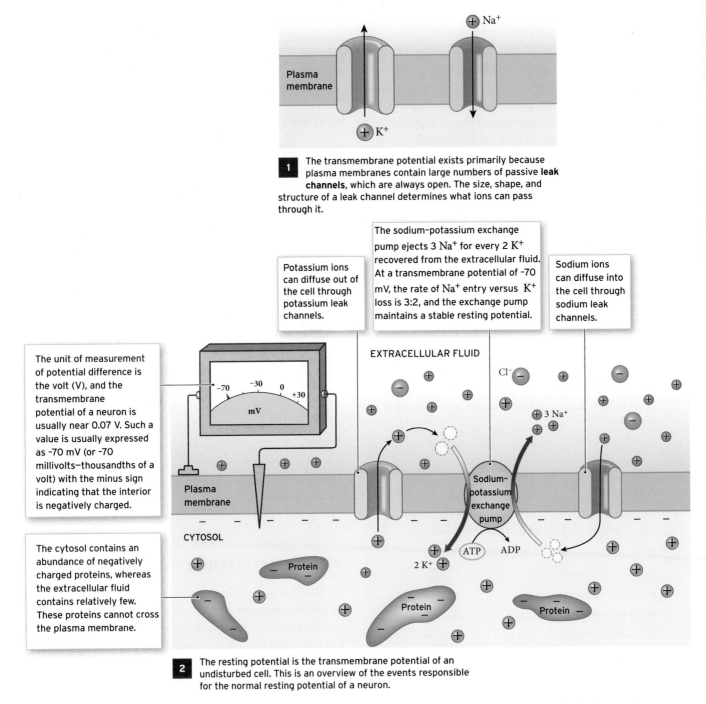

1 The transmembrane potential exists primarily because plasma membranes contain large numbers of passive **leak channels**, which are always open. The size, shape, and structure of a leak channel determines what ions can pass through it.

The sodium–potassium exchange pump ejects 3 Na$^+$ for every 2 K$^+$ recovered from the extracellular fluid. At a transmembrane potential of -70 mV, the rate of Na$^+$ entry versus K$^+$ loss is 3:2, and the exchange pump maintains a stable resting potential.

Potassium ions can diffuse out of the cell through potassium leak channels.

Sodium ions can diffuse into the cell through sodium leak channels.

The unit of measurement of potential difference is the volt (V), and the transmembrane potential of a neuron is usually near 0.07 V. Such a value is usually expressed as -70 mV (or -70 millivolts—thousandths of a volt) with the minus sign indicating that the interior is negatively charged.

The cytosol contains an abundance of negatively charged proteins, whereas the extracellular fluid contains relatively few. These proteins cannot cross the plasma membrane.

EXTRACELLULAR FLUID

Plasma membrane

CYTOSOL

2 The resting potential is the transmembrane potential of an undisturbed cell. This is an overview of the events responsible for the normal resting potential of a neuron.

Figure 4.7 Resting membrane potential and chemical gradients. (*Source*: Martini, F. H., Ober, J. and Nath, J. L. (2011) *Visual Anatomy and Physiology*, New York: Benjamin Cummings)

The Na$^+$-K$^+$ pump expels three Na$^+$ for every two K$^+$ brought into the cell, but in addition:

1. The plasma membrane is more 'leaky' to potassium ions than to sodium ions. Both ions will leak from high concentration to low concentration; however, more potassium ions will leak from the cell thereby increasing the potential difference (voltage) between the inside and outside of the cell.

2. There are many large negatively charged protein molecules and phosphate ions within the cell, which again increases the potential difference across the plasma membrane.

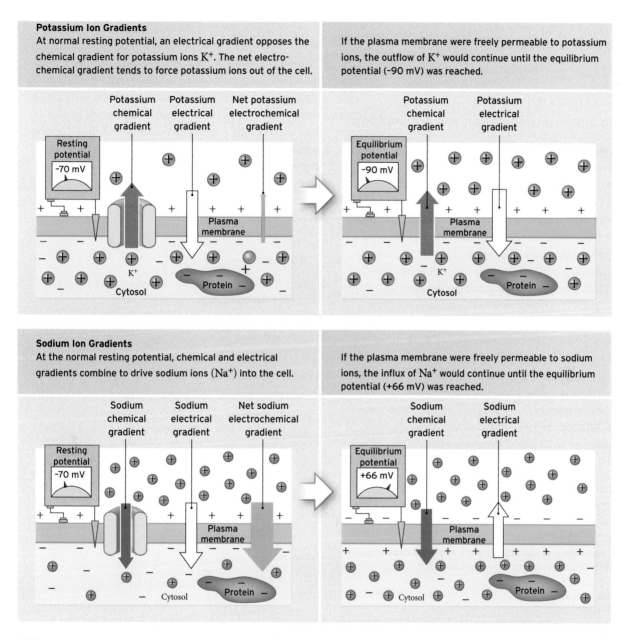

Potassium Ion Gradients
At normal resting potential, an electrical gradient opposes the chemical gradient for potassium ions K⁺. The net electro-chemical gradient tends to force potassium ions out of the cell.

If the plasma membrane were freely permeable to potassium ions, the outflow of K⁺ would continue until the equilibrium potential (-90 mV) was reached.

Sodium Ion Gradients
At the normal resting potential, chemical and electrical gradients combine to drive sodium ions (Na⁺) into the cell.

If the plasma membrane were freely permeable to sodium ions, the influx of Na⁺ would continue until the equilibrium potential (+66 mV) was reached.

3 Any ion's **chemical gradient** is the concentration gradient for that ion across the plasma membrane. The **electrical gradient** is created by the attraction between opposite charges, or the repulsion between like charges (+/+ or –/–). The two ions we need to be concerned with are potassium and sodium. At a transmembrane potential known as the **equilibrium potential**, the electrical and chemical gradients are equal and opposite, and there is no net movement of ions across the membrane.

Figure 4.7 *(continued)*

The negative ions immediately inside the plasma membrane are attracted to the positive ions on the outside of the cell and this creates a narrow band of ions either side of the membrane that have a relatively large difference in charge. This difference in charge between the inside and outside of the cell, the **resting membrane potential**, can be measured by a voltmeter and in most cells is around −70 mV. The negative sign indicates that the inside of the cell is negatively charged relative to the outside. Cells that maintain a resting membrane potential are said to be **polarised** (there is a difference in the electrical charge inside and outside the cell). Nervous and muscle tissue are able to use this potential difference to propagate an electrical current.

Knowledge integration question

Explain how a resting membrane potential is established.

Action potential generation and propagation

Although all cells have a resting membrane potential, it is only those with an excitable plasma membrane (muscle fibres and neurons) that are able to generate and propagate action potentials. When a stimulus reaches a neuron it changes the permeability of the plasma membrane and triggers the opening of special voltage-gated transmembrane protein channels. The Na^+ voltage-gated channels open and enable Na^+ to flood into the cell before they close again. The influx of Na^+ changes the electrical charge from -70 mV to around $+35$ mV and as a consequence the cell is said to be **depolarised** (Figure 4.8). This depolarisation is the actual action potential or nerve impulse. Once an action potential has been initiated, it is then self-propagating along the length of the axon. The action potential does not flow across the plasma membrane in one moment, especially as axons and muscle fibres can be quite long. Instead, the action potential moves down the membrane as a **wave of depolarisation**. As the action potential travels along an axon or muscle fibre it depolarises the next segment in the plasma membrane. As soon as the membrane has depolarised, the sodium voltage-gates are closed and potassium channels open and enable potassium ions to leave the cell. This action, along with the function of the Na^+-K^+ pump, returns the neuron or muscle fibre to its resting membrane potential and thus it has been **repolarised** (Figure 4.8). A repolarised cell is then ready to conduct a new action potential. The whole process of depolarisation and repolarisation, that is, the duration of an action potential, is very quick taking a thousandth of a second (1 msec or 0.001 sec).

Key point

Nerve impulses can travel to the brain (sensory neurons) or from the brain (motor neurons).

An action potential or nerve impulse is an electrical current propagated along the axon of neurons.

The initial change in electrical charge initiating an action potential is called depolarisation.

An action potential travels as a wave along a neuron axon or muscle fibre triggering the depolarisation of the next segment of the plasma membrane.

Generation of Action Potentials

Step 1: Depolarisation to threshold
- A graded depolarisation brings an area of excitable membrane to threshold (-60 mV).

Step 2: Activation of sodium channels and rapid depolarisation
- The voltage-gated sodium channels open (sodium channel activation).
- Sodium ions, driven by electrical attraction and the chemical gradient, flood into the cell.
- The transmembrane potential goes from -60 mV (the threshold level), toward $+30$ mV (the sodium equilibrium potential).

Step 3: Inactivation of sodium channels and activation of potassium channels
- The voltage-gated sodium channels close (sodium channel inactivation occurs) at $+30$ mV.
- The voltage-gated potassium channels are now open, and potassium ions diffuse out of the cell.
- Repolarization begins.

Step 4: Return to normal permeability
- The voltage-gated sodium channels regain their normal properties in 0.4-1.0 msec. The membrane is now capable of generating another action potential if a larger-than-normal stimulus is provided.
- The voltage-gated potassium channels begin closing at -70 mV. Because they do not all close at the same time, potassium loss continues and a temporary hyperpolarisation to approximately -90 mV (the potassium equilibrium potential) occurs.
- At the end of the relative refractory period, all voltage-gated channels have closed and the plasma membrane is back to its resting state.

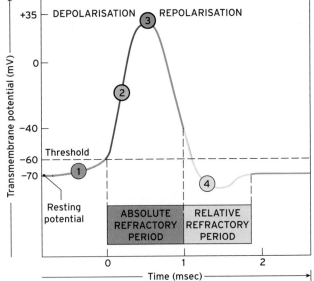

Figure 4.8 Action potential. (*Source*: Martini, F. H. and Nath, J. L. (2009) *Fundamentals of Anatomy and Physiology*, 8th edition, New York: Benjamin Cummings)

Nerve impulse conduction for unmyelinated neurons is conducted in this way, as a wave of depolarisation along the axon, and is called **continuous conduction**. The myelination of a neuron's axon, however, enables the action potential to 'jump' along the axon. The process of axon myelination is performed by Schwann cells, each of which is about 1mm in length. The gaps in myelination between the Schwann cells called nodes of Ranvier (see pp. 86 and 96). The insulating property of myelin means ions, and hence electrical currents, are only able to pass through the membrane at these nodes, thus an action potential in a myelinated neuron travels from one node of Ranvier to the next. The jumping of an action potential from node to node, called **saltatory conduction** from the Latin 'saltare' meaning to leap, greatly enhances the speed of nerve impulse conduction. This, along with axonal diameter differences, is the reason why nerve impulse conduction in Type A and B axons is faster than for Type C axons (refer to previous section on neuron structure for Types of axon). Figure 4.9 provides an illustration of how the conduction of action potentials takes place for myelinated and unmyelinated neurons.

Key point

Unmyelinated neurons carry action potentials by continuous conduction.

Myelinated neurons carry action potentials by saltatory conduction.

Knowledge integration question

Explain why saltatory conduction is more rapid than continuous conduction.

Central nervous system

The central nervous system is composed of the brain and the spinal cord which are enclosed by bony structures, the skull and the vertebral column. In addition to bones, the delicate tissues of the brain and spinal cord are protected by connective tissue membranes, adipose tissue and fluid-filled cavities. Three protective, connective tissue membranes surround the brain and spinal cord; the **dura mater, arachnoid mater** and **pia mater** which are known collectively as the **meninges** (see Figure 4.11). The outer layer of the meninges, the dura mater, is a dense connective tissue found

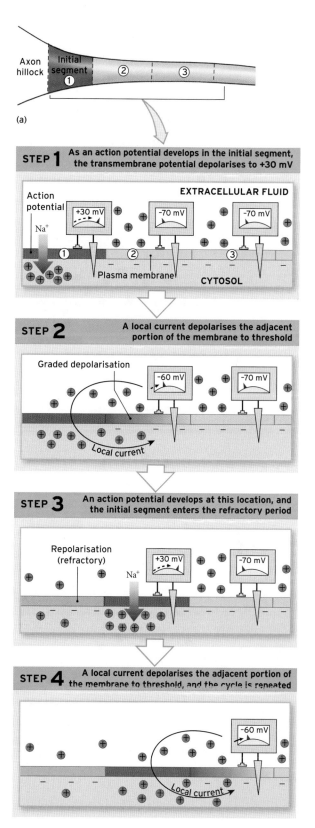

Figure 4.9 Nerve impulse conduction in unmyelinated (a) and myelinated (b) neurons. (*Source*: Martini, F. H. and Nath, J. L. (2009) *Fundamentals of Anatomy and Physiology*, 8th edition, New York: Benjamin Cummings)

(b)

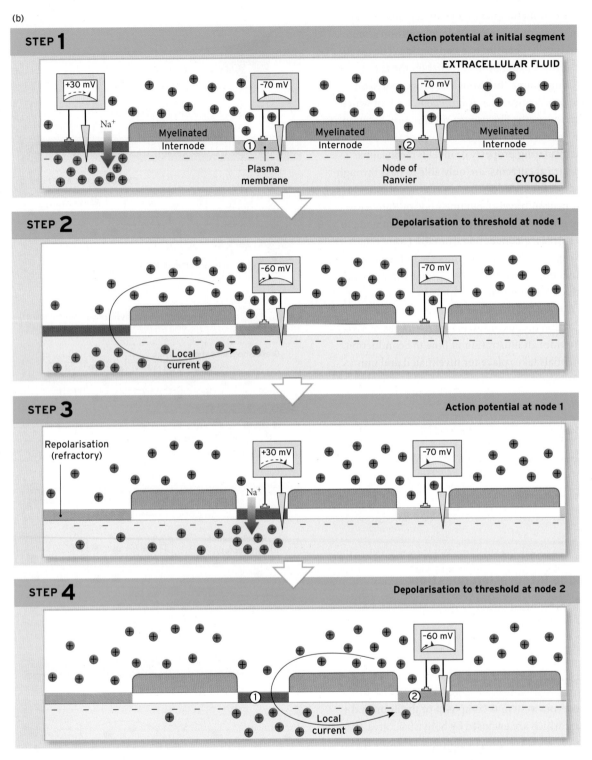

Figure 4.9 (continued)

immediately beneath the skull which covers the whole brain and, in a tube-like extension from the brain, the spinal cord. One difference in the meninges between the brain and the spinal cord is that the brain has two dura maters compared with only one protecting the spinal cord. Between the spinal dura mater and the vertebrae, within the epidural space, are connective tissue and fat as a second level of protection. A further difference between the brain and spinal cord is that no epidural space is found in the brain as the dura mater is fused to the periostium of the cranial bones.

The middle meningeal layer, the arachnoid mater, is attached to the inner surface of the dura mater. The sub-arachnoid space (between arachnoid and pia maters) is filled with cerebrospinal fluid (CSF) which is a clear liquid produced by the walls of the ventricles within the brain. In addition to acting as a shock absorber, the CSF plays an important role in regulating the extracellular environment of nerve cells, and provides the brain and spinal cord with nutrients and electrolytes. The pia mater, the innermost meningeal layer, sticks to the surface of the brain, following every contour. Blood vessels run along the surface of the pia mater, supplying the brain and spinal cord with nutrients and oxygen.

Unique to the brain is the **blood-brain barrier**, a vital protective mechanism to ensure a stable internal environment is maintained. The majority of capillaries in the brain are surrounded by the blood-brain barrier which functions to separate the general circulation from the neural tissue of the brain. This prevents the free flow of substances into the brain and is effective in protecting the brain from chemicals that might disrupt neural function, or from blood-borne bacterial infections.

A basic pattern of the distribution of matter in the CNS exists with slight variation depending on the region of the brain or spinal cord. In general, the central cavity is surrounded by **grey matter** with **white matter** lying externally. A slight variation on this is found in the cerebellum where an outer layer of gray matter exists which is known as the *cortex*. The grey matter contains neuronal cell bodies and their dendrites, whereas the white matter consists of myelinated neurons.

The brain

The human brain contains almost 97% of the body's neural tissue and typically weighs 1.5 kg (3 lb). There is a wide variability in brain size between individuals with no difference between genders when corrected for body mass. Although making up less than 3% of total body mass, the brain is comprised of around 100 billion neurons, and at rest uses up to 20% of oxygen and glucose consumed. It has a relatively high demand for oxygen because its neurons and neuroglia almost exclusively synthesise ATP through aerobic means, with glucose being the only nutrient it utilises as an energy source.

The brain is commonly divided into four regions, the brain stem (comprising the medulla oblongata, pons and midbrain) the cerebellum, the diencephalon (incorporates the thalamus, hypothalamus and the epithalamus) and the cerebrum. Figure 4.10 provides an illustration of the brain.

Key point

The brain is usually divided into the:

➤ Cerebrum

➤ Diencephalon (thalamus, hypothalamus and epithalamus)

➤ Cerebellum

➤ Brain-stem (medulla oblongata, pons and midbrain)

The **brain-stem** is a small, yet extremely important, part of the brain as it is responsible for providing a link between the spinal cord and the brain and it allows passage of all the sensory and motor nerve connections from the main part of the brain to the rest of the body. It controls autonomic processes that are independent of our consciousness, such as breathing, heart rate, blood vessel diameter and a variety of reflexes such as coughing, vomiting and sneezing. The brain stem is also vital for the regulation of the sleep cycle. The **cerebellum**, is very important to sports performers as it represents the brain's feedback centre. Its most well-known role is in controlling motor performance as it contributes to posture, balance, coordination, accurate timing and precision, and fine-tuning motor activity. The cerebellum judges movements made against planned movements and then makes adjustments as necessary. This is very important in the development of fine motor movements. The **diencephalon**, through the structures that in contains, plays numerous roles in the human body – it regulates the activity of the autonomic nervous system (hypothalamus), controls our circadian rhythms (body clock) (hypothalamus and epithalamus), regulates behaviour and emotion (hypothalamus), provides a relay of information to the cerebrum (thalamus), regulates body temperature (hypothalamus) and is involved in endocrine function (hypothalamus and pituitary gland – part of the epithalamus). The **cerebrum** is the largest, most well developed, region of the brain, accounting for 83% of total brain mass. It represents our *conscious mind*, directing volitional motor functions, processing sensory information and controlling higher cognitive functions such as language and communication, learning, memory, intelligence and personality.

Knowledge integration question

Why is the cerebellum important to athletes?

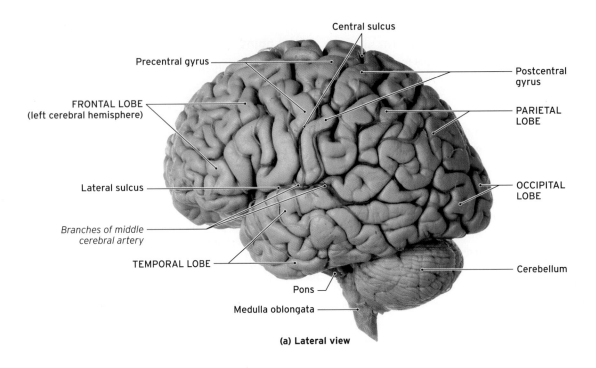

(a) Lateral view

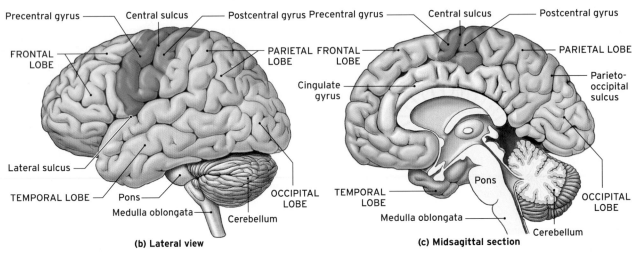

(b) Lateral view

(c) Midsagittal section

Figure 4.10 The structure of the brain.

The spinal cord

The spinal cord, illustrated in Figure 4.11, is on average 45 cm long and 1 cm wide. It is comprised of around 100 million neurons and is protected by a number of structures including the three protective meningeal sheaths, 33 vertebrae that form the vertebral column, surrounding fluids, connective tissue and fat (discussed at the start of this section). The vertebral column is divided into five regions, with a letter indicative of the region. Within each region, the vertebrae are numbered beginning with the uppermost; cervical ($C_1 - C_7$), thoracic ($T_1 - T_{12}$), lumbar ($L_1 - L_5$),

sacral ($S_1 - S_5$), and coccygeal ($C_1 - C_4$). In maturity, the vertebrae of the sacral and coccygeal regions are fused together, with no intervertebral discs.

The spinal cord has 31 pairs of spinal nerves that serve somatic and autonomic function roles for the rest of the body. On the basis of the origins of these spinal nerves, the spinal cord can be divided into 31 segments. Each segment is associated with a pair of **dorsal root ganglia** which contain the cell bodies of the sensory neurons which bring information to the CNS, with the axons forming the **dorsal roots**. In comparison, the axons of motor neurons that extend into the periphery and carry information from the

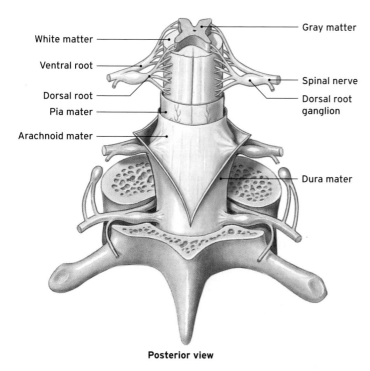

Figure 4.11 The structure of the spinal cord. (*Source*: Martini, F. H. and Nath, J. L. (2009) *Fundamentals of Anatomy and Physiology*, 8th edition, New York: Benjamin Cummings)

Posterior view

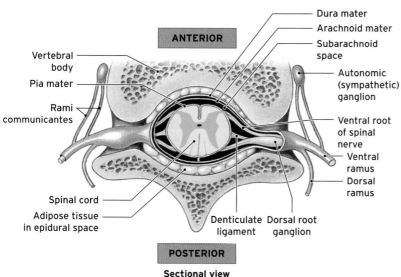

Sectional view

CNS, form the **ventral roots** with the cell bodies contained within the grey matter of the spinal cord. Distal to the dorsal root ganglia, the dorsal (sensory) and ventral (motor) roots are bound together into a single **spinal nerve**. The structure of the spinal cord, its protective tissues and spinal nerves are illustrated in Figure 4.11.

In the upper region of the vertebral column, spinal nerves leave the spinal cord directly, whereas, in the lower region, spinal nerves travel further down the vertebral column before exiting. This is because, at around the age of 4 years, the longitudinal growth of the spinal cord ceases.

However, as we continue to grow in height, the vertebral column continues to elongate. This results in the adult spinal cord extending only to the first or second lumbar vertebra, hence the origins of the sacral spinal nerves are actually in the upper lumbar region.

Peripheral nervous system

The PNS, which structurally includes the ganglia, sensory receptors and nerves, can be further divided into the somatic nervous and autonomic nervous systems. The

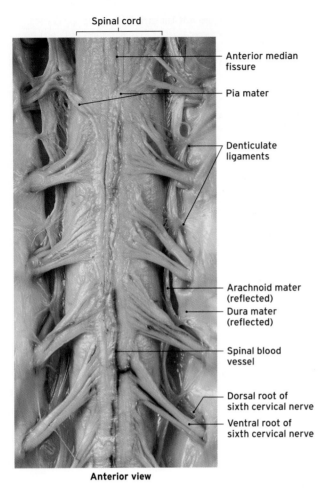

Spinal cord

- Anterior median fissure
- Pia mater
- Denticulate ligaments
- Arachnoid mater (reflected)
- Dura mater (reflected)
- Spinal blood vessel
- Dorsal root of sixth cervical nerve
- Ventral root of sixth cervical nerve

Anterior view

Figure 4.11 *(continued)*

somatic nervous system (SNS) is associated with the voluntary control of human movement via the contraction of skeletal muscle and is hence sometimes referred to as the voluntary system. The **autonomic nervous system (ANS)**, however, primarily functions below the level of consciousness and so is also known as the involuntary system. The ANS controls visceral functions, affecting blood vessel diameter, digestion, heart rate and breathing, to name but a few.

Somatic nervous system

The cranial and spinal nerves provide the afferent and efferent neuron pathways for the somatic and autonomic divisions. *Sensory neurons* for the somatic and autonomic systems have the same structure, and function in the same fashion, receiving information from receptors throughout the body and passing it to the CNS. At the CNS the sensory information is processed and a response generated. The efferent pathways are where structural and functional

differences between the autonomic and somatic nervous systems can be identified.

The somatic nervous system motor neurons comprise Type A axons, large diameter and myelinated, for fast innervation of the relevant skeletal muscle. The cell bodies of these neurons are located within the CNS and their axons form part of one of the 43 paired nerves that exit the CNS. Within the somatic nervous system a single motor neuron carries the nerve impulse from the CNS to the skeletal muscle fibres. Acetylcholine is the neurotransmitter released by the motor neuron and received by post-synaptic muscle receptors, thereby stimulating the muscle fibre to contract. In the somatic nervous system, excitation of a neuron will only lead to muscle contraction, that is, there are no inhibitory neurons.

Autonomic nervous system

In contrast to the somatic nervous system, two synapsed (linked by a synapse) neurons form the efferent pathway of the autonomic nervous system. In addition, there are two branches of efferent autonomic neuron, those that have a *sympathetic* effect (preparing the body for activity, e.g. increasing heart rate during exercise) and those that carry a *parasympathetic* response (restorative functions, e.g. decreasing heart rate). The first autonomic or **visceral** (pertaining to the internal organs) neuron has its cell body within the brain or spinal cord and conducts a nerve impulse to small clusters of neuron cell bodies called an **autonomic ganglion** (similar to ganglia described above). This type of visceral neuron is called a **pre-ganglionic neuron** because it is the neuron that conducts the autonomic response from the CNS to the autonomic ganglion. As was mentioned in the section on neurons (4.1.2 Nervous tissue) pre-ganglionic neurons normally have Type B axons and as a consequence nerve impulse conduction is slower than in somatic (motor) neurons. The second autonomic neuron, the **post-ganglionic neuron**, is usually a Type C fibre (unmyelinated) which carries impulses more slowly from the ganglion to the tissue where they have their effect. Figure 4.12 provides a diagrammatic representation of differences and similarities between sympathetic visceral, parasympathetic visceral and motor neurons.

Sympathetic division

The location of the autonomic ganglia, and therefore the lengths of the pre- and post-ganglionic fibres, differs between the sympathetic and parasympathetic divisions.

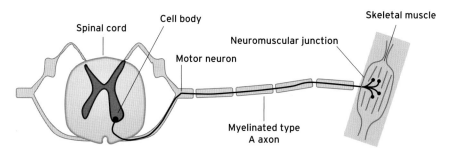

Figure 4.12 Somatic and autonomic efferent neuronal pathways.

(a) Motor neuron within the somatic nervous system

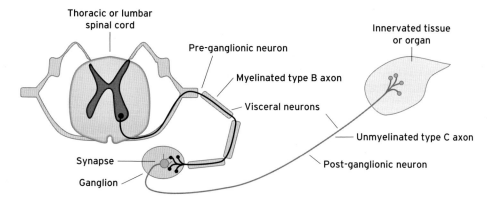

(b) Sympathetic visceral neuron within the autonomic nervous system

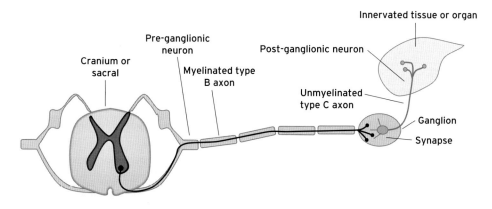

(c) Parasympathetic visceral neuron within the autonomic nervous system

Sympathetic pre-ganglionic neurons (myelinated Type B axons) have their cell bodies located only in the thoracic or lumbar regions of the spine and their axons originate from the spinal cord. There are three sympathetic autonomic ganglia which are located very close to the vertebral column, hence the pre-ganglionic neurons are short in length. In contrast, post-ganglionic neurons are unmyelinated (Type C axons) and much longer, emerging from the autonomic ganglia to complete the nerve impulse journey (see Figure 4.12). Similar to the somatic nervous system, the neurotransmitter of sympathetic pre-ganglionic fibres is acetylcholine; however, norepinephrine is released into the nerve-organ junction by post-ganglionic fibres.

Knowledge integration question

Explain the differences between the SNS and the ANS.

Parasympathetic division

Parasympathetic pre-ganglionic neurons originate only from cranial nerves or the sacral region of the spinal cord and connect with the parasympathetic autonomic ganglions. The *parasympathetic autonomic ganglia* are located close to or within the walls of the organ they innervate, so by the time the nerve impulse reaches the parasympathetic ganglion it has almost completed its journey. In contrast to the sympathetic system, therefore, the parasympathetic division has long pre-ganglionic neurons and short post-ganglionic neurons (see Figure 4.12). The pre- and post-ganglionic neurons of the parasympathetic system release acetylcholine from the axon terminals as the neurotransmitter.

Key point

The nervous system can be divided into the CNS (the brain and spinal cord) and the PNS (the nerves and ganglia outside the CNS).

The PNS is comprised of the:

➤ **somatic nervous system** (for control of skeletal muscles) over which we have control (the voluntary system).

➤ **autonomic nervous system** (for control of smooth muscle, cardiac muscle, glands and other tissues and organs) over which we do not consciously have control (involuntary system).

4.2 The endocrine system

The **endocrine system** is the body's second control system. Working alongside the nervous system, it is responsible for the regulation of the other systems within the body. Many life processes, such as growth, development and reproduction, are of a long-term nature, and it is these processes that are regulated by the endocrine system. Endocrine comes from the Greek, *endo* meaning inside and *crine* to secrete and the name underlies the system's function. Three elements are required for endocrine messaging, a *production organ* that secretes a *hormone* into the extracellular fluid and specific *target cells,* reached via the blood, upon which the hormone would take effect. A **hormone**, from the Greek 'hormaō' meaning to set in motion, is a chemical message that initiates a change in the function of the target cells. Each hormone is highly specific and impacts upon only the target cells for which it is intended. All cells are exposed to hormones but it is only those with the specific receptors for a particular hormone that respond to the changing levels of that hormone in the bloodstream. As hormones are transported in the bloodstream, target cells can be located

anywhere in the body, hence, the metabolic functioning of multiple tissues and organs can be simultaneously altered by a single hormone. An example of this is human growth hormone that alters the functioning of a wide number of cells within the body. Although the effects of hormones may be slow to initiate, they are prolonged in their response, generally continuing for a few days. It is thanks to the combination of hormones and neurons that the body is able to, in most circumstances, maintain or regain a state of homeostasis.

Key point

The endocrine system is the body's second control and regulation system.

Endocrine messaging includes:

➤ a production organ
➤ a hormone
➤ a target organ

Commonly mentioned hormones include adrenalin, insulin and testosterone.

There are two associated types of hormone producing cells that are sometimes included within the endocrine system, *paracrines* and *autocrines*. The inclusion of these chemical messengers is not strictly correct, however, for their hormones take effect close to (paracrines), or at (autocrines), the site of production, rather than travelling some distance within the body to take effect, as is the case with endocrines. Paracrines are local messengers and secrete hormones into the extracellular fluid around their cell with target cells very close and so consequently their hormones do not need to enter the bloodstream. Autocrines secrete hormones that have an effect on the same cell from which they are produced. For example the **eicosanoids** (fatty acid-based hormones), which exert control over many bodily functions, primarily immune function and inflammation, are released by nearly all cells and typically take their effect locally and therefore act as autocrines or paracrines. Normally, however, hormones are carried in the blood to the target cells, for example, erythropoietin (the hormone that stimulates erythrocyte production) is secreted from the kidneys and travels via the blood to the target cells in the bone marrow.

Endocrine organs

The organs of the endocrine system can be seen in Figure 4.13. The primary function of those within the

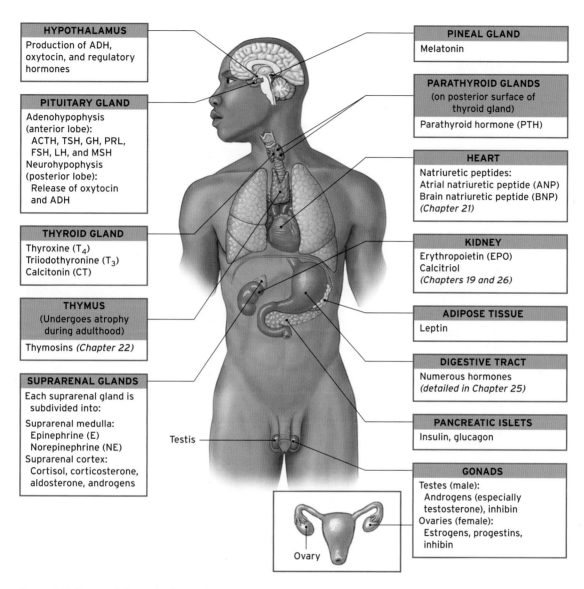

HYPOTHALAMUS
Production of ADH, oxytocin, and regulatory hormones

PITUITARY GLAND
Adenohypophysis (anterior lobe):
ACTH, TSH, GH, PRL, FSH, LH, and MSH
Neurohypophysis (posterior lobe):
Release of oxytocin and ADH

THYROID GLAND
Thyroxine (T_4)
Triiodothyronine (T_3)
Calcitonin (CT)

THYMUS
(Undergoes atrophy during adulthood)
Thymosins *(Chapter 22)*

SUPRARENAL GLANDS
Each suprarenal gland is subdivided into:
Suprarenal medulla:
Epinephrine (E)
Norepinephrine (NE)
Suprarenal cortex:
Cortisol, corticosterone, aldosterone, androgens

PINEAL GLAND
Melatonin

PARATHYROID GLANDS
(on posterior surface of thyroid gland)
Parathyroid hormone (PTH)

HEART
Natriuretic peptides:
Atrial natriuretic peptide (ANP)
Brain natriuretic peptide (BNP)
(Chapter 21)

KIDNEY
Erythropoietin (EPO)
Calcitriol
(Chapters 19 and 26)

ADIPOSE TISSUE
Leptin

DIGESTIVE TRACT
Numerous hormones
(detailed in Chapter 25)

PANCREATIC ISLETS
Insulin, glucagon

GONADS
Testes (male):
Androgens (especially testosterone), inhibin
Ovaries (female):
Estrogens, progestins, inhibin

Testis

Ovary

Figure 4.13 Organs of the endocrine system.

purple-headed boxes, such as the thyroid gland, is endocrine and so they are classified within the endocrine system. Other organs, however, such as the heart and kidneys, have a separate primary role in addition to their endocrine function. The total weight of the endocrine organs is relatively small, around 0.5 kg in an adult; however, their importance to the body as a control system is considerable. Organs with an endocrine function, examples of hormones they produce and target cells for each specific hormone are shown in Table 4.1. The hypothalamus represents the controlling mechanism for endocrine function, and along with the pituitary gland is responsible for the production of 16 hormones (nine from the hypothalamus and seven from the pituitary gland) which regulate growth, maturation, metabolism

and homeostatic balance. The hypothalamus is the interaction point between the endocrine and nervous system, for not only is it the driver of endocrine function, but it also controls autonomic nervous system functions. In its role within the nervous system it is responsible for controlling homeostatic processes such as body temperature, thirst and hunger. The hypothalamus integrates sensory information received from receptors throughout the body, and determines an endocrine and/or autonomic response as required. As a result of its dual nervous and endocrine system functions, the hypothalamus is referred to as a **neuroendocrine organ**

It has recently been shown that both adipose tissue (reviewed in Singla et al. 2010) and skeletal muscle (reviewed in Pedersen & Febbraio, 2008) have endocrine

Table 4.1 Organs with an endocrine function, their hormone and target cells for hormone effect.

Organ	Hormone	Function	Target cells
Hypothalamus	Releasing hormones Inhibiting hormones	Increase and decrease the functioning of the pituitary gland	Pituitary gland
Pituitary gland	Growth hormone	Stimulates growth and development of all body tissues	All cells
	Prolactin	Stimulates milk production in breast feeding mothers	Breasts
	Antidiuretic hormone	Plays a major role in reducing water excretion by kidneys	Kidneys
	Endorphins	Involved in providing pain relief for the brain	Brain
	Oxytocin	Assists during childbirth with the regulation of uterus contraction	Uterus
Pineal gland	Melatonin	Regulates sleep cycles by increasing the desire to sleep	Brain
Thyroid	Thyroxine	Increases metabolism and heart rate	All cells
	Calcitonin	Decreases blood levels of calcium and phosphate	Bones, kidneys
Parathyroid glands	Parathyroid hormone	Increases calcium levels in interstitial fluid and blood	Bones, kidneys small intestine
Thymus	Thymosin	Promotes and maintains immune function	All cells
Adrenal medulla	Adrenalin	Increases breakdown of glycogen and fats, heart rate, O_2 consumption	Most cells
	Noradrenalin	Increases lipid breakdown (lipolysis) and blood pressure	Most cells
Adrenal cortex	Aldosterone	Increases sodium retention and potassium excretion	Kidneys
	Cortisol	Anti-inflammatory and plays a role in control of metabolism	Most cells
Kidneys	Erythropoietin	Stimulates red blood cell (erythrocyte) production	Bone marrow
Pancreas	Insulin	Increases glucose uptake from the bloodstream	All cells
	Glucagon	Promotes release of glucose in to the bloodstream	All cells
	Somatostatin	Decreases glucagon and Insulin production	Pancreas
Gonads			
• Testes	Testosterone	Promotes muscle growth and development of male sex characteristics	Sex organs, muscles
• Ovaries	Oestrogen Progesterone	Promote development of female sex characteristics, regulate menstrual cycle and adipose tissue growth	Sex organs, adipocytes
• Placenta	Gonadotrophin	Stimulates testosterone production in the foetus - promoting growth	Foetal testes
• Platelets	Serotonin	Binds sites on sodium channels - promotes depolarisation	All cells

functions. In addition to its primary role as an energy store, adipose tissue has been found to be an important source of various hormones. Several of these hormones play important roles in weight control, such as leptin, resistin, visfatin and adiponectin. In 2005, Pedersen & Febbraio first suggested that skeletal muscle be termed an endocrine organ, due to the discovery that contracting skeletal muscle is a major source of the circulatory cytokine **interleukin-6**

(IL-6), an intercellular signalling molecule with a role in inflammation. The term 'myokines' is now commonly used to refer to substances (cytokines or other peptides) released by skeletal muscle during physical activity. It is thought that some myokines work in a hormone-like fashion, exerting effects in other tissues such as adipose tissue and the liver, whereas others will work in a paracrine or autocrine manner. The discovery of myokine release during exercise contributes to our understanding of why regular physical activity is important for the protection against a range of chronic diseases.

Function of hormones

Hormones regulate the functioning of the body by impacting upon processes such as growth, metabolism, reproduction, and circadian rhythms. There are two main groups of hormones based on chemical structure, those that are lipid (steroid) based and those that are protein-based (further classified as amino acid derivatives, peptide, polypeptide or protein hormones depending on their molecular size). Table 4.2 provides details of some of the most common hormones, their classification and the organ that produces them. The majority of hormones are produced by a host cell and secreted into the extracellular fluid and from there diffuse into the blood where they are carried to their target cells.

Lipid-based and protein-based hormones are both carried in the blood to their target cells. However, they differ as to the method by which they are transported and how they are received by their target cells. An illustration of lipid- and protein-derived hormone transport and message entry to a target cell is provided in Figure 4.14. As a result of their insolubility in water, lipid-based hormones attach to carrier proteins for transport within the blood. As they reach the target cell they disconnect from the carrier protein, which is left in the bloodstream to bind with other lipid-based hormones, and diffuse into the extracellular fluid surrounding the target cell. Upon reaching the plasma membrane of the target cell, lipid-based hormones diffuse into the cell and attach to an intracellular receptor on the nuclear membrane (Figure 4.14). In contrast, protein-based hormones (e.g. human growth hormone) travel unbound in the blood and, upon reaching the target cell, diffuse into the extracellular fluid and attach to extracellular receptors (a trans-membrane protein) on the surface of the target cell plasma membrane. The binding of a protein-based hormone to the receptor causes the release of a secondary messenger within the cell that stimulates the desired response (Figure 4.14). Cells typically have between 2,000–10,000 receptors for each hormone it requires as part of its functioning and regulation.

An example of hormone functioning can be found in the actions of glucagon and insulin, both of which are produced by the pancreas. The level of glucose within the bloodstream is regulated by the secretion of glucagon and insulin. The control process is carried out by way of

negative feedback. Following eating and the subsequent digestion of carbohydrates, blood glucose levels rise above normal creating a hyperglycaemic state which stimulates the β (beta) **cells** of the pancreas to produce insulin.

Table 4.2 Classification of some well-known hormones.

Hormone	Hormone classification	Produced by
Protein-based hormones		
Growth hormone	Protein	Pituitary gland
Insulin	Protein	Pancreas
Prolactin	Protein	Pituitary gland
Antidiuretic hormone	Polypeptide	Pituitary gland
Glucagon	Polypeptide	Pancreas
Somatostatin	Polypeptide	Pancreas
Endorphins	Polypeptide	Pituitary gland
Oxytocin	Polypeptide	Pituitary gland
Adrenalin	Amino acid derivative	Adrenal medulla
Noradrenalin	Amino acid derivative	Adrenal medulla
Serotonin	Amino acid derivative	Platelets
Melatonin	Amino acid derivative	Pineal gland
Thyroxine	Amino acid derivative	Thyroid
Erythropoietin	Glycoprotein	Kidneys
Parathyroid hormone	Glycoprotein	Parathyroid glands
Thyroid stimulating hormone	Glycoprotein	Pituitary gland
Lipid-based-hormones		
Testosterone	Steroid	Testes
Oestrogen	Steroid	Ovaries
Progesterone	Steroid	Ovaries
Aldosterone	Steroid	Adrenal cortex
Cortisol	Steroid	Adrenal cortex
Prostaglandins	Fatty acid derivative	All cells but RBC
Leukotrienes	Fatty acid derivative	All cells but RBC

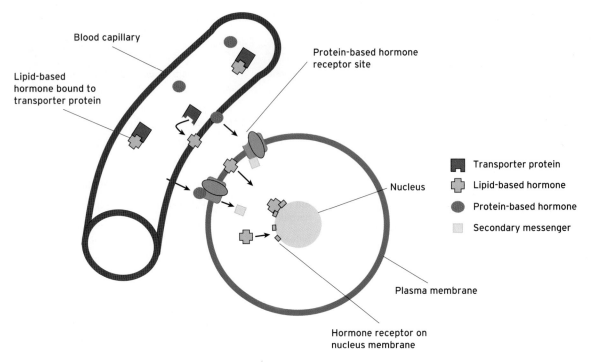

Figure 4.14 Processes through which lipid-based and protein-based hormones pass their message to the nucleus of a target cell.

Insulin diffuses into the blood and takes its effect on the many cells throughout the body, especially those of the liver and skeletal muscles, stimulating them to take up glucose and form glycogen (glycogenesis). As a result, the level of glucose in the blood decreases. This change is detected by receptors in the blood which relay information to the brain. When glucose levels return to normal there is no longer a need for insulin production and so the brain signals to the pancreas to discontinue insulin secretion (negative feedback). Glucagon, produced by pancreatic α (alpha) **cells**, is secreted at times of low blood glucose (hypoglycaemia). As blood glucose is used as an immediate energy source, levels will fall during a long training session. Detection of this change by the brain results in the stimulation of the pancreas to secrete glucagon which, following diffusion into the blood, takes effect on the hepatocytes of the liver. The liver, along with the muscles, is a major store of glycogen. When the muscles are exercising glucagon stimulates the liver to covert its glycogen back to glucose (glycogenolysis) and release it into the blood. Glucagon has an additional effect in the blood, for not only does it stimulate glycogenolysis, it also stimulates the conversion of lactic acid (produced during exercise) and amino acids to glucose through the process of gluconeogenesis in the liver. When blood glucose levels reach normal the secretion of glucagon is inhibited (negative feedback).

> ### Key point
>
> Hormones target specific cells and change the functioning of those cells.
>
> Hormones impact upon metabolism, growth, immune function, the body's internal environment and many other aspects of human functioning.

4.3 Acute responses to exercise

The metabolic requirements of the body at rest are low. These requirements, however, are greatly enhanced during exercise with the oxygen consumption of skeletal muscle increasing by up to 40-fold during intense exercise. In addition to the increased demand for oxygen, the active skeletal muscles must oxidise a greater amount of fuel for the generation of ATP required for muscle contraction, hence glucose and fats are mobilised from the body's stores. Many physiological responses within the body are altered during exercise to meet the increased metabolic demands, particularly of skeletal muscle. As we have discussed in this chapter, alterations to the body systems are under the control of both the nervous system and the endocrine system.

At the start of exercise, the sympathetic nervous system is the key driver of the physiological changes within the body, having immediate effects on the cardiovascular and respiratory systems, the details of which will be discussed in Chapter 6. The sympathetic nervous system also stimulates endocrine function resulting in the release of exercise-related hormones. These hormones provide a less immediate, but longer-enduring, reinforcement of stimulation initiated by the sympathetic nervous system. The hormonal response to exercise is mainly associated with increases in the cardiovascular response, metabolism and substrate availability through the increased release and action of the catecholamines (adrenaline and noradrenaline), thyroxine, cortisol, glucagon and human growth hormone. The roles of these hormones in the control of metabolism and substrate availability, particularly relating to skeletal muscle tissue, are discussed in Chapter 5 (The movement systems) while their role in the functioning of the cardiovascular system are discussed in Chapter 6 (The transport and exchange systems).

Key point

The alterations to body system function with exercise are under the control of the nervous system and the endocrine system, which work together to increase the transport and exchange of metabolites, and to increase fuel substrate availability.

Knowledge integration question

Describe what happens to your body at the start of exercise.

Check your recall
Fill in the missing words.

➤ The human body has two control and regulatory systems: the nervous system (immediate response) and the _____ _____ (slow, prolonged response).

➤ Under control of these systems, the body is able to maintain _____, a stable internal environment, required for cell survival.

➤ The _____ system functions in the control of metabolic activity, and initiates the breakdown of glycogen to glucose when blood glucose levels fall during prolonged exercise.

➤ The nervous system comprises of the brain, _____ _____, ganglia, nerves and sensory receptors.

➤ These components are often divided into the _____ nervous system (the brain and spinal cord) and the peripheral nervous system.

➤ The peripheral nervous system (PNS) can also be further divided into the _____ division, which carries information to the central nervous system (CNS), and the _____ division, which carries signals away from the CNS.

➤ Another useful distinction is to divide the nervous system into the _____ nervous system, over which we have conscious control, and the autonomic nervous system, which functions without our conscious control.

➤ The autonomic nervous system has _____ and _____ divisions, which speed up (_____) and slow down (_____) the body's autonomic responses.

➤ There are two types of cell that make up the nervous system: neurons and _____. The junction between two neurons is referred to as a _____.

➤ The electrical impulse in the pre-synaptic neuron triggers the release of a chemical messenger known as a _____ which is capable of crossing the synaptic cleft and in turn triggers the electrical impulse in the post-synaptic neuron.

➤ The endocrine system is the second _____ and regulation system for the human body.

➤ It involves the transmission of chemical messengers, called _____, through the blood.

➤ These can be either protein-based or _____-based messengers.

➤ The _____ provides a junction between the two communication systems as the controlling mechanism for the autonomic nervous system and endocrine functioning. This junction ensures that the two systems respond in harmony.

➤ The initiation of exercise induces a rapid increase in the _____ nervous activity. This is by the release of exercise-related _____ (adrenaline, noradrenaline, cortisol, human growth hormone, thyroxine, glucagon).

➤ Together, the _____ and _____ systems function to increase the transport and exchange of metabolites and to enhance the availability of fuel substrates.

Review questions

1. How are messages transmitted by the nervous system? How do electrical and chemical processes contribute to communication?

2. How do myelinated and unmyelinated neurons differ? What advantages do myelinated neurons have?

3. What is the difference in the function of neurons and neuroglia?

4. How is the resting membrane potential established?

5. Describe the propagation of an action potential along both a myelinated and unmyelinated axon.

6. What are the components of endocrine messaging?

7. What is the difference between endocrine, paracrine and autocrine signalling?

8. Name five hormones, their site of production and their target cells.

9. How is a lipid-based hormone transported from the organ of production to the target cells?

10. Describe the differences between the sympathetic and parasympathetic divisions.

Teach it!
In groups of three, choose one topic and teach it to the rest of the study group.

1. Explain, using a diagram, the divisions within the nervous system and the function of each component.

2. Explain how an action potential can arise and how it travels along a neuron.

3. Choosing one example, explain how a hormone can take its effect on cells within the body. Describe the components of endocrine messaging (for that hormone) and how it is regulated.

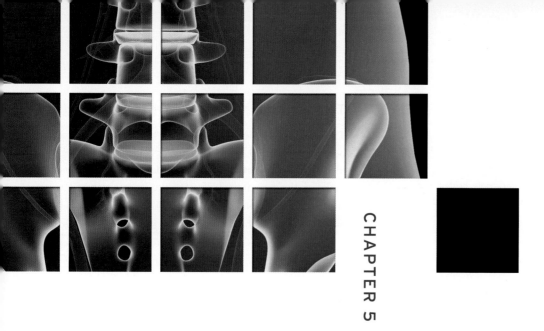

CHAPTER 5

The movement systems:
skeletal and muscular

Learning objectives

After reading, considering and discussing with a study partner the material in this chapter you should be able to:

➤ **discuss the functions of the skeletal system**

➤ **describe the structure of the different types of bones within the body**

➤ **explain the different types of joints found within the body**

➤ **identify the different types of muscle tissue**

➤ **summarise the gross and microscopic structure of muscle tissue**

➤ **teach others about the functioning of neuromuscular junctions**

➤ **summarise excitation-contraction coupling**

➤ **teach others the sliding filament theory and how this is thought to bring about muscular contraction**

➤ **highlight the differences between the different muscle fibre types**

➤ **describe the different types of muscular contraction**

The movement of the human body is elicited by the contraction of skeletal muscle pulling against a system of levers, the skeletal system. As we all know from everyday life and sports performance, the speed and force of a movement can vary depending on the situation. The structure and function of the skeletal system is covered in the first section of this chapter, followed by discussion of the muscular system, including muscle structure and muscular contraction, in section two. In the final section, the response of skeletal muscle to acute exercise, in relation to the increased demands for oxygen and fuel substrates, is covered.

5.1 The skeletal system

As we move on to cover the organ systems, the tables on the inside cover of the textbook may be helpful for learning the different anatomical terms and also their meaning. Understanding the language and the different directional terms used within anatomy will help greatly with learning about each of the systems. As was shown in Chapter 3 (Figure 3.1), organ systems, of which the skeletal system is one, are comprised of different organs that work closely together. The skeletal system includes the bones that form the skeleton and the joints, plus the cartilage and ligaments that stabilise and connect them. It typically represents around 20% of our total bodyweight. In common with the other 10 systems of the body, in its most basic units, the skeletal system is comprised of elements and molecules found within our diet. Along with carbon, hydrogen, oxygen and nitrogen, the elements calcium and phosphorus, as mentioned in Chapter 2, are vital minerals for the development of bones and together comprise two-thirds of their structure.

Key point

The body is composed of 206 bones which serve to support and protect other organs in the body.

Bones are a store of minerals and triglycerides ; they are also the production site for red and white blood cells and platelets.

The skeleton

The 206 bones which form the adult human skeleton can be seen in Figure 5.1. The skeleton is commonly divided into the **axial skeleton**, which includes the 80 bones that make up the core of the body (the skull, vertebrae and ribs), and the **appendicular skeleton**, which comprises the 126 bones that make up the pectoral girdle (shoulders),

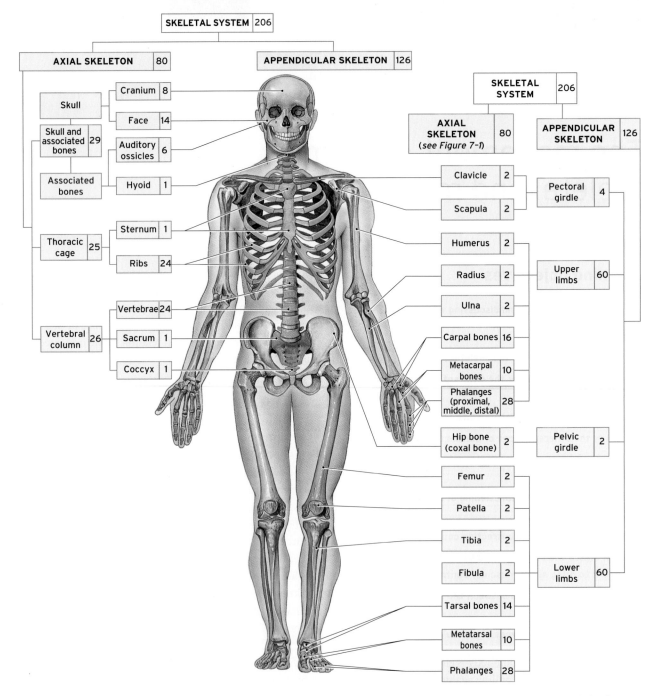

Figure 5.1 The human skeleton. (*Source*: Adapted from Figures 7.1 and 8.1, Martini, F. H. and Nath, J. L. (2009) *Fundamentals of Anatomy and Physiology*, 8th edition, New York: Benjamin Cummings)

pelvic girdle (hips) and four limbs. The skeletal system serves five main functions within the body:

- *Support*: To provide structural support for the body, including a framework for muscle attachment.
- *Protection*: The skeletal system provides protection for the soft tissues and organs of the body, for example, the thoracic cage protects the heart and lungs.
- *Movement*: Muscles, through their attachment via tendons to the skeleton, use bones as levers to bring about movement.
- *Storage*: The skeletal system provides a store for the mineral ions calcium and phosphate, and the yellow marrow within bone cavities serves as an additional triglyceride store.

- *Production*: The red marrow at the heart of bones is the production centre for red cells, white blood cells and platelets (the latter are involved in blood clotting).

Figure 5.2 illustrates the classification system for bones which is based on their shape. Bones are typically classified into five main types, *long bones* such as the humerus and femur, *short bones* like those of the wrist and the talus bone in the ankle, *flat bones* which include the ribs and sternum, *irregular bones* such as the vertebrae and *sesamoid bones* (shaped like sesame seeds) of which the patella is an example. In some textbooks sutural bones are identified as a sixth bone type.

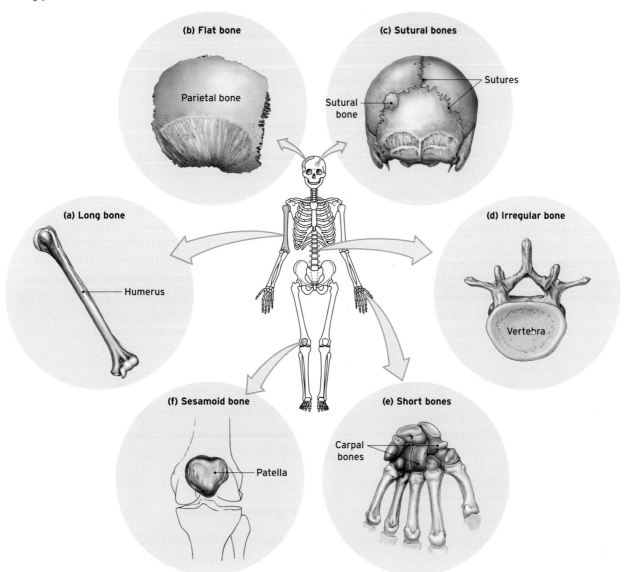

Figure 5.2 Classification of bones on the basis of shape. (*Source*: Martini, F. H. and Nath, J. L. (2009) *Fundamentals of Anatomy and Physiology*, 8th edition, New York: Benjamin Cummings)

The bones within the skeletal system do not have a uniform surface. When examined closely they have a large number of projections, depressions and openings within them that serve a variety of functions. Table 5.1 provides an overview of the main markings and shapes that can be found on bones. As can be seen from the table, the projections on bones provide sites for muscle and ligament attachment and are shaped to form the joints where bones meet. Bones are a living tissue and consequently have depressions and openings within them to enable the passage of blood vessels and nerves.

Bone physiology

The outward appearance of bone may suggest an inert material but, in the body, bone is a highly vascularised dynamic material that is continuously being remodelled dependent on several factors, including mechanical stresses and hormonal influences. Bone is a specialised, dense connective tissue which is relatively hard and lightweight. Its primary component is a mineral matrix of calcium phosphate (hydroxyapatite) crystals and bone cells (for more detail refer to Chapter 7 and the section on bone growth). The mineral matrix gives bone its rigidity and high compressive strength, however. On its own, bone would be brittle and unable to cope with pulling or torsional (twisting) forces. The combination of the mineral matrix with collagen, which makes up around 30% of bone, gives bone a degree of elasticity, reducing its brittleness.

Compact bone

Bone is deceptively light due to the numerous spaces within its structure. Depending on the size and distribution of these spaces, bone can be classified as either **compact** (dense) or **spongy** (trabecular, cancellous). Compact bone which has minimal gaps and spaces, accounts for 80% of the bone mass of an adult skeleton. It forms the hard outer regions of all bones, and the diaphysis (shaft) of long bones, and gives them a smooth, solid appearance. Compact bone is arranged in functional units called **osteons**, or **Haversian systems**, which consist of a central canal encircled by concentric rings (**lamellae**) of a hard intercellular substance. Small spaces (**lacunae**) exist between these rings and enclose **osteocytes** (mature bone cells). Nutrients and waste products are transported to and from osteocytes through a network of canals (**canaliculi**) connecting the lamellae. Compact bone provides strength and protection for bones and is a particular feature of long bones (see Figure 5.3).

Spongy bone

Spongy bone lies internally to compact bone and forms the remaining 20% of bone mass. However, its surface area is nearly ten times that of compact bone. The composition of spongy bone is similar to that of compact bone, but it is within the structural organisation of the bone that the two types differ. Spongy bone is an irregular lattice of thin plates of bone (**trabeculae**) (it has no functional unit) and contains many more gaps and spaces (sponge-like in its appearance) than compact bone (see Figure 5.3). The less dense nature of spongy bone allows bones to be lighter in weight, making them easier for muscles to move, while maintaining rigidity.

Long bone structure

The structure of a typical long bone, the humerus, is shown in Figure 5.3. It is constructed of compact and spongy bone. Compact bone is found on the outer surface, and within the diaphysis (shaft), of a long bone. Spongy bone is found within the epiphyses (heads) of the long bone, making the

Table 5.1 The topography of bones.

General Description	Anatomical Term	Definition
Elevations and projections (general)	Process	Any projection or bump
	Ramus	An extension of a bone making an angle with the rest of the structure
Processes formed where tendons or ligaments attach	Trochanter	A large, rough projection
	Tuberosity	A smaller, rough projection
	Tubercle	A small, rounded projection
	Crest	A prominent ridge
	Line	A low ridge
	Spine	A pointed or narrow process
Processes formed for articulation with adjacent bones	Head	The expanded articular end of an epiphysis, separated from the shaft by a neck
	Neck	
	Condyle	A rounded projection on the bone surface which is involved in articulation
	Trochlea	A smooth, rounded articular process
	Facet	A smooth, grooved articular process shaped like a pulley
		A small, flat articular surface
Depressions	Fossa	A shallow depression
	Sulcus	A narrow groove
Openings	Foramen	A rounded passageway for blood vessels or nerves
	Canal or Meatus	A passageway through the substance of a bone
	Fissure	An elongated cleft
	Sinus or Antrum	A chamber within a bone, normally filled with air

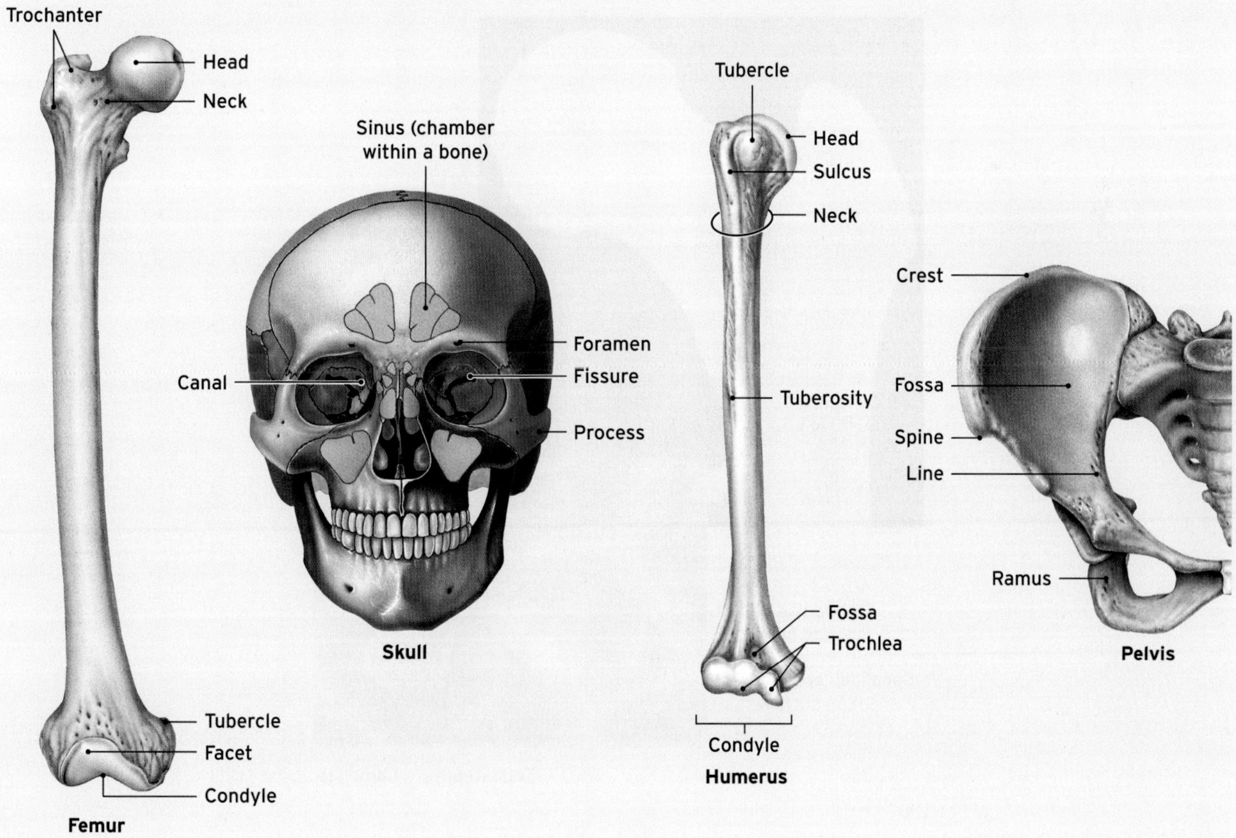

Trochanter
Head
Neck

Sinus (chamber within a bone)

Canal
Foramen
Fissure
Process

Skull

Tubercle
Head
Sulcus
Neck

Tuberosity

Fossa
Trochlea
Condyle

Humerus

Crest
Fossa
Spine
Line
Ramus

Pelvis

Tubercle
Facet
Condyle

Femur

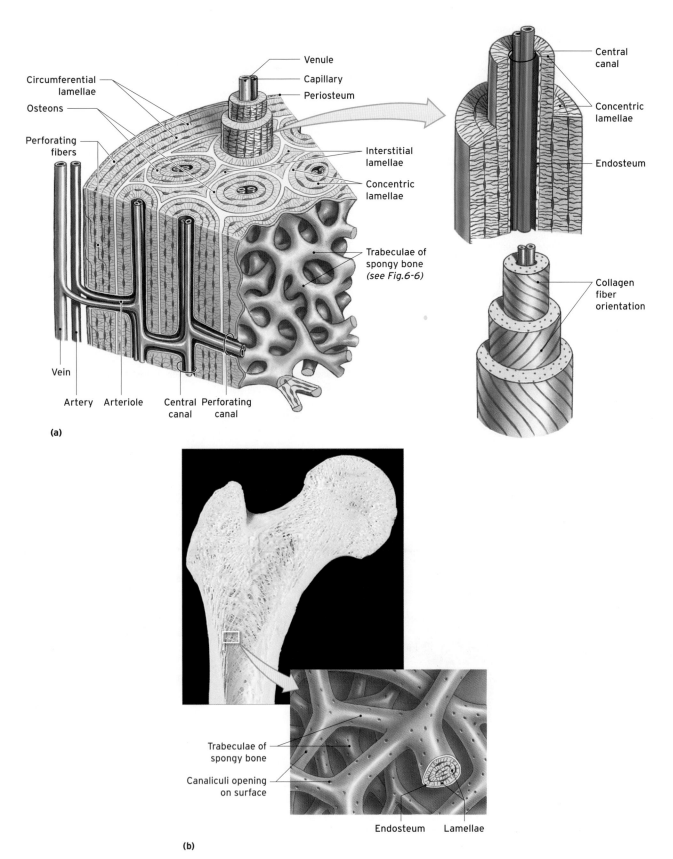

Figure 5.3 Structure of a long bone. (*Source*: Martini, F. H. and Nath, J. L. (2009) *Fundamentals of Anatomy and Physiology*, 8th edition, New York: Benjamin Cummings)

bone lighter and easier for muscles to move. Short, irregular and flat bones are made up in the main of spongy bone, surrounded by a thin layer of compact bone. The spaces in spongy bone contain the **red bone marrow**, where red blood cells, white blood cell and platelets are produced. The **yellow bone marrow**, where fat is stored in the form of triglycerides, is located within the **medullary cavity**, the central cavity within the diaphysis (bone shaft) of long bones. The medullary cavity is also the central tract for the passage of blood vessels to deliver blood to all parts of the bone. Each bone is surrounded by a connective tissue sheath, the **periosteum**, which protects the bone, helps with repair and presents the surface for ligament and tendon attachment. It is through the nutrient foramen in the periosteum that the blood vessels enter the diaphysis of the bone. For details of the three types of bone cell and bone growth, see Chapter 7.

Cartilage

Although much of the cartilage in the body is replaced by bone as the body develops, adults retain three types of cartilage which differ in composition according to their functions within the body (see Figure 5.4). **Hyaline cartilage** is the most common form of cartilage in the body and is comprised mainly of collagen. Collagen is a fibrous protein that gives this form of cartilage strength, toughness and smoothness. Hyaline cartilage is found at a variety of sites throughout the body including creating the articulating cartilage for joints. It also is the type of cartilage that forms the nose and the larynx as well as forming the joints between the sternum and the ribs. The cartilage that forms the ear and the epiglottis (flap that prevents food or fluid entering the lungs) is composed of **elastic cartilage** which is more flexible than hyaline cartilage due to the presence of the protein elastin. To help absorb the impact and loading on the body when jumping and landing and carrying heavy objects, a portion of the cartilage found in the knee and the cartilage forming the discs of the vertebrae consists of a specialised **fibrocartilage**. This form of cartilage, which is an intermediate cartilage, having a mix of the properties of hyaline and elastic cartilage, is strong but resistant to compression, such as that encountered when landing from a jump.

Joints

Joints or articulations are formed at the point where two or more bones come together, allowing movement and providing mechanical support. They can be classified either by their function or structure.

Classification of joints

Classification by function is based on the amount of movement, or range of motion, of the joint, with three subdivisions of function; **synarthroses** (*syn*, together and *arthros*, joint), **amphiarthroses** (*amyphi*, both sides) and **diarthroses** (*dia*, apart). Synarthrotic joints are extremely strong and located where movement is undesirable, for example the joints between skull bones or between the ribs and the sternum. An amphiarthrotic joint allows more movement than synarthrotic joints. However, it is still much less mobile, and much stronger, than a diarthrosis. The connection of the distal tibia and fibula by a ligament, and the articulation of vertebrae (separated by intervertebral discs) are examples of amphiarthrotic joints. The most freely moveable joints in the body are called diarthrotic, or more commonly, **synovial** joints. These joints are typically found at the ends of long bones and are discussed in more detail in the following sections.

When classified by structure, joints are distinguished by the tissues from which they are made and can be bony, fibrous, cartilaginous or synovial. Bony joints are rigid and completely immovable as two bones fuse together, as in the fusion of the epiphysis with the diaphysis of a long bone upon completion of longitudinal growth. In a fibrous joint the bones are joined by dense fibrous connective tissue and for cartilaginous joints the articulation between bones is made by either hyaline cartilage or a mixture of hyaline and fibrocartilage. Synovial joints are unique in that each articulation is contained within a fibrous capsule, the **articular capsule**, containing synovial fluid, and the articulating bones have a form of hyaline cartilage covering. It is this unique structure that enables synovial joints to move freely. Bony fusions and nearly all fibrous joints, such as the sutures (seams) found in the skull, are immovable synarthroses. Cartilaginous joints also tend not to allow movement although the pubic symphysis between the two pelvic bones is an example of a cartilaginous amphiarthrosis. Only synovial joints are freely moveable and are therefore examples of diarthroses.

Knowledge integration question

The skeletal system has a number of different functions. Explain how the different joint types can contribute to these functions.

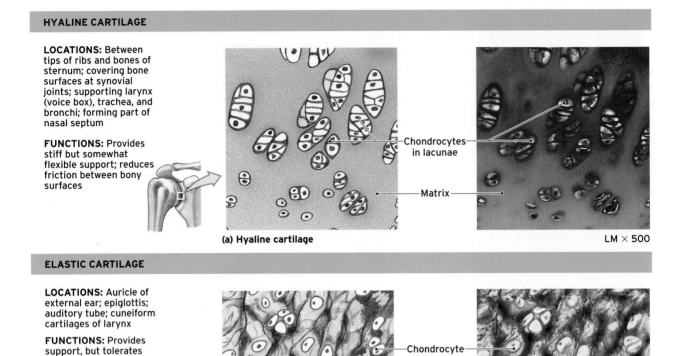

HYALINE CARTILAGE

LOCATIONS: Between tips of ribs and bones of sternum; covering bone surfaces at synovial joints; supporting larynx (voice box), trachea, and bronchi; forming part of nasal septum

FUNCTIONS: Provides stiff but somewhat flexible support; reduces friction between bony surfaces

Chondrocytes in lacunae

Matrix

(a) Hyaline cartilage

LM × 500

ELASTIC CARTILAGE

LOCATIONS: Auricle of external ear; epiglottis; auditory tube; cuneiform cartilages of larynx

FUNCTIONS: Provides support, but tolerates distortion without damage and returns to original shape

Chondrocyte in lacuna

Elastic fibers in matrix

(b) Elastic cartilage

LM × 358

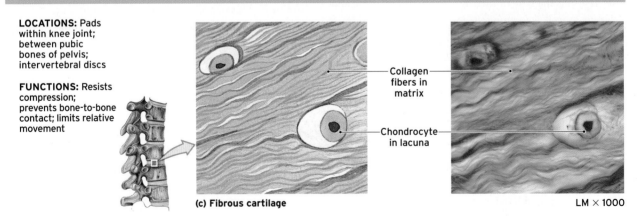

FIBROUS CARTILAGE

LOCATIONS: Pads within knee joint; between pubic bones of pelvis; intervertebral discs

FUNCTIONS: Resists compression; prevents bone-to-bone contact; limits relative movement

Collagen fibers in matrix

Chondrocyte in lacuna

(c) Fibrous cartilage

LM × 1000

Figure 5.4 Types of cartilage found in the human skeleton. (*Source*: Martini, F. H. and Nath, J. L. (2009) *Fundamentals of Anatomy and Physiology*, 8th edition, New York: Benjamin Cummings)

Synovial joints

Synovial articulation is central to the movement that skeletal muscles can bring about through contraction. There is a variety of synovial joints throughout the body that enable different degrees of movement, for example the elbow joint is less freely movable than the shoulder. As well as having a synovial cavity filled with fluid to lubricate and cushion the joint, and also articular cartilage on the bone ends, synovial joints have tendons and ligaments

Under normal conditions, the opposing bony surfaces within a synovial joint cannot contact one another, because these surfaces are covered by special articular cartilages, which are slick and smooth. This feature alone can reduce friction during movement at the joint. However, even when pressure is applied across a joint, the smooth articular cartilages do not touch one another, because they are separated by a thin film of synovial fluid within the joint cavity.

Components of Synovial Joints
Articular cartilages resemble hyaline cartilages elsewhere in the body. However, articular cartilages have no perichondrium, and the matrix contains more water than that of other cartilages.
The **joint capsule**, is dense and fibrous, and it may be reinforced with various accessory structures such as tendons or ligaments.
Synovial fluid within the joint cavity provides lubrication, cushions shocks, prevents abrasion, and supports the chondrocytes of the articular cartilages. Even in a large joint such as the knee, the total quantity of synovial fluid in a joint is normally less than 3 mL.

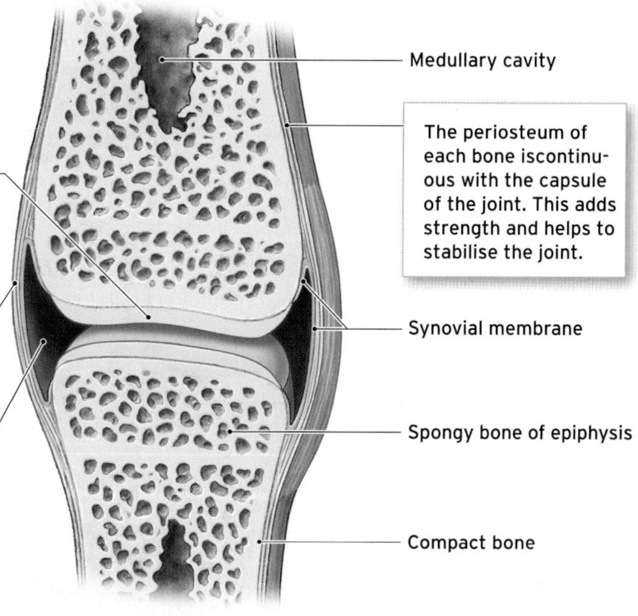

Medullary cavity

The periosteum of each bone iscontinuous with the capsule of the joint. This adds strength and helps to stabilise the joint.

Synovial membrane

Spongy bone of epiphysis

Compact bone

Figure 5.5 Generalised structure of a synovial joint.

to maintain their integrity. Figure 5.5 provides a generalised model of a synovial joint.

The different types of synovial joint are shown in Figure 5.6. **Gliding joints**, such as between the vertebrae in the spine or the sternoclavicular joint as illustrated, are formed when the flat surfaces of bones come together. The amount of movement in a gliding joint is minimal. The elbow, knee and ankle are examples of **hinge joints** that enable flexion and extension of the arm and leg along with dorsiflexion and plantar flexion of the foot. The atlanto-axial joint in the spine is an example of a **pivot joint** which enables the head to rotate and is formed between the odontoid peg or dens of the axis bone and the ring of the atlas. An example of **ellipsoid** or **condyloid joints** can be found between the arm and hand at the wrist which are called the radiocarpal joints. The wrist enables movement in two planes and is formed where a convex surface fits in to a concave surface.

A **saddle joint** can be found between the trapezium and first metacarpal in the thumb. In this joint the trapezium forms the saddle and the first metacarpal the 'rider's legs'. The joint allows the thumb to circumduct (move in a circle) but not rotate. The **ball and socket joints** of the shoulder and hip – pectoral and pelvic girdles – enable the greatest range of movement of any synovial joint. These joints enable abduction (moving limb away from midline), adduction (moving limb to midline), flexion, extension, circumduction and rotation. Examples of the different types of movement that can occur at a joint, such as flexion and extension, are provided in Appendix A.

The knee joint

A detailed illustration of the knee joint, the most complex joint in the body, is provided in Figure 5.7. The knee is in fact made up of three joints or articulations. One joint is formed between the patella and the femur and the other two are formed at the junctions of the lateral condyle and the medial condyle of the femur with the tibia. To facilitate smooth articulation, the condyles of the femur articulate on a combination of the lateral and medial **menisci** (fibrocartilage) of the tibia and the tibial articular cartilage (hyaline cartilage). The joint is held together by a complex arrangement of intracapsular and extracapsular ligaments and tendons. The anterior and posterior cruciate ligaments, which are contained within the synovial capsule, protect against forward and backward displacement of

TYPES OF SYNOVIAL JOINTS		MOVEMENT	EXAMPLES
Gliding joint 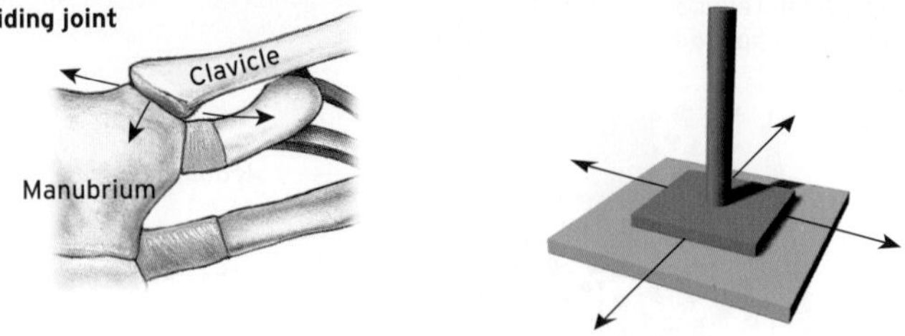 Clavicle, Manubrium		Slight nonaxial or multiaxial	• Acromioclavicular and claviculosternal joints • Intercarpal and intertarsal joints • Vertebrocostal joints • Sacroiliac joints
Hinge joint 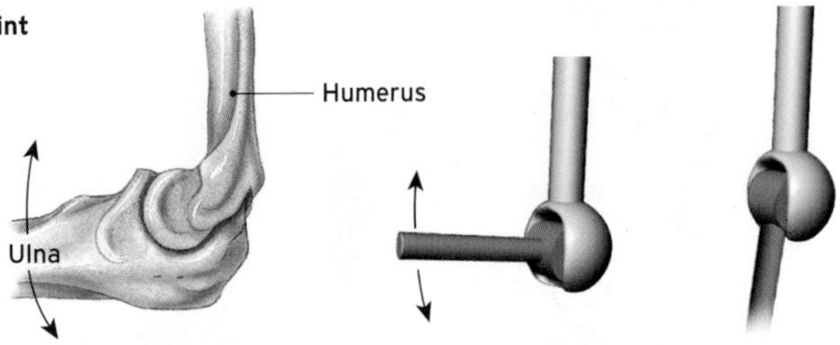 Humerus, Ulna		Monaxial	• Elbow joint • Knee joint • Ankle joint • Interphalangeal joint
Pivot joint 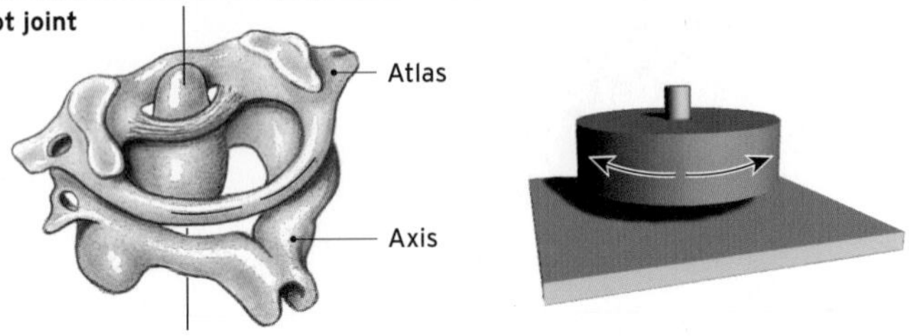 Atlas, Axis		Monaxial (rotation)	• Atlas/axis • Proximal radio-ulnar joint
Ellipsoid joint 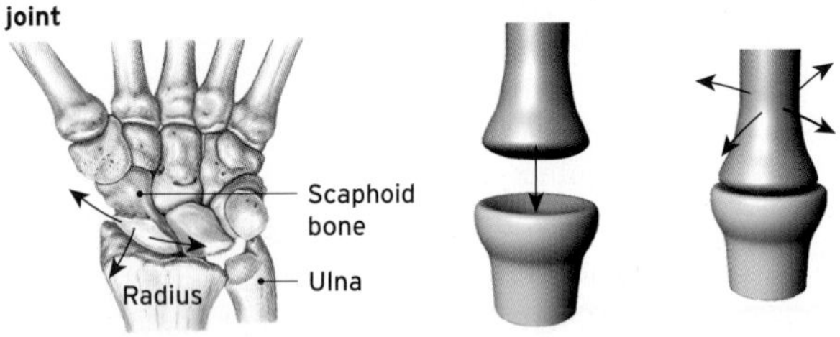 Scaphoid bone, Ulna, Radius		Biaxial	• Radiocarpal joint • Metacarpophalangeal joints 2–5 • Metatarsophalangeal joints
Saddle joint 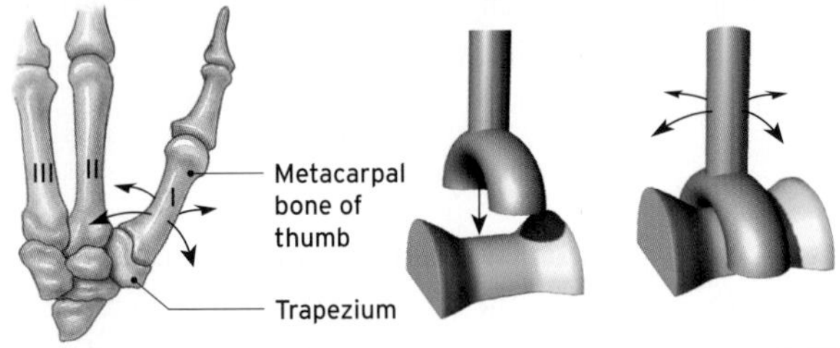 Metacarpal bone of thumb, Trapezium		Biaxial	• First carpometacarpal joint
Ball-and-socket joint 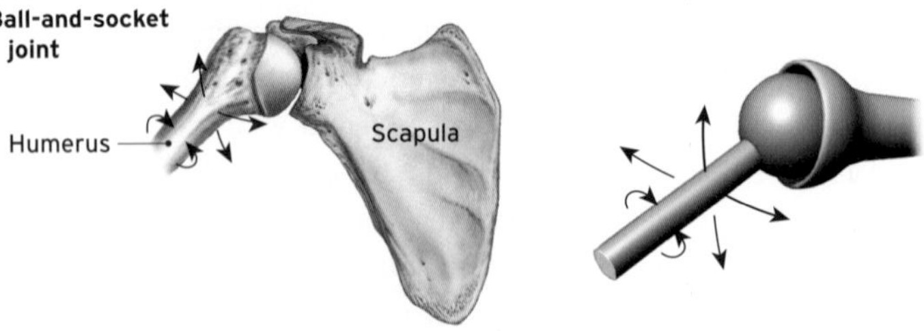 Humerus, Scapula		Triaxial	• Shoulder joint • Hip joint

This visual summary gives representative examples of the various anatomical classes of synovial joints based on the shapes of the articulating surfaces. It relates articular structure to simplified joint models and lists examples of each group of joints.

Figure 5.6 Types of synovial joint.

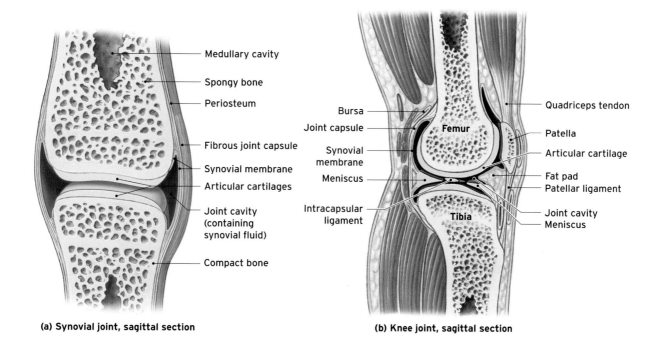

(a) Synovial joint, sagittal section

Medullary cavity
Spongy bone
Periosteum
Fibrous joint capsule
Synovial membrane
Articular cartilages
Joint cavity (containing synovial fluid)
Compact bone

(b) Knee joint, sagittal section

Bursa
Joint capsule
Synovial membrane
Meniscus
Intracapsular ligament
Femur
Tibia
Quadriceps tendon
Patella
Articular cartilage
Fat pad
Patellar ligament
Joint cavity
Meniscus

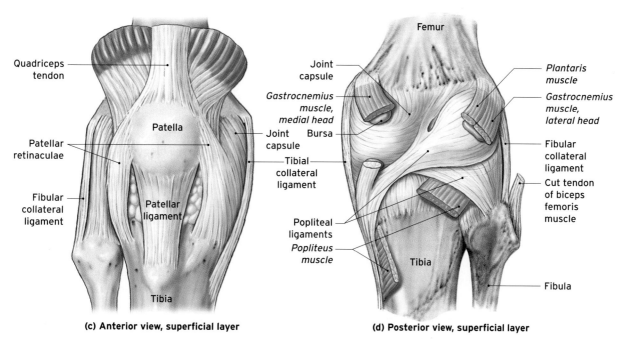

(c) Anterior view, superficial layer

Quadriceps tendon
Patellar retinaculae
Fibular collateral ligament
Patella
Patellar ligament
Tibia
Joint capsule
Tibial collateral ligament

(d) Posterior view, superficial layer

Femur
Joint capsule
Gastrocnemius muscle, medial head
Bursa
Popliteal ligaments
Popliteus muscle
Tibia
Plantaris muscle
Gastrocnemius muscle, lateral head
Fibular collateral ligament
Cut tendon of biceps femoris muscle
Fibula

Figure 5.7 Structure of the knee joint. (*Source*: Martini, F. H. and Nath, J. L. (2009) *Fundamentals of Anatomy and Physiology*, 8th edition, New York: Benjamin Cummings)

the tibia in relation to the femur, respectively. Outside the capsule and posterior to it, the joint is held together by the popliteal ligaments and the attachment of several muscles to the tibia and femur. On the anterior surface of the knee the quadriceps tendon, which encloses the patella, attaches to the tibia to further strengthen the joint. To the sides of the joint the tibial (medial) and fibular

(lateral) collateral ligaments protect against over rotation about the joint. Within the joint, around a dozen bursae (synovial-fluid-filled sacs) and fat pads provide further structural support and cushioning for the joint and help to further decrease friction between the bones. Together these structures enable flexion, extension and limited rotation.

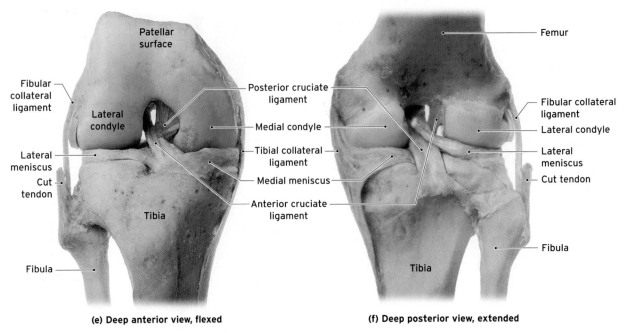

(e) Deep anterior view, flexed

(f) Deep posterior view, extended

Figure 5.7 *(continued)*

5.2 The muscular system

The skeletal and muscular systems are interrelated and are often known together as the **musculoskeletal system**. The attachment of muscles, across joints, to the bones of the skeleton allows for the movement of body parts upon muscle contraction. In addition to the importance for sports performance, a healthy musculoskeletal system helps to maintain a high quality of life, allowing us to complete our everyday tasks. This section of the chapter covers the different types of muscle tissue before focusing on the structure and function of skeletal muscle.

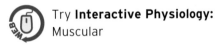

Try **Interactive Physiology:**
Muscular

Muscle tissue types and functions

Three types of muscle tissue can be found within the body: smooth, cardiac and skeletal muscle (Figure 5.8).

Muscle tissues, and the cells or fibres from which they are formed, are responsible for bringing about movement, whether it be movement of the body for playing sport, circulation of blood and nutrients around the body or the propulsion of foods through the digestive tract. The structure of each muscle tissue type differs according to its function. **Smooth muscle** is found throughout the body. It surrounds the blood vessels and airways and serves to assist with the passage of blood and air through the cardiovascular and respiratory systems. It is also part of the digestive tract walls where its contractions assist the movement of food along it. Smooth muscle, in common with cardiac muscle, is innervated by the autonomic nervous system and so we have little or no voluntary control over the contraction of these muscle groups. We cannot make the heart beat faster or push food through the digestive tract more quickly. **Cardiac muscle**, the muscle which forms the heart, is responsible for our heart beat and the subsequent pumping of blood and nutrients around the body. **Skeletal muscle** is the only muscle type that can be voluntarily contracted and is the form of tissue that enables bodily movement by contracting against the skeleton (hence the name). The human body is comprised of between 600 and 700 muscles which vary in size from 1 mm (such as those found attached to the bones of the ear) to 30 cm long in the sartorius muscle of the thigh.

Muscle Tissue

Several vital functions involve movement of one kind or another—movement of materials along the digestive tract, movement of blood around the cardiovascular system, or movement of the body from one place to another. Movement is produced by **muscle tissue**, which is specialized for contraction. There are three types of muscle tissue: skeletal muscle, cardiac muscle, and smooth muscle.

1 **Skeletal muscle tissue** is found in skeletal muscles, organs that also contain connective tissues and neural tissue. The cells are long, cylindrical, banded (**striated**), and have multiple nuclei (**multinucleate**).

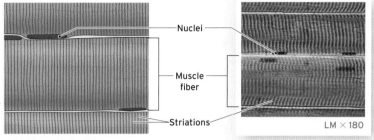

Nuclei

Muscle fiber

Striations

LM × 180

Skeletal muscles move or stabilise the position of the skeleton; guard entrances and exits to the digestive, respiratory, and urinary tracts; generate heat; and protect internal organs.

2 **Cardiac muscle tissue** is found only in the heart. The cells are short, branched, and striated, usually with a single nucleus; cells are interconnected at special-ised intercellular junctions called **intercalated discs.**

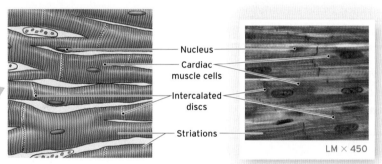

Nucleus

Cardiac muscle cells

Intercalated discs

Striations

LM × 450

Cardiac muscle moves blood and maintains blood pressure.

3 **Smooth muscle tissue** is found throughout the body. For example, smooth muscle is found in the skin, in the walls of blood vessels, and in many digestive, respiratory, urinary, and reproduc-tive organs. The cells are short, spindle-shaped, and nonstriated, with a single, central nucleus.

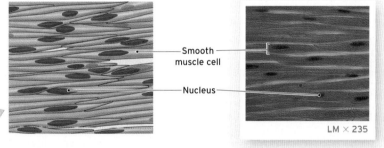
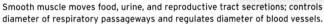

Smooth muscle cell

Nucleus

LM × 235

Smooth muscle moves food, urine, and reproductive tract secretions; controls diameter of respiratory passageways and regulates diameter of blood vessels.

Figure 5.8 The three types of muscle tissue.

Key point

There are three types of muscle tissue:

➤ skeletal

➤ smooth

➤ cardiac

Cardiac and skeletal muscle are **striated** (striped) in appearance, meaning they have microscopic light and dark patches within their structure. These striations are due to the specific arrangement of the proteins that enable muscular contraction. This will become clearer when the structure of skeletal muscle is discussed in the following section. As can be seen from Figure 5.8, smooth muscle is the only non-striated muscle tissue. While skeletal muscle tissue is multi-nucleate, due to its relatively long fibres, cardiac and smooth muscle fibres are shorter and have only one nucleus.

In addition to its role in movement, muscle tissue has several other functions. All are listed below.

- *movement* of both substances within the body (blood and food) and of the body as a whole.
- *stability* – the ability to stop the body moving to stabilise the body when standing or sitting.
- *storage* of oxygen and nutrients such as glycogen for energy production.
- *production of heat* – a by-product of energy-generating reactions that take place within muscle fibres, which serves to assist in the maintenance of body temperature.
- *protection* and *support* of vital organs, such as those in the abdomen, by the surrounding muscle tissue.
- *regulation* of sphincters at the entrance and exit of various tracts, such as the digestive and urinary tracts.

Skeletal muscle anatomy

When reading and talking about skeletal muscle many words are used that specifically relate to muscle. These are identified by the prefixes *myo*, meaning muscle, and *sarco* meaning flesh, which are commonly used for components of the muscular system. These prefixes let you know that a particular cellular component forms part of a muscle. Some examples include myoglobin, myofibre, myofibril, sarcomere, sarcoplasm and sarcolemma, all of which will be covered in the following sections.

Gross anatomy of skeletal muscle

Skeletal muscles are predominantly made up of skeletal muscle fibres, with blood vessels, nerve fibres, and connective tissue composing the remainder. As a very active organ requiring constant supplies of nutrients and oxygen, skeletal muscle is highly vascularised. The blood supply is also vital in the removal of waste products, a common one during high-intensity bouts of exercise being lactate. A skeletal muscle is served by a single nerve with the activity of each muscle fibre controlled by a neuron at the neuromuscular junction. The **epimysium** is a connective tissue sheath which surrounds the whole skeletal muscle. Within the muscle, groups of muscle fibres are bound together by the **perimysium** to form bundles called fascicles, within which each muscle fibre is protected by the **endomysium**. These three connective tissue sheaths are continuous with each

other and with the tendon or aponeurosis, that attaches the muscle to bone. These structures are illustrated in Figure 5.9. Upon muscle fibre contraction, a pulling force is transmitted from the sheaths, through the tendon, to the bone, resulting in movement.

The skeletal and muscular systems are either directly or indirectly connected. When directly connected, a muscle *epimysium* is fused directly with the bone's *periosteum*. Alternatively, an indirect connection is formed when the three layers of connective tissue surrounding each muscle form a tendon or aponeurosis that intermeshes with the skeletal periosteum. A **tendon** is a rope-like structure, whereas an **aponeurosis** is a flattened structure that enables connection over a wider area, which can include more than one bone.

Key point

The muscular and skeletal systems connect at tendons and aponeuroses.

Muscle fibre structure

Movement for sport performance is enabled due to the unique structure of skeletal muscle. Knowledge of the structure of muscle tissue, down to the microscopic level, is essential for understanding the physiology of muscular contraction. Muscular contraction is brought about at the cellular level through the interaction of specialised protein filaments within the muscle fibre, the cellular unit of muscular tissue.

Moving from the largest to smallest units, as can be seen in Figures 5.9 and 5.10, a *muscle* is made up of many hundreds or thousands of **fascicles**. Each fascicle contains anywhere from ten to hundreds of individual **muscle fibres** and each muscle fibre is made up of tiny **myofibrils** (little fibres) that run the length of the cell. Myofibrils enable muscular contraction through the arrangement of **myofilaments** (proteins) into specialised contraction units called **sarcomeres**. As already mentioned, a series of protective sheaths enclose each of these structures and together form the connection with the bone. Each muscle is enclosed within an epimysium, each fascicle within a perimysium and each muscle fibre by an endomysium. The **sarcolemma**, which encapsulates each muscle fibre, is contained within the endomysium that protects the muscle fibre. Unlike other cells, the nuclei and mitochondria in muscle fibres lie beneath the sarcolemma on the outside of the myofibrils.

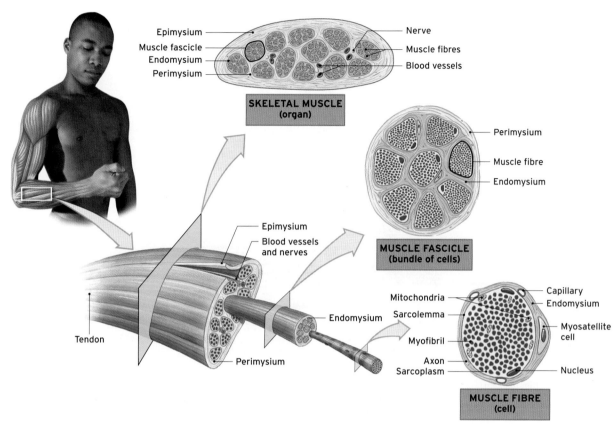

Figure 5.9 The structure of skeletal muscle. (*Source*: Martini, F. H. and Nath, J. L. (2009) *Fundamentals of Anatomy and Physiology*, 8th edition, New York: Benjamin Cummings)

Key point

The structure of a muscle can be broken down as follows:

Muscle – such as biceps to flex (bend) the arm, protected by epimysium

↓

Fascicle – groups of muscle fibres bound within the perimysium

↓

Muscle fibre (cell) – multinucleated fibres enclosed in the endomysium

↓

Myofibril – protein-based components that comprise the muscle fibre

↓

Sarcomere – contractile units within each myofibril

Sarcomeres – the contractile units of skeletal muscle

Each myofibril, the contractile fibre of the muscle cell, is composed of thousands of sarcomeres or contractile units. There are on average around 4,500 sarcomeres to every centimetre of a myofibril. The structure of a sarcomere is shown in Figure 5.10. Sarcomeres operate as individual contractile units, separated by **Z lines** or discs, and are comprised of over a dozen different proteins. The myofilaments, **actin** (thin) and **myosin** (thick), are the most common proteins found within the myofibril (refer to Figures 5.10 and 5.13). Other proteins found within the sarcomere that are important for contraction include **troponin** and **tropomyosin**. The structure and function of troponin and tropomyosin, in relation to actin, and how these proteins interact with myosin to bring about contraction, are described further in the following section. A further protein within each sarcomere is the large elastic protein **titin**, which runs the entire length of the sarcomere, holding the thick myosin filaments in place,

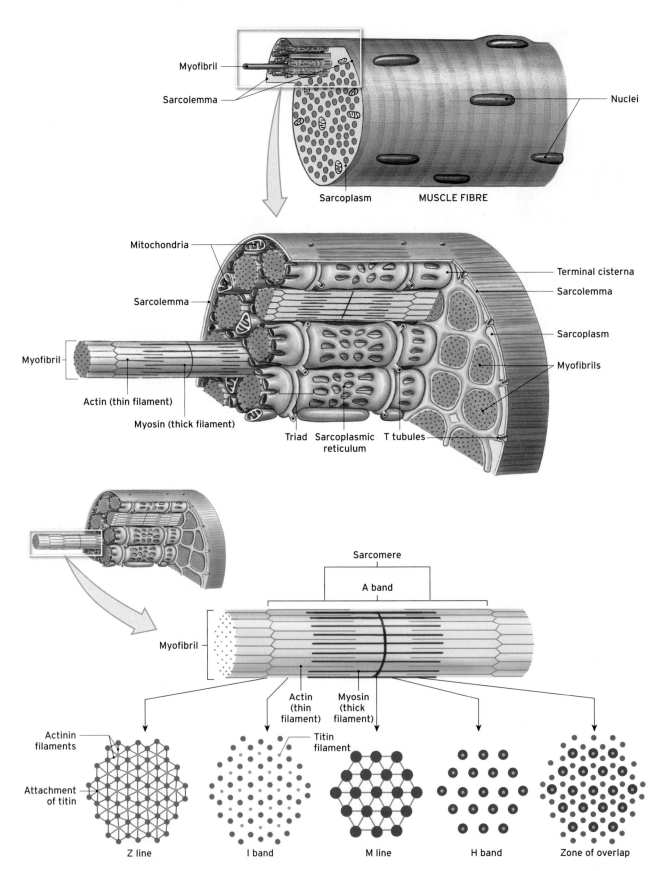

Figure 5.10 Myofibril structure. (*Source*: Martini, F. H. and Nath, J. L. (2009) *Fundamentals of Anatomy and Physiology*, 8th edition, New York: Benjamin Cummings)

and is thought to play an important role in the ability of muscle to be stretched without damage. **Desmin**, another sarcomere protein, is found to link adjacent Z lines, keeping them in place.

The sarcomeres in Figures 5.10 and 5.11 are shown at rest, with each part of the sarcomere labelled as a particular zone or band. As mentioned above, each sarcomere extends between two Z lines, with the **M line** representing the middle. The **I band** denotes the part of each sarcomere where only actin is present. The **A band** demarks the myosin filament location in each sarcomere, including the zone of overlap. The overlap between actin and myosin fibres at either end of the A band is essential for contraction. The **H zone** contains only myosin filaments, revealing the separation between the two sets of actin filaments attached to the Z lines at either end of a sarcomere. Sarcomere zones and bands are illustrated in Figure 5.10.

Knowledge integration question

Draw and describe the structure of a sarcomere.

The striated (striped) nature of skeletal muscle arises because of the presence of the thick myosin and the thin actin filaments. As can be seen from Figure 5.10, the *dark stripes* appear in the A band where both myosin and actin filaments are found, whereas the I bands form *lighter stripes* as they contain only the thinner actin filaments. Actin is a structural protein and forms the anchored part of the sarcomere, whereas myosin is a motor protein. The **Z lines** that separate sarcomeres are comprised of connective tissue within which the actin filaments are anchored.

The connective tissues of the Z lines form a thin dark stripe within the lighter I-bands.

 Try **Interactive Physiology:** Muscular: Anatomy review – skeletal muscle tissue

The tubular networks of muscle fibres

As illustrated in Figure 5.11, each myofibril is surrounded by two tubular networks, the **sarcoplasmic reticulum** (specialised endoplasmic reticulum) and the **T tubules**. The sarcoplasmic reticulum, as well as providing structure for the fibre, also stores and releases *calcium ions* which are essential to the process of muscular contraction. The network of tubules that runs from the sarcolemma, transversely across each muscle fibre, and encircles each sarcomere at the A band – I band junctions, is called the *transverse* or T tubules. As T tubules originate from an infolding of the sarcolemma, they are continuous with, and open to, the external environment of the cell. Consequently, each T tubule is filled with extracellular fluid. At the A band – I band junctions, sarcoplasmic reticulum is enlarged and forms a pair of **terminal cisternae**. As can be seen in Figure 5.11, it is between these terminal cisternae that the T tubule encircles the myofibril, forming triads (terminal cisterna, T tubule, terminal cisterna). The connection between T tubules and terminal cisternae at each triad, and their close proximity to individual myofibrils, are essential to the speed and coordination of muscular contraction.

 Try **Interactive Physiology:** Muscular: Anatomy review – skeletal muscle tissue

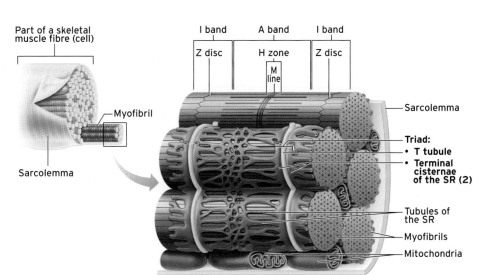

Figure 5.11 T tubules and sarcoplasmic reticulum (SR) encapsulating each myofibril. (*Source*: Martini, F. H. and Nath, J. L. (2009) *Fundamentals of Anatomy and Physiology*, 8th edition, New York: Benjamin Cummings)

Muscular contraction

Neural stimulus of muscle

To understand how muscular contraction is brought about, it is first important to understand how a muscle is *stimulated* to contract. Remember that nervous and muscle tissues are unique in that they are *excitable* – they can conduct an electrical current – hence stimulation of a muscle fibre at one point will rapidly lead to excitation of the whole fibre. The stimulus for muscular contraction comes from the nervous system, specifically motor neurons, and takes advantage of the excitable nature of these two tissues. When a muscular contraction is required for any movement, a nerve signal is sent to the necessary muscles to initiate the response. Once generated, a nerve impulse (or action potential) travels the length of a nerve very rapidly to reach the junction with the muscle fibres it innervates. At this junction, motor neurons divide into finger-like projections that enable one neuron to make contact with a number of muscle fibres.

A **motor unit** describes a motor neuron and all the muscle fibres it is responsible for innervating. Stimulation of a motor neuron, therefore, results in contraction of all the muscle fibres it innervates in an all-or-none fashion so they work together as a single unit. The size of motor units varies between muscles depending on the degree of control required by that muscle. Typically a nerve can stimulate anything from 6–10 individual muscle fibres for fine-control movements (such as muscles controlling the movement of the eye), to a thousand or more, for gross movements such as walking (for example, the gastrocnemius in the lower leg). Refer to Chapters 3 and 4 for detail on resting membrane potential, action potential initiation and propagation, respectively.

Neuromuscular junction

The junction between a neuron and the muscle it innervates is called the **neuromuscular junction**, and this is illustrated in Figure 5.12. The distance between the two types of tissues (the **synaptic cleft**) is very small, typically no more than 1–2 nm. Neuromuscular junctions are normally located in the middle of a muscle fibre to enable the action potential to travel the length of the fibre in the quickest time possible and to facilitate coordinated contraction. To stimulate the muscle fibres for which the neuron is responsible, the action potential must cross the synaptic cleft. The nerve does this by converting the electrical impulse that has travelled the length of the nerve fibre to a chemical message that can cross the extracellular fluid in the synaptic cleft. The arrival of the action potential at the *pre-synaptic terminal* stimulates the release of the neurotransmitter **acetylcholine (ACh)** from the vesicle stores shown in Figure 5.12. The sarcolemma of the muscle fibre located immediately beneath the axon terminal is highly folded (junctional folds), greatly increasing the surface area for acetylcholine receptors. The neuromuscular junction encompasses the pre-synaptic terminal, the synaptic cleft, and the junctional folds of the sarcolemma.

 Try **Interactive Physiology:**
Muscular: The neuromuscular junction

A close-up section of a neuron and muscle fibre within a neuromuscular junction is shown in Figure 5.12. The arrival of the action potential at the pre-synaptic terminal stimulates the acetylcholine (ACh) filled vesicles to fuse with the plasma membrane. The vesicles release their contents into the synaptic cleft via a process called **exocytosis** (the fusion of a vesicle with the plasma membrane to enable release of an intracellular substance to the extracellular space). The acetylcholine molecules diffuse across the synaptic cleft and bond with specialised muscle fibre receptor

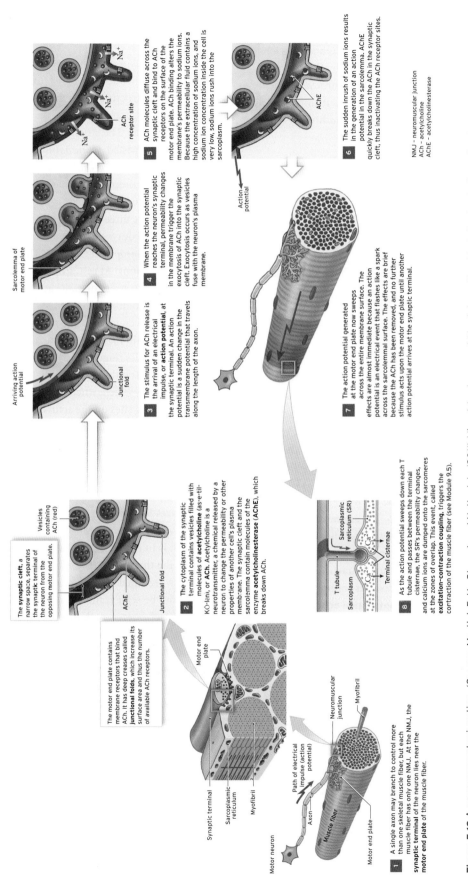

Figure 5.12 A neuromuscular junction. (*Source:* Martini, F. H., Ober, J. and Nath, J. L. (2011) *Visual Anatomy and Physiology*, New York: Benjamin Cummings)

proteins contained within the sarcolemma. This bond triggers depolarisation of the muscle fibre, which is associated with the conduction of an action potential. Once acetylcholine has completed its role it is catabolised by the enzyme **acetylcholinesterase** into its component parts, *acetyl acid* and *choline*. This catabolism is important as it stops further stimulation of the muscle without an additional nerve impulse being conducted from the CNS.

Key point

The neuromuscular junction is the point at which nervous and muscle tissue meet.

Neurons are not directly connected to the fibres they stimulate but form a junction.

The synaptic cleft is a small gap between the axon terminal and the motor endplate.

The axon terminal, synaptic cleft and motor endplate are referred to as the neuromuscular junction.

The influx of sodium ions associated with depolarisation is the trigger for muscular contraction. The mid-fibre location of neuromuscular junctions for most muscle fibres, along with the extracellular fluid-filled T tubules surrounding each myofibril, means that the action potential travels very quickly along the fibre. The arrival of the action potential to the triads is the starting point for muscular contraction. When a muscle fibre is at rest, the terminal cisternae of the sarcoplasmic reticulum sequester (store) the calcium ions which are essential for muscular contraction. The arrival of the action potential at the T tubules stimulates the terminal cisternae to release calcium ions into the **sarcoplasm**. It is the release of calcium ions that enables muscles to contract. This process of nervous stimulation leading to muscular contraction is sometimes referred to as **excitation-contraction coupling**.

Key point

An action potential propagates quickly down a muscle fibre and into the T tubules.

The arrival of an action potential at the T tubules stimulates the release of calcium.

The release of calcium from terminal cisternae enables muscular contraction.

Knowledge integration question

Explain how excitation (electrical stimulation) and muscular contraction are coupled.

The sliding filament theory of muscular contraction

The accepted model of muscular contraction, **sliding filament theory**, was first described by Huxley and Huxley in the 1950s. The structure of the main protein filaments involved in muscular contraction, actin and myosin, are shown in Figure 5.13. The structural actin filaments are comprised of two twisted *actin chains* with the protein **tropomyosin** wrapped around the length of the actin chain and a globular protein complex **troponin** (each of which is composed of different forms of troponin) bound to tropomyosin and actin. There are three forms of troponin; *troponin T* which binds to tropomyosin, *troponin I* which binds to the actin chain and *troponin C* which, when available, will bind with calcium ions. At rest, tropomyosin, a structural protein that helps to strengthen the actin filament, covers special myosin binding sites and stops the formation of **crossbridges** between myosin and actin. Myosin filaments are thicker than actin filaments and are comprised of around 200 *myosin molecules* (Figure 5.13). Each filament is formed from intertwined strands of myosin that form a long body and a myosin head, which, when possible, will bind with the myosin binding sites on the actin chains. Structurally, individual myosin molecules resemble two golf clubs twisted together. Extending from the club shaft (the rod of the myosin molecule) the club heads (myosin heads) will bind with actin-binding sites when possible to form crossbridges.

The arrangement of actin and myosin filaments can be seen in Figures 5.10 and 5.13 with their structure illustrated in the latter. In two dimensions the layout of the filaments appears as it is in Figure 5.10. However, it is important to visualise the three-dimensional structure of sarcomeres. A cross-sectional view across different sections of a sarcomere can be seen at the bottom of Figure 5.10. The structure of sarcomeres, with myosin filaments embedded between thinner actin filaments that are structurally attached to the Z lines, is what makes muscular contraction possible through the sliding of filaments.

Muscular contraction, as proposed within the sliding filament theory, begins with the release of calcium ions from the terminal cisternae. Figure 5.14 provides an illustration of the sequence of events in the sliding filament theory. The presence of calcium ions around the sarcomere enables the troponin C component of the troponin complex to bind with the available calcium ions. In binding with the calcium ions troponin C changes the shape of tropomyosin (which covers the active binding sites on the actin chain) and pulls it away from the myosin binding sites. This makes the binding sites on the actin filament available to bind with the myosin heads.

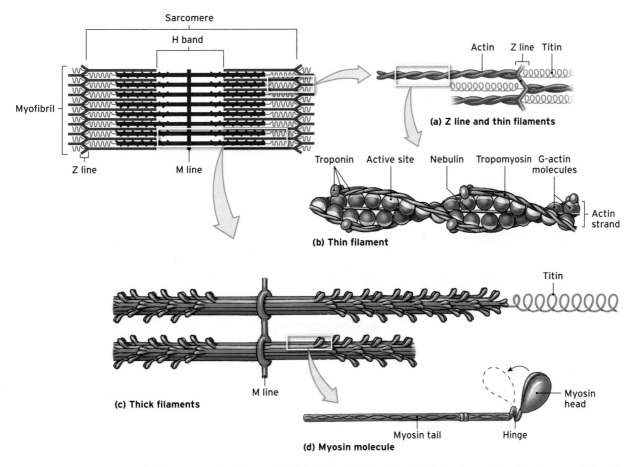

Figure 5.13 The structure of actin and myosin. (*Source*: Martini, F. H. and Nath, J. L. (2009) *Fundamentals of Anatomy and Physiology*, 8th edition, New York: Benjamin Cummings)

As well as the need for calcium ions to reveal the binding sites, energy, in the form of adenosine triphosphate (ATP), is required for muscular contraction to take place. As will be described in more detail later in this chapter, ATP is comprised of an adenosine molecule bonded to three phosphate groups. To release the energy stored within ATP a phosphate group has to be detached from the molecule, leaving adenosine diphosphate (ADP) and a phosphate group. The energy released provides the fuel for many processes within the body, including muscular contraction. Myosin heads store energy from the breakdown of ATP to ADP and retain the ADP and phosphate ion (Pi) attached to them as they form a *crossbridge* (binding with an active site on the actin filament). Myosin is now bound to the actin filament. The energy stored from the breakdown of the ATP molecule is then used by each myosin head to perform a 'powerstroke'. The myosin head *powerstroke* pulls the attached actin filament towards the

M line of the sarcomere and shortens its length. Through this action the actin slides along the myosin filament – hence *sliding filament theory*. During the powerstroke the ADP molecule and phosphate ion are released leaving the ATP binding site on the myosin head free to bind with another molecule of ATP. The binding of a new ATP molecule to the myosin head and its breakdown to ADP and Pi enables the myosin head to detach from the active binding site on the actin filament and leaves it 'cocked' ready to bind with another actin binding site (see Figure 5.14 for an illustration of this sequence of events). The crossbridge formation–powerstroke sequence continues many times during a contraction as long as sufficient calcium ions and ATP molecules remain available. Figure 5.15 shows the effect of muscular contraction and the sliding filaments on the size of a sarcomere. During muscular contraction the size of the I bands and H zone is decreased as the muscle shortens.

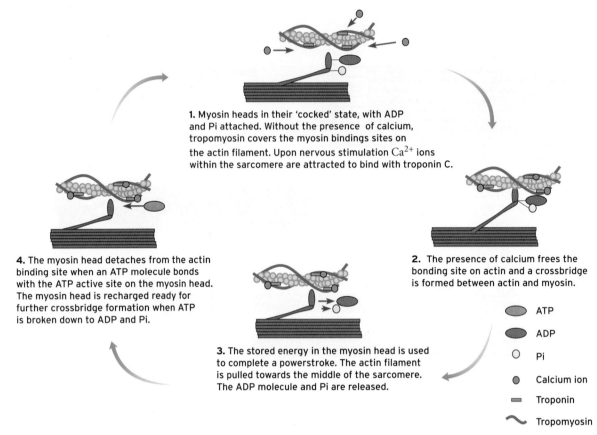

1. Myosin heads in their 'cocked' state, with ADP and Pi attached. Without the presence of calcium, tropomyosin covers the myosin bindings sites on the actin filament. Upon nervous stimulation Ca^{2+} ions within the sarcomere are attracted to bind with troponin C.

4. The myosin head detaches from the actin binding site when an ATP molecule bonds with the ATP active site on the myosin head. The myosin head is recharged ready for further crossbridge formation when ATP is broken down to ADP and Pi.

2. The presence of calcium frees the bonding site on actin and a crossbridge is formed between actin and myosin.

3. The stored energy in the myosin head is used to complete a powerstroke. The actin filament is pulled towards the middle of the sarcomere. The ADP molecule and Pi are released.

ATP

ADP

Pi

Calcium ion

Troponin

Tropomyosin

Figure 5.14 Sliding filament crossbridge-powerstroke cycle.

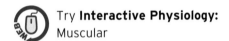 Try **Interactive Physiology:** Muscular

Key point

Muscular contraction is brought about through the release of calcium ions.

Calcium ions bind with troponin C to pull tropomyosin from the myosin binding sites.

This enables myosin heads to bind with actin.

Knowledge integration question

Explain the sliding filament theory of muscle contraction.

Development of tension in the muscle fibre

Upon stimulation, a muscle fibre is able to develop tension. The magnitude of this force is ultimately dependent upon the number of active cross-bridges. This is affected by two variables, the frequency of stimulation and the resting length of the fibre.

Frequency of stimulation

The mechanical response of a muscle fibre to a single action potential from its motor neuron is a contraction-relaxation sequence called a **muscle twitch** which can be divided into three phases: latent period, contraction phase and relaxation phase (see Figure 5.16a).

1. Following the stimulus, a **latent period** of a few milli-seconds occurs during which the stimulus spreads over the sarcolemma and down the T tubules, stimulating the release of Ca^{2+} from the terminal cisternae of the sarco-plasmic reticulum.

2. In the **contraction phase** muscle tension starts to develop and rises to a peak. This is due to the forma-tion of cross bridges as the elevated intracellular Ca^{2+} binds to troponin, unblocking the active sites on the actin filaments. As more active sites become available for myosin attachment, muscle tension rises to a peak.

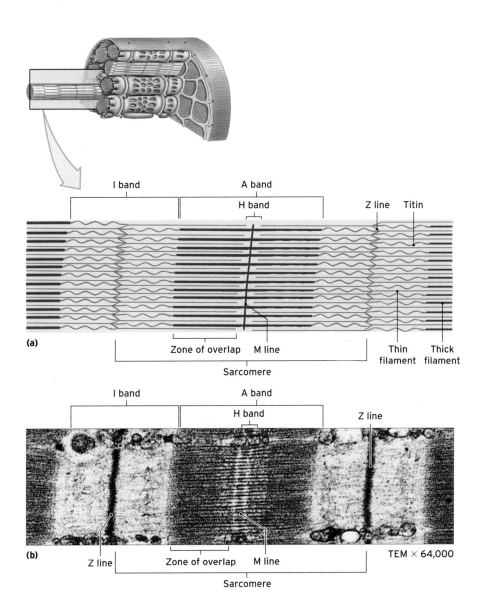

I band   A band

H band

Z line   Titin

(a)

Zone of overlap   M line

Thin filament   Thick filament

Sarcomere

I band   A band

H band

Z line

(b)

Z line   Zone of overlap   M line

TEM × 64,000

Sarcomere

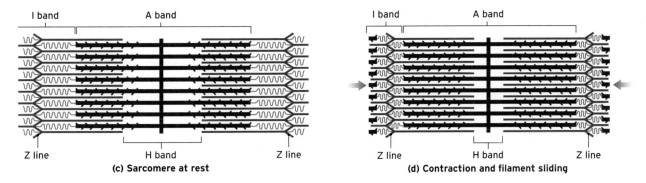

I band   A band

Z line   H band   Z line

(c) Sarcomere at rest

I band   A band

Z line   H band   Z line

(d) Contraction and filament sliding

Figure 5.15 (a) a longitudinal section of sarcomere, (b) same view for a sarcomere in a myofibril in the gastrocnemius muscle, (c) and (d) changes in appearance of sarcomere during contraction. Notice that the A band stays the same width, but I bands decrease in size. (*Source*: Martini, F. H. and Nath, J. L. (2009) *Fundamentals of Anatomy and Physiology*, 8th edition, New York: Benjamin Cummings)

The contraction phase is short-lived, lasting 10–100 milliseconds.

3. The *final* **relaxation** *phase* lasts 10–100 milliseconds. However, as can be seen in Figure 5.16, a muscle fibre contracts faster that it relaxes. The active transport of Ca^{2+} back into the sarcoplasmic reticulum allows tropomyosin to re-cover the actin active sites, resulting in a reduction of cross-bridges (because when myosin is released from actin in the cross-bridge cycle, it is unable to reattach to actin) and a fall in muscle fibre tension back to resting levels.

A muscle twitch can vary in duration from around 7.5–100 milliseconds depending on the muscle fibre type (Figure 5.16b), the internal and external environmental conditions, and other factors. Moving on to look at the effect of multiple action potentials on muscle fibre tension, bear in mind that the mechanical response of a muscle fibre is much longer than the electrical signal that generated it (~2 milliseconds), as is demonstrated in Figure 5.16.

In contrast to the sudden jerk-like contraction initiated by a single action potential, movements of our healthy muscles are smooth with a graded strength dependent on the demands placed on the muscle. These varied muscular contractions are referred to as **graded muscle responses**, with the smoothness and tension development affected by the frequency of stimulation.

When considering a pair of electrical stimuli delivered in quick succession, total tension developed in the muscle is greater than that following a single action potential, a phenomenon known as **temporal** or **wave summation** (Figure 5.17a). This occurs as the muscle remains partially contracted following the first stimulus when the second one arrives, resulting in an elevated intracellular Ca^{2+} level and hence greater cross-bridge cycling. The magnitude of the increased tension with summation is greater the shorter the interval between stimuli. This is due to elevated levels of intracellular Ca^{2+} as less and less time is available between stimuli for the sarcoplasmic reticulum to reclaim the Ca^{2+}.

Several stimuli in quick succession, but still allowing partial relaxation of the muscle fibre between stimuli, results in the progressive increase in muscle fibre tension (summation), the response of which is known as an **unfused** or **incomplete tetanus** (Figure 5.17b). When the stimulation frequency increases, muscle tension increases until a maximal tension is reached. At this stage the muscle has no time to relax between stimuli – there is no time for Ca^{2+} to be moved back into the sarcoplasmic reticulum before the next stimulus for Ca^{2+} release – resulting

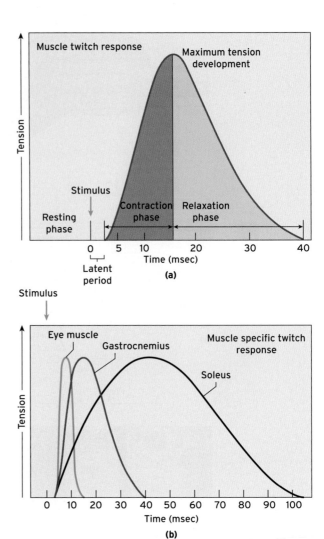

Figure 5.16 The general development of tension in a muscle twitch (a) and muscle specific twitch responses (b). (*Source*: Martini, F. H. and Nath, J. L. (2009) *Fundamentals of Anatomy and Physiology*, 8th edition, New York: Benjamin Cummings)

in a smooth, sustained contraction known as a **fused** or **complete tetanus** (Figure 5.17c). The occurrence of fused tetanus is uncommon in real life as maximal muscular activity inevitably leads to fatigue, with the muscle no longer able to contract, thus tension disappears.

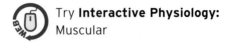 Try **Interactive Physiology:** Muscular

Resting length of muscle fibre

If you think back to the structure of a sarcomere (refer to Figure 5.10) it is clear that the resting length of a muscle fibre will determine the degree of overlap between the actin and myosin filaments. Upon stimulation, the amount of tension generated in a skeletal muscle fibre is dependent

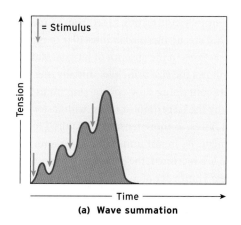

(a) Wave summation

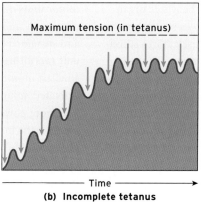

(b) Incomplete tetanus

Figure 5.17 The effect of stimulation frequency on muscle tension.

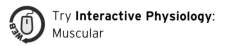

(c) Complete tetanus

on the number of cycling cross-bridges. Only myosin heads within the zone of overlap are able to bind to active sites and generate muscle tension, hence it is clear that the resting length of a muscle fibre will affect its tension-generating potential. In the situation where a muscle fibre, and hence sarcomeres, is greatly stretched and lengthened there will be little overlap of the myofilaments therefore few cross-bridges can be formed and minimal tension generated. Similarly, tension production is reduced when the muscle fibre is compressed and shortened as the actin filaments overlap in the middle of the sarcomere, interfering with the orientation and function of the myofilaments. A sarcomere functions most efficiently, with the muscle fibre producing the greatest force, when stimulated within a narrow range of lengths. In the body, resting sarcomeres are normally 75–130% of the optimal length as major compression or stretching of the skeletal muscle is normally prevented by the arrangement of the muscles, connective tissues and bones.

Try **Interactive Physiology**: Muscular

Key point

The degree of muscle fibre tension is dependent on the frequency of neural stimulation and the length of the resting muscle.

A single action potential elicits a muscle twitch – a single contraction-relaxation cycle. The tension developed is summated during repeated action potentials resulting in unfused tetanus.

When the frequency of stimulation is increased further, maximum tension is developed during a fused tetanus.

The development of muscle tension is also dependent on the degree of overlap of the muscle myofilaments.

Muscle fibres contract most forcefully when stimulated within an optimal range of resting lengths.

Development of tension in the skeletal muscle

It is now clear how individual skeletal muscle fibres generate tension and what factors alter the magnitude of that tension, but how do all the muscle fibres work together to produce skeletal muscle contractions at the whole organ level? The amount of tension produced by a skeletal muscle organ is dependent on the number of muscle fibres stimulated and the tension generated in these fibres. The tension generated in a skeletal muscle that exerts a pull on the tendon, and movement of the joint (if the tension is large enough), is the sum of the individual tensions of all the stimulated muscle fibres. Thus, control of the number of muscle fibres stimulated will dictate the tension generated by the muscle as a whole.

A brief review of the skeletal muscle and the control of its individual fibres will improve your understanding of how muscle contractions can vary in strength and can be maintained over a long duration without fatigue encroaching. A typical skeletal muscle contains thousands of muscle fibres – the contraction units of the muscle. A motor neuron and all the muscle fibres it innervates is known as a **motor unit**, whether it includes a few muscle fibres for fine control movements of the eye, or thousands of muscle fibres for the gross movements of the leg. Within a motor unit the muscle fibres are all of the same type, slow or fast twitch (see the following section), and are spread out within the muscle, intermingling with other motor units (Figure 5.18a). This mixing of motor unit muscle fibres means the direction of pull by the muscle on the tendon remains constant as more and more motor units are activated.

The signal from the CNS, via motor neurons, for a skeletal muscle to contract is very precise. The recruitment of motor units during muscle contraction is far from random, allowing a smooth but steady increase in muscular tension and sustained contractions in the absence of fatigue. **Motor unit recruitment** follows the size principle. Initially, the smallest motor units containing slow-contracting fibres are activated, followed by the larger motor units, with faster and more powerful fibres, as more tension is required to conduct the movement. As motor units with larger and larger muscle fibres are recruited, the generation of muscular force increases. This order of motor unit recruitment is important as it allows small gradual increases in muscle tension during weak contractions (like those for posture maintenance) and large increases in tension when forceful contractions are required during the vigorous movements involved in many sports.

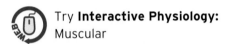 Try **Interactive Physiology:** Muscular

The stimulation of all motor units at once will generate a maximal muscle contraction. This situation in the body, however, is uncommon as muscle fibres quickly use up their energy reserves. During a sustained contraction motor units are activated asynchronously, that is on a rotational basis. While some are in tetanus, usually unfused, other motor units are resting and recovering before the next stimulation. This asynchronous recruitment allows for muscle contractions to be sustained with the prevention or delay of muscular fatigue (Figure 5.18b). Hence, when

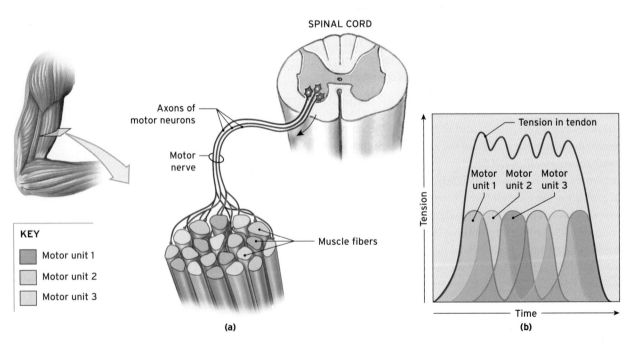

Figure 5.18 Motor unit arrangement and activity in a skeletal muscle.

our muscles are involved in sustained contractions they are producing less than maximal tension.

Finally, the force that a skeletal muscle is capable of generating is influenced by its cross-sectional area. Thicker muscle fibres contain more myofibrils and can therefore develop more tension. The response to strength training is muscle hypertrophy, that is an increase in the number of myofibrils and hence cross-sectional area of the muscle fibres, not an increase in muscle fibre number.

Key point

The magnitude of force generated by a contracting skeletal muscle can be increased by increasing the motor neuron action potential frequency or by the recruitment of more motor units.

Muscle fibre types

The strength, power and endurance for sports participation is provided by skeletal muscles. Just as there are different mechanisms for energy production, so there is a variety of muscle fibre types that can be recruited for muscular contraction. The muscle fibre types are differentiated by the predominant energy system each favours, and hence, rate of fibre contraction and susceptibility to fatigue. Two main distinctions have been made, type I (slow-twitch) and type II (fast-twitch) fibres. Type II fibres, however, can be further sub-divided and there are important distinctions between sub-types. The nature of these sub-types is important for muscle recruitment in power and power endurance sports, and also has implications for glycolytic and aerobic energy generation which are described in Chapters 10–12.

The identification of the two main muscle fibre types originates from early research into the structure and function of muscles. In the 19th Century researchers identified differences in muscle fibre types that were visible to the naked eye. In 1873 Louis Ranvier (1835–1922), who in other research identified the presence of a myelin sheath around nerve fibres (the gaps in the sheath, the nodes of Ranvier, being named after him), published a paper detailing structural differences in the white and red muscle tissue of rabbits and rays. This difference can be seen in chickens where the legs, which appear red in colour, comprise a higher proportion of type I fibres, whereas the breast and wings, which appear white, contain more type II fibres. The difference in colour between the two fibre types is due to the presence of a higher concentration of myoglobin (oxygen-binding protein) and increased capillarity within type I fibres.

Since this early research, new techniques have enabled researchers to identify further muscle fibre sub-divisions. Technical developments in the identification of muscle fibre proteins and enzyme presence through histochemistry, the study of the microscopic structure, and the chemistry of cells and tissues, led to the identification of a number of sub-divisions within type II fibres. For example, research in this field identified differences in the properties of adenosine triphosphatase (ATPase) in type I and type II fibres. This enzyme is responsible for the hydrolysis (catabolism) of ATP when it attaches to myosin heads, resulting in the release of myosin heads from actin binding sites and supplying the energy for muscular contraction. The form of ATPase differs for each muscle fibre type and it was these differences in properties of ATPase that enabled researchers to stain muscle tissue and identify additional fibre types. Figure 5.19 provides a photomicrograph of a microsection of muscle revealing the fibre types.

Sections of muscle tissue can be taken from humans or animals. Rat muscle tissue has been frequently studied in physiological research as its general properties are similar to human muscle. A muscle biopsy needle is used with humans to sample a small section of muscle tissue. Through histochemical staining the presence of three sub-divisions of type II muscle fibres have been identified in humans. These are commonly referred to as types IIa, IIx (also referred to as IIb) and IIc. Figure 5.19 shows type I fibres which are stained dark red, type IIa fibres stained pale red and type IIx fibres stained white. Type IIc occur

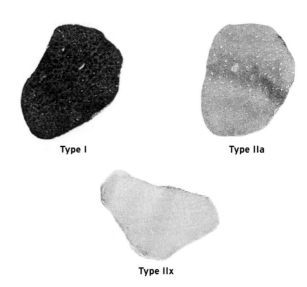

Figure 5.19 Microscopic cross section of a skeletal muscle. (*Source*: Martini, F. H. and Nath, J. L. (2009) *Fundamentals of Anatomy and Physiology*, 8th edition, New York: Benjamin Cummings)

less commonly in humans and are thought to account for only 1–2% of muscle fibres. Due to their rare occurrence and limits in our current knowledge about their function, we will concentrate on the structure and function of type I, type IIa and type IIx muscle fibres.

Knowledge integration question

Explain the similarities and differences between the different muscle fibre types.

It is worth mentioning two issues at this point. Firstly, the advent of **polyacrylamide gel electrophoresis** in the study of histochemistry has enabled further muscle fibre types to be identified. Gel electrophoresis, commonly carried out in biochemistry laboratories, enabled the separation of individual myosin filaments and further increased our understanding of their properties. Through this method up to nine muscle fibre types have been identified in the muscle tissue of rats and rabbits. Each of the muscle fibre types identified in humans can be found amongst the range of muscle fibres of rats. Secondly, although commonly called type IIb fibres in humans, research has indicated that the majority of these fibres are in fact type IIx fibres. Examination of rat muscle shows the presence of type IIx and IIb type fibres which have different properties including speed of contraction. Type IIb are slightly faster contracting than type IIx fibres. Comparison of human and rat muscle fibres has revealed that human type IIb fibres are actually structurally and functionally the same as type IIx fibres found in rat muscle. Consequently, they should be more correctly referred to as IIx fibres. In this textbook we will refer to type IIb fibres (as used by some textbooks) as type IIx which is more appropriate when discussing human muscle tissue. Over time a number of different systems have been developed by physiologists to refer to the different muscle fibre types. Table 5.2 provides details of several of these systems. The details provided here should be helpful when referring to additional readings.

The descriptors in Table 5.2 provide a very useful insight as to the properties of each fibre type. Type I, the slow oxidative fibres, contain slow-rate myosin ATPase and rely on oxidative (aerobic) mechanisms for energy generation. As a consequence, although type I fibres take twice as long to reach peak contraction (around 100 msec) and generate less force than type II fibres, they contain more myoglobin and mitochondria, have a richer blood supply and primarily rely on fat oxidation for their energy supply, making them much more resistant to fatigue. Many

Table 5.2 Terminology used to describe the various muscle fibre types.

Type I	Type IIa	Type IIx
Type I	Type IIa	Type IIx
Type I	Type IIa	Type IIb
Slow twitch	Fast twitch a	Fast twitch b
Slow oxidative (SO)	Fast oxidative glycolytic (FOG)	Fast glycolytic (FG)
Slow contraction (S)	Fast contraction, fatigue resistant (FR)	Fast contraction, fast fatigue (FF)

back and calf muscles are dominated by type I fibres as they almost continually contract to maintain an upright posture. Conversely, type IIx fibres, which contain fast-rate myosin ATPase, reach peak contraction quickly and can generate more force than type I fibres using anaerobic glycolytic metabolism for ATP synthesis (hence contain little myoglobin and few mitochondria, and have a limited blood supply) which means they fatigue relatively quickly. Due to their rapid fatigue rate, type IIx fibres are recruited for short periods during high-intensity, anaerobic activities. Type IIa fibres, also called fast oxidative glycolytic fibres, fall between type I and type IIx fibres with regard to many of their properties and functions. They are more fatigue-resistant than type IIx fibres, although less so than type I fibres, but can utilise both oxidative and glycolytic means for ATP synthesis. Table 5.3 provides a summary of the properties of each fibre type commonly found in human skeletal muscle.

Key point

Three main types of muscle fibre are identifiable in humans, with individuals differing in the proportion of each fibre type.

Type I contract more slowly than type II fibres and produce low relative force levels, but are fatigue-resistant.

Type IIa have a fast contraction speed with medium force production and fatigue more quickly than type I fibres.

Type IIx are capable of contracting at the highest speed, producing the highest levels of force but fatigue more quickly than type I or IIa fibres.

The recruitment of muscle fibres during exercise is dependent upon the intensity and duration of the exercise. When standing, where muscles have only to contract

Table 5.3 Properties of type I and type II muscle fibres.

Properties	Type I fibres	Type IIa fibres	Type IIx fibres
Appearance	Red	Pinkish	White
ATPase hydrolysis rate	Slow	Fast	Fast
Contraction speed	Slow	Fast	Fast
Contraction Force	Low	Medium	High
Fatigue resistance	High	Medium	Low
Oxidative capacity			
Myoglobin content	High	High	Low
Capillarisation	High	High	Low
Number of mitochondria	High	High	Low
Oxidative enzyme concentration	High	Medium	Low
Triglyceride content	High	Medium	Low
Glycolytic capacity			
Glycogen stores	Low	Medium	High
Glycolytic enzyme activity	Low	High	High
Phosphagen system capacity			
Phosphocreatine stores	Low	High	High
Creatine kinase stores	Low	Medium	High
Recruitment pattern			
Order	First recruited	Second recruited	Third recruited
Exercise intensity for recruitment	Low	Medium-high	High-maximal

against the forces of gravity, or during low-intensity exercise such as walking, type I fibres are recruited to provide the necessary muscular contractions. When the intensity of exercise is higher, for instance during activities such as jogging or steady-rate cycling or rowing, type I and IIa fibres are recruited. When all-out effort is required for power and power endurance sports, or for the finish of a race, all muscle fibre types are called upon to provide the necessary muscular contractions and force generation. The body, however, has protective mechanisms to avoid recruiting all motor units during maximal effort to avoid damage to muscle attachments and tendons. Consequently, in a maximal contraction we normally recruit up to 70% of the available muscle fibres at any one time. In situations of

grave danger there have been incidents of people being able to lift heavy weights to free a trapped person. It is thought that such capabilities, which often lead to major injury, are enabled through an emotionally driven maximal recruitment that overrides the normal protective mechanisms.

Key point

The speed of muscle fibre contraction or twitch is determined by the form of myosin ATPase present within the fibre.

Type II fibres have faster-acting ATPase than type I fibres, which results in a halving of the time to peak contraction when compared to slow-twitch fibres.

Each person normally has a mix of all human muscle fibre types, including type IIc. An average person's muscles are typically comprised of 50% type I, 30% type IIa, 19% type IIx and 1% type IIc fibres. The specific distribution of muscle fibre types varies according to the muscle's role within the body. The soleus, which is a postural muscle that requires low force contractions over long periods of time, is comprised of around 90% type I fibres. The muscles of the lower limbs tend to have relatively more type IIa than the muscles of the upper limbs which typically have a higher percentage of type IIx fibres.

Muscle fibre distribution is determined initially by individual genetic endowment and then by training, which mimics the nature versus nurture hypothesis. Are athletes drawn to a sport because of their genetic fibre type distribution or does the distribution alter as someone trains for a specific sport? The most likely answer, as with the nature versus nurture argument, lies somewhere in the middle. A certain level of genetic endowment is essential for high-level performance; however, training has been shown to alter the properties of an individual's muscle fibres. This ability of skeletal muscle to adapt both functionally and structurally in response to the stimulations imposed during training is known as **myoplasticity**, and is predominantly the result of changes in gene expression. These changes include alterations in the muscle fibre size, myosin heavy chain type, mitochondrial and capillary densities, oxidative enzyme activity and muscle fibre lipid content. Together, these alterations affect the function of the skeletal muscle through changes in the production of force, speed of contraction and resistance to fatigue.

Sedentary individuals tend to have around 50% type I and 50% type II fibres, whereas those involved in power sports tend to develop a higher percentage of type II fibres and those involved in endurance sports a higher percentage of type I fibres. The largest muscle fibres in trained individuals tend to be those which are most recruited during exercise. Endurance training has been shown to lead to a decrease in the size of type I fibres but a gradual shift in the properties of type IIx fibres towards those of type IIa fibres. Strength and power training, on the other hand, due to the all out nature of muscle recruitment, has been shown to increase the size of type I and II fibres and result in improvements in the anaerobic capacity of the trained muscle fibres.

Key point

Muscle fibre distribution can be determined through muscle biopsy and subsequent analysis of the cross-sectional fibre content.

Athletes in endurance sports such as marathon running and road cycling tend to have a higher distribution of type I fibres compared to those involved in strength and power sports.

Types of muscular contraction

Knowledge of the types of muscular contraction is useful for understanding muscle function as it pertains to training and sports performance. When a muscle moves as part of a contraction the load can be applied when the muscle is shortening which is a **concentric contraction** or when the muscle is lengthening known as an **eccentric contraction**. The difference between these two types of contraction can be illustrated using the bench press as an example. The push up of your maximum bench press would be brought about through the concentric contraction of the pectoral, front of deltoid and triceps muscles. If, for the next repetition you then added an additional 10 kg in weight you would not be able to lift the weight, but you could, using eccentric contraction of the same muscles, lower the weight to your chest, thereby training with a weight higher than your maximum. Eccentric contractions and training can be used as part of a strategy to increase the overload (supramaxially) to improve maximal lifting and adaptation. Research has shown that eccentric contractions improve muscle strength during concentric contraction, but they often result in increased post-exercise muscle soreness.

In the sport of rock climbing the nature of the sport means that there are many instances where the climber has to hold **isometric contractions** (*iso* meaning same and *metric* referring to length). Isometric contractions are ones where the muscle contracts; however, there is no muscle movement (shortening or lengthening). Each hold a climber takes with their hand involves an isometric contraction of the forearm muscles. The longer the climber remains holding a specific hold, and the tighter their grip on the hold, the greater the isometric contraction and the more quickly the muscle group will fatigue.

Isotonic and **isokinetic contractions** are associated with strength training and represent muscular contractions where the muscle moves against a resistance. In a weight training context *tonic* refers to load and *kinetic* to speed or work, thus they mean same-load and same-speed or work, respectively. An example of these terms can be drawn from a biceps curl. It is important to know that, as the biceps curls (the muscle shortens against the resistance) through its range of motion, the muscle is weakest at the start of the lift, when the biceps is fully extended and strongest once it gets past 90°. If an athlete performs a biceps curl with a 20 kg barbell the load remains the same throughout the lift (isotonic) as the bar moves to the chest. When performing an isokinetic contraction biceps curl an athlete would make the lift against a machine that can vary the load to ensure the muscle is contracting at the same speed, and hence performing the same relative work, throughout the range of motion. Special cams are used to decrease the load in the early part of the lift – where the biceps muscle is at its weakest – and increase the load as the biceps moves the load past 90°. This results in the relative work being the same throughout the lift – isokinetic. The use of isokinetic contractions, however, during everyday life and sporting activities is very rare, with the majority of our muscle contractions being isotonic or isometric.

In a **plyometric contraction**, *plyo* meaning variable or more and *metric* referring to muscle length, the muscle varies in length as it makes its contraction. In the context of weight training a plyometric contraction is made where the muscle is pre-tensioned prior to the actual lift or movement to increase the force generated. The use of plyometric contraction will improve the power of a movement. A plyometric contraction uses an eccentric contraction (pre-tensioning) to bring about a more powerful concentric contraction. The pre-tensioning of the muscle adds an eccentric stretch to the muscle and makes it recoil like a spring as well as making a muscular contraction. If the recoil of the muscle is timed with the start of the concentric contraction the result is increased force generation. An example of this can be seen in long jump. In the final strides before take-off a high-level long jumper will 'sink' into the jump, thereby pre-tensing the muscles. In doing this the jumper will increase the force generated in the take-off and improve the distance jumped. They are making a plyometric contraction or movement.

Muscles and movement

As already discussed, muscles bring about movement by contracting and leveraging against their attachments to bones. To bring about movement, the muscular contraction and bone operate as levers, with a *load, effort* and balance point or *fulcrum*. Within the body it is possible to find examples of first, second and third order levers through the varied attachment of muscles and bones. Figure 5.20 provides an example of each type of lever. *First order levers* have the fulcrum in the middle, *second order levers* have the load in the middle and *third order levers* have the effort in the middle. First order levers can produce a mechanism advantage or disadvantage, depending on whether the fulcrum is closer to the load or effort. The closer the fulcrum is to the load, the greater the mechanical advantage. Second order levers always produce a mechanical advantage and third order levers a mechanical disadvantage.

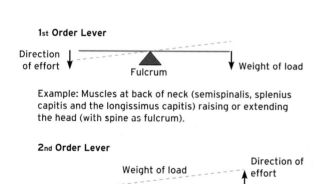

1st Order Lever

Example: Muscles at back of neck (semispinalis, splenius capitis and the longissimus capitis) raising or extending the head (with spine as fulcrum).

2nd Order Lever

Example: Calf muscle (gastrocnemius) raising the body (with ball of foot as the fulcrum).

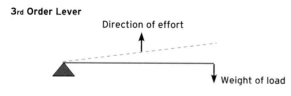

3rd Order Lever

Example: Biceps muscle flexing the arm with a load in the hand (elbow as fulcrum).

Figure 5.20 Levers created between muscles and bones.

The points of attachment of a muscle are called the origin and insertion. The **muscle origin** is normally the point of attachment on the bone that does not move and the **muscle insertion** is the attachment to the bone that moves. For example, the origin of the biceps muscle is on the scapula and the attachment is on the radius of the lower arm (which moves). Muscles are normally arranged in antagonistic pairs such that they have the opposite effect of each other. Taking the biceps as an example again, when bending (flexing) the arm the biceps forms the **prime mover** or **agonist** and the triceps is the **antagonist**. When straightening the arm the roles are reversed and the triceps are the agonist and the biceps becomes the antagonist.

Major skeletal muscles in the body

The major muscles of the body can be seen from the anterior and posterior views of the body shown in Figure 5.21. As there are 600–700 muscles within the body, with varying locations and functions: it is unrealistic to learn them all. The major muscles and their functions in the body that would be useful for you, as a future PE teacher, sports coach or exercise physiologist, to know are summarised in Table 5.4 These primarily include muscles of the limbs, shoulders and body core. The arms and legs, as with everyday life, are involved in all sports as their muscles allow actions such as walking, running, jumping, swinging, throwing, pitching and bowling. The core muscles (abdominal and back) play a vital role in stabilising the body during any movement or activity. Some of the major muscles in the body, along with their functions, are presented in Table 5.4 and covered in the following sections. In Table 5.5 the origins and insertions for each of these muscles are described. After this, the differing fascicular arrangements of muscles are discussed.

Leg muscles

The leg can be divided into the upper (thigh) and lower leg with, anterior and posterior compartments. The major muscle of the anterior thigh is the quadriceps femoris which arises from four separate heads (origins) but has a common insertion tendon, the quadriceps tendon. The insertion of the quadriceps tendon is into the patella, and then via the patellar ligament, into the tibial tuberosity. The

(a)

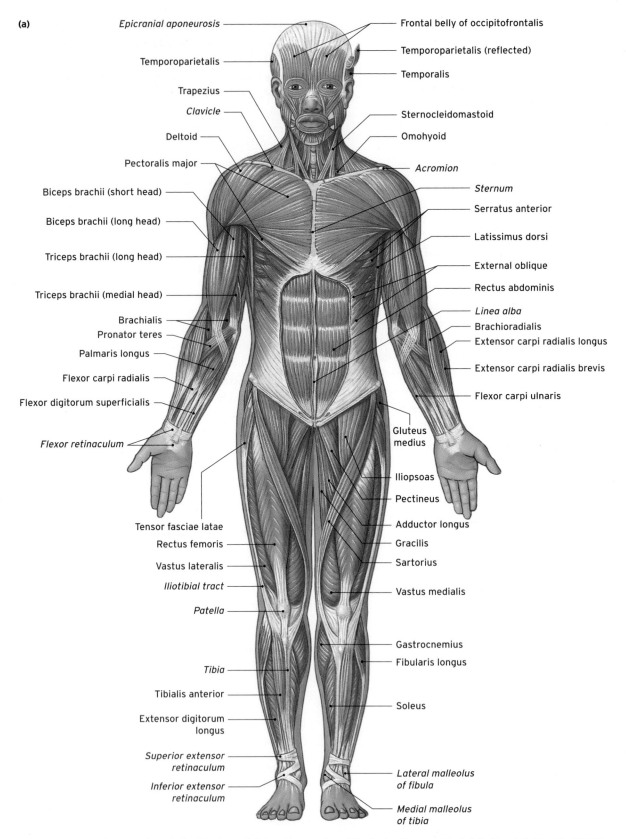

Epicranial aponeurosis — Frontal belly of occipitofrontalis

Temporoparietalis — Temporoparietalis (reflected)

Temporalis

Trapezius

Clavicle — Sternocleidomastoid

Deltoid — Omohyoid

Pectoralis major — Acromion

Biceps brachii (short head) — Sternum

Biceps brachii (long head) — Serratus anterior

Triceps brachii (long head) — Latissimus dorsi

Triceps brachii (medial head) — External oblique

Rectus abdominis

Brachialis — Linea alba

Pronator teres — Brachioradialis

Palmaris longus — Extensor carpi radialis longus

Flexor carpi radialis — Extensor carpi radialis brevis

Flexor digitorum superficialis — Flexor carpi ulnaris

Flexor retinaculum

Gluteus medius

Iliopsoas

Pectineus

Adductor longus

Tensor fasciae latae — Gracilis

Rectus femoris — Sartorius

Vastus lateralis

Iliotibial tract — Vastus medialis

Patella

Gastrocnemius

Fibularis longus

Tibia

Tibialis anterior — Soleus

Extensor digitorum longus

Superior extensor retinaculum

Inferior extensor retinaculum — Lateral malleolus of fibula

Medial malleolus of tibia

Figure 5.21 Anterior (a) and posterior (b) views of the major muscles of the body. (*Source*: Martini, F. H. and Nath, J. L. (2009) *Fundamentals of Anatomy and Physiology*, 8th edition, New York: Benjamin Cummings)

(b)

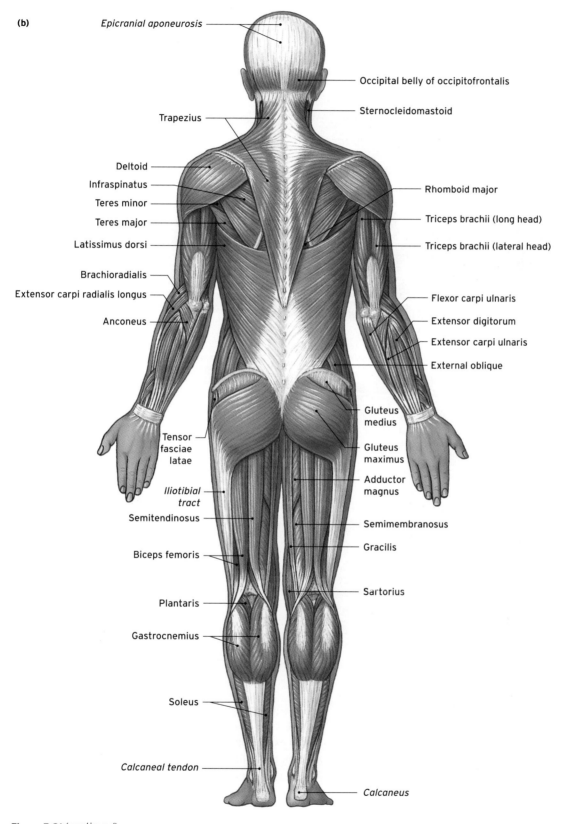

Figure 5.21 *(continued)*

Figure 5.21 (*continued*)

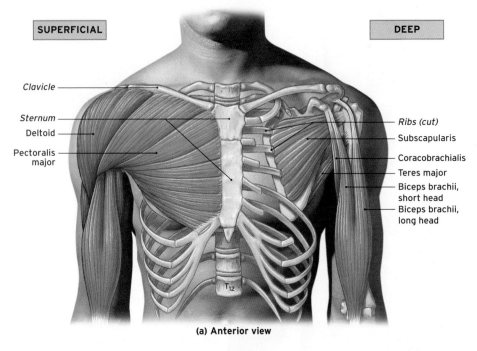

SUPERFICIAL

DEEP

Clavicle

Sternum

Deltoid

Pectoralis
major

Ribs (cut)

Subscapularis

Coracobrachialis

Teres major

Biceps brachii,
short head

Biceps brachii,
long head

T$_{12}$

(a) Anterior view

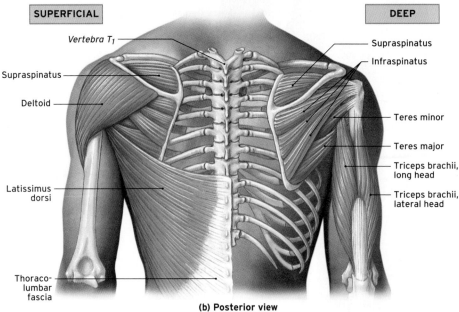

SUPERFICIAL

DEEP

Vertebra T$_1$

Supraspinatus

Infraspinatus

Supraspinatus

Deltoid

Teres minor

Teres major

Triceps brachii,
long head

Latissimus
dorsi

Triceps brachii,
lateral head

Thoraco-
lumbar
fascia

(b) Posterior view

four muscles of the quadriceps group are the rectus femoris, vastus lateralis, vastus medialis and vastus intermedius. The quadriceps muscle spans the knee joint and is a powerful knee extensor which is involved in many sporting activities which include running, jumping and climbing. In terms of health, it is important to limit the loss of quadriceps strength as it is responsible for the ability to stand up.

The hamstrings form the major muscles of the posterior thigh. This group of muscles includes the biceps femoris (careful not to confuse with the biceps brachii of the arm),

semitendinosus and semimembranosus. Crossing both hip and knee joints, the hamstrings are prime movers of both thigh **extension** and knee **flexion**. All three muscles originate at the ischial tuberosity of the pelvic bone but have separate insertions.

The major muscles in the lower leg are the tibialis anterior on the anterior aspect and the soleus and gastrocnemius muscles form the posterior 'calf' of the lower leg. These muscles span the ankle joint and promote **dorsiflexion** and **plantar flexion** of the foot, respectively.

Table 5.4 Some important muscles and their actions.

Muscle name	Muscle action
Movement of the thigh, leg and foot	
Quadriceps:	
Rectus femoris	Extension at knee, flexion at hip
Vastus lateralis	Extension at knee
Vastus medialis	Extension at knee
Vastus intermedius	Extension at knee
Hamstrings:	
Biceps femoris	Flexion of the knee, extension and lateral rotation at the hip
Semitendinosus	Flexion of the knee, extension and medial rotation at the hip
Semimembranosus	Flexion of the knee, extension and medial rotation at the hip
Tibialis anterior	Dorsiflexion of the foot
Soleus	Plantar flexion of the foot
Gastrocnemius	Plantar flexion of the foot
Movement of the arm and shoulder	
Biceps brachii	Flexion of the arm
Brachialis	Flexion of the arm
Triceps brachii	Extension of the arm
Pectoralis major	Flexion, adduction and medial rotation at the shoulder
Lattisimus dorsi	Extension, adduction and medial rotation at the shoulder
Deltoid	Abduction of shoulder (anterior part: flexion and medial rotation; posterior part: extension and lateral rotation)
Muscles of the rotator cuff	
Supraspinatus	Stabilises shoulder joint and initiates abduction
Infraspinatus	Stabilises shoulder joint and laterally rotates humerus
Teres minor	Stabilises shoulder joint and laterally rotates humerus
Subscapularis	Stabilises shoulder joint and medially rotates humerus
Muscles for core stability	
Rectus abdominis	Flexion of the spine
Internal obliques	Flexes spine and aids in trunk rotation and lateral flexion
External obliques	Flexes spine and aids in trunk rotation and lateral flexion
Erector spinae:	
Iliocostalis	Extension of the spine
Longissimus	Extends and laterally flexes spine; extends head and turns face
Spinalis	Extends spine and neck

Arm and shoulder muscles

Flexion of the elbow is primarily controlled jointly by the biceps brachii and the brachialis, two muscles in the anterior compartment of the upper arm. Forearm extension is elicited by the major muscle in the posterior upper arm, the triceps brachii. Movement of the arm (humerus) occurs at the freely-moveable ball-and-socket shoulder joint, the most flexible but least stable joint in the body. The prime movers of the shoulder joint are the pectoralis major (chest), latissimus dorsi (back) and deltoid (shoulder) muscles. The rotator cuff muscles (supraspinatus, infraspinatus, teres minor and subscapularis), commonly heard of through injuries, primarily function to reinforce the shoulder joint capsule and prevent dislocation. In addition, they act as synergists in the angular and rotational movements of the arm.

Core stability

The abdominal muscles (rectus abdominus, internal obliques and external obliques) function to flex and rotate the spine whereas the erector spinae muscles of the back are prime movers of back extension. The combined contraction

Table 5.5 The origins and insertions of some important muscles.

Muscle name	Origin and insertion
Movement of the thigh, leg and foot	
Quadriceps:	
Rectus femoris	**Origin** - anterior inferior iliac spine and superior margin of acetabelum **Insertion** - patella and tibial tuberosity via patellar ligament
Vastus lateralis	**Origin** - greater trochanter, intertrochanteric line, linea aspera **Insertion** - patella and tibial tuberosity via patellar ligament
Vastus medialis	**Origin** - linea aspera, intertrochanteric and medial supracondylar lines **Insertion** - patella and tibial tuberosity via patellar ligament
Vastus intermedius	**Origin** - anterior and lateral surfaces of proximal femur shaft **Insertion** - patella and tibial tuberosity via patellar ligament
Hamstrings:	
Biceps femoris	**Origin** - ischial tuberosity (long head), linea aspera, lateral supracondylar line and distal femur (short head) **Insertion** - head of fibula and lateral condyle of tibia
Semitendinosus	**Origin** - ischial tuberosity **Insertion** - medial aspect of upper tibial shaft
Semimembranosus	**Origin** - ischial tuberosity **Insertion** - medial condyle of tibia and lateral condyle of femur
Tibialis anterior	**Origin** - lateral condyle and upper two-thirds of tibial shaft and interosseous membrane **Insertion** - inferior surface of medial cuneiform and first metatarsal bone
Soleus	**Origin** - superior tibia, fibula and interosseous membrane **Insertion** - posterior calcaneus
Gastrocnemius	**Origin** - medial and lateral condyles of femur **Insertion** - posterior calcaneus
Movement of the arm and shoulder	
Biceps brachii	**Origin** - supraglenoid tubercle and lip of glenoid cavity (long head) and coracoid process (short head) **Insertion** - radial tuberosity
Brachialis	**Origin** - anterior of distal humerus **Insertion** - coronoid process of ulna and capsule of elbow joint
Triceps brachii	**Origin** - infraglenoid tubercle of scapula (long head), posterior shaft of humerus (lateral head) and posterior humeral shaft distal to radial groove (medial head) **Insertion** - olecranon process of ulna
Pectoralis major	**Origin** - medial clavicle, sternum, cartilage of ribs 1–6 and aponeurosis of external oblique muscle **Insertion** - intertubercular sulcus and greater tubercle of humerus
Lattisimus dorsi	**Origin** - inferior thoracic and all lumbar vertebrae, lower 4 ribs and iliac crest **Insertion** - intertubercular sulcus of humerus
Deltoid	**Origin** - Clavicle, acromion and spine of scapula **Insertion** - deltoid tuberosity of humerus
Muscles of the rotator cuff	
Supraspinatus	**Origin** - supraspinous fossa of scapula **Insertion** - superior edge of greater tubercle of humerus
Infraspinatus	**Origin** - infraspinous fossa of scapula **Insertion** - greater tubercle of humerus inferior to insertion of supraspinatus
Teres minor	**Origin** - lateral border of dorsal scapular **Insertion** - greater tubercle of humerus inferior to insertion of infraspinatus
Subscapularis	**Origin** - subscapular foss of scapula **Insertion** - lesser tubercle of humerus

Table 5.5 (continued)

Muscle name	Origin and insertion
Muscles for core stability	
Rectus abdominis	**Origin** - pubic crest and symphysis **Insertion** - costal cartilages (ribs 5-7) and xiphoid process
Internal obliques	**Origin** - lumbar fascia and iliac crest **Insertion** - linea alba, pubic crest, last 4 ribs and costal margin
External obliques	**Origin** - lower 8 ribs **Insertion** - linea alba, pubic crest, pubic tubercle and iliac crest
Erector spinae: Iliocostalis	**Origin** - iliac crest; inferior 6 ribs; superior thoracic vertebrae **Insertion** - angles of ribs; transverse processes of cervical vertebrae (C4-6)
Longissimus	**Origin** - transverse processes of lumbar through cervical vertebrae **Insertion** - transverse processes of thoracic or cervical vertebrae; ribs superior to origin
Spinalis	**Origin** - spinal processes of upper lumbar and lower thoracic vertebrae **Insertion** - spinous process of upper thoracic and cervical vertebrae

of the abdominal muscles and the back muscles helps to splint the entire body trunk. Having a strong core is very important in the prevention of injuries, whether sport-related or from everyday tasks such as lifting a heavy load.

Fascicle arrangement

As well as being classified individually by name, muscles can be classified by the arrangement of the muscle fascicles. The four differing organisations of fascicles are depicted in Figure 5.22. The majority of muscles in the body have a parallel arrangement of fascicles in relation to the long axis of the muscle. **Parallel muscles** are varied, however, in terms of their shape with some being flat with broad attachments (aponeuroses) at each end and others plump and cylindrical with tendons for attachment. Those with a cylindrical shape have a central body, also known as the belly. The biceps brachii in the upper arm is a classic example of a cylindrical parallel muscle with the belly becoming prominent upon contraction and shortening of the muscle. A skeletal muscle fibre has the capacity to shorten by approximately 30%, hence, due to the arrangement of the fascicles in a parallel muscle, the whole muscle is also able to shorten to the same degree. The number of myofibrils within a parallel muscle is the major determinant of the total tension that can be generated during muscular contraction.

In a **convergent muscle**, the fascicles spread out like a fan over a broad area with a common attachment site at the apex. The most obvious example in the body is the pectoralis muscles of the chest. As the fascicles are arranged in slightly differing directions, the direction of pull of the muscle can be varied by stimulating different portions of it. If the whole muscle is stimulated to contract, however, the tension developed would be less than that of a parallel muscle of a similar size, due to the differing angles of pull compared with all pulling in the same direction.

A **pennate** muscle has fascicles that attach obliquely, at a common angle, to the tendon. Due to the angular arrangement, and hence direction of pull of the muscle fibres, contraction of a pennate muscle is unable to reduce its length to the same degree as a parallel muscle. A greater number of myofibrils, however, are found in pennate muscles allowing for a greater development of muscular tension. Pennate muscles, therefore, generally allow a higher force production but a smaller range of movement. Depending on the location of the fascicles in relation to the tendon, a pennate muscle may be classified as *unipennate*, *bipennate* or *multipennate*. A muscle is unipennate when all muscle fibres are on one side of the tendon and bipennate when on both sides of the tendon. Bipennate muscles are much more common, with the rectus femoris muscle of the thigh being a well-known example. In some cases the tendon branches within a pennate muscle and is known as multipennate, for example the deltoid muscle of the shoulder.

The final arrangement of muscle fascicles is in a circular fashion around an opening or recess, known as a **circular muscle** or **sphincter**. The orbicularis oris muscle of the mouth is an example of a circular muscle we see every day, with the size of the opening decreasing as the muscle contracts. The function of circular muscles is to control the entrance and release of substances with several sphincters found along the digestive and urinary tracts.

Fascicle Organisation

1 In a **parallel muscle**, such as the biceps brachii, the fascicles are parallel to the long axis of the muscle. Most of the skeletal muscles in the body are parallel muscles. Some are flat bands with broad attachments (aponeuroses) at each end; others are plump and cylindrical, with tendons at one or both ends. The muscle has a central **body**, also known as the belly. A skeletal muscle fibre can contract until it has shortened by roughly 30 percent. Because the muscle fibres in a parallel muscle are parallel to the long axis of the muscle, when those fibres contract together, the entire muscle shortens by about 30 percent. The tension developed during this contraction depends on the total number of myofibrils the muscle contains.

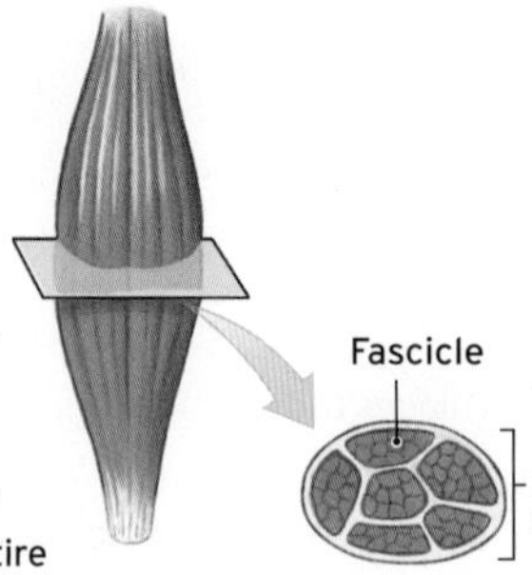

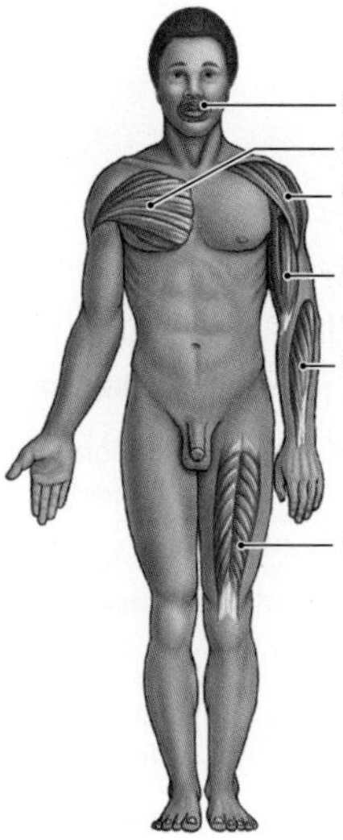

2 In a **convergent muscle**, such as the pectoralis major, muscle fascicles extending over a broad area converge on a common attachment site. A convergent muscle is versatile, because the stimulation of different portions of the muscle can change the direction of pull. However, when the entire muscle contracts, the muscle fibres do not pull as hard on the attachment site as would a parallel muscle of the same size.

Fascicle
Body (belly)

Base of muscle
Tendon

(4)
(2)
(3c)
(1)
(3a)
(3b)

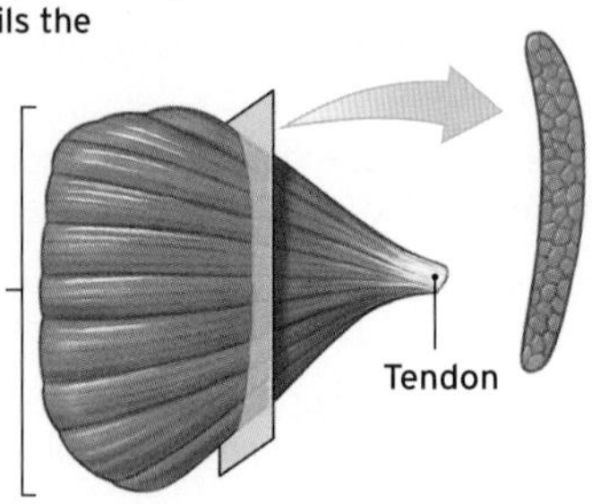

3 In a **pennate muscle** (penna, feather), the fascicles form a common angle with the tendon. Because the muscle fibers pull at an angle, contracting pennate muscles do not move their tendons as far as parallel muscles do. But a pennate muscle contains more muscle fibres—and thus more myofibrils— than does a parallel muscle of the same size, so it produces more tension.

ⓐ Extensor digitorum muscle **ⓑ** Rectus femoris muscle **ⓒ** Deltoid muscle

Extended tendon

Tendons

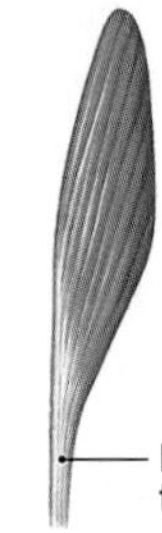

If all the muscle fibers are on the same side of the tendon, the pennate muscle is **unipennate**.

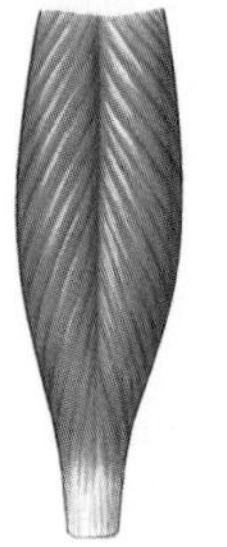

If a pennate muscle has fibers on both sides of the tendon, it is called **bipennate**.

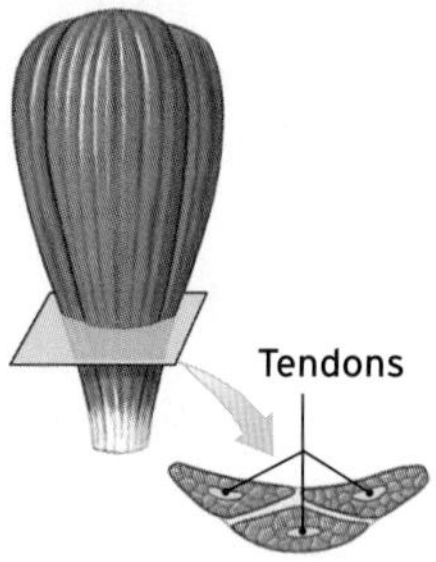

If the tendon branches within a pennate muscle, the muscle is said to be **multipennate**.

4 In a **circular muscle**, or **sphincter** (SFINK-ter), the fascicles are concentrically arranged around an opening or a recess. When the muscle contracts, the diameter of the opening decreases.

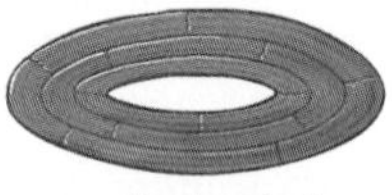

Contracted

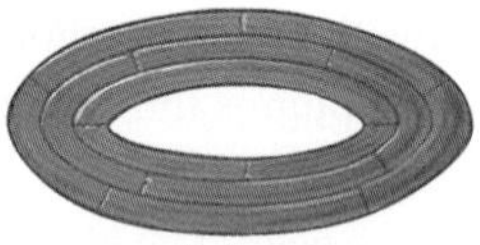

Relaxed

Figure 5.22 Fascicular structural arrangements of skeletal muscle tissue.

Key point

The human body contains 600–700 muscles which are attached to the skeleton at two positions, the origin and insertion.

These muscles work in pairs, with one contracting (the prime mover or agonist) while the other relaxes (antagonist).

It is through the contraction of the muscles exerting a force on the bones (levers) of the skeletal system that produces every movement we make, whether in everyday life or sporting performance.

The magnitude and direction of force created by muscular contraction varies depending on the fascicular arrangement of the muscle.

5.3 Acute responses to exercise

As discussed in the previous chapter, the increased rate of metabolism and hence increased demand for fuel of skeletal muscle tissue is controlled by the nervous and endocrine systems. Skeletal muscle tissue is under the control of the somatic (voluntary) division of the nervous system which plays an immediate role in the production of the faster, and more forceful, contractions required during exercise. The rate of skeletal muscle metabolism is increased through the action of the hormones thyroxine, adrenaline and noradrenaline, during increasing intensities of exercise.

A further function of the endocrine system during exercise is to increase the availability of fuel substrates to support the increased metabolism. The hormones glucagon, adrenaline and noradrenaline stimulate the liver to release glucose into the blood through the processes of **glycogenolysis** (breakdown of glycogen to glucose) and **gluconeogenesis** (formation of glucose from noncarbohydrate molecules such as amino acids). Cortisol also enhances glucose availability through its stimulation of amino acid gluconeogenesis. Carbohydrate stores in the form of glucose and glycogen, unlike the body's fat stores, are limited in supply and as a consequence a number of hormones stimulate the catabolism of fats and amino acids to promote glycogen sparing. These hormones also stimulate the catabolism of fat as an energy source when glucose levels are low, such as during endurance activities. The hormones adrenalin, noradrenaline, cortisol, human growth hormone and glucagon all increase the activation of the enzyme **hormone-sensitive lipase** which is the key enzyme in the mobilisation of fats for metabolism by the process of **lipolysis**. Through their general stimulatory effect on metabolic rate, thyroxine, adrenaline and noradrenaline serve to enhance the catabolism of fats through β **oxidation**. Lipolysis, fat catabolism and β oxidation are discussed in more detail in Chapter 12.

Check your recall
Fill in the missing words.

➤ Together, the skeletal and muscular systems are the _____ systems of the body.

➤ The bones, acting as _____, allow the contraction of muscles across joints to result in movement.

➤ Muscles are also responsible for the _____ movement of substances along tracts, such as the digestive and urinary tracts, and the life-supplying beating of the heart and blood circulation around the body.

The skeletal system

➤ The skeletal system provides the basic structure and _____ for the human body.

➤ The skeletal system consists of bones, cartilage and _____.

➤ The skeletal system has five main functions: support, protection of the soft tissues, a role in movement, _____ of minerals and triglycerides and the production of some blood components.

➤ In contrast to its inert appearance, bone is a highly vascularised dynamic material that is continuously being remodelled by the function of _____ (bone-forming cells) and osteoclasts (_____ cells).

➤ Bone has numerous spaces within its structure and can be classified as compact (minimal spaces) or _____ (many spaces).

➤ A protective, connective tissue sheath called the _____, surrounds each bone and provides the site for ligament and tendon attachment.

➤ Joints are formed where two or more _____ come together.

➤ They can be classified by the range of motion or the _____ of the joint.

➤ _____ joints are the most freely moveable joints in the body, and are hence central to body movement brought about through skeletal muscle contraction.

➤ They are surrounded by an articular capsule which contains _____ fluid, aiding lubrication and cushioning of the joint.

➤ The articulating surfaces of the bones are covered with _____ cartilage, aiding smooth articulation of the bones.

➤ These joints are held together and supported by complex arrangements of _____, tendons and muscles.

Muscular system

➤ The muscular system is responsible for movement, stabilisation of posture, _____ production and the storage of both oxygen and nutrients.

➤ Both blood and _____ are moved within the body by the muscular system.

➤ Together with the _____ system, the muscular system allows the movement of the body as a whole.

➤ There are _____ types of muscle tissue in the human body.

➤ _____ muscle is the only muscle type that can be voluntarily contracted.

➤ Smooth muscle and cardiac muscle are under the control of the _____ nervous system.

➤ _____ muscle is found in the digestive tract and surrounds blood vessels and the airways.

➤ _____ muscle is the main tissue from which the heart is formed.

➤ The plasma membrane of a muscle fibre is referred to as the _____ and surrounds a specialised cytoplasm known as the sarcoplasm.

➤ Oxygen is stored within the sarcoplasm by _____.

➤ Muscle fibres are grouped together into fascicles and fascicles are bound together to form _____.

➤ Each muscle fibre contains tiny fibres called _____ (the contractile fibres of the cell).

➤ These _____ are formed from specialised protein filaments (myofilaments) arranged in contractile units called _____.

➤ Together with troponin and tropomyosin, actin and _____ enable contraction of the muscle fibre.

➤ Actin fibres provide a framework within which the _____ fibres slide.

➤ Myosin heads bind to sites on the actin forming _____.

➤ The breakdown of ATP provides energy that the myosin head stores and then uses to perform a 'powerstroke' which pulls the actin filament towards the middle of the _____ thus shortening the overall length.

➤ The binding of a new ATP molecule to the myosin head allows it to release the _____ filament and become 'cocked'.

➤ Essentially the filaments _____ along each other to shorten or lengthen the sarcomere and it is for this reason that it is referred to as the _____ _____ theory of muscle contraction.

➤ If a number of action potentials arrive in quick succession, the muscle fibre tension progressively *summates* and the mechanical response is called a _____.

➤ The tetanus may be _____, at lower rates of stimulation with oscillating tension (most common situation in the body), or _____, as the frequency of stimulation rises to produce a smooth development of tension.

➤ At the level of the whole skeletal muscle, tension can be increased by the recruitment of additional _____ _____, following the size principle.

➤ The strength of a muscle is positively related to its cross-sectional area. A greater cross-sectional area is due to larger muscle fibres, and hence more _____, increasing the capacity to generate force.

➤ This underlies the process of muscle _____, the muscle's response to strength training.

➤ Whilst muscle fibres are often divided into _____ and type II there are in fact important subdivisions.

➤ Type II fibres can be divided into three further types designated by physiologists as type IIa, _____ and type IIc.

➤ In fact, research has shown the vast majority of type II muscle fibres in human muscle tissue to be type IIa and type IIx (rather than type _____ as commonly reported).

➤ Type I fibres are described as slow _____ fibres which rely on aerobic energy pathways.

➤ Type IIx fibres generate greater _____ than type I fibres and use the fast-rate glycolytic pathway which means they fatigue far more quickly.

➤ Type IIa fibres are an _____ fibre also referred to as fast oxidative glycolytic fibres as they use both oxidative and glycolytic pathways for energy production and lie in between type I and type IIx fibres for speed and force of contraction.

➤ Muscles can contract in _____ different ways.

➤ When a muscle applying force shortens the contraction is said to be _____.

➤ In an _____ contraction the muscle applying force lengthens (for instance in lowering or braking actions).

➤ If the muscle applying force remains in a constant length the contraction is described as _____.

➤ In any contraction the working muscle is referred to as the prime mover or _____. Normally muscles are arranged in pairs with the opposing muscle being referred to as the _____.

➤ An isotonic contraction is made against a
_____ load.

➤ A resistance machine with cams, however, might be designed
to provide a load that varies throughout the movement so
that force production within the muscle is constant. This
type of contraction is described as _____.

➤ Some exercises require a bouncing action in order to pre-
tension a muscle before a concentric contraction and these
are referred to as _____ contractions.

➤ In addition to being classified individually by name,
skeletal muscles can be classified according to their
_____ arrangement.

➤ There are four main arrangements: parallel, convergent,
pennate and _____.

Review questions

1. What are the two divisions of the skeleton and what bones
are included in each division?

2. In terms of composition, structure and function, what
are the similarities and differences between spongy and
compact bone?

3. Name the three types of cartilage in the body and discuss
their locations and functions.

4. Describe the anatomy of a typical synovial joint and name
an example of such a joint.

5. Name the three types of muscle tissue and describe the
microscopic differences between the types.

6. What is the contractile unit of skeletal muscle and what
factors relating to it affect the generation of tension within
a muscle fibre?

7. What factors affect the development of tension in a skeletal
muscle as a whole?

8. Describe how the motor neuron action potential is transferred to the skeletal muscle fibre across the neuromuscular
junction.

9. What is excitation–contraction coupling and what processes are involved?

10. How might the composition of a sport performer's muscle
fibres impact on the types of activity they perform best in?

11. What is the controversy over designating the third common group of fibres in human muscle 'Type IIx'?

12. How do isometric, isotonic and plyometric muscular contractions differ? Describe an example of each of these types
of contraction.

Teach it!
In groups of three, choose one topic and
teach it to the rest of the study group.

1. Describe how an action potential crosses from a neuron to
a muscle.

2. Explain, with reference to excitation–contraction coupling,
how a muscle contraction is initiated.

3. Explain, using diagrams, how muscular contraction is
brought about as described in the sliding filament theory.

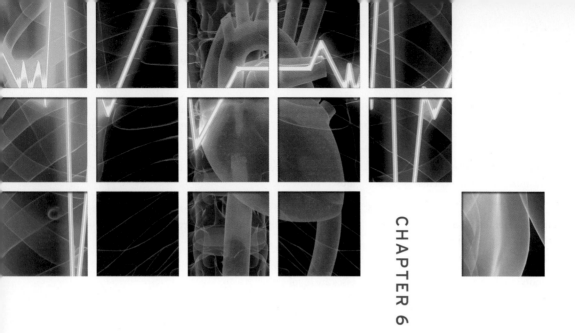

The transport and exchange systems:
respiratory and cardiovascular

Learning objectives

After reading, considering and discussing with a study partner the material in this chapter you should be able to:

➤ describe the structure and function of the respiratory system

➤ summarise how pulmonary ventilation occurs

➤ describe the control mechanisms for pulmonary ventilation

➤ explain how pulmonary gaseous exchange takes place

➤ identify a range of pulmonary function tests

➤ explain how VO_2 and VCO_2 are measured and calculated

➤ discuss the components of the cardiovascular system including their structure and function

➤ distinguish between the components of blood

➤ highlight the immune function of the cardiovascular system

➤ summarise the key aspects of an ECG trace

➤ explain the complete pathway in cardiovascular circulation including passage through the heart

➤ teach others about how blood pressure is measured and what the readings mean

All cells in the body require a constant supply of oxygen and nutrients for survival, and a means in which to remove the waste products of metabolism, the demands of which increase with exercise. The respiratory system functions to oxygenate the blood flowing through the lungs, while removing the waste product carbon dioxide. The cardiovascular system then takes this oxygenated blood and pumps it around the body. As discussed in Chapter 2, nutrients from the digestive system enter the bloodstream and are transported, along with the oxygen, to all cells of the body. During the passage of blood through the tissues, oxygen and nutrients enter cells, while carbon dioxide and other waste products move into the blood for removal. The interrelated functions of the respiratory and cardiovascular systems mean that, should either system fail, the body will become starved of oxygen and survival will no longer be possible.

6.1 The respiratory system

The primary role of the respiratory system is to facilitate the exchange of oxygen and carbon dioxide between the air and the internal cells of the body. Oxygen is essential for producing energy which is a requirement of every cell in the body. Carbon dioxide, a waste product of energy production, must be removed from the body to sustain life. In addition, the tissues of the respiratory system have an important role in smell, speech, coughing, hiccuping, yawning, sneezing and the Valsalva manoeuvre.

Respiration

The respiratory system supplies the oxygen required for **cellular respiration**. This refers to the use of oxygen by cells of the body to sustain life and results in the production of energy, water and carbon dioxide. Oxygen is the most important substance for sustaining life because of its role in respiration. It reaches the cells through three stages of *ventilation* or gas exchange. **Pulmonary ventilation** or *breathing* enables oxygen to enter the lungs and carbon dioxide to be expelled. **Alveolar ventilation** enables oxygen brought into the lungs via pulmonary ventilation to diffuse into the bloodstream and carbon dioxide to be exchanged. Once within the bloodstream, oxygen is transported to cells throughout the body. The final form of gas exchange, **cellular ventilation**, enables oxygen to diffuse

across the plasma membrane and enter the cell for use within cellular respiration, and carbon dioxide to move from the tissue cells into the blood for eventual removal from the body by the lungs.

Knowledge integration question

Explain the differences between pulmonary, alveolar and cellular ventilation.

Key point

The respiratory system transports oxygen into the body for cellular respiration.

Anatomy of the respiratory system

The major organs within the respiratory system are shown in Figure 6.1 starting from the mouth and nasal cavities

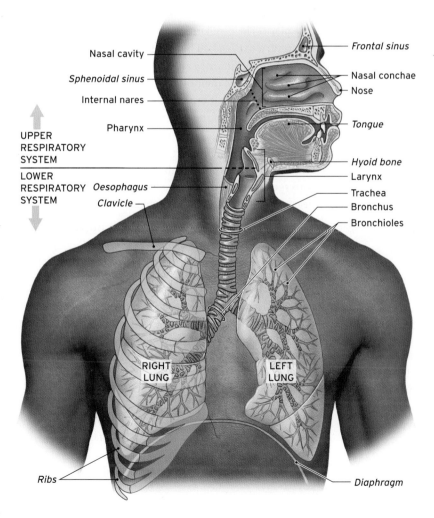

Figure 6.1 Major organs within the respiratory system. (*Source*: Martini, F. H. and Nath, J. L. (2009) *Fundamentals of Anatomy and Physiology*, 8th edition, New York: Benjamin Cummings)

leading down the trachea (windpipe), branching in to two bronchi, to reach the lungs. The respiratory tract continues to subdivide within the lungs creating lobes in each lung and each of these lobes is comprised of lobules. Each lobe has its own secondary bronchi, and lobules are formed by further branching of the respiratory tract. Due to the presence of the heart on the left side of the body the left lung has only two lobes, whereas the right lung is comprised of three lobes and is therefore slightly bigger (about 10%) than the left. Within the lungs, the respiratory tract finally leads to the alveoli, which are the terminal structures of the respiratory tract.

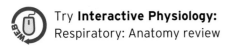 Try **Interactive Physiology:**
Respiratory: Anatomy review

Zones of the respiratory system

The respiratory tract is most commonly divided in to two zones. The **conducting zone** (Figure 6.1), passes air to the sites of gas exchange; this includes the nose, mouth, pharynx (throat), larynx (voice box), trachea (windpipe), bronchi, bronchioles and terminal bronchioles. The **respiratory zone** (Figure 6.2), is the site of gas exchange, and comprises the respiratory bronchioles, alveolar ducts, alveolar sacs and the alveoli. Air reaching the alveoli from the trachea typically passes through 25 branches, starting with the division of the trachea into the left and right bronchi, before ultimately reaching the alveoli.

> **Key point**
>
> The respiratory system can be divided into the conducting and respiratory zones.

The *Pleurae*

The left and right lungs are contained within a **pleural sac**, a serous membrane that folds back on itself forming a two layered structure. The pleural sac is composed of the **parietal** *pleura* (outer membrane lining the thoracic wall and diaphragm) and the **visceral** *pleura* (inner membrane covering the lungs) with the gap between the membranes known as the **pleural cavity**. The pleural cavity is filled by **pleural fluid**, which is largely comprised of water, the special properties of which are vital for the functioning of pleural fluid. The fluid's surface tension ensures the two membranes stick together, but also allows for the sliding

of the membranes across each other during pulmonary ventilation. Due to the surface tension, and the fact the parietal pleura is attached to the thoracic wall and the diaphragm, the lungs expand and recoil when the thoracic volume increases and decreases with breathing. By way of analogy, the dual function of pleural fluid can be likened to placing water between two microscope glass slides. The slides would be difficult to pull apart because of the surface attraction, but would be easy to slide between your fingers.

Blood supply of the lungs

Pulmonary exchange takes place between the lungs and the pulmonary blood vessels. The pulmonary arteries supply deoxygenated blood which is pumped from the right ventricle of the heart to the lungs. The pulmonary artery leaves the heart and divides into a left and right branch supplying blood to the left and right lung respectively. The pulmonary arteries then branch into smaller vessels that lead to the tiny capillaries that surround each alveolus and enable gaseous exchange to take place. The capillaries lead to four pulmonary veins that return oxygenated blood to the left atrium of the heart before its journey around the rest of the body. The lungs receive their own supply of oxygenated blood via the right and left bronchial arteries (branches from the aorta) as part of the systemic blood flow. This supply enables the lung cells to obtain the oxygen necessary to sustain their functioning as well as facilitating the removal of carbon dioxide through gaseous exchange. The deoxygenated blood from the lung tissue is returned to the heart via the bronchial veins, which flow into the superior vena cava.

Mechanics of pulmonary ventilation

Pulmonary ventilation comprises inspirations (inhalations) and expirations (exhalations). At rest inspiration is achieved through *active* mechanisms whereas expiration is *passive* and completed through the relaxation of the muscles involved in inhalation.

> **Key point**
>
> Pulmonary ventilation or breathing consists of:
>
> *Inspirations* – breathing in, inhalation
> *Expirations* – breathing out, exhalation

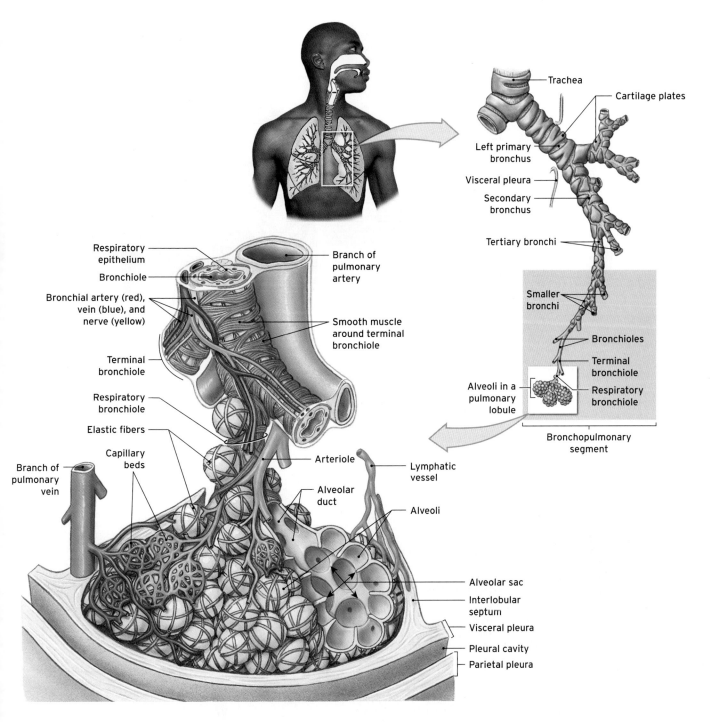

Figure 6.2 The structure of alveoli. (*Source*: Martini, F. H. and Nath, J. L. (2009) *Fundamentals of Anatomy and Physiology*, 8th edition, New York: Benjamin Cummings)

Inspiratory and expiratory muscles

The muscles involved in inspiration and expiration are shown in Figure 6.3. Each inspiration is brought about through two mechanisms. Firstly, the **diaphragm** and the **external intercostals** (primary inspiratory muscles) contract causing the rib cage to rise and the diaphragm to flatten which serve to increase the volume of the thoracic cavity and hence, as discussed above, the lungs. Secondly, the increased lung volume decreases air pressure within the lungs, causing air to rush into the body thus equalising the pressure.

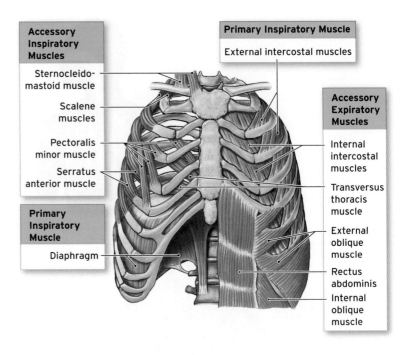

Accessory Inspiratory Muscles

Sternocleido-mastoid muscle

Scalene muscles

Pectoralis minor muscle

Serratus anterior muscle

Primary Inspiratory Muscle

Diaphragm

Primary Inspiratory Muscle

External intercostal muscles

Accessory Expiratory Muscles

Internal intercostal muscles

Transversus thoracis muscle

External oblique muscle

Rectus abdominis

Internal oblique muscle

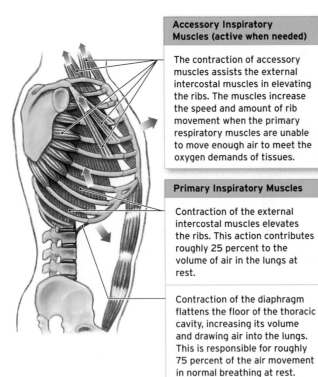

Accessory Inspiratory Muscles (active when needed)

The contraction of accessory muscles assists the external intercostal muscles in elevating the ribs. The muscles increase the speed and amount of rib movement when the primary respiratory muscles are unable to move enough air to meet the oxygen demands of tissues.

Primary Inspiratory Muscles

Contraction of the external intercostal muscles elevates the ribs. This action contributes roughly 25 percent to the volume of air in the lungs at rest.

Contraction of the diaphragm flattens the floor of the thoracic cavity, increasing its volume and drawing air into the lungs. This is responsible for roughly 75 percent of the air movement in normal breathing at rest.

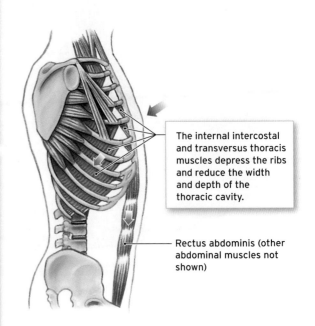

The internal intercostal and transversus thoracis muscles depress the ribs and reduce the width and depth of the thoracic cavity.

Rectus abdominis (other abdominal muscles not shown)

Figure 6.3 Muscles involved in pulmonary ventilation.

At rest, around 0.5 L of air is exchanged during each inspiration and expiration. During exercise up to six times this volume (3.0 L) can be exchanged. As a result of the ebb and flow of air from the body, the amount in each breath is known as the **tidal volume** (V_T). The increase in tidal volume during exercise is enabled through the recruitment of accessory inspiratory muscles and a switch from passive to active expiration. During exercise the *sternocleidomastoid*, *scalene*, *pectoralis minor* and the *serratus anterior* muscles add to the force of contraction resulting in a further increase in the lung volume with each inspiration. This causes an increased differential between the air pressure in the lungs and that outside the body and, as a consequence, more air enters the lungs with each inhalation. The passive mechanism of exhalation at rest, resulting from the return of the elastic inspiratory muscle fibres, is enhanced by the contraction of the *internal intercostals, transversus thoracis* and *abdominal muscles* during exercise. The abdominal muscles involved are the external oblique, rectus abdominis, internal oblique and transversus abdominus. In addition to the increased depth of breathing (tidal volume), exercise also results in an increase in the rate of breathing (**respiratory frequency**). At rest, each respiratory cycle takes around 5 s (2 s for inspiration and 3 s for expiration) resulting in a respiratory frequency (R_f) of 12 breaths·min^{-1}.

 Try **Interactive Physiology:**
Respiratory: Pulmonary ventilation

Minute ventilation

The tidal volume and respiratory frequency can be multiplied to calculate the **minute ventilation** ($\dot{V}$ or $\dot{V}_E$), the amount of air inspired or expired each minute ($\dot{V}_E = V_T \times R_f$). Typically $\dot{V}_E$ at rest is around 6 L·min^{-1} ($\dot{V}_E = 0.5$ L $\times$ 12). During exercise, when the demand for oxygen to supply the working muscles increases dramatically, both tidal volume and respiratory frequency can be increased to meet demand. At maximal levels tidal volume can rise to 3.0 L·breath^{-1}, and the respiratory frequency to 60 breaths·min^{-1} for experienced endurance athletes such as marathon runners and cross-country skiers. Minute ventilation volumes can therefore rise from around 6 L·min^{-1} at rest, to 180 L·min^{-1} during maximal exercise. Changes in the depth and frequency of breathing are controlled by the respiratory centre.

Control of pulmonary ventilation

The rate and depth of breathing is controlled by respiratory centres located in the medulla oblongata and the pons (both of which form part of the brain stem). Cranial afferent nerves deliver sensory information to the CNS from chemoreceptors located in three positions in the body: (i) within the brain stem that detect changes in the partial pressure of carbon dioxide (PCO_2) and H$^+$ concentration in cerebral spinal fluid and blood, (ii) in the aorta (artery) and (iii) common carotid arteries which, along with the receptors in the aorta, detect changes in PCO_2, partial pressure of oxygen (PO_2) and H$^+$ concentrations in the blood.

Although the sensory neurons pick up information about the PO_2 in the blood, the respiratory centre is more sensitive and responsive to changes in levels of CO_2 in the blood and as such PCO_2 is the more important stimulus to increase breathing rate and/or depth. It is for this reason that free-divers hyperventilate (breathe very rapidly) before diving. By hyperventilating prior to a dive they reduce the PCO_2 in the blood and this decreases the drive to inspire air and means they can hold their breath for longer. The extended breathhold required for such dives, however, can result in decreased oxygen levels (PO_2) in the blood causing a blackout during the dive and resultant drowning. Chemoreceptors in all three locations respond to changes in H$^+$ concentration in the blood. Carbon dioxide, produced within cells, quickly combines with water in the blood to form carbonic acid (H_2CO_3) which dissociates to HCO_3^- (bicarbonate) and H$^+$. As a result, H$^+$ concentration is related to the concentration of carbon dioxide in the body. Indeed, as CO_2 accumulates in the brain during exercise, it is the increase in H^+ concentration from carbonic acid dissociation that is detected by the localised chemoreceptors which stimulate an increase in R_f and V_T.

Cranial sensory nerves relay information about PCO_2, PO_2 and H^+ concentrations to four areas in the brain stem. During breathing at rest the *inspiratory area*, located in the medulla oblongata, controls the rate and depth of breathing for inspiration and expiration. The inspiratory area stimulates the external intercostals and diaphragm to contract for two seconds. When this stimulus is removed (for three seconds) these muscle relax and expiration takes place. During exercise when active expiration is required, the *expiratory area*, also located in the medulla oblongata, sends nerve impulses to stimulate the internal intercostals, transversus thoracis and the abdominal muscles to contract. The *pneumotaxic* and *apneustic* centres, found within the Pons, are responsible during exercise for shortening the duration of inspiration and deepening breathing respectively.

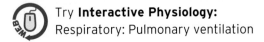

Try **Interactive Physiology:**
Respiratory: Pulmonary ventilation

Knowledge integration question

Explain how the brain triggers and alters breathing rate.

Pulmonary gas exchange

Gaseous exchange between the alveoli and the capillaries is enabled through the unique structure of their cell membranes. The structure of each, and the way in which they interconnect, enables gaseous exchange to take place as illustrated in Figure 6.4.

Alveoli and the role of surfactant

Alveoli are grape-like structures that have two layers. The outer layer is a protective membrane and the inner layer, the wall of an alveolus is comprised of two types of epithelial cells. *Type I* alveolar cells, which form the main structure of the wall, are interspersed with *Type II* cells, which help to maintain the structure of each alveolus by secreting an alveolar fluid which is largely composed of water but also contains **surfactant**. Surfactant is chiefly composed of lipoproteins and phospholipids and is essential to gaseous exchange.

The secreted alveolar fluid lines the inner surface of the alveolar walls. If composed solely of water, alveolar fluid would result in the collapse of alveoli between breaths due to its high surface tension. The surfactant within the alveolar fluid, however, reduces the surface tension, as lipids and water do not mix well, maintaining the alveolar structure during pulmonary ventilation. *Macrophages* are a third type of alveolar cell; they serve an immune function and maintain the gaseous exchange surfaces by removing debris from the alveoli.

Gas exchange

As can be seen from Figure 6.4, alveoli are surrounded by an intricate network of capillaries. Gaseous exchange takes place across the **respiratory membrane** formed between the capillaries and the alveoli. This consists of the cellular walls of the alveoli and capillaries bound together by their fused protective basement membranes. Despite the complexity of the respiratory membrane, which is required to protect and maintain the integrity of the alveoli and capillaries, the structure is very thin. The membrane is 15 times thinner than a sheet of tissue paper, enabling gaseous exchange to proceed very rapidly. The unique structure of the lungs, which are thought to be comprised of over 300 million alveoli, means there is a vast surface area available for gaseous exchange between the alveoli and the millions of capillaries that surround them. This surface area is around 75 m^2, almost the equivalent of a singles badminton court.

Gaseous exchange takes place by diffusion, the flow of gases across the respiratory membrane from high to low concentration. Through this process, carbon dioxide which is in higher concentration in the capillaries, diffuses into the alveoli while oxygen, in higher concentration in the alveoli, diffuses into the capillaries. The concentration of a gas is measured by its *partial pressure*, first described by the English scientist John Dalton and subsequently known as Dalton's law. Table 6.1 shows the percentage and partial pressure of each of the gases and water vapour in atmospheric air. Dalton's law states that the total pressure of a mixture of gases (such as that found in air) is equivalent to the sum of the partial pressures of each of the gases. The partial pressure of oxygen (PO_2) needs to be higher in the alveolar air than in the blood for oxygen to diffuse into the bloodstream. Similarly, if the partial pressure of carbon dioxide (PCO_2) is higher in the bloodstream than in the alveoli carbon dioxide will diffuse into the alveolar space.

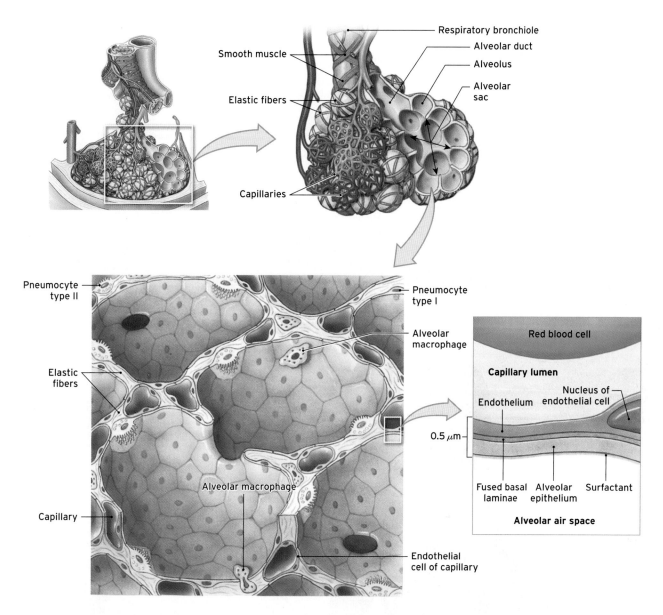

Figure 6.4 Section through an alveolus depicting gaseous exchange. (*Source*: Martini, F. H. and Nath, J. L. (2009) *Fundamentals of Anatomy and Physiology*, 8th edition, New York: Benjamin Cummings)

Table 6.1 The partial pressures of the main gases and water vapour in air.

Air constituent	% concentration	Calculation	Partial pressure
Nitrogen*	78.63	(78.63 ÷ 100) × 760	597.6 mmHg
Oxygen	20.93	(20.93 ÷ 100) × 760	159.1 mmHg
Carbon dioxide	0.04	(0.04 ÷ 100) × 760	0.3 mmHg
Water vapour**	0.4	(0.4 ÷ 100) × 760	3 mmHg
Total pressure	**100 %**		**760 mmHg***

*The percentage concentration for nitrogen includes other trace gases found in air, but not involved in respiration, such as argon.
**Water vapour in air is referred to as humidity and varies according to time and location, the figure of 0.4 % is a typical example.
*** 760 mmHg represents mean atmospheric pressure at sea level.

The oxygen cascade

The partial pressures of the respiratory gases, oxygen and carbon dioxide, differ between alveolar and atmospheric air, as shown in Table 6.2 and Figure 6.5. When air enters the mouth it is immediately saturated with water vapour and as a consequence the partial pressure of water (PH_2O) rises from 3.0 mmHg to 47 mmHg. This results in a drop in the PO_2 to 149 mmHg because, when air enters the trachea, oxygen comprises 20.93% of 713 mmHg pressure (760−47 mmHg for water vapour). As the percentage of CO_2 in inspired air is so small the increased PH_2O in the trachea has a negligible effect on PCO_2 (0.3 mmHg to 0.28 mmHg). There is a second drop in the PO_2 and an increase in the PCO_2 as air reaches the alveoli due to the constant diffusion of gases between the blood and alveoli. The continual movement of oxygen out of, and carbon dioxide into, the alveoli results in the percentage of oxygen being lower and carbon dioxide being higher (around 14.5% and 5.5% respectively). Despite the drop in

Table 6.2 Changes in PCO_2 and PO_2 between atmospheric and alveolar air (mmHg).

Air constituent	Atmospheric air	Tracheal air	Alveolar air	Pulmonary*
Nitrogen	597.6	563.49	570.41	N/A
Oxygen	159.1	149.23	103.38	40
Carbon dioxide	0.3	0.28	39.21	46
Water vapour	3.0	47.0	47.0	N/A
Total pressure	**760**	760	760	N/A

* The partial pressures in the last column are for oxygen and carbon dioxide in pulmonary capillary blood. At sea level nitrogen is not normally absorbed into the blood and water vapour does not take part in the respiratory process.

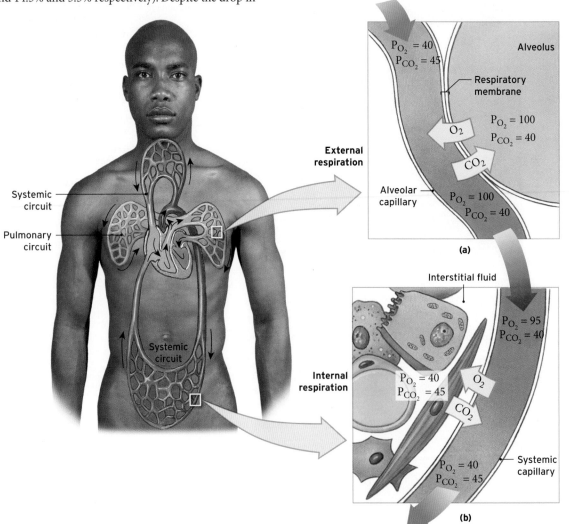

Figure 6.5 Oxygen and carbon dioxide partial pressure changes from inspired air to alveoli (a) and to body tissues (b). (*Source*: Martini, F. H. and Nath, J. L. (2009) *Fundamentals of Anatomy and Physiology*, 8th edition, New York: Benjamin Cummings)

PO_2 as it makes its journey from the atmosphere to the alveoli, oxygen molecules are able to diffuse across the respiratory membrane because the PO_2 in the bloodstream is lower than that in the alveolar space, at around 40 mmHg (see Figure 6.5). Carbon dioxide, on the other hand, diffuses into the alveoli from the bloodstream because the PCO_2 in the bloodstream is around 7 mmHg higher which, although lower than the differential for oxygen, is still sufficient for CO_2 to cross the respiratory membrane.

The fall in the PO_2 from 159 mmHg to around 100 mmHg as air moves from the atmosphere to the alveoli, is known as the **oxygen cascade** and is an important aspect of altitude physiology. As you gain altitude the atmospheric pressure falls resulting in a decrease in the PO_2, which, when ascending to extreme altitudes, can affect the ability of oxygen to diffuse into the blood.

Key point

Gaseous exchange takes place across the respiratory membrane which is formed between the alveoli walls and the walls of the capillaries that surround them.

To facilitate diffusion of gases the respiratory membrane is very thin which enables oxygen and carbon dioxide to pass easily between the blood and alveoli.

Measurement of pulmonary ventilation

For physiologists and medical staff the movement of air from the lungs, and the component gases in expired air, can reveal much about human functioning. The resting measurements of lung volumes, along with analysis of the gas composition of expired air, are frequently recorded in research and clinical settings. In addition, the analysis of expired air samples collected during exercise is a common measurement made by exercise physiologists to assess aerobic fitness.

Pulmonary function tests

A spirometer, diagrammed in Figure 6.6a, can be used to assess basic pulmonary function by measuring the static lung volumes (illustrated in Figure 6.7). Average total lung capacity for a male is around 6 L and approximately 4.2 L for females. Gender differences in lung volumes and capacities tend to be due to the smaller physical size of females. The spirometer, and the spirogram trace it creates, records a wide variety of lung volumes including total lung capacity.

Spirometry is commonly used to assess changes in respiratory function, particularly for the identification of pulmonary disorders. In addition to the measurement

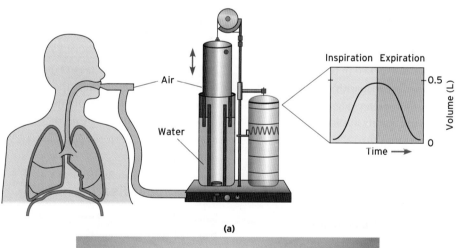

(a)

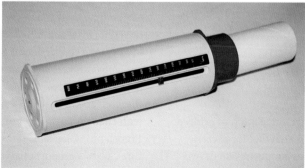

(b)

Figure 6.6 Spirometer (a) and peak flow meter (b). (*Source:* (b) Simon Fryer)

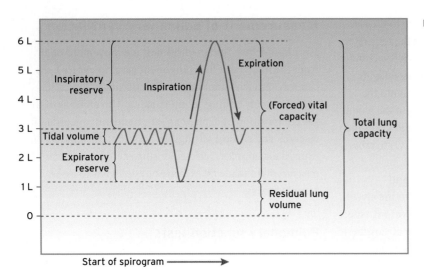

Figure 6.7 Lung volumes.

of minute ventilation, spirometry is commonly used to determine an individual's **forced vital capacity** (FVC) and **forced expiratory volume** (FEV). The FVC is a measure of the voluntary capacity of the lungs which involves maximal inhalation followed by the forceful exhalation of as much air as possible, as rapidly as possible. The forced expiratory volume in one second (FEV_1) measures lung efficiency. The volume of air expired in the first second is recorded and shown as a percentage of the total FVC. The higher the percentage of their FVC a person can exhale in one second the more efficient their lungs. In those with healthy lungs, around 80% of FVC can be expelled in the first second, with much lower volumes in those with obstructive pulmonary disease. A peak flow meter (Figure 6.6b) – cheaper, simpler and more readily available in the laboratory and clinical settings than a spirometer – is now more commonly used for the measurement of FEV_1.

Knowledge integration question

Explain the difference between FVC and FEV_1. Why is it necessary to measure FVC in order to calculate FEV_1?

Analysis of expired air

Measurement of the volume and composition of expired air represents a fundamental research tool for exercise physiologists. Figure 6.8 provides an illustration of two methods of sampling expired air; the traditional Douglas

bag method, and the current computer-based online sampling. During online gas analysis, the computer can record real-time breath-by-breath data with the volume of oxygen consumed ($\dot{V}O_2$) and the volume of carbon dioxide produced ($\dot{V}CO_2$) calculated almost instantaneously by the programme software.

The Douglas bag method involves the analysis of collected gas samples after test completion. A gas analyser is used to measure the percentage of oxygen remaining in the expired air sample and the percentage of carbon dioxide present. These percentages are known as the fraction of expired oxygen (F_EO_2) and the fraction of expired carbon dioxide (F_ECO_2) respectively. After the analysis of gas composition, the Douglas bag is emptied using a gas meter to measure the total volume of air expired during the test. From these results, it is possible to calculate the $\dot{V}_E$ (expired gas volume), $\dot{V}O_2$ and the $\dot{V}CO_2$ during the test.

Gas standardisation

The gas collected in any experiment through the Douglas bag method of gas collection must be standardised before any comparisons can be made with previously collected data or results from a different laboratory. This standardisation involves the conversion of gas volume collected at *ambient temperature and pressure saturated* (ATPS) to *standard temperature and pressure dry* (STPD). The need to make this conversion is due to the fact that gas volume varies with changing temperature and pressure. Jacques Charles, a French physiologist, identified that an increase in temperature causes a proportional increase in the volume of a gas (Charles' Law), and Robert Boyle showed that the volume

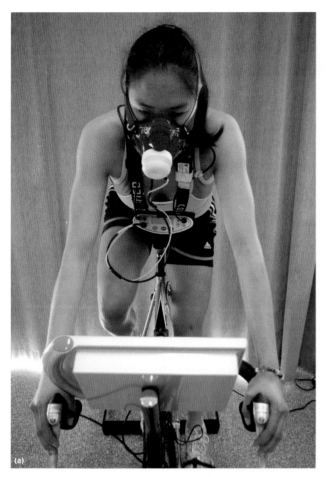
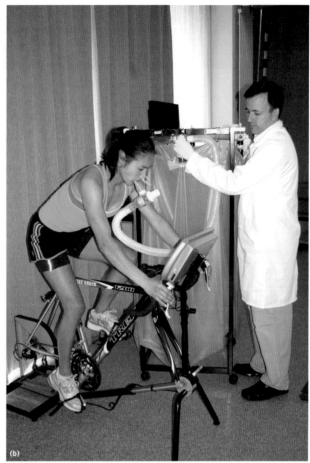

Figure 6.8 Online (a) and Douglas bag (b) gas analysis equipment (*Source*: Simon Fryer)

of a gas varies inversely with pressure (Boyle's Law). Finally, the humidity in the air and the *water saturation* that occurs while air is in the lungs will increase any gas volume. The dry component of STPD takes account of water saturation and provides a dry air conversion which makes an STPD gas collection comparable with data from anywhere in the world, providing those data are also converted to STPD. Consequently, collecting a gas sample from one individual completing the same amount of work in different environmental conditions, would reveal different expired gas volumes before conversion to STPD.

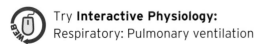 Try **Interactive Physiology:** Respiratory: Pulmonary ventilation

The conversion to STPD changes a gas volume to that which would have been recorded at 0°C and at 760 mmHg

(sea level). The conversion of a gas volume from ATPS to STPD can be calculated by equation, or more simply through the use of a correction factor table, such as the one in Appendix 2. In the example of STPD conversion shown below the correction factor was 0.898; this was found by looking down the barometric pressure column to the row for 760 mmHg and then across to the 22°C temperature column. By multiplying the gas volume by the correction factor the expired air volume can be found, as shown on next page.

Once the $\dot{V}_E$ STPD has been found it is possible to calculate the $\dot{V}O_2$ and $\dot{V}CO_2$ for an expired air gas sample. In its most straightforward format the volume of oxygen consumed ($\dot{V}O_2$) is simply the volume of oxygen in inspired air ($\dot{V}O_{2I}$) minus the volume of oxygen in expired air ($\dot{V}O_{2E}$):

$$\dot{V}O_2 = \dot{V}O_{2I} - \dot{V}O_{2E}$$

From an expired air sample the volume of expired oxygen is not known. However, it can be calculated from the F_EO_2

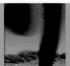

CALCULATION

Calculation of STPD gas volume from ATPS

In a laboratory a 60 second expired gas sample was collected from a runner during a treadmill running test. The laboratory temperature was 22°C and the barometric pressure was 760 mmHg on the day the data was collected.

The gas volume at ATPS was 82.5 L. The correction factor for the temperature and pressure during this experiment using the table in Appendix 2 is 0.898. The conversion of the minute ventilation ($\dot{V}_E$), or expired gas volume, to STPD is as follows:

$$\dot{V}_E \text{ STPD} = \dot{V}_E \text{ ATPS} \times \text{correction factor}$$

$$= 82.5 \times 0.898$$

$$= 74.085 \text{ L}$$

$$\dot{V}_E \text{ STPD} = \underline{74.1 \text{ L·min}^{-1}}$$

reading taken from the gas analyser. The calculation of $\dot{V}O_{2\,E}$ from F_EO_2 would then be as follows:

$$\dot{V}O_{2E} = (\dot{V}_I \times F_IO_2) - (\dot{V}_E \times F_EO_2)$$

A problem with this equation is that the volume of inspired air ($\dot{V}_I$) cannot be determined from an expired air sample. Early physiologists assessed both $\dot{V}_I$ and $\dot{V}_E$ and found that the number of molecules of oxygen consumed during metabolism is not replaced by an equivalent number of molecules of carbon dioxide produced. As a consequence, the gas volume in expired air was smaller than the volume of air inspired.

The **Haldane transformation** was named after the Scottish physiologist John Haldane, but originally developed some 20 years earlier by the German physiologists August Geppert and Nathan Zuntz. This transformation makes an allowance for the change in volume between inspired and expired gas samples and has enabled physiologists to calculate $\dot{V}O_2$ without the need for measurement of $\dot{V}_I$ or the nitrogen content in expired air. Geppert, Zuntz and Haldane recognised that with the drop in total gas volume the relative percentage of nitrogen in an expired air sample increased. They determined that, as nitrogen remained unchanged during metabolism, the same concentration of nitrogen became a larger percentage of a smaller gas volume. The change in the relative percentage of nitrogen forms the basis for the Haldane transformation. From an original series of equations, a single calculation for the

determination of $\dot{V}O_2$ from an expired air sample now constitutes the Haldane transformation.

$$\dot{V}O_2 = \dot{V}_E \times [\{[1 - (F_EO_2 + F_ECO_2)] \times 0.265\} - F_EO_2]$$

Although the brackets make this formula look a little complicated, the following calculation boxes show the Haldane transformation equation broken down into stages to help your understanding.

In the age of technology, however, computer programs are available to convert gas data from ATPS to STPD and run the data through the Haldane transformation to calculate the $\dot{V}O_2$ for an expired air sample without the need for hand calculation. It is useful though to know how the end gas volumes are calculated for a fuller understanding of the conversion of gas volumes to STPD and the Haldane transformation. It is very easy to enter data into a computer without having an understanding of the products of the computations. Following an example through can help you to realise how the results from a computer program are calculated.

Knowledge integration question

Explain why gases are converted from ATPS to STPD.

The $\dot{V}CO_2$ produced during exercise is more simply identified than $\dot{V}O_2$ due to the very small content of carbon dioxide in inspired air (i.e. the majority of the $\dot{V}CO_2$ in an

CALCULATION

Steps in the calculation of $\dot{V}O_2$ from expired gas samples based on the Haldane transformation:

$$\dot{V}O_2 = \dot{V}_E \times [\{[1 - (F_EO_2 + F_ECO_2)] \times 0.265\} - F_EO_2]$$

For simplicity, the equation can be broken down into the following steps (a–d) before the final calculation of $\dot{V}O_2$:

$$\dot{V}O_2 = \overbrace{(F_EO_2 + F_ECO_2)}^{a}$$

$$= \overbrace{[1 - a]}^{b}$$

$$= \overbrace{\{b \times 0.265\}}^{c}$$

$$= \overbrace{[c - F_EO_2]}^{d}$$

The final step and identification of $\dot{V}O_2$: $\dot{V}O_2 = \dot{V}_E \times d$

The calculation of $\dot{V}O_2$ and $\dot{V}CO_2$ using example data can be found on page 164.

expired gas sample is the product of cellular respiration). The amount of carbon dioxide in the air around us represents around 0.04% (0.04 expressed as a fraction = 0.04/100 or more simply 0.0004) of the total volume. As a result the $\dot{V}CO_2$ can be calculated by subtracting the amount of carbon dioxide that was already in the inspired air from that found in the expired gas sample to determine how much was produced by the body:

$$\dot{V}CO_2 = \dot{V}_E \times (F_ECO_2 - 0.0004)$$

Key point

The capacity and functioning of lungs can be measured through the use of spirometers and peak flow meters.

In addition, expired air samples can be collected to provide details about the $\dot{V}O_2$, the $\dot{V}CO_2$ and $\dot{V}_E$ at rest or during exercise.

Pulmonary ventilation and exercise

The use of gas analysis techniques can be employed to examine the effects of exercise on oxygen consumption,

carbon dioxide production and minute ventilation. From this fundamental data collection method, a number of measures have been developed for assessing exercise performance. Perhaps the most commonly reported of these measures is the **maximal oxygen uptake** ($\dot{V}O_{2max}$) which has traditionally been the measure of aerobic fitness and is described in more detail in Chapter 12. The **anaerobic threshold**, the transition between aerobic and anaerobic exercise (see Chapter 11), can be estimated from $\dot{V}O_2$, $\dot{V}CO_2$ and $\dot{V}_E$ data. The **respiratory exchange ratio** (RER) provides physiologists with information about the food-stuff that is providing the main energy source for exercise. At low exercise intensities, lipids, as part of aerobic energy production, form the main fuel source for exercise: as the intensity rises, the body will rely more heavily upon gly-colysis (carbohydrates) as an anaerobic method for energy production. This shift in fuels from lipids to glucose can be derived from the ratio of $\dot{V}CO_2$ produced to $\dot{V}O_2$ con-sumed. The calculation on page 165 shows the RERs for the saturated lipid palmitic acid and glucose. The RER for fats is 0.7 and the RER for glucose is 1.0. During the transition from low-intensity work to high-intensity work the RER moves from 0.7 closer to 1.0. An RER of 0.85 provides an

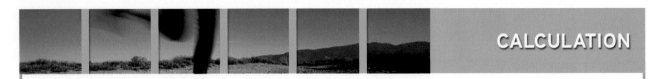

CALCULATION

Calculation of $\dot{V}O_2$ and $\dot{V}CO_2$

Using the example from the STPD calculation for the runner during the treadmill running test the $\dot{V}_E$ was 74.1 L·min^{-1}, the $F_EO_2 = 17.4\%$ (or 0.174 as a fraction) and $F_ECO_2 = 4.1\%$ (or 0.041 as a fraction).

An example calculation of $\dot{V}O_2$ from an expired gas sample based on the Haldane transformation:

$$\dot{V}O_2 = \dot{V}_E \times [\{[1 - (F_EO_2 + F_ECO_2)] \times 0.265\} - F_EO_2]$$

$$\dot{V}O_2 = \overbrace{(0.174 + 0.041)}^{a} = 0.215$$

$$= \overbrace{[1 - 0.215]}^{b} = 0.785$$

$$= \overbrace{\{0.785 \times 0.265\}}^{c} = 0.208$$

$$= \overbrace{[0.208 - 0.174]}^{d} = 0.038$$

The final step and identification of $\dot{V}O_2$ in this example:

$$\dot{V}O_2 = 74.1 \times 0.034$$

$$= 2.5194 \text{ or } \underline{2.52 \text{ L·min}^{-1}}$$

The calculation of $\dot{V}CO_2$ from an expired gas sample:

$$\dot{V}CO_2 = \dot{V}_E \times (F_ECO_2 - 0.0004)$$

$$\dot{V}CO_2 = \dot{V}_E \times (F_ECO_2 - F_ICO_2)$$

$$= 74.1 \times (0.041 - 0.0004)$$

$$= 74.1 \times 0.0406$$

$$= 3.00846 \text{ or } \underline{3.01 \text{ L·min}^{-1}}$$

indicator that mixed fuels are being used – fats and carbohydrates are jointly providing the energy for work.

At rest the RER is sometimes referred to as the **respiratory quotient** (RQ) which is calculated in exactly the same way. The RQ was first developed in the early 20th century, before the term RER came into use, to identify the predominant fuel for metabolism. Since the early research into RQ it has been discovered that during exercise carbon dioxide is produced from additional sources as well as from macronutrient catabolism. As a consequence, during exercise, the term RQ was replaced with RER to recognise the possible influence of non-marconutrient produced CO_2 to the expired $\dot{V}CO_2$. In a similar way,

further research has indicated that during exercise protein can provide up to 10% of the necessary fuel. Protein catabolism has an RQ of around 0.83, although the RER cannot distinguish protein from fat or carbohydrate. As a result, RER is generally thought of as a non-protein RER – the relatively small contribution of protein to metabolism means that it is generally ignored in exercise physiology.

Knowledge integration question

Explain the difference between the RQ and RER.

CALCULATION

Calculation of RER from $\dot{V}CO_2$ and $\dot{V}O_2$ data

Lipid oxidation:

Palmitic acid $C_{16}H_{32}O_2$

$$C_{16}H_{32}O_2 + 23O_2 \longrightarrow 16CO_2 + 16H_2O + 105 \text{ ATP}$$

$RER = 16CO_2{:}23O_2 = 16 \div 23 = \underline{0.7}$

Glucose oxidation:

Glucose $C_6H_{12}O_6$

$$C_6H_{12}O_6 + 6O_2 \longrightarrow 6CO_2 + 6H_2O + 30 \text{ ATP}$$

$REP = 6CO_2{:}6O_2 = 6 \div 6 = \underline{1.0}$

Valsalva manoeuvre

In this section on pulmonary ventilation and exercise, particularly in the case of strength training for sports, it is useful to consider the effects of the Valsalva manoeuvre. The **Valsalva manoeuvre** was first described by an Italian anatomist, Antonio Valsalva. In a sporting context the Valsalva manoeuvre can be used to stabilise the thoracic and abdominal cavities, to augment the action of the chest muscles and increase strength during heavy lifting. After a full inhalation the performer closes the glottis (the opening between the vocal folds of the larynx) and at the same time contracts the respiratory muscles and additional abdominal muscles. The net result of this is a fixation of the chest and abdomen cavities and a great increase in the intra-abdominal and intra-thoracic pressures. The performer uses this pressure to enhance the strength response for a lift. The danger from the Valsalva manoeuvre comes from the increased pressure which can cause the great veins within the abdominal and thoracic cavities to collapse, greatly reducing venous return and causing a drop in blood pressure that can lead to a performer seeing spots before their eyes or fainting. While commonly used in some weight-lifting activities the Valsalva manoeuvre is potentially dangerous.

6.2 The cardiovascular system

The **cardiovascular system**, the body's main transport mechanism, comprises three components: *blood* (4–6 L) which is pumped by the *heart* round the *vascular system* (a continuous circuit of vessels through which blood flows). From very early in development the cardiovascular system is required for transport and as a consequence the heart is the first functional organ in the body. The primary functions of the cardiovascular system are to *transport* nutrients and hormones to cells and waste products from cells for removal from the body, to help *maintain* body temperature and to assist in the *prevention* of infection. In Chapter 5 the muscular system was described, with a focus on skeletal muscle tissue. The cardiovascular system includes organs that comprise the other two forms of muscle tissue. The heart is comprised of *cardiac muscle tissue* which enables the heart to beat continuously, without fatigue, around 40,000,000 times per year and therefore between 300–350 billion times in an average life time, while the blood vessels contain *smooth muscle tissue* that assists the heart in moving blood around the body.

Blood

Adult males and females carry an average of 5–6 L and 4–5 L of blood respectively. Taking an average blood volume of 5 L, the volume of blood in the different parts of the circulatory system at any one time is approximately: 0.6 L in the lungs, 3 L in the systemic venous circulation, and 1.4 L in the heart, systemic arteries, arterioles and capillaries. Within the different tissues of the body, blood is redistributed depending on their activity levels. During strenuous exercise in a hot environment, for example, blood is in high demand by both the active skeletal muscles (for delivery of nutrients and removal of waste) and the skin (for dissipation of heat), with minimal blood transported to the less active tissues. The functions of blood are similar to those of the cardiovascular system as a whole:

- To enable *transport* by carrying hormones, nutrients and waste products either in solution or combined with cells which form part of the blood.
- To enable *heat transfer* for cooling or conservation purposes.
- To carry cells, proteins and solutes which perform major roles in *immune function, minimising blood loss,* and *maintaining blood pH.*

Knowledge integration question

Speculate as to how the blood can transfer heat to decrease core body temperature.

Blood components

The blood represents on average 8% of the total body mass and is normally around 55% plasma and 45% cellular components. The cellular components include *erythrocytes* (red blood cells), *leukocytes* (white blood cells) and *platelets* (thrombocytes) which are all developed in the bone marrow. Blood **plasma**, which is around 91% water, carries plasma proteins and other solutes in solution, while cellular components are transported in suspension. Blood can be spun and separated into its component parts by centrifugation, as illustrated in Figure 6.9. Centrifuging blood is employed clinically to examine the **haematocrit**, the packed cell volume in relation to the plasma volume, which is normally around 42% for females and 47% for males. After centrifugation, the leukocytes and platelets can normally be clearly identified as a 'buffy' coat between the red cells (RBCs) and the yellowish plasma. Blood is slightly sticky to touch, tastes slightly metallic and due to its cellular components is denser that water.

Key point

Haematocrit refers to the ratio of the volume of RBCs to the total volume of blood.

Plasma

The largest component of the blood is plasma. Healthy males and females at rest have plasma volumes of 2.8–3 L and around 2.4 L, respectively.

As shown in Figure 6.9, plasma is comprised of over 90% water, 7% plasma proteins and 2% additional solutes such as electrolyte ions, nutrients, gases, enzymes, hormones and waste products. The electrolytes include sodium (the principal cation), potassium, chloride (the principal anion) and bicarbonate. A wide range of macronutrients and micronutrients are carried in solution by plasma along with the gases oxygen and carbon dioxide. Waste products carried primarily by the plasma include those to be excreted by the lungs and through the urinary system. The main plasma proteins, synthesised in the liver, include *albumin* which serves as a carrier protein for fat-soluble hormones and fatty acids, *globulins* which are involved in immune function and also serve as fat-soluble vitamin carriers, and *fibrinogen,* an essential component of the blood clotting process.

Erythrocytes

Erythrocytes are the most common type of blood cell and represent around a third of all human body cells.

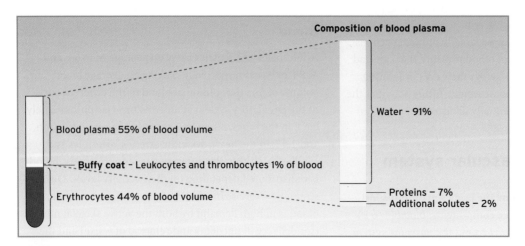

Figure 6.9 Major components of centrifuged blood.

They are very numerous with around 5×10^9 (5 billion) red blood cells in every millilitre of blood, each having a life cycle of around 120 days. The life cycle for an erythrocyte is limited by the stresses placed on the plasma membrane during its journey through the narrow capillaries of the vascular system. As a consequence, erythrocytes have to be replaced at a rate of about 2 million cells every second, which represents about 1% of all blood cells being replaced each day. As was mentioned in the section on cells, the specialised oxygen and carbon dioxide carrying function of red blood cells requires a unique structure that is established during their development in the bone marrow. During their development, erythrocytes eliminate many of their organelles to create more room for haemoglobin molecules and hence enhance their oxygen-carrying capacity. This is another reason why the life cycle of erythrocytes is limited, for by removing other organelles, they become incapable of repairing damage to their structures.

Each erythrocyte contains in the region of 280 million haemoglobin molecules and each one of those can hold up to four oxygen molecules. Each haemoglobin molecule contains four protein-based polypeptides which combine to form the protein globin. Attached to each of the four polypeptides chains is a haem unit which is a ring-like structure that contains an iron ion (Fe^{2+}) at its centre. It is this Fe^{2+} to which each oxygen molecule binds during transport in the blood. In addition to its specialised structure to maximise oxygen transport, the bi-concave shape of erythrocytes (Figure 6.10) greatly increases the surface area to volume ratio and hence enhances the diffusion rate of oxygen across the plasma membrane.

Knowledge integration question

Explain why red blood cells are so well equipped for transporting oxygen.

Leukocytes

The blood carries far fewer **leukocytes** than erythrocytes, around 7 million per millilitre of blood; however, their role is vital to the protection of our body against disease. Leukocytes are commonly divided into two types, those with and those without visible (under a light microscope) granules within the cytoplasm. Figure 6.11 illustrates three types of **granular leukocyte** – neutrophils, eosinophils and basophils, and two forms of **agranular leukocyte** – lymphocytes and monocytes. The relative percentage of each leukocyte in whole blood is shown in Figure 6.12.

Neutrophils represent about 65% of the leukocytes and their key role is to ingest and destroy bacteria, a process known as **phagocytosis**, as the first line of defense against infection. Eosinophils, are much rarer than neutrophils, comprising around 3% of leukocytes and their role is primarily based around releasing enzymes to fight against parasitic worms such as roundworms and flatworms. Eosinophils hunt in packs and when they corner a parasitic worm they surround it, releasing their digestive enzymes on to the surface of the worm. In addition, eosinophils have antihistamine properties, playing an important role for people with allergies. The rarest leukocytes, representing ≤1%, are the histamine-producing basophils which release this substance at a site of inflammation to attract other leukocytes and to stimulate vasodilation.

Lymphocytes, the most common agranulocyte are found within the blood but, more commonly, within the tissues of the lymphatic (immune) system. Nevertheless, they are the second most common leukocyte (25% of total) in the blood where their role involves producing immunoglobulins (antibodies) which are used to identify and neutralise bacteria and viruses. Monocytes, the largest type of leukocyte (around 6% of total leukocytes), are carried in the blood to sites of infection where they leave the blood to enter the infected tissue where they phagocytise pathogens. Monocytes play additional roles in antigen presentation (capturing antigens and presenting them to lymphocytes to activate an immune response against the antigen) and cytokine release. Cytokines are signalling molecules with a wide variety of immunomodulatory functions.

The lifespan of a leukocyte is determined by the health of the individual. In a healthy person they can live months and even years. When someone is ill, however, they survive for a matter of days. As well as fighting bacterial and viral infection, white blood cells protect against fungal infections and fight against chronic diseases such as tuberculosis.

Platelets

Platelets, or thrombocytes, are formed by budding off from the cytoplasm of megakaryocytes in the red bone marrow. During their development in the bone marrow, megakaryocytes fragment into around 2,500 smaller subcellular units. These units are called platelets, each with its own plasma membrane within which it stores a wide range of chemicals including ATP, glycogen and serotonin.

1 The human body contains an enormous number of red blood cells (RBCs). A standard blood test—the **red blood cell count**—reports the number of RBCs per microliter (μL) of whole blood. In adult males, 1 μL, or 1 cubic millimeter (mm³), of whole blood contains 4.5-6.3 million RBCs; in adult females, 1 μL contains 4.2-5.5 million. A single drop of whole blood contains approximately 260 million RBCs, and the blood of an average adult has 25 trillion RBCs. RBCs thus account for roughly one-third of all cells in the human body.

2 Each RBC is a biconcave disc with a thin central region and a thicker outer margin.

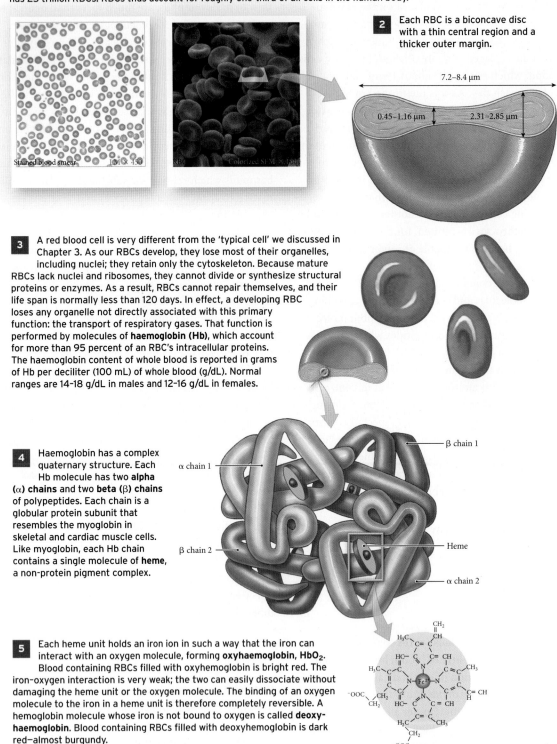

Stained blood smear   LM × 450

RBC   Colorized SEM × 1800

7.2–8.4 μm

0.45–1.16 μm   2.31–2.85 μm

3 A red blood cell is very different from the 'typical cell' we discussed in Chapter 3. As our RBCs develop, they lose most of their organelles, including nuclei; they retain only the cytoskeleton. Because mature RBCs lack nuclei and ribosomes, they cannot divide or synthesize structural proteins or enzymes. As a result, RBCs cannot repair themselves, and their life span is normally less than 120 days. In effect, a developing RBC loses any organelle not directly associated with this primary function: the transport of respiratory gases. That function is performed by molecules of **haemoglobin (Hb)**, which account for more than 95 percent of an RBC's intracellular proteins. The haemoglobin content of whole blood is reported in grams of Hb per deciliter (100 mL) of whole blood (g/dL). Normal ranges are 14-18 g/dL in males and 12-16 g/dL in females.

β chain 1

α chain 1

4 Haemoglobin has a complex quaternary structure. Each Hb molecule has two **alpha (α) chains** and two **beta (β) chains** of polypeptides. Each chain is a globular protein subunit that resembles the myoglobin in skeletal and cardiac muscle cells. Like myoglobin, each Hb chain contains a single molecule of **heme**, a non-protein pigment complex.

β chain 2

Heme

α chain 2

5 Each heme unit holds an iron ion in such a way that the iron can interact with an oxygen molecule, forming **oxyhaemoglobin, HbO_2**. Blood containing RBCs filled with oxyhemoglobin is bright red. The iron-oxygen interaction is very weak; the two can easily dissociate without damaging the heme unit or the oxygen molecule. The binding of an oxygen molecule to the iron in a heme unit is therefore completely reversible. A hemoglobin molecule whose iron is not bound to oxygen is called **deoxyhaemoglobin**. Blood containing RBCs filled with deoxyhemoglobin is dark red—almost burgundy.

Heme

Each red blood cell contains about 280 million Hb molecules. Because a Hb molecule contains four heme units, each RBC can potentially carry more than a billion molecules of oxygen at a time. Roughly 98.5% of the oxygen carried by the blood travels through the bloodstream bound to Hb molecules inside RBCs; the rest is dissolved in the plasma.

Figure 6.10 Structure of an erythrocyte, haemoglobin and haem units.

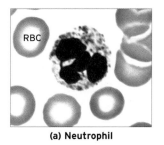

(a) Neutrophil

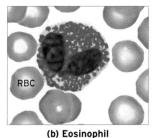

(b) Eosinophil

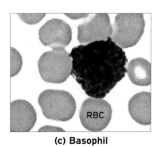

(c) Basophil

Figure 6.11 The structure of granular (a–c) and agranular (d and e) leukocytes. (*Source*: Martini, F. H. and Nath, J. L. (2009) *Fundamentals of Anatomy and Physiology*, 8th edition, New York: Benjamin Cummings)

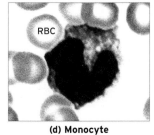

(d) Monocyte

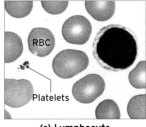

(e) Lymphocyte

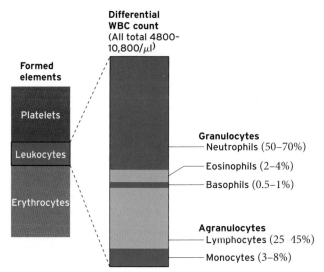

Figure 6.12 Relative percentage of leukocytes in whole blood.

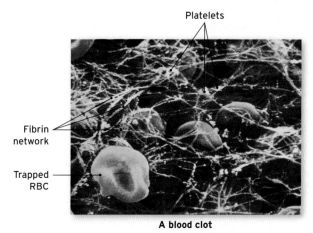

A blood clot

Figure 6.13 Electron micrograph showing erythrocytes trapped in a fibrin mesh (*Source*: Martini, F. H. and Nath, J. L. (2009) *Fundamentals of Anatomy and Physiology*, 8th edition, New York: Benjamin Cummings)

There are normally around 250 million platelets found in each millilitre of blood. The primary role of platelets is blood clot formation to stop blood loss following trauma to a blood vessel. Arriving at the site of an injury, platelets stick to the side of the wound and create a platelet plug which seals the wound. They are assisted in this role by the blood-borne enzyme, thrombin, which converts the plasma protein fibrinogen to fibrin. Fibrin threads interact with the platelets to create a fibrin mesh which encapsulates the platelets and seal the wound. An illustration of erythrocytes trapped in a fibrin mesh is shown in Figure 6.13.

Key point

The cellular contents of blood include:

➤ Erythrocytes – red blood cells

➤ Leukocytes – white blood cells

➤ Thrombocytes – platelets

Gas transport in the blood

The link between the respiratory and cardiovascular systems lies in the transport of oxygen and carbon dioxide.

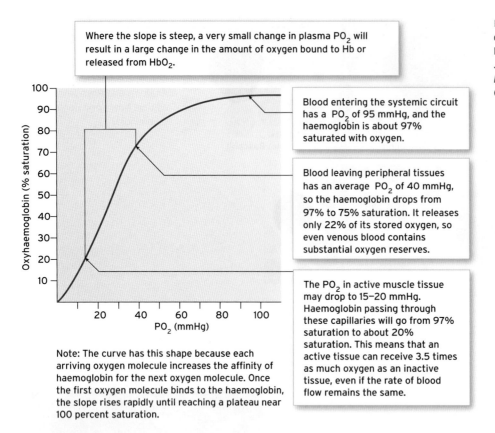

Where the slope is steep, a very small change in plasma PO_2 will result in a large change in the amount of oxygen bound to Hb or released from HbO_2.

Blood entering the systemic circuit has a PO_2 of 95 mmHg, and the haemoglobin is about 97% saturated with oxygen.

Blood leaving peripheral tissues has an average PO_2 of 40 mmHg, so the haemoglobin drops from 97% to 75% saturation. It releases only 22% of its stored oxygen, so even venous blood contains substantial oxygen reserves.

The PO_2 in active muscle tissue may drop to 15–20 mmHg. Haemoglobin passing through these capillaries will go from 97% saturation to about 20% saturation. This means that an active tissue can receive 3.5 times as much oxygen as an inactive tissue, even if the rate of blood flow remains the same.

Note: The curve has this shape because each arriving oxygen molecule increases the affinity of haemoglobin for the next oxygen molecule. Once the first oxygen molecule binds to the haemoglobin, the slope rises rapidly until reaching a plateau near 100 percent saturation.

Figure 6.14 The oxyhaemoglobin dissociation curve. (*Source*: Martini, F. H., Ober, J. and Nath, J. L. (2011) *Visual Anatomy and Physiology*, New York: Benjamin Cummings)

As oxygen diffuses from the lungs into the blood for transport to the cells, carbon dioxide, produced by cells and transported within the blood, diffuses from the blood to the lungs for removal from the body.

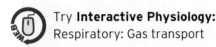 Try **Interactive Physiology:**
Respiratory: Gas transport

Oxygen transport

Due primarily to the vast number of haemoglobin molecules within each red blood cell, fully oxygenated blood is able to transport 20 mL oxygen per dL of blood. Oxygen is either bound with haemoglobin, specifically to the iron ions of the haem units to form oxyhaemoglobin (98.5%) or dissolved in the blood plasma (1.5%). The 1.5% found in the plasma is involved with the control of breathing and heart rate. It is the concentration levels of oxygen in the plasma that is detected by chemoreceptors in the common carotid artery and relayed to the brain.

Oxyhaemoglobin dissociation curve

When oxygen molecules are bound to all four iron ions, a haemoglobin molecule is 100% saturated, and 50% saturated if only two iron ions are bound to oxygen. In the body, this saturation of haemoglobin is dependent on the partial pressure of oxygen (PO_2), which, as we know from above, differs between the alveoli ($PO_2 = 100$ mmHg) and systemic tissues ($PO_2 = 40$ mmHg). This relationship between haemoglobin saturation and PO_2 is known as the oxyhaemoglobin dissociation curve, and is illustrated in Figure 6.14. The S-shape of the curve reflects the fact that when haemoglobin binds an oxygen molecule its affinity to bind a subsequent oxygen molecule is enhanced, explaining the steep portion of the curve. At a high PO_2, such as when the blood picks up oxygen from the lungs, haemoglobin approaches its maximal saturation and is unable to bind many more oxygen molecules, hence the curve plateaus. When the blood passes through resting systemic tissues and oxygen diffuses into the cells PO_2 falls from 100 mmHg to less than 40 mmHg. As can be seen in Figure 6.14, this fall in PO_2 means the blood leaving the tissues is around 75% saturated. In comparison to tissue at rest, exercise increases the cellular demand for oxygen and, due to a fall in PO_2 to around 15 mmHg, haemoglobin is left only 25% saturated.

Carbon dioxide transport

Carbon dioxide is transported in the blood combined with haemoglobin to form carbaminohaemoglobin (20%), dissolved in the plasma (5%), or, most commonly, as bicarbonate ions, a product of the hydration of carbon dioxide as shown below.

$$CO_2 + H_2O \xrightleftharpoons[]{\text{carbonic anhydrase}} H^+ + HCO_3-$$

This reversible reaction is catalysed by the enzyme carbonic anhydrase and forms carbonic acid which immediately dissociates into hydrogen and bicarbonate ions. Just as dissolved oxygen is detected by sensory chemoreceptors, the dissolved CO_2 and the presence of H^+, through the dissociation of carbonic acid, are detected by sensory bodies in the aorta and common carotid arteries. The pH of blood (the ratio of acidity to alkalinity of a solution ranging from 0–14 with 7 being neutral) is around 7.4 so it is very slightly alkaline. However, when exercise intensity is above 50% of maximum the blood pH levels begins to decrease (i.e. blood becomes more acidic). This is due to an enhanced release of H^+ into the blood.

Key point

Blood is comprised of 55% plasma and 45% cellular components.

Plasma, which is largely composed of water, carries plasma proteins and a range of additional solutes essential for life or requiring removal from the body.

Knowledge integration question

Explain how oxygen and carbon dioxide are transported in the blood.

The heart

The heart is the first functional organ to commence activity during development and it continues to beat around 40 million times a year, without fatigue, throughout our lives. Each day it pumps around 370 litres of blood around the body. The heart, which weighs less than half a kilogram and is about the size of a fist, is situated near the midline of the body resting on the diaphragm and is protected by the sternum and rib cage. It is located so that two-thirds of its volume is on the left side of midline with a downward diagonal orientation. It is for this reason that the left lung is slightly smaller than the right and has two lobes instead of three. Figure 6.15 shows a representation of the heart – note that the heart is always drawn from the perspective of a person looking out from the page such that the left side of

the heart appears on the right side of the page as you look into the textbook.

Anatomy of the heart

The heart is protected and stabilised by an outer membrane known as the **pericardium**. **Cardiac muscle**, or **myocardium**, forms the wall of the heart, within which four chambers are found; the superior left and right **atria**, and the larger, inferior left and right **ventricles**. The left and right sides of the heart are separated by the interatrial and interventricular septa, which separate the atria and ventricles respectively. The atria are the collecting chambers of the heart with the right atrium receiving deoxygenated blood from the superior and inferior vena cavae (the great veins) and the coronary sinus (which returns blood from the heart's own blood circulation). At the same time, oxygenated blood from the four pulmonary veins (coming from the lungs) is returned to the left atrium. During the first contraction of the heart blood is pumped from the atria to the ventricles and then, upon the second contraction, from the ventricles round the body. **Atrioventricular (AV) valves** are found at the junction of the atria and ventricles, preventing back flow of the blood into the atria during ventricular contraction. The **tricuspid valve**, between the right atrium and right ventricle, has three cusps while the **bicuspid** or **mitral valve**, between the left atrium and left ventricle, has two flaps. In addition to closing the AV valves, the increased pressure during ventricular contraction opens the **aortic** and **pulmonary (semilunar) valves**. When the heart relaxes and pressure falls, blood flows backwards toward the heart but, due to their cusp-like structure, the semilunar valves close, ensuring the blood flow continues in a one-way direction. The right ventricle pumps blood via the pulmonary arteries round the **pulmonary circuit**, which carries blood to and from the lungs. The blood supplied to the rest of the body is pumped from the left ventricle into the aorta and round the **systemic circuit**. As the left ventricle is required to generate a much greater pressure that the right ventricle, due to the greater distance the blood has to travel round the systemic circuit, the wall of the left ventricle is approximately three times thicker than that of the right. This anatomical difference between the ventricles is illustrated in Figure 6.16.

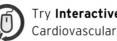 Try **Interactive Physiology:**
Cardiovascular: Anatomy review – the heart

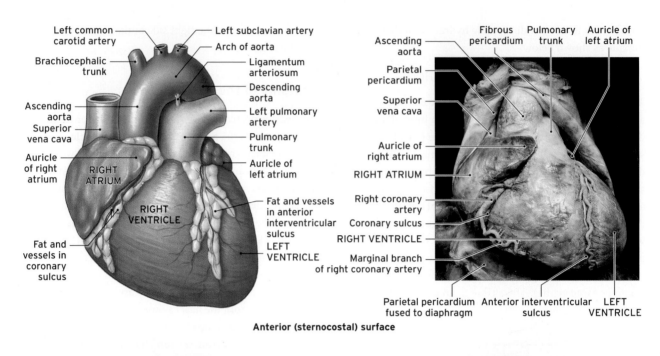

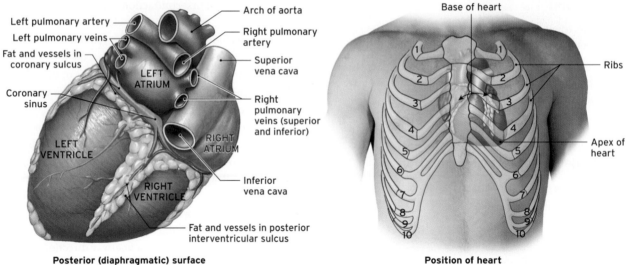

Figure 6.15 The structure of the heart. (*Source*: Martini, F. H. and Nath, J. L. (2009) *Fundamentals of Anatomy and Physiology*, 8th edition, New York: Benjamin Cummings)

The journey of blood through the heart and around the body

The heart actually consists of two pumps (right and left) which contract in unison to supply the pulmonary and systemic circuits. To understand the pathway of blood through the heart and round the body, we will look at the journey of a single red blood cell round a complete circuit of the cardiovascular system.

In sequence, a deoxygenated red blood cell returning from the leg would enter the right atrium from the inferior vena cava pass through the tricuspid valve and into the right ventricle. After contraction of the right ventricle it would be ejected into the pulmonary truck and then pass to either the left or right pulmonary artery and onwards to the capillaries of the lungs. The same red blood cell, having been oxygenated at the lungs, would return to the heart via one of the four pulmonary veins and pass into the left atrium. From the left atrium the erythrocyte would pass into the left ventricle where, upon ventricular contraction, it would be ejected into the aorta and onwards into the systemic circulation to supply oxygen to another tissue or

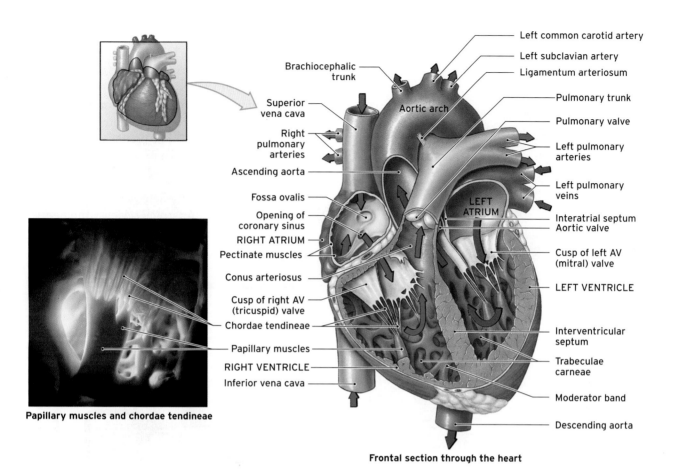

Left common carotid artery

Left subclavian artery

Ligamentum arteriosum

Brachiocephalic trunk

Aortic arch

Pulmonary trunk

Pulmonary valve

Superior vena cava

Right pulmonary arteries

Left pulmonary arteries

LEFT ATRIUM

Left pulmonary veins

Ascending aorta

Interatrial septum

Aortic valve

Fossa ovalis

Opening of coronary sinus

RIGHT ATRIUM

Pectinate muscles

Cusp of left AV (mitral) valve

Conus arteriosus

LEFT VENTRICLE

Cusp of right AV (tricuspid) valve

Chordae tendineae

Interventricular septum

Papillary muscles

Trabeculae carneae

RIGHT VENTRICLE

Inferior vena cava

Moderator band

Descending aorta

Papillary muscles and chordae tendineae

Frontal section through the heart

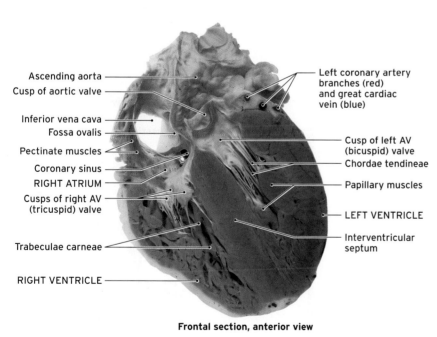

Ascending aorta

Cusp of aortic valve

Left coronary artery branches (red) and great cardiac vein (blue)

Inferior vena cava

Fossa ovalis

Pectinate muscles

Cusp of left AV (bicuspid) valve

Chordae tendineae

Coronary sinus

RIGHT ATRIUM

Papillary muscles

Cusps of right AV (tricuspid) valve

LEFT VENTRICLE

Trabeculae carneae

Interventricular septum

RIGHT VENTRICLE

Frontal section, anterior view

Figure 6.15 (*continued*)

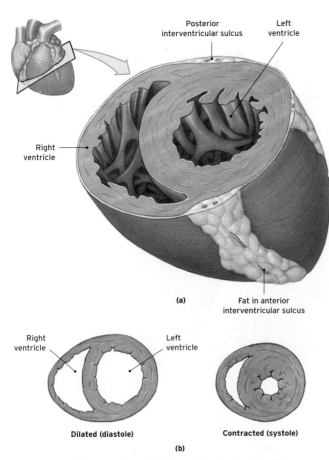

Figure 6.16 Cross section of the heart illustrating the difference in ventricular wall thickness (a) and the influence of cardiac muscle contraction on the two ventricles (b). (*Source*: Martini, F. H. and Nath, J. L. (2009) *Fundamentals of Anatomy and Physiology*, 8th edition, New York: Benjamin Cummings)

organ in the body. This journey of a red blood cell through the heart and round the pulmonary and systemic circulations is depicted in Figure 6.17.

Knowledge integration question

Explain the transport of a red blood cell through the heart commencing at the right atrium.

Cardiac muscle fibres

The muscle of the heart, known as **cardiac muscle** or **myocardium**, is similar to skeletal muscle in that they are both striated and contract by the sliding filament mechanism. Here, the similarity ends. Cardiac muscle fibres are short, branched and contain a single centrally located nucleus. The fibres are arranged in a network to facilitate co-ordinated contraction, and act as a single unit in terms

of both structure and function. The plasma membranes of adjacent fibres interlock to form **intercalated discs**, an identifying feature of cardiac muscle. At an intercalated disc, **desmosomes** structurally join fibres together preventing separation during contraction, whereas **gap junctions** allow action potentials to spread across fibres and transfer the force of contraction. The myocardium, therefore, behaves as a single coordinated unit.

Try **Interactive Physiology:**
Cardiovascular: Anatomy review – the heart

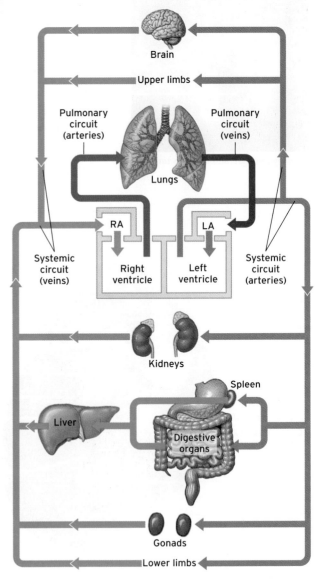

Figure 6.17 The journey of blood round the vascular system. (*Source*: Martini, F. H. and Nath, J. L. (2009) *Fundamentals of Anatomy and Physiology*, 8th edition, New York: Benjamin Cummings)

Key point

The heart is a four-chamber pump, comprised of cardiac muscle tissue, responsible for delivering blood to the lungs and every tissue and organ of the body.

The heart is functional from very early on in foetal development and beats continually throughout life.

The left side of the heart is responsible for delivering blood to the systemic circulation and the right for the transit of blood to the lungs via the pulmonary circulation.

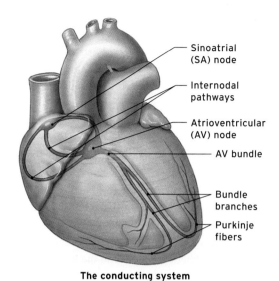

The conducting system

Figure 6.18 Conduction system within the heart. (*Source:* Martini, F. H. and Nath, J. L. (2009) *Fundamentals of Anatomy and Physiology*, 8th edition, New York: Benjamin Cummings)

The heart sounds

As was mentioned earlier the heart is comprised of two pumps. The heart's double pump can be thought of in two ways. *Firstly,* deoxygenated blood pumped into the right ventricle supplies blood to the lungs and the left side supplies oxygenated blood to systemic circulation. *Secondly,* the heart contracts in a '*1-2*' fashion, which can be inferred from the sounds heard when using Doppler ultrasound echocardiography (which makes it possible to listen to the sounds of the heart). During echocardiography the contraction of the heart appears as a 'lub-dup' sound. The '*1*' or 'lub', the first sound, is created by the closure of the atrioventricular valves at the start of a ventricular contraction (after completion of atrial contraction) and the '2', or dup phase of contraction, represents the end of the ventricular contraction and the closure of the semi-lunar valves in the pulmonary trunk and aorta, which stop blood flowing back into the ventricles (after which the atria will begin to contract again to fill the ventricles).

The contraction of the heart

Control of contraction of the heart is brought about by nervous stimulation and is triggered by two nerve bodies, the **sinoatrial node** (SA node) and the **atrioventricular node** (AV node). The conduction system for the heart is shown in Figure 6.18. The SA node works as the pacemaker for the heart and the SA and AV nodes together provide the conduction system for the contraction of atria and ventricles.

The SA node, situated on the right atrial wall, stimulates autorhythmic contraction of the heart. This means that even without nervous stimulation from the autonomic nervous system the SA node, as the heart's pacemaker, propagates contraction of the heart at rate of around

100 beats per minute. Nervous stimulation of the SA node via the parasympathetic division slows the natural rhythm of the SA node to around 70–75 beats per minute and the effects of the sympathetic nervous system and the release of the hormone adrenalin during exercise can increase SA node rhythm to an individual's maximum heart rate. The SA node triggers an action potential through the muscle fibres of the atria causing them to contract and eject blood into the ventricles of the heart. The spread of the action potential through the atria reaches the AV node and this triggers the release of an action potential through the **atrioventricular bundle (bundle of His)** to the **Purkinje fibres**. The *Purkinje fibres* propagate the action potential to the ventricular cardiac muscle initiating contraction from the apex of the heart. The location of the Purkinje fibres and the nature of cardiac muscle fibres result in a twisting-squeezing contraction by the ventricles, ejecting blood from within. The steps involved in the spread of stimulation across the heart are illustrated in Figure 6.19a.

 Try **Interactive Physiology:**
Cardiovascular: Intrinsic conduction system

Heart rate recording

An **electrocardiograph** can be employed to detect the electrical stimulation of the heart and the trace it creates, called an **electrocardiogram** (ECG), can be interpreted by cardiologists, exercise physiologists and clinicians to assess the functioning of the heart. Figure 6.19 provides a representation of an ECG.

The ECG trace is normally described according to the three common deflections in the trace, the P wave, QRS complex and T wave. The *P wave* represents the depolarisation of the atria, i.e. the spreading of an electrical impulse from the SA node that stimulates the atria to contract. The *QRS complex* depicts the depolarisation of the ventricles propagated from the AV node via the Purkinje fibres to the ventricular muscle fibres. The *T wave* represents the repolarisation of the ventricles ready for the next contraction. The repolarisation of the atria which takes place during the depolarisation of the ventricles is masked by the QRS complex and as such does not form an identifiable trace on an ECG. The period between the P and the R wave, called the *P-R interval,* represents the time for the atria to contract and then begin to relax (R is used rather than Q for this interval because the Q wave is often small). The same phase for the ventricles, from the start of contraction to the start of relaxation is known as the *Q-T interval.* The contraction phase of the cardiac cycle is known as systole and the relaxation phase as diastole.

Knowledge integration question

Explain what is happening on the ECG trace shown in Figure 6.19.

In a medical setting a great deal of information can be gleaned from an ECG. The size of each of the waves and the time taken for each can be interpreted to identify problems with heart function. As part of the detection of heart dysfunction an exercise ECG can be completed to examine the cardiac cycle under physiological stress. The stress of exercise can reveal changes in wave traces and arrhythmias that might not be present in a resting ECG. Irrespective of any heart dysfunction, during exercise the cardiac cycle will shorten with a corresponding increase in heart rate. As a consequence of this, the gaps between electrical events will decrease, for instance the T-P interval (the gap between the end of ventricular repolarisation and atrial depolarisation), will shorten as heart rate increases. Abnormal ECGs are relatively common in highly trained athletes due to the physiological hypertrophy of the left ventricle. Great care, however, must be taken when interpreting an ECG as it is very difficult, even by the most experienced cardiologists, to differentiate between this physiological thickening of the myocardial wall compared to that of hypertrophic cardiomyopathy (thickening of heart muscle caused by disease).

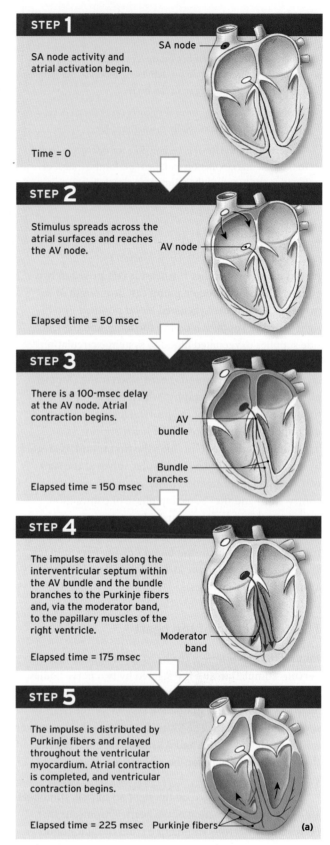

STEP 1

SA node activity and atrial activation begin.

SA node

Time = 0

STEP 2

Stimulus spreads across the atrial surfaces and reaches the AV node.

AV node

Elapsed time = 50 msec

STEP 3

There is a 100-msec delay at the AV node. Atrial contraction begins.

AV bundle

Bundle branches

Elapsed time = 150 msec

STEP 4

The impulse travels along the interventricular septum within the AV bundle and the bundle branches to the Purkinje fibers and, via the moderator band, to the papillary muscles of the right ventricle.

Moderator band

Elapsed time = 175 msec

STEP 5

The impulse is distributed by Purkinje fibers and relayed throughout the ventricular myocardium. Atrial contraction is completed, and ventricular contraction begins.

Elapsed time = 225 msec   Purkinje fibers   (a)

Figure 6.19 The steps involved in the spread of an action potential across the heart (a) and an illustration of the recording of the heart's electrical activity on an ECG (b).

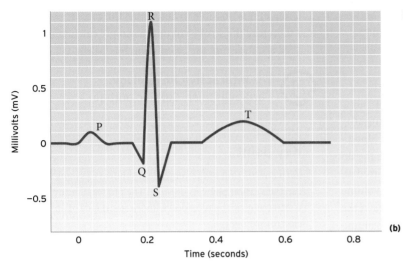

Figure 6.19 (*continued*)

(b)

At rest a complete cardiac cycle, that is from P wave to P wave, normally takes about 0.8 seconds for a person with a heart rate (HR) of 75 beats per minute ($60 \div 0.8 = 75$ beats per minute). As well as identification of the phases in a cardiac cycle an ECG can be used to determine heart rate. An ECG heart rate is normally calculated by counting the number of R waves in a given time or by the number of squares between R waves. **Tachycardia**, normally defined as a HR above 100 beats per minute can be cause by rises in body temperature during illness, or other sympathetic responses. **Bradycardia**, a resting HR below 60 beats per minute, is often detected in athletes who have a higher stroke volume (amount of blood ejected in one ventricular contraction) due to the trained increase in ventricular wall thickness, or could be related to illness.

In a sporting context HR is normally determined by telemetry through the use of a heart rate monitor. Heart rate monitors, such as the one in Figure 6.20, still rely on the electrical activity of the heart that determines the rate of contraction, but only display the HR rather than any information about the cardiac cycle phase as would be revealed in an

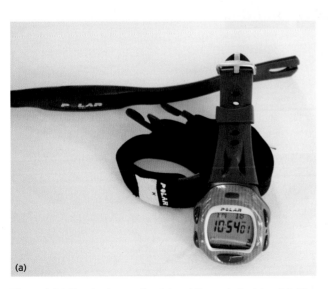

(a)

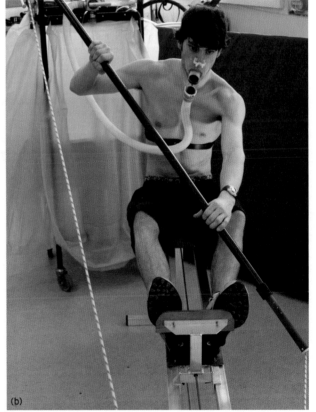

(b)

Figure 6.20 Heart rate monitor (a) and its use in training (b). (*Source*: (b) Nicky Norris)

ECG. Nevertheless, because of the close relationship between HR and exercise intensity, heart rate monitors provide an excellent method of monitoring effort during training.

Cardiac output

A further measure of cardiac function, is cardiac output ($\dot{Q}$). Cardiac output represents the total amount of blood ejected from the left ventricle in one minute (hence the dot above the Q which indicates the parameter is measured at a rate per minute) and is determined by the stroke volume (SV) and heart rate (HR). The problem which arises in the calculation of cardiac output is the fact that stroke volume, the amount of blood ejected in one contraction of the left ventricle, is difficult to measure. In contrast, as discussed in the previous section, HR is readily determined using a heart rate monitor. Stroke volume is theoretically determined by the difference in the volume of blood in the left ventricle by the end of the diastole (*end-diastolic volume – EDV*) and the amount of blood left in the chamber at the end of the systole (*end-systolic volume – ESV*). To directly measure SV and $\dot{Q}$, invasive techniques would be required. Due to the unacceptability of these invasive techniques, a number of indirect methods have been devised to calculate $\dot{Q}$. The most widely accepted of these was first proposed by Adolf Fick in 1870. Fick noted that by determining the amount of oxygen consumed by an individual in one minute and the difference between the oxygen content in a known amount of arterial and venous blood (the a-$\bar{v}$ O_2 difference) it is possible to determine the cardiac output and therefore the stroke volume. Example calculations of $\dot{Q}$ and SV are shown in the calculation box below.

 Try **Interactive Physiology:**
Cardiovascular: Cardiac output

Key point

Each contraction of the ventricles is known as systole, each relaxation phase as diastole. The phases in heart contraction can be recorded with the assistance of an electrocardiograph.

The ejection of blood from the ventricles is known as the stroke volume (SV) and the total volume ejected in one minute as the cardiac output ($\dot{Q}$), which is the product of the SV and the number of times the ventricles contract per minute (HR).

Vascular system

The vascular system is comprised of the various blood vessels that form a complete system to transport blood to and from the heart. Early physiologists believed the blood ebbed and flowed from the heart and it was not until the work of William Harvey in 1628 that the true circulatory nature of blood flow was discovered. The main vessels of the vascular system include the arteries, arterioles, capillaries, venules and veins. Figure 6.21 shows the main

CALCULATION

Equations

$\dot{Q}$ = SV × HR

SV = EDV − ESV

$\dot{Q}$ = [$\dot{V}O_2$ ÷ a-$\bar{v}$ O_2 difference] × 100   Fick Equation

Example for an individual with a resting HR of 75 beats·min^{-1}, a $\dot{V}O_2$ of 250 mL·min^{-1} and an a-$\bar{v}$ O_2 difference of 5 mL:

$\dot{Q}$ = [250 ÷ 5] × 100

$\dot{Q}$ = 5,000 mL or 5 L of blood

$\dot{Q}$ = SV × HR   so   SV = $\dot{Q}$ ÷ HR

SV = 5,000 mL ÷ 75

SV = 66 mL

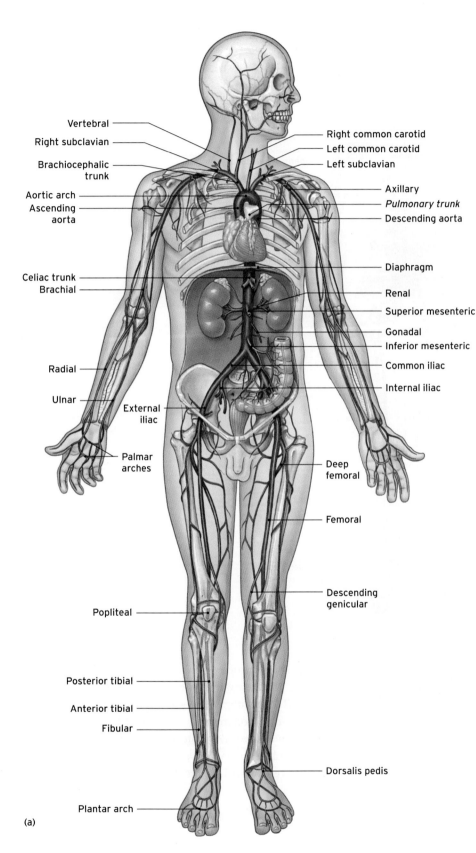

Figure 6.21 Main vessels of blood circulation; arteries (a) and veins (b). (*Source*: Martini, F. H. and Nath, J. L. (2009) *Fundamentals of Anatomy and Physiology*, 8th edition, New York: Benjamin Cummings)

Vertebral

Right subclavian

Brachiocephalic trunk

Aortic arch

Ascending aorta

Celiac trunk

Brachial

Radial

Ulnar

External iliac

Palmar arches

Popliteal

Posterior tibial

Anterior tibial

Fibular

Plantar arch

Right common carotid

Left common carotid

Left subclavian

Axillary

Pulmonary trunk

Descending aorta

Diaphragm

Renal

Superior mesenteric

Gonadal

Inferior mesenteric

Common iliac

Internal iliac

Deep femoral

Femoral

Descending genicular

Dorsalis pedis

(a)

Figure 6.21 (continued)

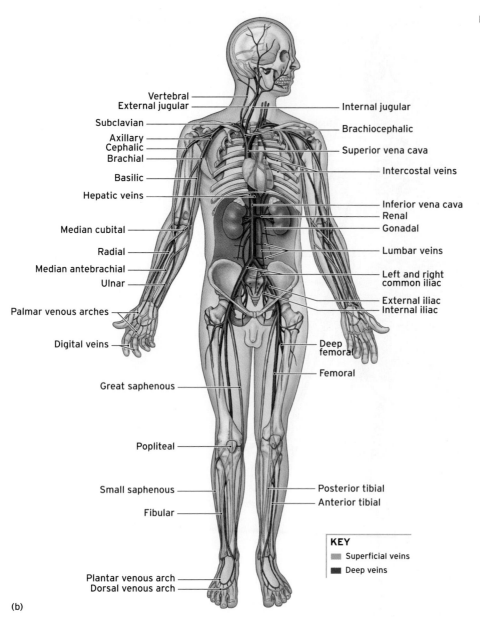

Vertebral
External jugular
Subclavian
Axillary
Cephalic
Brachial
Basilic
Hepatic veins
Median cubital
Radial
Median antebrachial
Ulnar
Palmar venous arches
Digital veins
Great saphenous
Popliteal
Small saphenous
Fibular
Plantar venous arch
Dorsal venous arch

Internal jugular
Brachiocephalic
Superior vena cava
Intercostal veins
Inferior vena cava
Renal
Gonadal
Lumbar veins
Left and right
common iliac
External iliac
Internal iliac
Deep femoral
Femoral
Posterior tibial
Anterior tibial

KEY
Superficial veins
Deep veins

(b)

circulatory routes, with the aorta being the main artery from which all other arteries flow and the main veins being the superior and inferior vena cavae.

Arteries and arterioles carry blood away from the heart to the capillary networks that form the gaseous and nutrient/waste product exchange beds for the cells of the body. Venules and veins, receiving blood from the capillaries return blood to the right atrium of the heart. Arteries always carry blood *away* from the heart, while veins carry blood *to* the heart. In general, arteries carry oxygenated blood (blood that has been supplied with oxygen from the lungs) and veins carry deoxygenated blood (blood which has had some of its oxygen removed by the tissues of the

body). The exceptions to this rule are the pulmonary vessels; the pulmonary arteries carry deoxygenated blood from the heart to the lungs for oxygenation and the pulmonary veins return blood from the lungs to the left atrium (as can be seen in Figure 6.17). Note, however, that the pulmonary arteries still carry blood *away* from the heart and the pulmonary veins carry blood *to* the heart.

Structure of blood vessels

There are five basic subgroups of blood vessels; arteries, arterioles, capillaries, venules and veins. The walls of these vessels enclose the inside space through which blood flows, commonly known as the vessel **lumen**. Blood vessel walls are composed of three distinct layers; the *tunica intima*, *tunica media* and *tunica externa* (also known as tunica adventitia) (Figure 6.22). The layer surrounding the vessel lumen, the tunica intima, minimises resistance to blood flow as it provides a smooth surface. The tunica media is composed primarily of smooth muscle and elastin

and hence, plays a pivotal role in the **vasoconstriction** (reduction in lumen diameter) and **vasodilation** (increase in lumen diameter) of blood vessels. This middle layer provides the mechanical strength of the blood vessel. The external layer, the tunica externa, is a collagen fibre protective layer which also functions to attach the vessel to surrounding structures.

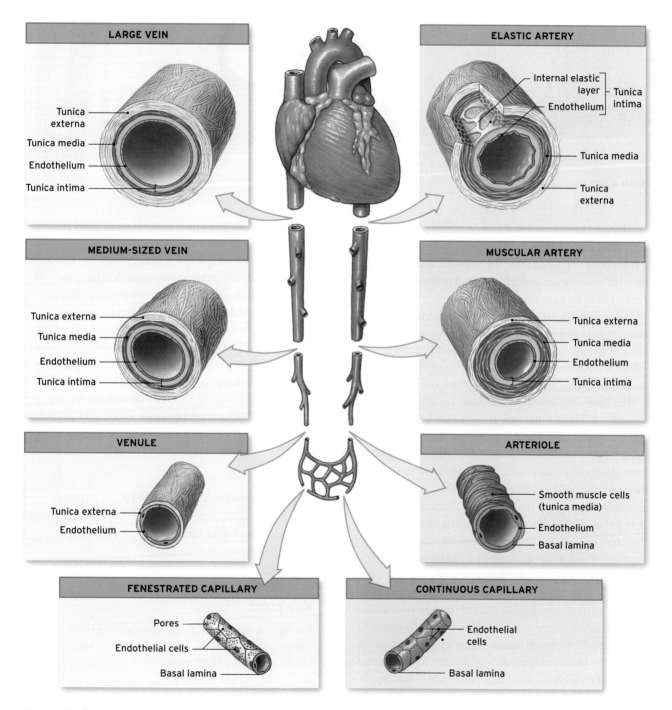

Figure 6.22 Generalised structure of arteries, veins and capillaries. (*Source*: Martini, F. H. and Nath, J. L. (2009) *Fundamentals of Anatomy and Physiology*, 8th edition, New York: Benjamin Cummings)

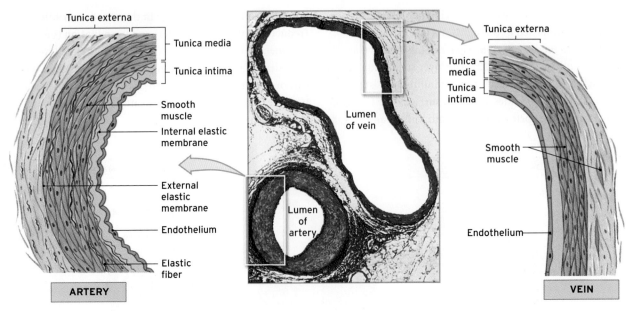

Figure 6.22 (continued)

The structures of arteries and veins differ to suit their individual roles. Arteries are the primary distribution vessels transporting blood from the heart around the body, whereas veins merge and return blood to the heart. In general, arteries have thicker walls, a smaller relative lumen and contain a greater proportion of smooth muscle and elastic tissues than veins. The smooth muscle within the walls of arteries and veins assists the movement of blood within the vessels. The differences in vessel structure are illustrated in Figure 6.22.

The large arteries leaving the heart are subjected to large pressures as blood is pumped from the left ventricle round the systemic circuit. These arteries, commonly referred to as *elastic arteries*, have the largest diameter and contain the most elastin of all the vessels. The large diameter reduces the resistance to blood flow while the elastin allows the arteries to stretch and recoil helping to smoothe the flow of blood as it leaves the heart. Elastic arteries empty into muscular arteries, the primary role of which is to efficiently transport blood to the multiple vascular beds. Muscular artery walls contain the thickest tunica media of all vessels, with less elastin but more smooth muscle compared to elastic arteries. The strong, thick walls of these arteries allow them to resist collapse at joints where they are subjected to bending. The smooth muscle tissue within the arterioles enables the vessels to dramatically alter the lumen diameter to control blood flow. Arterioles pass blood to the capillaries, the site of gas exchange. Due to this function of capillaries, their walls are very thin consisting simply of a single layer of endothelial cells on a basement membrane (no smooth muscle) across which nutrients and waste products can easily move.

Capillaries reunite to form venules which are, also very thin-walled and similar to capillaries in that fluid and cells can move easily across their walls. Venules then join to form the veins of the body. Although similar in structure to arteries, the walls in veins are much thinner relative to the lumen diameter, and as such are more distensible and can accommodate a fairly large blood volume (up to 65% of total blood volume) at any one time. The larger veins in the limbs are unique in that they contain valves (see Figure 6.22), allowing blood to move up the vein toward the heart while preventing back flow due to gravitational forces.

 Try **Interactive Physiology:**
Cardiovascular: Anatomy review blood-vessel structure and function

Key point

The vascular system is a closed network of arteries that take blood away from the heart, and veins that return blood to the right and left atria.

The function of the vascular system is to serve as the transport network enabling blood to circulate to every tissue in the body.

Control of blood vessel diameter

Blood vessels are under both intrinsic and extrinsic control. The intrinsic control is the response of the smooth muscle to local factors such as stretch, temperature, and chemicals (such as CO_2 and H^+). A reduction in blood vessel diameter, vasoconstriction, and resultant decrease in blood flow is promoted in cold temperatures and in response to rises in oxygen levels or decreases in CO_2 and H^+ ions. In contrast, vasodilation increases blood flow by relaxation of the smooth muscle, and is triggered by warm temperatures, decreases in oxygen levels, or increases in CO_2 and H^+ ions. Extrinsic control by the autonomic nervous system and endocrine system is the primary regulator of the major arteries (except the aorta) and veins. Arterioles and small veins are under both intrinsic and extrinsic control, whereas the lack of smooth muscle in capillaries means their diameters are not regulated.

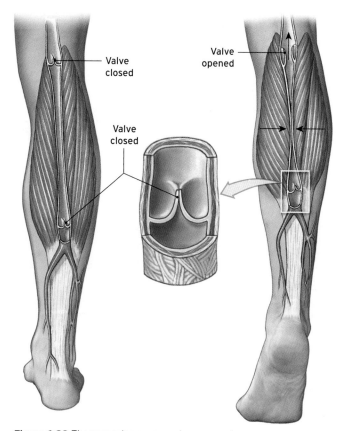

Figure 6.23 The muscular pump and venous valves.

The muscular pump

Blood leaves the heart under pressure imparted by each contraction of the heart. Arteries carry blood under pressure and blood flows to the capillaries as a result of this pressure. At rest during each heart beat (contraction), the pressure in the arterial system normally rises to 120 mmHg. As blood flows further from the heart the pressure decreases to such an extent that by the time blood enters the veins the internal pressure is as low as 18 mmHg. Without alternative assistive processes, venous return would be seriously compromised. Venous return is assisted by an active pump brought about by the contraction of skeletal muscles which squeeze blood with veins (Figure 6.23). This mechanism is called the **muscular pump**.

Enhancement of venous return by the muscular pump is enabled due to the presence of one-way valves within veins, which prevent blood 'leaking' back through the valve (Figure 6.23). In this way, as a skeletal muscle contracts, blood is forced through venous valves in a one-way direction back towards the heart. In addition to these mechanisms, the pressure created in the abdomen and thoracic regions by respiration places a further squeeze on veins, known as the respiratory pump, enhancing venous return.

Despite these methods of venous return, at rest over 60% of the total blood volume is contained within the veins. As such the veins represent a significant blood store. During rest, when the parasympathetic nervous system is the predominant neural control, much of the blood is directed to the liver, kidneys and digestive tract (after a meal) with perhaps only 15% being directed to the active muscles. During exercise, when the sympathetic nervous system triggers responses in the body, up to 80% of systemic blood flow can be redirected to the skeletal muscles. In addition to the redirection of arterial blood flow, exercise aids the return of blood in the large veins of the legs to the heart through the muscular pumping action of the skeletal muscles. Adequate venous return is important to ensure there is sufficient blood to pump round the systemic circulation for the delivery of oxygen and nutrients to the working muscles.

The nature of venous pooling at rest makes the employment of a cool-down strategy after exercise all the more important. If an athlete finishes exercise without a cool-down, waste products produced by the exercising muscles will pool in the veins of the legs. Completing an active cool-down and utilising the muscular pump will facilitate the removal of waste products from the blood for catabolism, re-synthesis or excretion from the body.

> ## Key point
>
> Blood leaves the heart under pressure created by each contraction (heartbeat) and flows to the capillaries for gaseous exchange and transfer of nutrients and waste products.
>
> By the time blood reaches the veins it is under much less pressure so the presence of valves within the vessels, combined with the operation of the muscular and respiratory pumps, aids the return of blood to the heart.

Blood pressure

As was described above, each contraction of the heart ejects blood from the left ventricle to the aorta and systemic circulation. Each surge of blood places pressure on the walls of the arteries and it is this arterial pressure that physiologists and clinicians measure when they take blood pressure. The equipment used to measure blood pressure, a sphygmomanometer, and the process of taking a blood pressure reading, are illustrated in Figure 6.24.

During blood pressure measurement at rest, the pressure cuff is placed round the upper arm, as in Figure 6.24, and normally inflated to around 200 mmHg which is a sufficient pressure to stop blood flow in the artery. The sounding end of the stethoscope is placed over the brachial artery at the point of the antecubital fossa (the hollow at the front of the elbow joint) and the pressure slowly

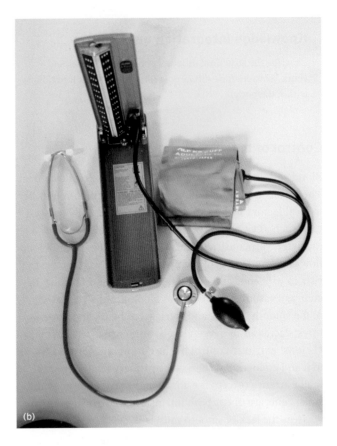
(b)

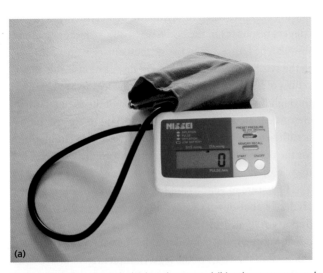
(a)

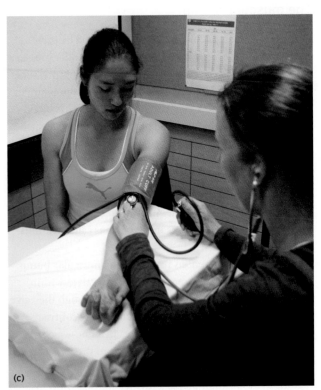
(c)

Figure 6.24 An automated (a) and a manual (b) sphygmomanometer and its use (c). (*Source*: Simon Fryer)

released from the cuff. It is useful when practising taking blood pressure to find the brachial artery pulse by palpating and then marking this point with a pen, prior to applying the stethoscope. The pressure in the cuff is sufficient to continue to halt the flow of blood until the pressure falls to around 120 mmHg. At or close to this point in the assessment of normal blood pressure, a first surge of blood is able to push through the artery, making a sound like a 'pop' in the stethoscope ear pieces. This point forms the reading for **systolic blood pressure**. The popping sound continues in the ear pieces as the pressure in the cuff continues to fall, and if you watch the mercury column on the sphygmomanometer you can observe blips in the meniscus that coincide with the pops you hear. When the pressure in the cuff falls to around 80 mmHg the blood is able to pass through the artery without any obstruction. This point, when the sounds disappear, is termed the **diastolic pressure**. The diastolic pressure represents the lowest level of pressure in the vascular system, in between the contractions of the heart when the walls of the arteries have recoiled after the stretch induced by the contraction. A blood pressure reading is normally given as systolic pressure 'over' diastolic pressure such that a normal blood pressure reading would be spoken as '120 over 80' or written 120/80. A blood pressure reading is used by clinicians as an initial examination of the health of the vascular system.

Hypertension (high blood pressure) normally occurs from a narrowing and or hardening of the arteries which both function to increase the resistance of the vessel. This means the heart has to beat harder to pass blood through the vascular system and as a consequence resting blood pressure readings are higher. This increase in pressure can be seen when you place a thumb over the end of a hosepipe to spray water out. The occlusion of the hosepipe causes an increase in the pressure on the water which then travels further. As discussed in the following section, systolic blood pressure will rise naturally during exercise in response to the heart contracting harder to increase the flow of blood to the active muscles. This is a normal response to exercise. However, in contrast, the diastolic pressure of a healthy individual normally remains close to its resting value.

 Try **Interactive Physiology:**
Cardiovascular: Measuring of blood pressure; Factors that affect blood pressure; Blood pressure regulation; Autoregulation dynamics

> **Key point**
>
> The movement of blood around the body can be detected by palpating a pulse in arteries that run close to the surface of the skin.
>
> The pressure under which blood flows can be determined using a sphygmomanometer.

6.3 Acute responses to exercise

Upon the initiation of exercise, regardless of its intensity, the nervous and endocrine systems alter the functioning of the respiratory and cardiovascular systems to meet the demands of exercise. Following a general increase in functioning at the onset of exercise, a specific response of the transport and exchange systems is determined by the intensity and duration of exercise.

The sympathetic nervous system is the key driver of the physiological changes within the body at the start of exercise. Sympathetic stimulation causes a relaxation of the lung airways and an increased breathing rate and depth. This will enhance the volume of gas exchange between the lungs and the blood. Heart rate and stroke volume, and hence cardiac output, will increase with the majority of blood supplying the active skeletal muscles as visceral organ (such as the stomach, kidneys and intestine) blood flow is reduced through the vasoconstriction of their blood vessels. The sympathetic nervous system will also stimulate endocrine function resulting in the release of exercise-related hormones, which, as discussed below, play major roles in the control of the cardiovascular system. One of the main functions of the nervous and endocrine systems during exercise is to increase the transport and exchange of metabolites to match the demands of elevated metabolism.

Respiratory system

The onset of exercise stimulates an increase in the depth and rate of breathing, a response that is controlled by the medulla oblongata and the pons (each located in the brain stem). This increase in neural stimulation is thought to result from a combination of simultaneous activation of skeletal muscles and the respiratory centre, psychological stimuli, and signalling from the propriocepters in moving skeletal muscles and joints. The increase in ventilation allows a greater exchange of oxygen and carbon dioxide in the lungs, a crucial response as the skeletal muscle demand for oxygen, and the carbon dioxide production, are increased with exercise. This increase in ventilation due to the enhanced metabolic needs of skeletal muscle is known as **hyperpnea**.

As discussed in section 6.1, the primary driver for increases in respiration is the level of CO_2 and when higher levels are detected it creates a strong stimulus for increases in depth and rate of breathing. The onset of exercise increases the levels of CO_2 and H^+ and decreases the level of O_2 in the blood. Recent research has also suggested that rises in plasma K^+ concentration may also serve as a stimulus for increased respiration rates. Chemoreceptors in the brain, aorta and common carotid arteries detect these changes and relay this information to the respiratory centre in the brainstem driver.

Cardiovascular system

The cardiovascular response to exercise begins before the exercise commences with an anticipatory rise in heart rate and blood flow. Research suggests that the rate of the anticipatory rise in heart rate is related to the intensity of the exercise ahead. The greater the intensity of the exercise the higher the anticipatory heart rate response. For example, the anticipatory rise in heart rate for a 100 m sprint would be higher than that for aerobic endurance sports. The cardiovascular responses to exercise involve alterations in cardiac output and blood flow.

The heart's output, introduced previously in this chapter, is the product of stroke volume and heart rate. In other words the cardiac output is determined by how much blood is ejected from the heart with each contraction (SV) and how many times the heart beats per minute (HR). Increases in heart rate are initially stimulated by the sympathetic division of the central nervous system and subsequently jointly by the action of the CNS and the hormones adrenaline and noradrenaline. At low exercise intensities, below 50% of $\dot{V}O_{2max}$, increases in cardiac output are brought about through rises in the heart rate and stroke volume. Stroke volume is thought to increase due to the effects of two mechanisms. The first mechanism, known as the *Frank–Starling Law*, suggests that the increased venous return brought about through exercise results in an increased filling of the ventricles, placing an additional stretch on the ventricular cardiac muscle. This pre-stretching is thought to create a stronger contraction and therefore result in an increased stroke volume. The second proposed mechanism suggests that increases in electrical stimulation of the myocardium brought about through the demands of exercise result in an increase in the *strength of ventricular contractions* and a consequential rise

in SV. Adrenaline and noradrenaline reinforce the CNS-driven increases in stroke volume by further increasing the myocardial contractility. Both mechanisms of increasing SV are thought to operate during exercise, although research has determined that increases in SV are limited, and while SV may increase during exercises at intensities up to around 50% of maximum, SV appears to plateau above this intensity and may even decrease as a result of continually decreasing filling times between contractions. Further increases in cardiac output during exercise above 50% of $\dot{V}O_{2max}$ are therefore the result of rises in heart rate up to a maximum of around 220 beats per minute minus age for each individual.

The increased force of ventricular contraction and greater stroke volume function to elevate systolic blood pressure during exercise, the magnitude of which is related to exercise intensity. In contrast, diastolic pressure is little affected during dynamic exercise and may even decline due to the vasodilation of skeletal muscle arterioles. The mean arterial pressure therefore, may rise only slightly, or potentially decline.

Increases in blood flow to the muscles are brought about through an increased venous return and by alteration in blood circulation. At rest skeletal muscles receive around 15% of the total blood flow; during exercise this can increase to 80% of the total volume. The onset of exercise increases the skeletal pump thereby increasing venous return and total blood flow. Central nervous and hormonal stimulation jointly bring about vasoconstriction and vasodilation to redirect blood flow to the working muscles. Vasodilation occurs in the arteries supplying the working muscles, the brain and the heart during exercise, whereas vasoconstriction is increased in the visceral arteries (supplying the organs of the abdomen). Reduced blood flow to the stomach and the intestine inhibits digestion, while the reduction to the kidneys results in a drop in urine production, which helps to maintain hydration and consequently blood volume.

An almost immediate decrease in plasma volume occurs with the onset of exercise as the elevated blood pressure within the arteries forces some fluid from the blood vessels into the interstitial fluid. Prolonged exercise can lead to a further fall in plasma volume as intramuscular osmotic pressure (the tendency of water to move into a more concentrated solution) rises thus moving fluid from the plasma into the muscle fibres and interstitial space. Additionally, should an individual become dehydrated during an exercise bout, fluid loss from the interstitial space will result in a fluid shift out of the intravascular space. This haemoconcentration with acute exercise is a transient response.

Knowledge integration question

Explain the main changes in functioning of the respiratory and cardiovascular systems brought about through the body's response to exercise.

Key point

Even before the start of exercise, and subsequently in response to exercise, the body makes a number of alterations in functioning to maintain homeostasis. The alterations in cardiovascular and respiratory function, driven by sympathetic nervous stimulation, result in enhanced transport and exchange of metabolites.

Check your recall
Fill in the missing words.

Respiratory system

➤ The main function of the respiratory system is to facilitate the exchange of oxygen and _____ between the surrounding air and the body's cells.

➤ Oxygen reaches the cells of the body through three stages: pulmonary ventilation (breathing), alveolar ventilation (oxygen diffusion into the blood stream) and finally _____ ventilation (the diffusion of oxygen across the plasma membrane into the cell).

➤ The respiratory tract is generally divided into two zones, the conducting zone and the _____ zone.

➤ At rest, the contraction of the external intercostals and _____ results in inspiration and expiration occurs during the relaxation of these muscles.

➤ During exercise active expiration is required and this is achieved through the contraction of the internal intercostals, _____ and abdominals.

➤ The amount and type of work that an athlete is performing can be inferred from _____ _____ carried out during (on-line system) or after (Douglas bag method) exercise.

➤ _____ _____ _____ or $\dot{V}O_{2max}$ has traditionally been viewed as the gold standard measurement for aerobic fitness and is an assessment of the body's ability to utilise oxygen for energy generation during exercise.

➤ The _____ _____ _____ (VCO_2/VO_2) allows physiologists to assess which fuels (lipids or carbohydrates) are being utilised for energy production.

Cardiovascular system

➤ The cardiovascular system is comprised of three components: the vascular system, the heart and _____.

➤ The cardiovascular system performs a number of important functions: it is a transport system for nutrients, waste products and hormones. It also plays a key role in _____ regulation and contributes to the functioning of the immune system.

Blood

➤ Blood is comprised of plasma and _____ components including red and white blood cells and platelets.

➤ Plasma is _____-based but also has proteins and other water-soluble components dissolved within it.

➤ Red blood cells (erythrocytes) contain _____ and provide the main oxygen transport facility of the blood.

➤ White blood cells (leukocytes) are part of the _____ system and are responsible for fighting viral, bacterial and fungal infections.

➤ There are five types of white blood cell, three of which appear granular and two which appear _____.

➤ Platelets (thrombocytes), together with the protein fibrinogen, provide the blood with its _____ ability.

Heart

➤ The heart is constructed from a unique kind of muscle tissue called _____ muscle which is able to function continuously without fatigue.

➤ The atrium and ventricle on the right side of the heart are responsible for collecting and pumping blood to the _____ (pulmonary circulation).

➤ The atrium and ventricle on the left supply the rest of the body (_____ circulation).

Vascular system

➤ The vascular system contains _____ muscle which assists the heart in moving blood around the body.

➤ The main vessels of the vascular system are arteries, _____, capillaries, venules and veins.

➤ Arteries and arterioles carry blood away from the _____ to other tissues.

➤ _____ networks are the areas where gaseous and nutrient exchange take place. Venules and _____ carry blood from the tissues back to the heart.

➤ Arteries have thicker walls and a _____ diameter lumen.

➤ Veins have one-way _____ which, along with the skeletal muscle and respiratory pumps, facilitate the return of blood back to the heart.

➤ Arterioles help control blood flow by actively increasing (_____) or decreasing (_____) lumen diameter.

Acute responses to exercise

➤ The sympathetic nervous system will increase the rate and _____ of respiration as well as increase heart rate.

➤ The hormones adrenaline and _____ also contribute to the elevated heart rate and stroke volume with exercise and play a role in the regulation of blood flow.

➤ During the onset of exercise the levels of carbon dioxide (CO_2) and H^+ _____ and the level of oxygen (O_2) decreases.

➤ These changes are detected by _____ in the brain, aorta and carotid arteries and relayed to the respiratory centre.

➤ The increase in _____ _____ is the main driver for increases in respiration.

➤ Cardiovascular responses to exercise begin prior to the exercise itself in an _____ response which is related to the intensity of the expected exercise.

➤ The increases in blood flow and circulation with exercise favour the _____ muscles.

➤ At rest muscles receive 15% of the blood flow but this can increase to _____ % during exercise.

Review questions

1. How do the muscles involved in respiration differ between rest and exercise?

2. During respiration what is meant by the term tidal volume? Describe the changes in respiration that occur when exercising hard.

3. Explain the oxygen cascade from the air to the alveoli.

4. Why do physiologists convert the volume of gases collected to standard temperature and pressure dry (STPD)? What is the standard temperature (°C) and pressure (mmHg) for gases?

5. Draw and label a diagram of the heart, explain how the heart operates as a pump to move blood around the body.

6. Describe the different types of vessels within the vascular system.

7. Why are there two sounds every time the human heart beats? What processes occur during each of these sounds?

8. The heart's natural rhythm, dictated by the pacemaker, is around 100 beats per minute. How is the heart rate decreased or increased during rest or exercise?

9. Why are blood CO_2 levels important during exercise? What is the role of this respiratory driver?

10. Explain the response of the body's transport systems to exercise.

Teach it!

In groups of three, choose one topic and teach it to the rest of the study group.

1. Explain gaseous exchange.

2. Explain what the two numbers in a blood pressure reading mean – how they are measured and what is happening within the body when a reading is taken.

3. Describe the pathway of a red blood cell on a complete circuit from and to the right big toe.

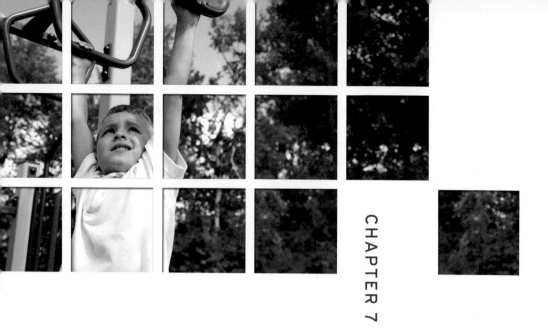

Physical and functional growth and development

Learning objectives

After reading, considering and discussing with a study partner the material in this chapter you should be able to:

➤ describe in detail the general pattern of human physical growth

➤ highlight gender differences in the general pattern and extent of physical growth to maturity

➤ describe the nature of skeletal growth

➤ explain growth and development within the muscular system

➤ highlight the key changes in the cardiovascular system during growth

➤ summarise the changes in aerobic and anaerobic fitness that occur during maturation

The human body changes greatly, both physically and functionally, from newborn to adulthood with influences of both a genetic and environmental nature involved. Growth and development are gradual, continuous processes infiltrated by two periods of rapid change: early infancy and adolescence. Although all healthy humans follow the same general pattern of physical growth, there are individual variations in the extent of growth and the timing of growth stages. You may remember from your youth, or from having seen children playing in a group or competing on the sports field, that despite being of a similar chronological age, there may be a dramatic variation in height and physical presence. This is due to the individual differences in the timing of puberty, with the early maturers experiencing a greater height gain than those that are still to mature. It is clear that when sports are segregated into chronological age groups, and puberty is approaching, the greater physical size and strength of early maturers gives them a substantial advantage in terms of athletic performance.

Following rapid growth in the first couple of years of life, the most dynamic period of post-natal growth is the adolescent growth spurt which is one of the milestones of puberty. This period involves the release of growth hormone and the sex hormones which stimulate a cascade of events including the acceleration of bone and muscle maturation, alterations in body composition and the development of secondary sexual characteristics, with the extent, timing and rate of these changes being gender-specific. It is during puberty that the most significant gains in height and weight, and subsequent increases in lung and heart masses, occur, in both males and females. In addition to the physical changes during growth, an enhanced functional capacity of the cardiorespiratory system also becomes evident.

This chapter examines physical changes during growth (height and weight, the skeletal and muscular systems, and the cardiorespiratory system) alongside functional changes of the muscles, the heart and the lungs. Following this, the development of anaerobic and aerobic fitness, along with training adaptations, are considered.

7.1 Physical growth

The overall growth of the body from newborn to adulthood follows a pattern of growth called a sigmoid curve (S-shaped). This pattern involves rapid growth after birth, particularly within the first year of life. A gradual and steady growth occurs during childhood followed by rapid growth during early adolescence after which growth plateaus as adult dimensions are obtained. Despite following a similar pattern of growth, the timing of growth changes, and the rate at which growth occurs, are highly variable between individuals.

Anthropometry (Greek meaning: 'anthropos' = man; 'metry' = measure) involves a variety of measurements of both the whole body and its individual parts, in order to understand human physical variation and to track changes during growth. These measurements include height, weight, skinfold thicknesses, segment lengths, skeletal breadths, as well as limb and head

circumferences. This chapter will focus on the measurement and growth changes of height, weight, and body composition, with consideration also given to the body mass index ratio. Height and weight both show diurnal variation (variation within the day) hence it is important to measure these variables at the same time of day, best in the early morning; this allows meaningful comparison with standard growth curves, or if repeated measures are to be taken across time.

Growth patterns of height and weight

Stature, or standing height, is the most common measure of growth. It is a composite measure of leg, trunk, neck and head lengths, and is determined with the use of a stadiometer which records the distance from the floor to the top of the head. For the greatest accuracy, readings are taken without socks and shoes, using a sliding measure board. Body weight is a measure of body mass, and reflects changes in lean body tissues and adipose (fat) tissues. Physical activity and nutrition, through their effects on skeletal muscle mass and fat deposition, can have strong extrinsic influences on body weight.

The increases in both height and weight follow the sigmoid curve of growth (Figure 7.1). As is illustrated in Figure 7.1, the first year of life after birth involves a large increase in height and weight, followed by a slower but steady increase during childhood. A large, rapid

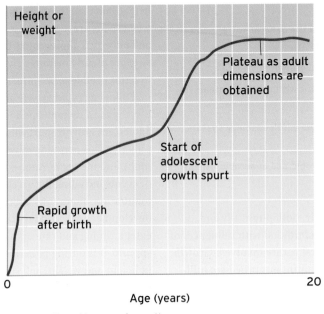

Figure 7.1 Sigmoid curve of growth.

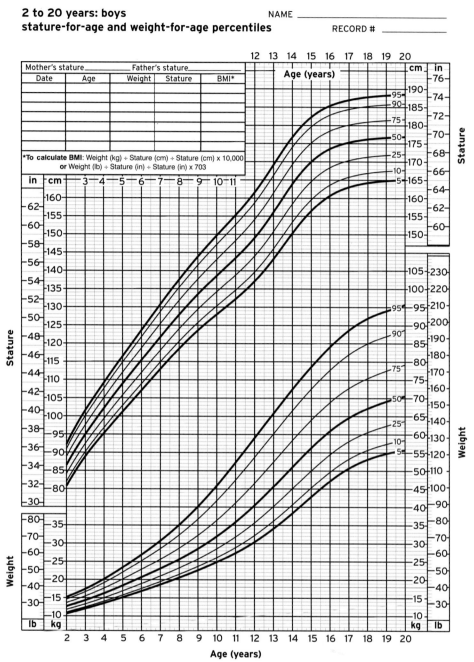

2 to 20 years: boys
stature-for-age and weight-for-age percentiles

NAME _____

RECORD # _____

Figure 7.2 Stature and weight for age percentiles of American boys (2-20 years of age). (*Source*: Developed by the National Center for Health Statistics in collaboration with the National Center for Chronic Disease Prevention and Health Promotion. (2000). www.cdc.gov/growthcharts.)

increase in both height and weight occurs during early adolescence which then slows down and levels off as adult height and weight are attained. These graphs are known as distance curves which convey the extent of change in absolute height or weight with increasing age. The variability in the extent of growth in stature and weight in boys (Figure 7.2) and girls (Figure 7.3) is illustrated with percentile charts, with the 50th percentile representing the average size. The increase in height during infancy and childhood is primarily due to growth in leg and trunk lengths, with the legs contributing a greater proportion. In contrast, growth of the trunk is largely responsible for increased height during late adolescence and adulthood. Due to the increases in stature and weight with growth,

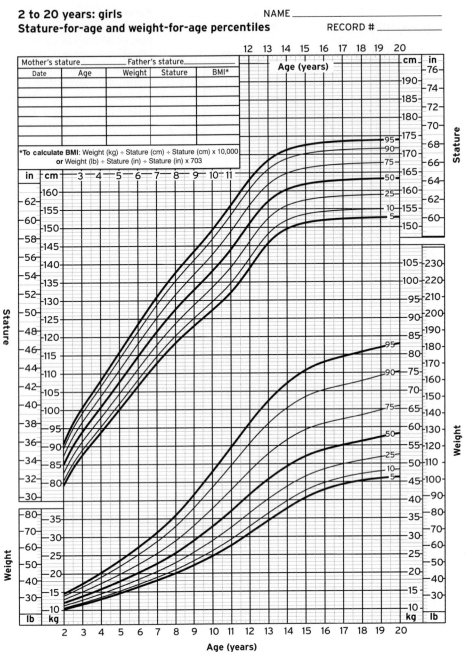

2 to 20 years: girls
Stature-for-age and weight-for-age percentiles

NAME _____

RECORD # _____

Figure 7.3 Stature and weight for age percentiles of American girls (2-20 years of age). (*Source*: Developed by the National Center for Health Statistics in collaboration with the National Center for Chronic Disease Prevention and Health Promotion. (2000) www.cdc.gov/growthcharts)

earlier maturing boys tend to be taller and heavier than those that mature later, with the earlier change in body shape and size advantageous for the participation in a wide variety of sports.

Key point

Height and weight follow a similar pattern of growth: the sigmoid curve.

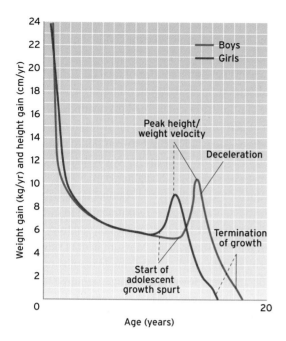

Figure 7.4 Velocity curves for the stature of British children. (*Source*: 'Growth and maturation during adolescence', James M. Tanner, *Nutrition Reviews* 39 (2): 43-55, 1981)

The slope of the distance graph indicates the *rate* of growth, with a steep slope indicating a rapid change in growth. An easier way of visually identifying the periods of rapid growth, however, is illustrated by velocity curves (Figure 7.4). A falling line on a velocity curve is indicative of a slowing rate of growth, and a peak illustrates a change in the rate of growth from faster to slower.

Following the rapid increase in growth during the first few years of life, the peak velocity of overall growth occurs during the adolescent growth spurt. These points of growth for height and weight can be clearly identified on the velocity curves and are generally known as peak height velocity (PHV) and peak weight velocity (PWV). The rates of growth of stature and weight differ during childhood. The height of the child increases, but at a constantly slower rate, reaching its lowest rate of growth increase prior to the adolescent growth spurt. In contrast, the rate of weight gain gradually increases from the age of three years until the point of rapid increase during the growth spurt.

Gender differences

The extent and timing of growth are gender-specific. During childhood, the height (5–6 cm/yr) and weight (2.5 kg/yr) of boys and girls increase at approximately the same rate. Gender differences, however, become strikingly clear during adolescence, the first main difference being the earlier onset of the growth spurt in females (9 years of age) compared to males (11 years of age).

Girls demonstrate a fairly rapid increase in height from 10.5 to 13 years of age, and a PHV of 8 cm/yr occurring at 11.5–12 years and a total gain in height of around 25 cm across the pubertal period. Following the growth spurt the rate of height increase steadily falls with adult stature attained around 16 years of age. In contrast, boys reach PHV at a later age (13.5–14 years) but experience a higher rate of growth (9 cm/yr) resulting in a 28 cm height gain across the growth period. Following PHV, the rate of height growth declines with little further growth from around 18 years of age (Figure 7.4). Some individuals (males and females), however, may continue to increase slightly in height during the third decade of life. These stages in the velocity of stature growth are demonstrated in Figure 7.4. The later onset of the growth spurt in males allows for around two years more growth than females. This, combined with the higher PHV in males, accounts for the adult height difference of 10–13 cm between adult males and females. In addition to the adolescent growth spurt, some children experience a mid-growth spurt around 7 years of age, although the increase in height is not as dramatic as that during the adolescent spurt.

Key point

Adult males tend to be 10–13 cm taller than females due to their longer growth period and higher peak height velocity.

Similar to height, significant weight gains occur during the adolescent growth spurt, with around 50% of adult body weight gained during this growth period. The rapid increase in weight which occurs during adolescence is similar to the height curve, except that PWV occurs later than PHV, and growth in weight generally continues for longer. In girls, PWV occurs 3.5–10 months following PHV with the most rapid gain in weight (8.3 kg/yr) occurring between 12 and 13 years of age. As with the growth in height, males begin the rapid increase in weight gain later than girls and increase weight to a greater extent. The PWV in boys (9 kg/yr) is higher than girls and occurs 2.5–5 months after their PHV. The increase in body weight due to growth appears to cease in females around 17 years of age; however, the growth of weight in males continues beyond 18 years. As mentioned previously, body weight is greatly influenced by physical activity levels and dietary intake, therefore, weight has the potential to fluctuate greatly throughout adult life. It is clear that the promotion of physical activity and healthy eating from an early age is important to help reduce the incidence of obesity in children.

Key point

Body weight is significantly influenced by physical activity and dietary intake throughout life.

The development of body composition

In contrast to body weight, a composite measure of all body tissues, body composition divides the body into fat-free, or lean body mass (LBM) and fat mass (FM). It is common to use LBM as an estimation of skeletal muscle mass. However, it is important to realise that LBM also includes water and other non-fat tissues such as bone, connective tissue, and the body organs. The physiological response to exercise is significantly related to body composition, as LBM (skeletal muscle mass) is responsible for body movements, whereas body fat is an additional weight that needs to be supported and moved by the LBM. Body fat, therefore, has a negative influence on performance. It is important to identify the changes in body composition during growth to allow for the accurate interpretation of exercise responses. Additionally, the increasing incidence of childhood obesity and its link to chronic disease and life-long obesity are current major health concerns. Body composition is, therefore, a common measure in large research studies as an indicator of health-related fitness.

Measurement of body composition

Several techniques can be used for the estimation of body composition: underwater weighing, subcutaneous skinfolds, body mass index, dual-energy X-ray absorptiometry and bioelectrical impedance are some of the most commonly used. Underwater weighing has often been referred to as the 'gold standard' method to measure fat. This method of estimation uses body density, the ratio of body weight to body volume, as a reflection of body fat content (density of fat is lower than that of lean tissue). Body volume is determined by the displacement of water by full body submersion in a water tank (Figure 7.5a). This

method, however, is time-consuming, is limited to research settings, and is not recommended for children due to the complete submersion in water.

Subcutaneous fat is an indicator of total fat, hence skinfold thicknesses measured with calipers (Figure 7.5b) at single or multiple sites can be used in equations for the estimation of percentage body fat or the determination of fat distribution. The relationship between skinfolds and body fat, however, varies with age hence child-specific equations have been derived (Slaughter et al., 1988). For the estimation of total body fat and regional fat distribution in children and adolescents, it is recommended to measure the triceps, subscapular and abdominal skinfold thicknesses (Lohman & Going, 2006). Measurement of skinfold thicknesses is a relatively cheap and simple method of body composition analysis. However, training is required to ensure accurate and reproducible measurement.

Currently in research, the most common methods used for the analysis of body composition are dual-energy X-ray absorptiometry (DXA) and bioelectrical impedance analysis (BIA). As a scanning method, DXA can be used to estimate both LBM and FM, and both regional and total body composition. The body composition of subjects over a wide range of ages and body sizes can be analysed, however, due to the cost of the procedure and the size of the machine (Figure 7.5c), its use is limited to research settings. Utilising the fact that electric currents pass more easily through lean tissue (high water content) than fat tissue (very low water content), BIA captures the resistance between conductors to provide a measure of body fat. It is a simple, portable and quick method which involves standing on a small machine with bare feet and, depending on the particular machine used, holding a grip in each hand (Figure 7.5d). For these reasons, BIA has become a very popular method of body composition analysis which can be readily used in the field for the measurement of large subject numbers. A downfall is that several factors, such as temperature, exercise and hydration status, that are difficult to control in the field, can result in measurement error.

The body mass index (BMI) is an expression of body weight relative to stature and is useful for distinguishing between underweight, normal weight and overweight individuals.

$$BMI = body\ weight\ (kg)/height^2\ (m)$$

BMI relates well to percentage body fat and is easy to calculate, hence it is commonly used as a marker of overweight or obesity in many research studies. During growth, however, BMI is an inadequate marker of body composition. When using BMI it is assumed that a greater value is

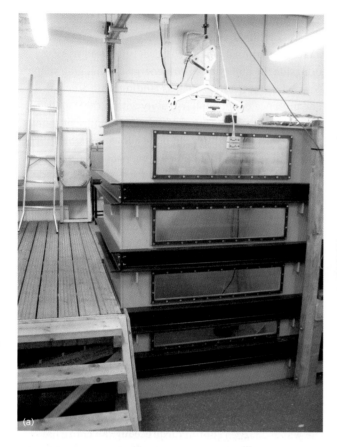

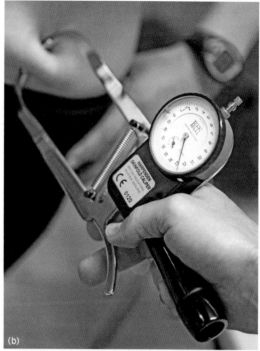

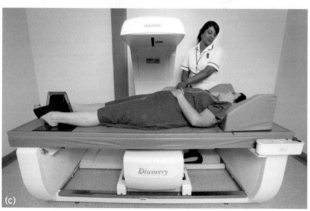

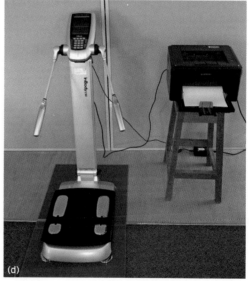

Figure 7.5 Equipment used for the determination of body composition by (a) underwater weighing, (b) skinfold thickness measurement, (c) dual-energy X-ray absorptiometry and (d) bioelectrical impedance analysis.

related to a higher proportion of body fat. During growth, however, the BMI increases as a result of a greater lean mass rather than fat mass, particularly in boys (Maynard et al., 2001; Wells, 2000).

Knowledge integration question

Explain why using BMI might misrepresent a person's body composition during the growth period.

Key points

Body composition:

Divides the body into lean body mass (LBM) and fat mass (FM)

A variety of techniques can be used for its estimation:

➤ Laboratory – underwater weighing, DXA, BIA

➤ Field – subcutaneous skinfolds, BMI

Gender differences in body composition

Changes in body composition during growth are gender-related, with gender differences accentuated during adolescence. During childhood, similar increases in FM and LBM occur, but females tend to have a greater FM and lower LBM than males (Hills & Byrne, 2010). Upon reaching the growth spurt, LBM in males increases at a faster rate due to the increase in muscle mass associated with elevated testosterone during this period of growth. This gender difference results in the LBM of adult males being approximately 150% greater than that of females (Hills & Byrne, 2010). In contrast to males, hormonal influences in females result in little muscle growth and the accumulation of adipose tissue during the growth spurt, hence LBM plateaus around 15 years of age (~5 years earlier than in males) while FM continues to rise, amplifying the gender differences.

Gender differences are also clear in percentage body fat during growth. From the age of around three years, females consistently demonstrate a greater percentage body fat compared with males. A gradual decline in both genders occurs during early childhood, following which percentage body fat steadily rises from eight years of age throughout adolescence in females. Little change occurs in males until puberty when the development of muscle tissue (LBM) is reflected in a decrease in percentage fat from around 16% to 12–14% of total body mass.

In addition to total body fat, the distribution of body fat changes during growth with an increase in trunk and abdominal fat. The identification of changes in fat distribution is therefore important as abdominal fatness is associated with disease risk factors (Sardinha & Teixeira, 2005).

Key point

Due to hormonal changes, males increase lean body mass whereas females lay down more fat during the adolescent growth spurt.

7.2 Development of the skeletal system

Healthy bone development is brought about through a unique balance between strength and lightness, along with rigidity and flexibility, achieved through its unique composition and structural design. Its rigid mineral matrix combined with elastic collagen allows it to withstand gravitational and mechanical (muscle) forces, alongside the ability to absorb energy by changing shape during impact loading, such as landing from a height. The presence of a medullary cavity within the diaphysis of long bones, along with the cancellous nature of spongy bone, results in a lightweight bone allowing mobility. The normal development of bone during childhood and adolescence is important, not only in these younger years of life, but also in later years by helping to reduce the occurrence of fractures and the development of osteoporosis. Sport-specific training has become common in children and adolescents. Great debate and concern exists over the safety of early specific training due to the continuing growth of the bones. This will be discussed in more detail in section 7.5 'Anaerobic and aerobic fitness and training'.

In utero, a cartilage 'model' of the skeleton is initially laid down by week 6 of gestation. Bone tissue begins to develop from this time; however, the process of ossification is not complete until the third decade of life. The human skeleton may merely appear to be a rigid supporting structure, but it is in fact a dynamic tissue which changes continuously during the entire life span. These changes are influenced by both genetics and external factors (mechanical stresses, hormones, nutrition). During childhood and adolescence the longitudinal growth of the long bones is reflected in increasing stature (height). In contrast, other skeletal developments (bone mineral content, bone mineral density and strength) occur due to the continuous remodeling and renewal of bone and are not directly observable. These continual changes to the physical properties of bone occur not only during childhood and adolescence, but also during adulthood.

Key points

Bone is a dynamic tissue which is continuously being remodelled and renewed.

Bone development is influenced by genetics, mechanical stress, hormones and nutrition.

The growth of long bones

Nearly all bones begin life as cartilage. Both are forms of connective tissue but cartilage is more elastic in nature and therefore less rigid. During the formation of cartilage, **chondroblasts** (cartilage forming cells) become entrapped in their own network or matrix and develop into **chondrocytes** (cartilage cells). Most of the skeletal cartilage is replaced by bone as the body develops in a process called **ossification**. Three types of bone cell are involved in the growth, repair and remodeling of bone tissue. In a similar fashion to cartilage, bone-forming **osteoblasts**, which combine calcium and phosphorus to produce **hydroxyapatite crystals** (the mineralised form of bone), become **osteocytes** when entrapped in their own mineral network. **Osteoclasts** (from the Greek words for bone and broken), the third form of bone cell, are responsible for the removal and resorption of unwanted bone or the breakdown of bone when the minerals are required elsewhere in the body. While osteocytes are trapped within the matrix of the bone, osteoclasts, which are large multinucleated cells, are free to move along the bone surface as they remove and repair damaged sections of the bone matrix.

During development long bone growth begins within the **diaphysis** and later, around the time of birth, secondary ossification centres appear in the proximal and distal epiphyses. The cartilage that remains between the primary and secondary ossification centres is called the **epiphyseal plate** or **growth plate**. The general structure of a long bone is shown in Chapter 5 (Figure 5.3). At the epiphyseal plate, new cartilage is continuously formed and then mineralised to form bone,

resulting in an increase in the length of the bone (Figure 7.6). As the increase in long bone length is reflected in increased body height, the growth of the skeleton approximately follows the growth curve for height (refer to Figure 7.1).

At the end of adolescence the formation of new cartilage slows until the epiphyseal plates are entirely replaced by bone tissue. This fusion of the epiphysis and the diaphysis, leaving only the **epiphyseal line** (refer to Figure 5.3), symbolises the end of longitudinal bone growth. The majority of epiphyseal plates are fully ossified by the age of 18 or 19 years; however, great individual variation occurs. Children of the same chronological age may have a skeletal age which varies by three or more years. Also, as females mature earlier than males, their epiphyseal plates tend to close at an earlier chronological age. This was demonstrated by Hansman (1962) who found the epiphyseal plate in the head of the humerus to close at an average age of 15.5 years in females compared with 18.1 years in males.

Knowledge integration question

Explain how differences in epiphyseal plate closure affects total height gain for males and females.

Although the longitudinal growth of bones is finite, the thickness of bones can continue to increase if put under stress, such as that encountered during weight-bearing activities. The growth in diameter of long bones occurs by **appositional growth**, with osteoblasts beneath the periosteum laying down new bone on the external bone surface. Simultaneously, old layers of bone are removed from the inside of the bone (the wall of the medullary cavity) but at a slightly slower rate, allowing the bone to increase in thickness and strength, yet maintain its light weight.

Key point

Longitudinal bone growth occurs at the epiphyseal plate, the cartilaginous region between the diaphysis and epiphysis.

The thickness of bone increases by appositional growth.

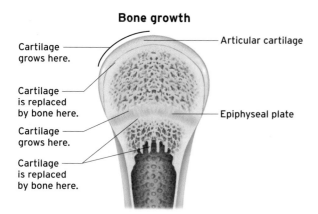

Bone growth

Cartilage grows here.

Articular cartilage

Cartilage is replaced by bone here.

Cartilage grows here.

Epiphyseal plate

Cartilage is replaced by bone here.

Figure 7.6 A schematic illustration of long bone growth.

The development of the physical properties of bone

Several parameters of bone are measured as indicators of bone strength. These include bone mineral content (BMC), bone mineral density (BMD), bone cross-sectional area (bCSA) and cortical thickness. Mineral content (measured in grams) can be reported as a total-body value or that for a particular bone. The ratio of BMC to bone CSA or volume is referred to as areal BMD (aBMD $g \cdot cm^{-2}$) or volumetric BMD (vBMD $g \cdot cm^{-3}$), respectively. During bone analysis, the total width of the bone and the width of the medullary cavity (refer to Figure 5.3) are measured, allowing for the calculation of the cortical thickness (cortical thickness = total width − medullary cavity width). The most common tool used for the measurement of a wide variety of bone parameters is densitometry, which functions by measuring radiation absorption by the skeleton. A more recent development for bone assessment utilises ultrasound which does not involve radiation; however, cortical thickness is not able to be assessed.

The increase in bone size during growth is accompanied by an increase in bone mass and bone strength. The modeling and remodeling of bone during growth function to optimise strength and minimise mass, by depositing bone where it is needed (area under the most stress) and removing it from where it is not needed. Bone strength is now regarded as the most critical property of bone rather than its mass (Schönau, 2006; Schönau & O'Fricke, 2008). Age-dependent increases in bone cross-sectional area and cortical thickness have been demonstrated during childhood and adolescence, with these parameters being suggested as the most important factors of bone strength (De Schepper et al., 1996; Schönau, 1998). The cortical thickness has been shown to be slightly higher in boys than girls with a greater increase in boys from around 14 years of age (De Schepper et al., 1996). The cortical thickness in boys and girls is illustrated in relation to age in Figure 7.7.

Bone mineral content

As bone grows, and the cortical thickness increases, the total bone mineral content (BMC) increases. This change in BMC with growth has been demonstrated in a variety of locations (such as the hip, lumbar spine, head, arms and legs) and also as total body values, with boys in general exhibiting greater BMC compared with girls (Gutin et al.,

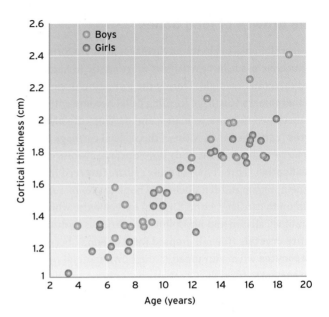

Figure 7.7 The development of bone cortical thickness in girls and boys. (*Source*: Adapted from de Schepper et al. (1996))

2011; Kriemler et al., 2008; Maynard et al., 1998). This gender difference in BMC has been suggested to be related to a difference in the sensitivity of the male and female bone to exercise stress (Kriemler et al., 2008).

Bone mineral density

Bone mineral density (BMD), often referred to simply as bone density, represents the bone mineral content relative to the outer bone area or volume, as mentioned above. The density of bone mineral is assessed by dual-energy X-ray absorptiometry (DXA) which reports an areal value ($g \cdot cm^{-2}$) for BMD. During the measurement of aBMD, a two-dimensional image of a three-dimensional structure is produced. As the depth of the bone remains unknown, a larger bone with a greater depth (as occurs with increasing age) will be reported as having a greater areal density as more photons emitted during densitometry will be attenuated by the greater mineral content of the larger bone. Volumetric BMD ($g \cdot cm^{-3}$), however, can be calculated from the areal value by taking bone dimensions into account. As the greater amount of mineral in a larger bone is dispersed in a larger bone volume, vBMD remains relatively unchanged with growth. It is clear that care must be taken when interpreting BMD data reported in the literature as aBMD and vBMD demonstrate differing responses to growth and development.

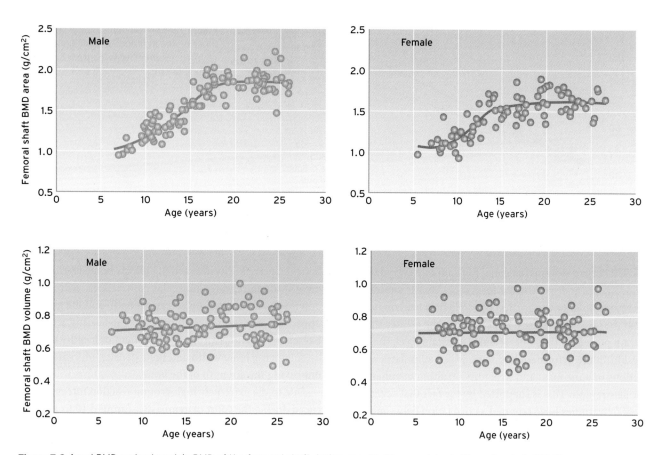

Figure 7.8 Areal BMD and volumetric BMD of the femoral shaft during growth. (*Source*: Adapted from Lu et al. (1996))

A common misconception is that as bone grows it becomes denser. This stems from the reports of increasing aBMD during childhood and adolescence in both males and females (Boot et al., 1997; Kriemler et al., 2008; Lu et al., 1996; Maynard et al., 1998). Both genders have been shown to exhibit a similar increase in mean total-body aBMD until the age of 14 years, following which the increase in males was greater than that of females (Maynard et al., 1998). The main predictor of aBMD during the end of adolescence is LBM, independent of gender. Between the ages of 15 and 18 years, however, muscular fitness, contributes more to the aBMD of males than females (Fonseca et al., 2008). It is clear, therefore, that exercise participation and a healthy diet (refer to Chapter 2 for dietary information), through their influence on LBM and muscular fitness, play important roles in the growth of healthy bones.

In contrast to areal density, the vBMD of long bones is less dependent on age and growth variables (Lu et al., 1996). The change in vBMD with growth appears to vary between sites, with a relatively stable vBMD of the femoral shaft and neck (males 5–27 years of age), but a small increase in the vBMD of the radius and lumbar spine from childhood to adolescence in both males and females (Boot

et al., 1997; De Schepper et al., 1996; Lu et al., 1996). The differing responses of the areal and volumetric femoral shaft bone mineral densities during growth are illustrated for both boys and girls in Figure 7.8.

Key point

Growth results in a larger skeleton, with minimal change in volumetric bone mineral density.

Knowledge integration question

Describe the differences in bone mineral density prior to and after puberty.

Roles of muscle strength, physical activity and nutrition on bone growth

The muscle/bone strength relationship

The discussion of the musculoskeletal system in Chapter 5 outlined the synchronous function of the muscular and

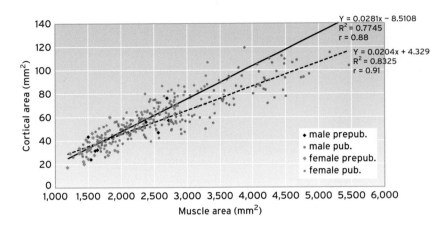

Figure 7.9 Cortical bone area in relation to muscle area in prepubertal and pubertal children. (*Source*: Adapted from Schönau et al. (2000))

skeletal organ systems, essential for both our everyday movements and sporting performance. Muscle contraction is responsible for the greatest physiological load on bone, and the larger the muscle force applied, the greater the strain placed on the bone. If above a certain level, the strain results in the deformation of bone which stimulates adaptations in bone mass and structure, resulting in enhanced bone strength. This is supported by the fact that several research studies have reported a correlation between an index of muscle strength (mCSA, grip strength) and an index of bone strength (bCSA, cortical thickness, BMC) (Heinonen et al., 2001; Schönau et al., 1998; 2000; 2004).

A good correlation ($r^2 = 0.77$) was found between radial muscle area (index of muscle strength) and cortical area (index of bone strength) in children, adolescents and adults (aged 6 to 22 years) (Schönau et al., 2000). This relationship was found to be similar across gender prior to puberty; however, the cortical area became greater in comparison to the muscle area in girls after puberty (Figure 7.9). It was subsequently found that the increased oestrogen level in females at puberty was responsible for an increase in bone mass, although this was not reflected in additional bone strength (Schönau et al., 2004). In contrast to its positive effects on cortical area, muscular strength (grip strength) has no effect on the volumetric bone density of the distal radius (Schönau, 1998).

Key point

The strength of bone is adapted to muscle strength.

The role of physical activity in bone growth

In addition to physical maturity, environmental factors such as physical activity and nutrition are known to affect

bone properties. Physical activity affects bone development through repeated muscular contractions, with potentially an elevated muscular strength, and the ground impact forces experienced during weight-bearing activities. Exercise is essential for the development of healthy bones, by enhancing bone width and bone density, ultimately improving the strength of the bone.

Due to the extremely high ground reaction forces experienced during the sport of gymnastics (around 10 to 15 times body weight), much research has used this sport to identify the effects of impact activities on bone accrual. Many studies on gymnasts have identified an increased bone accrual in girls during the peripubertal years compared with active controls (Bass et al., 1998; Courteix et al., 1999; Gero et al., 2005; Laing et al., 2002; Nickols-Richardson et al., 2000; Nurmi-Lawton et al., 2004). Retrospective studies have suggested that this positive effect of gymnastics on bone structure is maintained into later life, with former gymnasts having a 5–22% greater aBMD than non-gymnasts (Bass et al., 1998; Kirchner et al., 1996; Kudlac et al., 2004). This was supported by a recent three-year longitudinal study which found childhood gymnastics to produce positive skeletal adaptations (in aBMD, BMC and cortical area) that were maintained for at least two years from the cessation of gymnastics involvement and menarche (Scerpella et al., 2010). They also reported, however, that continued involvement in gymnastics during adolescence yielded additional benefits. In addition to gymnastics, high-intensity, intermittent loading of the bones has been shown to produce an osteogenic effect, suggesting that short bursts of explosive exercise, such as skipping and jumping, are effective for bone development (Kemper, 2000).

The influence of exercise on bone growth is sport-specific as the bone adapts to the mechanical strain placed upon it. For example, racquet sports enhance the BMD of the dominant arm (Watson, 1974), gymnastics improves the health of the arm, leg and hip bones (Gero et al., 2005), while activities such as soccer (Calbet et al., 2001; Falk et al., 2010; Magnusson et al., 2001; Söderman et al., 2000; Vicente-Rodriguez et al., 2004) promote the health of the lower-limb bones. In contrast, non-weight-bearing sports such as swimming and water polo have been found to have no effect on aBMD in children or adults (Andreoli et al., 2001; Duncan et al., 2002; Lima et al., 2001). It is important, therefore, to promote weight-bearing activities during growth to aid the development of healthy, strong bones.

Although high-impact weight-bearing sports such as gymnastics and soccer have been found to be beneficial in the accrual of bone, is there any benefit of general physical activity on the properties of bone? The good news is that children do not have to be involved in high levels of training for a specific sport to yield these benefits. Total habitual physical activity and the time spent in vigorous physical activity have been found to increase BMC in boys, but not girls, potentially due to a greater sensitivity of bone to physical loading in boys (Baptista et al., 2011; Kriemler et al., 2008). In addition, habitual physical activity has been found to be positively correlated with lumbar spine aBMD, but not with vBMD (Boot et al., 1997). While greater habitual physical activity appears to improve BMC in prepubertal boys, lean body mass (as an index of muscle forces) has been found to be the main predictor of bone size and/or mineralisation in children (8–10 years of age) and adolescents (15–18 years of age) of both genders (Baptista et al., 2011; Fonseca et al., 2008).

Nutrition and bone growth

The mineral matrix of bone is formed mostly by calcium hydroxyapatite, and for this reason calcium is an important nutrient in our diet, especially during periods of bone growth during childhood and adolescence. It has been shown that, in addition to age, factors affecting BMC are calcium intake and vigorous physical activity (Gutin et al., 2011). Although calcium plays an important role in the development of healthy bones, it has been suggested that physical training has a greater effect on bone properties than nutritional factors such as calcium intake (Falk et al., 2007). As suggested by Falk et al., (2007), however, it is possible that deficient calcium intake during growth may not affect bone properties until later in life. It is currently thought that for physical activity to exert its optimal effect on bone development an adequate intake of calcium may be required (Harvey et al., 2011).

Key point

During childhood, a combination of physical activity and calcium intake are essential for the optimal growth of bones.

7.3 Development of the muscular system

The growth of skeletal muscles during childhood and adolescence is interlinked with the growth and development of the skeletal system and hence is essential to maintain the ability to pull efficiently on the growing bones, initiating body movement. The increase in muscle size during growth is linked with enhanced muscular strength. However, other factors, such as muscle composition or neural control, may also be involved in the production of force. The enhanced muscular strength due to growth and development is important for not only sports performance, but also health-related fitness. Low levels of muscular fitness (including both strength and endurance) have been associated with high cardiovascular disease risk factors (Garcia-Artero et al., 2007), hence, the importance of monitoring it throughout childhood and adolescence is clear.

Skeletal muscle growth

The growth of muscle *in utero* occurs via both **hyperplasia** (an increase in the number of muscle fibres) and **hypertrophy** (an increase in muscle fibre size). Shortly following birth, the number of muscle fibres is fixed, with postnatal muscle growth occurring primarily by hypertrophy. This was demonstrated by the examination of cross sections of autopsied whole human vastus lateralis muscle, where no change in muscle fibre number was found from 5 to 37 years of age (Lexell et al., 1992).

Key point

Following birth, muscle growth occurs primarily via hypertrophy.

Muscle fibre growth

The length and diameter of muscle fibres increase during growth. The increase in length is brought about by the addition of sarcomeres at muscle-tendon junctions and also the lengthening of existing sarcomeres (Malina & Bouchard, 1991). The process of hypertrophy during growth is stimulated by the release of certain hormones (growth hormone, testosterone and insulin growth factor 1 (IGF-1)) which have anabolic properties. They stimulate the synthesis of new contractile proteins which are incorporated into the existing myofibrils. It is the dramatic increase in testosterone during adolescence, however, that has the greatest influence on muscle growth in males. The extent of hypertrophy during childhood may vary between muscle groups (Aherne et al., 1971; Bowden & Goyer, 1960), potentially as a result of the differing forces subjected on each muscle during growth. Muscle fibre diameter increases from birth, with around 50% of adult values reached by around the age of five years (Colling-Saltin, 1980). Further, the mean fibre size of the vastus lateralis muscle has been estimated to more than double from the age of five years to full maturity (Lexell et al., 1992). Peak muscle fibre diameter is reached during adolescence in females, but continues to increase into early adulthood in males (Oertel, 1988).

Muscle mass and cross-sectional area

The increase in muscle fibre size during growth is reflected in a rise in total muscle mass and muscle cross-sectional area (mCSA). Total muscle mass is most commonly estimated in children from the measurement of urinary creatinine, a muscle metabolite. The change in estimated muscle mass is illustrated in Figure 7.10. The graph demonstrates a linear increase in muscle mass for both males and females until the onset of puberty, with males having a slightly greater muscle

mass than females. From this time, around the age of 12 years, the gender difference in muscle mass becomes magnified with a rapid increase in males which starts to plateau around 20 years of age. In contrast, muscle mass of females continues to increase gradually until around 15 years of age.

The large gender difference in muscle mass that occurs during adolescence is related to the high androgen levels, particularly testosterone, initiated during puberty in males. In addition, it has been suggested that the greater increase in muscle mass in males may also be related to the fact that from the age of 9–10 years they participate in more high-intensity activities than females (Thomas et al., 1991), with the higher stresses placed on the muscle resulting in greater levels of hypertrophy.

The contribution of body regions to total muscle mass differs during growth as suggested by an increased contribution of lower extremity musculature to the total body value. During childhood, and in particular adolescence, males have proportionally more upper-body muscle mass than females, a gender difference which persists through adulthood.

As expected, the increased muscle fibre size during growth also results in an increased muscle volume and mCSA. The mCSA is the physical property of muscle that is focused on in the literature due to its relationship with muscle mass and the fact that it can be measured non-invasively (magnetic resonance imaging, computed tomography, dual X-ray absorptiometry). Muscle CSA (*vastus lateralis*) has been shown to more than double in males from the age of 5 to 25 years (Lexell et al., 1992).

The mCSA of the lower leg and arm muscles increases in both males and females from childhood to adolescence (Deighan et al., 2006; Kanehisa et al., 1995b; Tonson et al., 2008). Males start to demonstrate a greater mCSA than females during adolescence which continues through to young adulthood (Deighan et al., 2006; Kanehisa et al., 1995b). The growth of mCSA tends to plateau around 20 years of age in males, while female mCSA tends to level off around 16 years of age, reflective of the growth pattern of muscle mass.

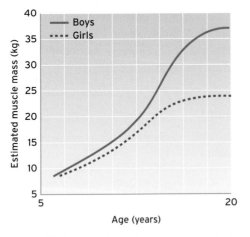

Figure 7.10 An illustration of muscle mass changes during childhood and adolescence.

Key point

Muscle fibre growth is reflected in elevated muscle mass, muscle cross-sectional area and muscle volume.

Development of muscular strength

Muscular strength is the amount of force that can be generated during a single maximal contraction. Strength is an important component of health-related physical fitness which allows us to perform life's daily activities efficiently, in addition to being crucial for optimal performance in a wide variety of sports. It allows for good posture, the prevention of injuries, and sporting success. The development of strength is similar on both sides of the body with reports of either a slightly stronger dominant side (Molenaar et al., 2010) or no effect of dominance on muscular strength (Butterfield et al., 2009; Mathiowetz et al., 1986).

Muscle strength of children and adolescents is commonly measured with the use of hand-held dynamometers as the equipment is portable and easily used in the child's natural environment. A common measure of isometric strength in children is grip strength which also gives an estimation of upper-body strength (Payne & Isaacs, 2008) and appears to reflect the overall strength development of both boys and girls during childhood (Blimkie et al., 1989). More detailed measures of both isometric and isokinetic strength and muscular activity can be made with an isokinetic dynamometer in the laboratory, although this equipment holds limitations for the large research studies required to monitor growth and development due to the cost and lack of portability.

General pattern of muscular strength development

It is well established that absolute muscle strength increases during growth from childhood to adulthood (Ahmad et al., 2006; Butterfield et al., 2009; Cohen et al., 2010; Falk et al., 2009a, 2009b). The development of strength has been shown to be related to muscle size, with developmental curves for muscle strength following the same general shape as those for muscle mass (refer to Figure 7.10). Isometric and isokinetic strength show similar developments during childhood and adolescence (Butterfield et al., 2009; Mathiowetz et al., 1986; Molenaar et al., 2010; De Ste Croix et al., 2003, 2009; Seger & Thorstensson, 2000). Strength increases with age in both genders, although males exhibit greater absolute strength values at all ages. Prior to the onset of puberty the gender difference is small and it is around the age of 12 years that the strength of males increases at a faster rate than that of females. This pattern of strength development is illustrated in Figure 7.11 which depicts the relationship between grip strength and

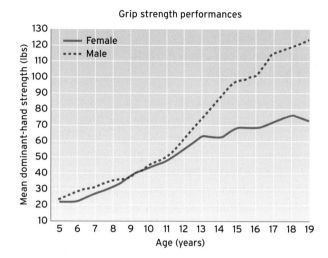

Figure 7.11 The dominant hand strength of males and females during childhood and adolescence. (*Source*: Adapted from Butterfield et al. (2009)).

age (5 to 19 years). Although a large gender difference in grip strength (a marker of arm strength) exists, this is generally smaller when comparing trunk or leg strength.

The greater increase in muscular strength of males during and following puberty is related to the elevated levels of androgens (male sex hormones), particularly testosterone, and resultant increase in muscle mass. At the same developmental age, the increase in female body weight is related to an increase in fat levels due to the effects of oestrogen. Therefore, when muscular strength is reported relative to body mass, although the gender difference is reduced, males are generally still stronger as females have greater fat and less lean body mass, resulting in less strength per unit of body weight. If reported relative to LBM, however, there is a considerable reduction in the absolute gender differences in strength.

Key points

Muscular strength increases with age in males and females.

Males are stronger at all ages with the gender difference becoming most obvious from around 12 years of age. This is primarily due to the higher testosterone levels in males during puberty.

There are two mechanisms through which muscular strength is primarily increased;

1. muscle hypertrophy (increased mCSA), and
2. improved neuromuscular activation that allows the recruitment of more motor units and hence muscle fibres.

The role of each of these mechanisms is discussed below.

Relationship between muscle size and strength

It is commonly assumed that when a muscle visually increases in size (muscle hypertrophy) the strength of the muscle is enhanced. It is those with large muscles that compete in events such as the shot putt, weightlifting, gymnastics and the World's Strongest Man. The large muscles of Mariusz Pudzianowski, five-time winner of the title of World's Strongest Man, are shown in Figure 7.12a. The strength of Jacko Gill, shot putt World Youth Champion 2011, is also illustrated (Figure 7.12b)

During growth from childhood to adulthood, mCSA has been shown to increase in both males and females, with a greater increase in males (Deighan et al., 2006; Kanehisa et al., 1995b). This increase in mCSA is associated with an increase in muscular strength (Falk et al., 2009a, 2009b; Kanehisa et al., 1995a, 1995b; Tonson et al., 2008; Wood et al., 2006). However, is the increase in muscular strength during growth solely related to the increase in muscle size? It would appear not. Kanehisa et al. (1995a) reported that pre- or early-pubertal children develop strength at a greater rate than the concurrent increase in muscle size, similar to the finding that resistance training in pre-pubertal children can improve muscular strength in the absence of muscle hypertrophy (Blimkie, 1993; Ozmun et al., 1994). In addition, when maximal muscle force is normalised to body mass or mCSA, lower values are generally found in children compared to adults (Falk et al., 2009b; Grosset et al., 2008; Lambertz et al., 2003; Tonson et al., 2008; Wood et al., 2006). Together, these findings suggest that factors other than muscle size must be involved in the development of muscular strength.

Key point

The bigger the muscle, the stronger the muscle.

Muscle composition and contractile properties: effects on muscular strength

Characteristics of skeletal muscle tissue other than physical size that may contribute to enhanced strength during childhood and adolescence, are the fibre type proportions

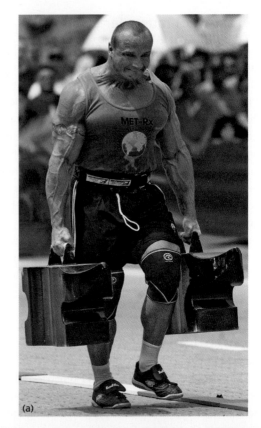

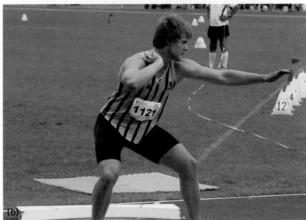

Figure 7.12 (a) Mariusz Pudzianowski, five-time winner of the World's Strongest Man title. (*Source*: Getty Images) (b) Jacko Gill, World Youth shot putt champion 2011. (*Source*: Didier Poppe)

and contractile properties of the fibres. Alongside the increase in muscle fibre size with growth is a functional development of the fibre population. Children have a higher proportion of type I fibres with the proportion of type II fibres increasing through to late adolescence when adult proportions are attained (Glenmark et al., 1994; Lexell et al., 1992). As type II fibres are fast-twitch fibres capable of generating a greater force than type I fibres, the fibre composition of skeletal muscle may play a role in the increase in muscular force during growth and development. This is still debatable, however, as other studies have reported little change in the proportion of type I and type II muscle fibres with increasing age (Lexell, 1995). As different adult muscles contain varying proportions of type I and type II fibres, the change in fibre type proportions during growth, and subsequent influence on muscle strength, may be muscle-dependent.

A further factor potentially involved in the development of muscular strength is the **muscle-specific tension**, the force produced per unit area of muscle. An increased muscle-specific tension during growth could potentially contribute to the overall increase in muscular strength. Recent research, however, has demonstrated that muscle-specific tension in pre-pubertal children is either similar to or greater than adults, suggesting no role of muscle-specific tension in the development of muscular strength (O'Brien et al., 2010; Morse et al., 2008).

Neuromuscular influences on muscular strength

It is widely accepted that neuromuscular differences between children and adults are partially responsible for the greater muscular strength exhibited by adults. With the use of an isokinetic dynamometer (Figure 7.13), great detail regarding the activation of the muscle and development of force can be established. The ability to activate the neuromuscular system is lower in pre-pubertal boys compared with adults (Belanger & McComas, 1989; Cohen et al., 2010; Grosset et al., 2008; O'Brien et al.,

2009). In addition, it has been suggested that children are less able to recruit, or utilise, their higher-threshold motor units (in elbow flexors), that is those comprised primarily of type II fibres, which are recruited last during maximal muscle activation (Falk et al., 2009b). An earlier study, however, found children as young as six years of age able to fully activate the ankle dorsiflexor muscles (Belanger & McComas, 1989). These contrasting findings may relate to the differing functions of the arm and lower-limb muscles. The lower limbs are perhaps more continuously used by children, with the muscles more regularly experiencing maximal contractions, than the arms. It may be, therefore, that the development of muscle activation occurs at an earlier age in the lower-limb muscles compared with those of the arm. A further indication of neuromuscular differences between children and adults is the lower ability of children to coordinate their motor activity (Gibbs et al., 1997).

Further neuromuscular variables, including rate of torque development (RTD) and muscle activation have been shown to be lower in children compared with adults, while electromechanical delay (EMD–the delay between neural stimulation and development of muscle tension) and time to reach peak RTD are longer (Cohen et al., 2010; Falk et al., 2009b). The longer EMD is a reflection of lower excitation–contraction coupling, muscle fibre conduction velocity, and muscle-tendon stiffness (Cavanagh & Komi, 1979; Halin et al., 2003) all of which influence the force generated during muscular contraction.

The force measured during a muscular contraction is the net force produced by the simultaneous activation (coactivation) of the muscles on both sides of the joint; these are the agonist and antagonist muscles. A decreased level of coactivation from childhood to adulthood could therefore partially explain the increase in muscular strength with growth. During walking and running the coactivation of the knee muscles has been shown to be higher in children compared with adolescents (Frost et al., 1997). However, further studies using isokinetic dynamometry have failed to find an age difference in the coactivation of the elbow or knee muscles during isokinetic, concentric or eccentric contractions producing flexion or extension of the joint (Bassa et al., 2005; Falk et al., 2009b; Kellis & Unnithan, 1999). The cyclic actions of walking and running, used in everyday life, may stimulate a different pattern of agonist and antagonist muscle activation compared with knee extension and flexion on an isokinetic dynamometer, potentially explaining the equivocal findings.

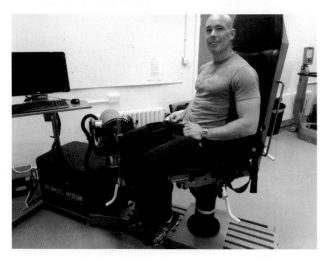

Figure 7.13 An isokinetic dynamometer. (*Source*: Dr Susan Dewhurst)

Key point

Neuromuscular differences between adults and children are partially responsible for the increase in muscular strength with increasing age.

Development of muscular endurance

Muscular endurance refers to the ability of a muscle or muscle group to perform repeated contractions or to maintain a contraction for a predetermined period of time. It is clear that muscular endurance is vital for everyday tasks such as walking, hanging out washing or gardening, and plays a major role in the majority of sports. Repeated contractions are commonly measured in children through field tests involving activities such as sit-ups, push-ups, pull-ups and chin-ups. In general, boys and girls make gradual improvements in most muscle endurance activities during childhood, with boys slightly outperforming girls. A larger gender difference is generally then found during adolescence with males outperforming females in most endurance fitness tests.

Abdominal endurance (as measured by number of bent-knee sit-ups in 60 seconds) during childhood is similar between genders, with a slightly higher endurance in boys starting from 8 years of age. Around the age of 12 years males start to make more significant gains in abdominal endurance and the gender difference becomes exaggerated during adolescence (Figure 7.14). As with strength, larger gender differences occur in the muscular endurance of the upper body.

In activities such as the flexed-arm-hang females consistently perform weakly with a small gradual improvement in endurance during childhood and adolescence. In contrast, the upper-body muscular endurance of males gradually increases up to 10–12 years of age, following which a more rapid increase occurs (Figure 7.15). The absolute level of muscular endurance, as depicted in Figures 7.14 and 7.15, is greater in adults than children; however, when reported relative to body mass, the muscular endurance of children often approaches or exceeds that of adults (Figure 7.16).

Key points

Males outperform females in tests of muscular endurance.

Larger gender differences occur in the muscular strength and endurance of the upper body compared with the lower body.

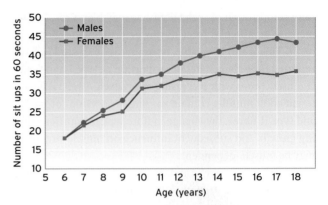

Figure 7.14 Growth changes in abdominal endurance in males and females. (*Source*: Adapted from Thomas et al. (1991))

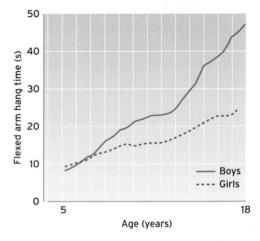

Figure 7.15 The development of upper-body muscular endurance in males and females, 5–18 years.

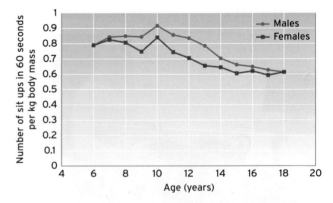

Figure 7.16 Relative muscular endurance during childhood and adolescence. (*Source*: Adapted from Thomas et al. (1991))

The minimal increase in muscular endurance in females during adolescence is likely due to several factors. From the start of puberty, oestrogen levels are elevated which results in an increase in the proportion of fat to body composition.

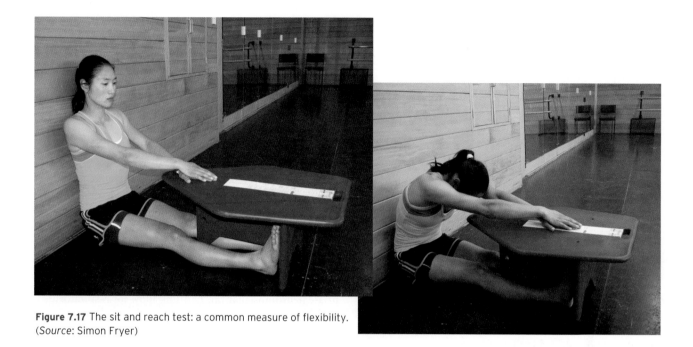

Figure 7.17 The sit and reach test: a common measure of flexibility. (*Source*: Simon Fryer)

This increase in fat, alongside the lower muscle mass in girls, could be responsible for the lower endurance performance compared with boys. Unfortunately, girls tend to be less encouraged than boys to be active, and have been found to adopt a more sedentary lifestyle around puberty. Research indicates that a number of different reasons have been cited for this change including issues such as wanting to avoid sweating and showers, a lack of role models and not liking the traditional sports that are often offered in schools. This reduction in activity levels may coincide with the plateau in their motor abilities.

Flexibility

The importance of flexibility within life, whether it may include elite sports performance or physical activity for health benefits, is now widely recognised and is considered an essential component of physical fitness and performance. The flexibility of an individual relates to the available range of motion at a joint. This is determined by the arrangement of muscles and ligaments, and the articulation of the bones at a joint and is hence joint-specific. When thinking of flexibility, activities commonly thought of are gymnastics, dancing and ice-skating. As often demonstrated in these sports, individuals can bend their bodies to extents that many of us could only dream of replicating. It is clear that a high level of flexibility is required for performing these sports. However, these levels may be

over and above that required for the safe and successful performance of other sports providing that '… the necessary body positions can be comfortably achieved' (Corbin & Noble, 1980). It is important as a sports coach to identify the level of flexibility required in a given sport before deciding on the amount of flexibility training to include within an individual's programme and on which joints the training should focus.

The most common general measure of flexibility in children is that of the hamstrings and lower back. It is measured with the use of the sit-and-reach test developed in 1952 by Wells & Dillon. This test, as illustrated in Figure 7.17, involves sitting on the floor with straight legs, extending the arms and reaching forward along the measuring scale on the sit-and-reach box.

The change in flexibility with growth and development does not follow the same general pattern as that of muscular strength and endurance. Firstly, females consistently demonstrate a greater level of flexibility than males from the age of 5 to 18 years, as measured by the sit-and-reach test. Little improvement in flexibility occurs during childhood in girls, following which an improvement is seen up to 15 years of age with little change thereafter. In contrast, boys become less flexible from 5 through to 12 years of age, following which an improved flexibility is demonstrated through to 18 years of age. This unique pattern of growth for flexibility (using the sit and reach test) is likely due to the changes in leg and trunk lengths that occur during growth. A greater increase in trunk length than lower

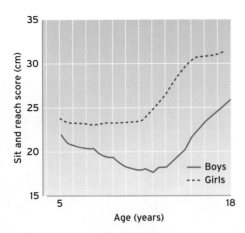

Figure 7.18 The development of flexibility in males and females, 5–18 years.

leg length would be advantageous in this test as a greater reach could be made. The development of flexibility during growth is demonstrated in Figure 7.18.

Knowledge integration question

Explain the problems associated with using the sit-and-reach test as a composite measure of flexibility.

Key points

Females are consistently more flexible than males.

During the growing years, flexibility is affected by the differing rates of leg length and trunk growth.

7.4 Cardiorespiratory development

Life 'in utero' is a completely different environment to the one we know and live in. Surrounded by fluid, the fetus is entirely dependent upon the placenta for gas exchange, nutrition and waste removal. The sudden entrance to our environment, and the loss of placental blood supply at birth, are responsible for major alterations in the cardiovascular and respiratory systems for the newborn as it strives to adjust to extra-uterine life. Growth and development of the cardiorespiratory system continues during childhood and adolescence and is vital for the maintenance of nutrient delivery and waste removal from all cells of the body as an individual grows in mass and stature from newborn to adulthood. Knowledge of the cardiorespiratory system changes during growth helps us to understand the changing responses to exercise as an individual grows.

'In utero'

During fetal life, a miniature cardiovascular system is fully developed by 11 weeks of gestation. The arrangement of the circulatory system is such that the two sides of the heart work in parallel (in contrast to the series arrangement in the adult) and three shunts are present which allow blood to bypass organs with little or no function. For example, only about 10–15% of the fetal circulation passes through the lungs. Fetal lungs are unsuitable for gas exchange as they are filled with amniotic fluid and blood constituents. Despite this, the respiratory centres of the brain and appropriate neuromuscular mechanisms allow for respiratory movements in fetal lungs. The site of fetal gas exchange is the placenta which connects the maternal and fetal circulations via the umbilical vein and arteries. The umbilical vein carries oxygen and nutrients from the mother's circulation to the fetus, whereas the umbilical arteries transport venous blood from the fetus to the placenta for reoxygenation and for the removal of waste products into the maternal circulation.

A simplified plan of the fully developed fetal cardiovascular system is illustrated in Figure 7.19 and the location and function of the three circulatory shunts are described below:

1. *The foramen ovale* A one-way gap between the heart atria allowing blood to pass from the right to the left atrium, reducing the amount of blood going from the right ventricle to the non-functional lungs.

2. *The ductus arteriosus* A direct link between the pulmonary artery and the aorta, again reducing blood flow to the lungs.

3. *The ductus venosus* Permits blood flow from the umbilical vein to the right atrium (via the inferior vena cava), providing the fetus with maternal oxygen and nutrition.

At birth

At birth, the occlusion of the umbilical cord and the initiation of breathing result in many circulatory and respiratory changes and the resultant closure of the three circulatory shunts. As the fetus passes along the birth canal the thorax is compressed, expelling the majority of amniotic fluid

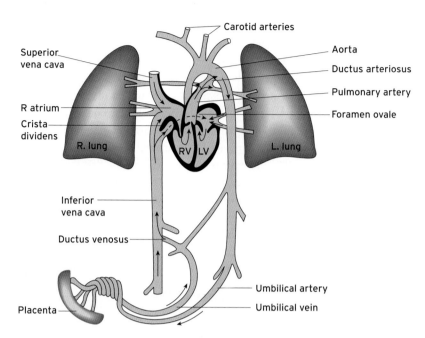

Carotid arteries
Superior vena cava
Aorta
Ductus arteriosus
Pulmonary artery
R atrium
Foramen ovale
Crista dividens
R. lung
L. lung
RV LV
Inferior vena cava
Ductus venosus
Umbilical artery
Umbilical vein
Placenta

Figure 7.19 A simplified illustration of the foetal cardiovascular system.

from the lungs. The expansion of the lungs, as the newborn takes its first breaths, reduces pulmonary vascular resistance and elevates systemic blood pressure, resulting in an increased blood flow through the pulmonary (lung) vessels. Secondly, with the occlusion of the umbilical cord, blood pressure in the left atrium rises above that in the right atrium, responsible for the closure of the foramen ovale. An increase in systemic, and hence aortic, pressure allows blood to flow along the pulmonary artery, with the eventual full closure of the ductus arteriosus. Failure of the foramen ovale and/or the ductus arteriosus to close properly at birth may lead to paediatric heart complications. The ductus venosus is generally closed at birth, with full elimination by around two weeks of age.

Knowledge integration question

What are the differences in gaseous exchange between the fetus (before birth) and the newborn (after birth)?

Postnatal growth and development

Physical cardiovascular changes

Cardiac muscle grows by both **hyperplasia** (increased number of cells) and **hypertrophy** (increased cell size).

During fetal life the left and right sides of the heart have approximately the same volume. Following birth, however, the left ventricle grows more rapidly than the right as the left ventricle has to work harder to pump blood round the high-resistance systemic circuit compared with the lower resistance pulmonary circuit which is supplied by the right ventricle. This results in the progressive hypertrophy of the left ventricle, with the wall reaching adult proportions of two to three times thicker than the right ventricle by around seven years of age. The heart increases in size until maturity, with growth generally following the sigmoid pattern of whole-body growth (refer to Figure 7.1). This relationship is particularly apparent during the adolescent growth spurt, with the ratio of heart volume to body mass remaining relatively constant between the ages of 8 and 18 years (Bouchard et al., 1977). There is very little gender difference in heart size until puberty, after which the male heart is around 15% larger, even when the greater body mass of males is taken into consideration.

Alongside the growth of the heart and the body, blood volume increases by more than tenfold from birth (300-400 mL) to adulthood (~5000 mL), with its expansion following the general pattern of body mass growth. During adolescence, and continuing into adulthood, the mean blood volume of males becomes higher than that of females due to both expanded plasma volume and greater cell content. With the increase in heart size and blood volume, a proportional growth of the blood vessels ensures the continued efficient supply of nutrients to the cells of the body.

Functional changes of the cardiovascular system

In addition to the physical size of the heart, changes in functional characteristics of the heart occur during growth which can be indicated by changes in parameters such as heart rate, stroke volume and cardiac output. Basal, or resting, heart rate (measured when an individual is resting lying down but remains awake) gradually falls from ~140 beats·min^{-1} following birth to ~60 beats·min^{-1} in late adolescence. A gender difference in basal heart rate is not apparent during early childhood; however, by around the age of 10 years basal HR is 3–5 beats·min^{-1} higher in girls. This gender difference continues throughout adolescence with an average basal HR of 57–60 beats·min^{-1} in males and 62–63 beats·min^{-1} in females upon reaching young adulthood.

During growth, the energy requirements of an individual increase and these must be matched by an elevated cardiac output (newborn ~0.5 L·min^{-1}, young adult male ~5 L·min^{-1}). As basal HR falls with growth, the increase in cardiac output is the result of an increase in stroke volume (newborn 3–4 mL, young male adult ~60 mL); remember, cardiac output = SV × HR (refer to section 6.2 Cardiovascular system for more details). As may be expected, the increase in resting SV during childhood is associated with the increase in left ventricular size.

Key points

Increases in heart size follow a similar pattern to whole-body growth. It is similar in males and females during childhood, following which the male heart is ~15% larger.

Resting cardiac output is elevated due to an increased stroke volume during growth.

Physical respiratory changes

Fetal lung development, including formation of the bronchial tree, development of alveoli and the formation of the alveoli-capillary interface (the site of postnatal gas exchange), is generally complete shortly after the 26th fetal week. Following birth, lung tissue grows considerably, almost in proportion to the growth in stature. The small mass of the newborn lungs (60–70 g) increases by approximately twenty-fold before the attainment of maturity. In contrast, the increase in the number of alveoli is complete by around eight years of age with around 20 million in the newborn compared with around 300 million at eight years. The increase in lung size during the first three years of life is primarily due to the increased number of alveoli. Following the growth of the lung tissue, adults are able to inhale much more air per gram of tissue than the newborn (adult 8–10 mL air·g of tissue^{-1}; newborn ~3 mL air·g of tissue^{-1}).

Functional changes of the respiratory system

The breathing frequency, or respiratory rate, of newborns is extremely rapid, around 40 breaths·min^{-1}. This rate gradually falls by around half in the first five to six years of life (~22 breaths·min^{-1}). During childhood and adolescence, a slight fall in breathing frequency occurs with levels stabilising at 16–17 breaths·min^{-1} by young adulthood.

Respiratory volumes and capacities of the growing child increase in proportion to the increase in stature, independent of gender. This indicates that, in conjunction with the increase in lung mass during growth, there is an increase in the total volume of the lungs. The total volume of air that can be utilised during breathing (vital capacity), and the speed at which the air can be expelled from the lungs following full inspiration (FEV$_1$) are also enhanced during growth. From around the age of 13 years and 15 years, in girls and boys respectively, the rate at which lung function develops falls and plateaus in young adulthood in both genders (Hibbert et al., 1995).

Key points

Lung growth is almost in proportion to the growth in stature.

Breathing rate falls while respiratory volumes and capacities increase during growth.

Development of cardiorespiratory responses to submaximal exercise

The transport of oxygen from the ambient air to the active muscle cells by the pulmonary and cardiac systems, at a specific exercise-intensity-dependent rate, is crucial during aerobic exercise. The growth of the heart and the lungs, alongside elevated blood volume, haemoglobin concentration, and stroke volume, may therefore result in differing cardiorespiratory responses to submaximal exercise between children and adults. Increases in breathing rate and tidal volume, and heart rate and stroke volume, are synchronous in ensuring a greater delivery of oxygen to the muscles. These responses to the onset of exercise occur in all individuals, independent of age, but what adaptations occur in the exercise response during the growing years?

The cardiorespiratory response to an acute exercise bout is not only dependent upon the intensity and duration of exercise, but also on developmental stage. At the same absolute exercise intensity (e.g. cycling at 30 watts (W) or running at $12 \, km \cdot h^{-1}$), heart rate and breathing rate during steady-state sub-maximal exercise fall during growth. Despite this maturational change in sub-maximal heart rate, oxygen consumption and cardiac output are relatively unaffected by age, hence an elevated SV, accompanying heart growth, is likely to be responsible for the fall in HR. The majority of cardiovascular responses to exercise are similar between boys and girls. A gender difference is apparent, however, in sub-maximal exercise HR, with girls exhibiting higher heart rates than boys, likely due to their smaller heart and lower SV. A further difference between children and adults is that, at the same level of $\dot{V}O_2$, children are able to extract more oxygen from the blood than adults, that is, they have a higher arteriovenous difference in oxygen content (a-vO_2 difference). The timing of the attainment of the adult pattern of cardiovascular responses to exercise remains to be determined.

Key points

During submaximal exercise of the same absolute intensity, cardiac output is unaffected during growth hence the increase in SV (accompanying increase in heart size) is accompanied by a fall in HR.

Girls' HR is higher than boys due to a smaller heart and lower SV.

At the same absolute exercise intensity, absolute tidal volume (V_T) and minute ventilation ($\dot{V}_E$) increase with growth, whereas relative V_T (per kg body mass) remains constant, and, due to the lower breathing rate, relative $\dot{V}_E$ also drops. During exercise of the same relative intensity, absolute $\dot{V}_E$ increases in males but remains stable in females while breathing rate falls and tidal volume increases in both males and females. Children demonstrate a lower ventilatory efficiency compared to adolescents, as reflected by a higher ventilatory equivalent for oxygen ($\dot{V}_E/VO_2$), indicative of an improved ventilatory control with growth. This lower ventilatory efficiency in children is likely due to the fact that they have more rapid, shallow breathing than adults, resulting in lower alveolar ventilation.

Key point

Ventilatory control is improved with growth.

7.5 Anaerobic and aerobic fitness and training

As discussed in the previous sections, many physical and functional changes of the body occur during growth and development, hence it is not surprising that the performances of children in anaerobic and aerobic activities, and their adaptations to training, differ to those of the adult. Although the energy systems are touched on in the following discussion, full information on anaerobic and aerobic metabolism, and the utilisation of the different systems in a wide variety of sports, is found in section two of this book (Chapters 8–13).

Anaerobic fitness

Habitual physical activity in children is highly dominated by short bursts of vigorous activity, hence children are heavily reliant on anaerobic metabolism for their energy supply. In addition, children involved in organised sport are commonly drawn to those involving an anaerobic component. Intermittent sports, such as soccer, rugby football, basketball, netball, field hockey and ice hockey, involve low-intensity periods interspersed with short bouts of high-intensity, sometimes maximal, efforts. It is clear that activity during everyday life and organised sport in children is highly dependent on anaerobic glycolysis. Knowledge on how anaerobic capacity changes during growth, taking gender differences into consideration, is therefore important when planning activities or training sessions for children or adolescents.

Maturation of anaerobic fitness

In the field, the change in anaerobic fitness from child-hood to young adulthood is commonly monitored with jump (squat jump, vertical jump, standing horizontal jump) or sprint (30–50 metres) tests. The anaerobic performance of children improves with age in both males and females. In general, from the age of 10 years, males outperform females with the gender difference increasing during adolescence. In females, no further improvement in 50-yard sprint time is found from around 14 years of age; however, the increase in performance in males is still evident at 18 years. A similar finding is found for the 30-yard sprint, as shown in Figure 7.20.

Due to the ease of application and low cost, field tests are used for the determination of anaerobic fitness in large research studies. Peak and mean power outputs, as determined in field tests, show significant correlation with results from laboratory tests (Davies & Young, 1984; Dore et al., 2008; Van Praagh et al., 1990).

The most common measures of anaerobic fitness as measured in the laboratory are peak power output (PPO), mean power output (MPO) and fatigue resistance (FR). These variables are generally identified using a *maximal* test involving cycle ergometry or isokinetic dynamometry. However, running and jumping protocols have also been utilised. To obtain accurate power results, the subject must perform maximally for the full duration of the test. A

popular test of anaerobic fitness in children is a 30-second maximal cycling test known as the Wingate Anaerobic Test (WAnT). For full details on the WAnT refer to Chapter 10, section 10.2. Irrespective of the protocol used, peak power is normally elicited within the first 5 seconds of exercise, whereas the mean anaerobic power is calculated as the total work done divided by the total time. Fatigue resistance, a measure of buffering capacity, is generally calculated as the percentage decline in peak power, peak torque or total work, following repeated bouts of maximal exercise. This variable is in contrast to the fatigue index (FI), calculated as the decline in power output during a single bout of maximal exercise, which is discussed as a gauge of anaerobic capacity in Chapter 10. For a review of both field and laboratory tests of anaerobic performance refer to Van Praagh & Doré (2002).

Peak and mean power outputs

As would be expected due to the increase in body size and muscle mass with age, absolute peak and mean power outputs are enhanced during growth (Armstrong et al., 2000, 2001; Bar-Or, 1983; Dore et al., 2005; Martin et al., 2004; McNarry et al., 2011; Ratel et al., 2004). During the childhood years, little gender difference in absolute PPO and MPO exists whereas, from around 14 years of age, the effects of the enhanced musculature of males becomes apparent and a large gender difference is found by the end of adolescence (Blimkie et al., 1988; Dipla et al., 2009; Doré et al., 2005; Martin et al., 2004). This gender difference is demonstrated for cycling peak power in Figure 7.21.

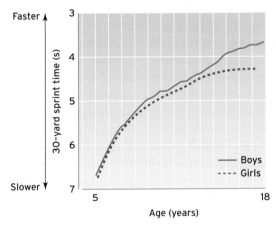

Figure 7.20 Mean 30-yard sprint time from a running start during the growth of males and females.

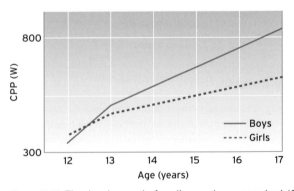

Figure 7.21 The development of cycling peak power output (CPP) in males and females. (*Source*: drawn from data in Table 1 of Armstrong et al. (2001) *British Journal of Sports Medicine* 35: 118-24)

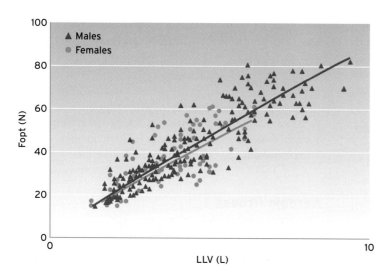

Figure 7.22 The force (Fopt) at peak power relative to lean leg volume (LLV) in males and females. (*Source:* Adapted from Martin et al. (2004))

The increase in physical size and muscle mass with growth, however, is not solely responsible for the improved PPO and MPO, as when normalised for body weight (Bar-Or, 1983; Duché et al., 1992; Falgairette et al., 1991; Saavedra et al., 1991), lean body mass (Mercier et al., 1992; Saavedra et al., 1991) or lean leg volume (Doré et al., 2005; Martin et al., 2004; Ratel et al., 2004; Van Praagh et al., 1990), anaerobic fitness continues to improve with age, particularly in males (Figure 7.22).

> **Key points**
>
> Tests of anaerobic fitness:
>
> ➤ Field – jump and sprint tests
> ➤ Laboratory – cycle ergometer or isokinetic dynamometer tests
>
> Anaerobic performance improves during growth. From around 14 years old, males have a greater anaerobic fitness than females.

Fatigue resistance and recovery

As mentioned at the start of this section, a wide variety of sports are of an intermittent nature, involving short, sporadic bouts of high-intensity activity. It is clear that the ability to resist fatigue during these bouts of activity, and to recover rapidly following them, is essential for optimal sports performance. The rates of fatigue and recovery are related to biological maturation (De Ste Croix et al., 2009; Dipla et al., 2009; Ratel et al., 2004, 2006) and are important aspects of neuromuscular function. The effect of growth on fatigue and recovery rates provides important information on the capacities of the energy systems.

The ability to resist fatigue falls from childhood to adulthood. This helps to explain why children have the ability to run around sporadically for long periods of time and we, as adults, struggle to keep up! While the reduction in fatigue resistance continues from childhood through adolescence to adulthood in males, the adult fatigue resistance profile is reached by mid puberty in females (Dipla et al., 2009). The fall in fatigue resistance during growth is related to the enhanced anaerobic capacity of the muscle, as demonstrated by increased muscle power and blood lactate concentration immediately following exercise (Dipla et al., 2009). Accompanying their greater resistance to fatigue is the ability of children to recover faster following anaerobic activity compared to adolescents and adults (Ratel et al., 2002). This is due to the higher muscle oxidative activity of children compared to adults which enhances the rate of creatine phosphate regeneration and allows the faster re-establishment of peak muscle power.

> **Key points**
>
> Children have a greater resistance to fatigue and recover faster from anaerobic activity compared to adolescents and adults.

Determinants of anaerobic fitness

Factors that may play a role in the increasing anaerobic fitness during childhood and adolescence include muscle structure, muscle metabolism, fatigue resistance, hormonal and neuromuscular factors. As type IIx fibres are the fast-contracting, glycolytic fibres, an increase in the number (Kotzamanidou et al., 2005) and size (Van Praagh & Doré, 2002) of type IIx fibres during male growth may contribute to the age and gender difference in power output during adolescence. Additionally, the neural activation of type II motor units may not be optimal in children compared with adolescents and adults (Halin et al., 2003).

An improved glycolytic function during growth is at least partly responsible for the corresponding enhancement of anaerobic performance. Increased exercise blood lactate levels and enzyme activity, and a lowered relative anaerobic threshold with increasing age, are all indicative of an improved anaerobic capacity. Originally, muscle biopsies were required to directly analyse muscle metabolites and distinguish differences in energy metabolism. However, these studies were sparse due to the invasive nature of the technique. For many years, therefore, blood lactate concentration has been used regularly as an indicator of muscle glycolysis. Blood lactate levels following anaerobic exercise gradually increase during the growth period, supportive of an improved glycolytic function with growth. Consideration, however, must be given to the fact that blood lactate concentration is a reflection of the balance between its production and removal, although the limited biopsy information available suggests the blood level reflects the changes at the muscle level (Eriksson et al., 1973). It is commonly reported that a reduced glycolytic capacity in children during high-intensity exercise is partly due to a lower activity of enzymes involved in the glycolytic pathway. Indeed, the available data from limited muscle biopsy studies suggests a lower enzyme activity in children both at rest (Eriksson et al., 1973) and during intense exercise (Berg & Keul, 1988).

The advent of nuclear magnetic resonance spectroscopy (NMRS) now provides a safe, non-invasive means of monitoring muscle metabolism, which has supported the data showing that there are metabolic changes across maturation with children having a lower glycolytic capacity than adults (Zanconato et al., 1993; Kuno et al., 1995). During intense exercise, the use of NMRS has reported a smaller reduction in the intramuscular pH of children and adolescents compared with adults, consistent with the findings of lower muscle and blood lactate concentrations in children compared with adults following high-intensity exercise.

The improvement in anaerobic function during growth has also been suggested to be due to hormonal changes, such as increases in IGF-1 and testosterone during puberty. Additionally, it has been suggested that high-intensity exercise may induce a lower sympathetic response, and hence lower adrenaline level, in adolescents compared with adults. As a potential stimulator of glycolysis (refer to Chapter 10), a greater adrenaline level in adults may be partly responsible for the improvement in anaerobic function during growth. Finally, neuromuscular changes such

as improved motor coordination may be involved in the development of anaerobic fitness (Van Praagh, 2000).

Key point

The improved anaerobic performance with growth is related to improved glycolytic function: greater activity of glycolytic enzymes, increased lactate concentration, decreased intramuscular pH, increased adrenaline.

Aerobic fitness

The energy required for prolonged, endurance-type activities is predominantly supplied by aerobic metabolism or oxidative phosphorylation, involving three distinct steps: macronutrient-specific pathway, the Krebs cycle and the electron transport chain (ETC). For more detail on the steps involved in aerobic metabolism, and information regarding sports which primarily utilise this energy system, refer to Chapters 11 and 12. As the efficient delivery of oxygen to the active muscles is crucial during aerobic exercise, the cardiorespiratory system plays a vital role.

Although the play pattern of children, and that of many childhood sports, was described previously as being heavily reliant on the anaerobic system, the low-intensity recovery periods, in addition to general everyday activities such as walking, are fuelled primarily by aerobic metabolism. Also, children often participate in school sports, such as cross-country running, or even specialise in prolonged endurance activities (e.g. marathon running) at an early age. Aerobic fitness, often referred to as cardio-respiratory fitness, is regarded as a general marker of health with low levels in children associated with increased cardiovascular disease risk (Anderssen et al., 2007; Eiberg et al., 2005; Eisenmann et al., 2005; Janz et al., 2002). Unfortunately, children are now less physically active, have a greater percentage body fat and lower cardio-respiratory endurance compared with those of 25 years ago (Sziva et al., 2009). As yet, however, there is no convincing evidence that this fall in cardio-respiratory endurance translates to a fall in $\dot{V}O_{2peak}$ (Armstrong et al., 2011). Measures of aerobic fitness during childhood tend to predict aerobic fitness during puberty (Janz & Mahoney, 1997). The role of aerobic metabolism and the importance of aerobic fitness during growth are therefore clear.

Maturation of aerobic fitness

Maximal aerobic power ($\dot{V}O_{2max}$) is the highest rate at which the body can utilise oxygen for energy production, and is accepted as the best single indicator of aerobic fitness of children and adolescents. In adults, $\dot{V}O_{2max}$ is associated with a plateau in oxygen uptake despite an increase in exercise intensity. This levelling-off of $\dot{V}O_2$, however, is often not observed in children and adolescents during a maximal test, despite them exhibiting a similar $\dot{V}O_2$, HR, RER or post-exercise blood lactate concentration to those that experienced a $\dot{V}O_2$ plateau. For this reason, $\dot{V}O_{2max}$ is commonly reported as peak oxygen uptake ($\dot{V}O_{2peak}$) in the paediatric years, and will thus be referred to as such in the current section.

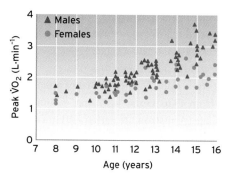

Figure 7.23 Peak oxygen uptake during childhood and adolescence. (*Source*: Adapted from Armstrong & McManus (2010))

Knowledge integration question

What reasons might be behind the common absence of a plateau in $\dot{V}O_2$ observed during maximal aerobic power tests for children?

Aerobic fitness can be measured in the field or in the laboratory, and involves a progressive exercise test to voluntary exhaustion. Field tests of aerobic fitness are indirect estimations of $\dot{V}O_{2peak}$ as gas analysis is not conducted and some form of prediction equation is involved. A commonly used field test for the indirect estimation of $\dot{V}O_{2peak}$ is the 20-metre Multistage Shuttle Run Test (Bleep or Beep test) (Léger et al., 1988) which involves 1-minute stages of continuous, incremental 20-metre shuttle running. Used in many fitness batteries worldwide, the test is easily administered, requires minimal equipment, and is relatively low-cost, enabling the simultaneous testing of large numbers in a school setting. Although suitable for estimating group $\dot{V}O_{2peak}$, the accuracy of its use for individual $\dot{V}O_{2peak}$ predictions in children (Melo et al., 2011) and adolescents (Ruiz et al., 2009) remains questionable. In contrast to field tests, $\dot{V}O_{2peak}$ can be directly measured in the laboratory with online gas analysis using cycle ergometry, treadmill or rowing ergometry protocols.

It is generally accepted that aerobic fitness increases with age and is greater in males than females, with the gender difference progressively increasing during puberty (Armstrong et al., 2011). From the age of 8 to 16 years, $\dot{V}O_{2peak}$ is enhanced in boys and girls by 150% and 80%, respectively. These changes during growth are well illustrated in Figure 7.23. From the age of 12 years, female aerobic fitness plateaus whereas that of males continues to rise, hence the magnification of gender difference during adolescence. A longitudinal study found a 70% increase in boys' $\dot{V}O_{2peak}$ from 12 to 17 years of age. This improvement in aerobic fitness was lower than that of anaerobic

markers (PPO 121%, MPO 113%) indicating that anaerobic metabolism increases to a greater extent than aerobic metabolism during growth (Armstrong et al., 2001).

It has been suggested that a range of 40–60% of the variation in maximal aerobic power is due to genetic factors (Bouchard et al., 1986). The remaining variation could relate to a wide variety of factors including body size, body composition, cardiovascular system growth and function, lung growth and function, habitual physical activity levels, or neuromuscular factors which, alongside $\dot{V}O_{2peak}$, also change during the growth period.

Key points

The best indicator of aerobic fitness in children is $\dot{V}O_{2peak}$ – can be indirectly estimated in the field (Multistage Shuttle Run Test) or directly measured in the laboratory.

Aerobic fitness increases with age. Boys demonstrate a higher $\dot{V}O_{2peak}$ than girls with the gender difference increasing during puberty.

In addition to $\dot{V}O_{2peak}$, running endurance, as a marker of aerobic fitness, has been shown to improve from 7 to 11 years of age, although, due to changes in lifestyle, running endurance has fallen over the last 25 years (Sziva et al., 2009). This confirms that the roles of physical educators and sports coaches in the promotion of physical activity and organised sport participation are vital in the attempt to improve the health and fitness of children, our future adults.

Body mass and composition

During childhood and adolescence, peak oxygen uptake is highly correlated with body size and hence, to determine the independent effects of a variety of variables, $\dot{V}O_{2peak}$ is often reported relative to body mass ($mL \cdot kg^{-1}min^{-1}$). When expressed as a relative value, $\dot{V}O_{2peak}$ remains fairly stable from childhood through to adolescence in males ($48–50\ mL \cdot kg^{-1} \cdot min^{-1}$), whereas that of females progressively falls from 45 to 35 $mL \cdot kg^{-1} \cdot min^{-1}$ from 8 to 16 years of age (Armstrong & Barker, 2011; Krahenbuhl et al., 1985; Mota et al., 2002). This gender difference is likely due to the fact that body mass is inclusive of fat mass and body composition differences exist between boys and girls. The greater muscle mass of males, and greater fat mass of females suggest that $\dot{V}O_{2peak}$ values should be reported relative to a measure reflecting muscle mass, such as lean body mass or leg volume. Indeed, lean body mass has been found to be a major predictor of aerobic fitness in childhood and adolescence (Armstrong & Welsman, 2001; Dencker et al., 2007). Supporting these findings, relative $\dot{V}O_{2peak}$ has been found to be inversely associated with percentage body fat (Mota et al., 2002) and BMI (Butterfield et al., 2008) in children and adolescents. Despite these links with aerobic fitness, body composition does not fully account for the gender differences in $\dot{V}O_{2peak}$, suggesting additional factors are involved in the development of $\dot{V}O_{2peak}$.

It is currently recognised that reporting $\dot{V}O_{2peak}$ relative to body mass in the attempt to remove the influence of body size is not an appropriate method. With the use of more complex scaling (allometric scaling), Welsman et al. (1996) reported a progressive increase in $\dot{V}O_{2peak}$ from childhood to adulthood in males, whereas females' $\dot{V}O_{2peak}$ increased from childhood to adolescence following which it remained stable. From late childhood $\dot{V}O_{2peak}$ is consistently higher in males than females, with the gender difference becoming more distinct during adolescence. The best method of scaling for $\dot{V}O_{2peak}$, to optimise our understanding of $\dot{V}O_{2peak}$ changes with growth and maturation, remains equivocal.

Cardiovascular system growth and function

Growth and development of the cardiovascular system during childhood and adolescence is vital for maintaining the delivery of oxygen to the increasing muscle mass of the growing body. Improvement in the delivery of oxygen to the muscle cells by the cardiorespiratory system, rather than enhanced utilisation of oxygen by the muscle cells, is responsible for the increase in $\dot{V}O_{2peak}$.

Heart rate

Peak HR, as determined during a $\dot{V}O_{2peak}$ test, remains constant throughout childhood and adolescence (195–205 bpm), with no difference between males and females. This indicates that the improved aerobic fitness during maturation is not a result of improved oxygen delivery to the muscles via an increased heart rate. It is important to recognise at this stage, that due to its stability across the growing years, equations commonly used in the prediction of adult HR_{peak} (for example, 220 minus age) are not appropriate for children or adolescents.

Cardiac output and stroke volume

The cardiac output, the volume of blood pumped round the body in a set time ($L \cdot min^{-1}$), represents the functional capacity of the circulatory system. The increased size of the heart during growth allows for a greater maximal cardiac output which follows a similar pattern of development to $\dot{V}O_{2peak}$. As HR_{peak} remains stable during the growing years an enhanced maximal stroke volume allows for the elevation in maximal cardiac output. The greater heart size (and hence stroke volume and cardiac output capacities) with growth is a predictor of aerobic fitness in children and adolescents, with a more powerful prediction apparent in males (Dencker et al., 2007; Janz & Mahoney, 1997).

Blood characteristics

The increases in blood volume and haemoglobin concentration during growth are closely related to body mass growth, with higher levels found in males. As the transport mechanisms of oxygen from the lungs to the muscle cells, blood volume and haemoglobin concentration have the potential to play a major role in aerobic fitness. Gender differences in haemoglobin concentration start to emerge at puberty with males having higher levels than girls, therefore, it is possible that aerobic performance may also be influenced by haemoglobin concentration from the start of adolescence.

The lack of change in relative $\dot{V}O_{2peak}$ during growth suggests blood volume and haemoglobin concentration play no role in the maturation of aerobic fitness. The lack of relationship between aerobic fitness and blood characteristics with age may be due to the observation that children and adolescents have a greater ability to unload oxygen at the muscle tissue than adults (Armstrong & Welsman, 2000).

Lung growth and function

The increase in lung size with growth, along with the improved respiratory volumes and capacities, may play a positive role in aerobic fitness as the first link in the transport of oxygen from the environment to the muscle cells. Maximal breathing rate can reach as high as 60 breaths·min^{-1} in children compared with 30–40 breaths·min^{-1} in adults. Despite this, lung function (FEV$_1$ and vital capacity) has no relation to $\dot{V}O_{2peak}$ (Dencker et al., 2007), hence it appears that the respiratory system is able to present the blood with a more than adequate supply of oxygen during maximal exercise. The aerobic fitness of healthy children and adolescents is not limited by $\dot{V}_E$ (Armstrong & Welsman, 2007).

Habitual physical activity

From around the age of six years, boys are generally more active than girls. It is possible that these gender differences in energy expenditure may translate into similar differences in aerobic fitness. Due to the sporadic nature of physical activity in children, however, a link between habitual physical activity and $\dot{V}O_{2peak}$ may not be expected. The measure of physical activity found to be most closely related to $\dot{V}O_{2peak}$ is time spent in vigorous activity. However, a subsequent study showed only a modest relationship between daily vigorous activity duration and $\dot{V}O_{2peak}$ (Dencker et al., 2006, 2007). This finding is not surprising as the physical activity patterns of children reveal that the intensity and duration of physical activity required to improve $\dot{V}O_{2peak}$ are rarely experienced, hence maturation of aerobic fitness alongside gender differences are unlikely to be attributable to differences in habitual physical activity. A recent meta-analysis concluded that there is no meaningful relationship between aerobic fitness and habitual physical activity (Armstrong et al., 2011).

Neuromuscular factors

Increasing $\dot{V}O_{2peak}$ with age is likely related to neuromuscular factors. The improvement of motor skills and coordination will allow the growing child to develop more economical and efficient exercise patterns, reducing some potential limitations of $\dot{V}O_{2peak}$.

Key point

Improved $\dot{V}O_{2peak}$ with growth is related to increased body size, increased heart size (SV and cardiac output) and improved motor skills and coordination.

Aerobic fitness and endurance performance

A high $\dot{V}O_{2peak}$ is a prerequisite of elite performance in many sports, hence an improvement in aerobic fitness is commonly assumed to be reflected in an improved endurance performance. Remember, however, that although absolute $\dot{V}O_{2peak}$ improves with age, when expressed relative to body mass or LBM, little change is seen in $\dot{V}O_{2peak}$ in males and a gradual decline occurs in females. Despite this, endurance performance improves greatly during growth. Several methods of determining endurance performance are commonly used in children, the most common being the time taken to run/bike/swim etc. a specified distance. This endurance model simulates the reality of athletic events such as track or cross-country races, cycle racing, swimming competitions, to name but a few. Two further popular protocols for the measurement of endurance performance are the distance completed in a set time (e.g. 9 or 12 minutes) and the time to exhaustion during exercise of an increasing intensity. Independent of the method used, endurance performance is greatly improved during childhood with males consistently outperforming females. An improved endurance occurs in males throughout adolescence, whereas performance deteriorates in females from around the age of 13 years. It is clear that $\dot{V}O_{2peak}$ is not the best predictor of a child's endurance performance. This, therefore, raises the question – what factors are responsible for the improved endurance performance during the growing years?

Key point

Even in the absence of an improvement in relative $\dot{V}O_{2peak}$, endurance performance is improved during childhood.

Exercise economy

The improved submaximal exercise economy (lower $\dot{V}O_2$ per kg body mass) during growth, and hence diminished relative exercise intensity, plays an important role in the improved endurance performance. The enhanced exercise economy in older children would, therefore, be expected to translate to performing at a faster speed, or at the same speed for a longer duration.

Blood lactate accumulation

Lactate is a by-product of fast-rate glycolysis, which diffuses from the muscle into the blood and can be used as an indicator of aerobic fitness. Three reference values are

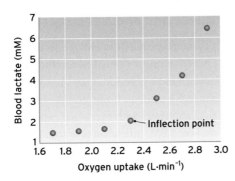

Figure 7.24 Blood lactate increases during incremental exercise in relation to oxygen uptake. (*Source*: Adapted from Armstrong & Welsman (2007))

commonly used as indicators of aerobic fitness: the lactate threshold (LT), the ventilatory or anaerobic threshold (AT) and the maximal lactate steady state (MLSS). The first observable increase in blood lactate concentration during a progressive, incremental exercise test is the LT which is widely accepted as a predictor of endurance performance in adults. The change in lactate with increasing exercise intensity is demonstrated in Figure 7.24, where a clear inflection of lactate can be seen at an oxygen uptake of 2.3 L·min^{-1}. The AT occurs at a similar timepoint to the LT during incremental exercise, and is hence often used as a non-invasive alternative to the LT. At the AT the volume of carbon dioxide production ($\dot{V}CO_2$) increases relatively faster than the rise in oxygen consumption ($\dot{V}O_2$) which is observed as an inflection in $\dot{V}_E$ (refer to Chapter 10, 'Fatigue in anaerobic endurance sports', for further details). The MLSS is the highest exercise intensity that can be sustained with no concurrent accumulation of blood lactate.

Blood lactate accumulates to a lower level in children than adults, during both submaximal and maximal exercise, reflective of their lower glycolytic capacity. LT reported as a percentage of $\dot{V}O_{2peak}$ is well-established as a measure of aerobic fitness and endurance performance and, alongside AT, occurs at a higher relative exercise intensity in children compared with adults. Consequently, the MLSS in children tends to occur at a higher percentage of $\dot{V}O_{2peak}$, but lower absolute lactate concentration, than adults, although a recent study indicates that MLSS is independent of age (Beneke et al., 2009). LT and MLSS are common tools used for designing and monitoring training programmes, but individual responses must be determined due to the large variation reported between individuals. Comparison of the literature on the accumulation of lactate in children should be made with the consideration that the determination of LT differs between studies. Some define the LT as a fixed blood lactate concentration (2, 2.5 or

4 mmol·L^{-1}) whereas others use the inflection point of the LT curve (see Figure 7.24).

$\dot{V}O_2$ kinetics as a component of aerobic fitness

The commencement of aerobic exercise initiates an increase in $\dot{V}O_2$ as the elevated muscle contraction is primarily dependent on the aerobic generation of energy. Aerobic metabolism, however, is comparatively slow to adapt to the demands of exercise hence the initial supply of energy is from the muscles' ATP stores and the anaerobic regeneration of ATP via the phosphocreatine (PCr) and glycolytic pathways. The rate at which $\dot{V}O_2$ increases, therefore, is important to minimise the breakdown of PCr and anaerobic glycolysis within the muscle.

There are three phases in the oxygen uptake kinetics with the exponential second phase, referred to as the primary component, being the time during which $\dot{V}O_2$ is elevated to the steady-state value due to the increased oxygen consumption of the muscles. Prior to obtaining steady state $\dot{V}O_2$, aerobic metabolism does not fully meet the energy requirements of the muscle, hence anaerobic pathways are utilised. During moderate (below LT) and heavy (between LT and MLSS) intensity exercise, children exhibit a faster increase in $\dot{V}O_2$ to reach steady state (primary time constant) compared to adults, indicative of a smaller oxygen deficit which is thought to be due to a greater mitochondrial capacity for aerobic metabolism (Armstrong et al., 2011; Armstrong & Welsman, 2007). A gender difference exists in the $\dot{V}O_2$ kinetics of heavy exercise, with a faster response in boys. As multiple changes in exercise intensity, and hence $\dot{V}O_2$, occur during children's play and sporting activities, $\dot{V}O_2$ kinetics are important in terms of limiting anaerobic metabolism.

Physical training and growth
Controversies and concerns

As discussed in the previous sections of this chapter, children are not merely miniature adults. Their physical size, body composition, and physiological responses to exercise are all influenced by growth. Due to these differences it is not surprising that much controversy surrounds the appropriateness of the involvement of the growing child in physical training programmes. Many Olympic sporting bodies have selection processes that attempt to identify potential in children for an elite future in the sport. This can lead to early specialisation in sport with the initiation of specific, intensive training. There are several drawbacks of this early focus on a single sport. Participation in a wide variety of activities, which is important for the development of a wide range of motor skills, is lost. Due to the volume and repetitiveness of specific training, injury risk is higher during a period when the tissues are still growing. Premature drop-out may occur due to psychological burnout or, when reached, it may be identified that the adult physique is inappropriate for the sport in which they specialised as a child.

Concerns regarding the suitability and safety of high-level training in children and adolescents have therefore been raised. What effect does this type of training have on the growth and development of the body at this critical time in life? Is there potential to affect the timing of maturation, or could the rate of growth be negatively influenced?

Growth and reproductive health

It has been found that, for the majority of sports, participation does not appear to negatively influence pubertal timing or linear growth rate (Baxter-Jones et al., 2003; Roemmich et al., 2001), although some controversy still remains (Caine et al., 2001). Problems may occur in sports where weight control is essential for performance, such as gymnastics and wrestling. In addition to the intensive training, these athletes have the added burden of a negative energy balance, that is, an energy expenditure exceeding the intake. If under-nutrition is substantial, and is combined with heavy training, growth may be suppressed and puberty delayed. In this situation, the delayed activity of oestrogen in girls can result in the permanent under-mineralisation of the skeleton, potentially causing problems throughout life. This situation, however, is a rare occurrence in young athletes. Delayed menarche can occur in female athletes, particularly those participating in sports such as gymnastics, dancing and swimming. This has been found to be partially due to genetic factors; however, it is likely that intensive training is also involved.

The under-nutrition and menstrual dysfunction encountered by some female athletes may lead to premature osteoporosis, with these three conditions forming what is known as the 'female athlete triad' (see Chapter 11, 'The female athlete triad', for further details). The majority of research on the female athlete triad is on young adults, with few studies on adolescents. Although the literature is sparse, considerable numbers of female high school athletes show signs of disordered eating, menstrual dysfunction and low bone mass (Hoch et al., 2009; Nichols et al., 2006). As this time of life is the main period of growth, when bone increases greatly in length and strength, the existence of the female athlete triad in these adolescent girls is of great concern.

Key point

Early specialisation in sport is unlikely to delay the onset of puberty or impair the rate of height increase.

Sports involving weight control – under-nutrition combined with heavy training may suppress growth and delay menarche; it can also lead to premature osteoporosis.

Strength training

The suitability of strength training during childhood and adolescence has been questioned in the past. The concern was that the excessive forces placed on the bones might cause harm to the epiphyseal plates, the regions of bone growth. A 14-week resistance training programme, however, was found to cause no damage to epiphyses, bone or muscle, indicating that supervised strength training is safe and effective in pre-pubertal boys (Weltman et al., 1986). Following consideration of the available literature, it has been agreed by several North American organisations (Canadian Society for Exercise Physiology, American Academy of Paediatrics, American College of Sports Medicine, National Strength and Conditioning Association) that strength training is safe and can be beneficial for pre-pubescent children, so long as their training is individualised, monitored and supervised by qualified personnel, takes place using suitable training equipment and lifts are performed with the correct techniques at all times. In contrast to the concerns raised, an increase in muscular strength via resistance training may help to stabilise the growing skeleton and reduce the likelihood of injuries. In situations where resistance training is strictly supervised and proper techniques are used fewer injuries occur compared to during other sports or general play at school. Using exercise equipment at home, however, in an unsupervised setting can lead to an increased risk of injury in children and adolescents. Despite strength training being deemed safe during growth, participation in power lifting, body building and maximal lifts is not recommended until physical and skeletal maturity is reached.

Knowledge integration question

Why can training with weights offer a safe alternative to bodyweight exercises?

Although deemed effective and safe, does resistance training transfer to an improved athletic performance? A very recent meta-analysis has demonstrated just that; the motor performance of children and adolescents is enhanced by resistance training, with younger children and non-athletes demonstrating greater gains (Behringer et al., 2011).

Key point

Strength training is deemed safe for pre-pubertal children provided that:

➤ Sessions are individualised, monitored and supervised

➤ Suitable equipment is used

➤ Correct techniques are learnt and used at all times

Extreme endurance training – marathon running

To carry out research in children into the physiological effects of training for, and participating in, marathons is unethical, hence there is no literature to support, or refute, the safety of such activities. The risk of injury is directly related to the amount of time spent running, therefore, considering the hours spent training for and competing in marathons, combined with the physical changes occurring during growth, the risk of injury is likely to be high in children and adolescents. There are, however, obvious benefits of endurance training such as the reduced risk of cardiovascular disease. In the absence of scientific literature, it has been suggested that children should not be actively encouraged to participate in marathon running, and whether event organisers should allow children to compete is still an area of controversy.

Response to anaerobic training

Muscle strength, power and speed play critical roles in a wide variety of sports, hence, due to the early specialisation in sport, high-intensity and resistance training are common components of child and adolescent training programmes. So how effective are these methods of training in children and adolescents and what physiological mechanisms are involved?

Resistance training

Muscular strength, as tested in both the field and the laboratory, is enhanced in pre-pubertal children through appropriate resistance training, over and above that expected due to growth and development. The magnitude of strength increase is related to the volume of training, involving the combination of intensity, frequency and duration of sessions (Bencke et al., 2002; Faigenbaum

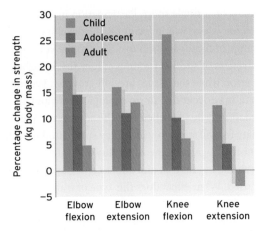

Figure 7.25 Trainability of relative muscular strength during childhood, adolescence and adulthood. (*Source*: Adapted from Gom Van Praagh (ed.) (1998))

et al., 2009; Ratel, 2011). Despite the lack of muscle hypertrophy prior to puberty, relative strength gains (% change above initial level) during childhood are similar to, or greater than, those found during adolescence and adulthood although, as expected, absolute strength gains are smaller in children (Blimkie, 1992; Falk & Tenenbaum, 1996; Lillegard et al., 1997; Pfeiffer & Francis, 1986; Ratel, 2011). It is currently believed that the effectiveness of strength training is similar in boys and girls during childhood, although little research has addressed this topic. The trainability of relative muscular strength in children, adolescents and adults is illustrated in Figure 7.25.

In general, a resistance programme for children lasting 8–20 weeks will enhance relative muscular strength by 10–40%, although an increase of as much as 74% following an eight-week resistance programme has been reported (Faigenbaum et al., 2009). Similar to adults, the effectiveness of strength training in children appears to be primarily dependent on a sufficient training intensity and volume, although the optimal training volume remains to be determined. In children, a high-repetition, moderate load resistance training programme appears to elicit greater muscular strength gains in children than lower-repetition, higher load programmes. This may be due to the fact that the mechanisms behind child strength gains are of a neuromuscular nature rather than related to muscle size (see below), with high repetitions providing a longer stimulus to the neural system. Faigenbaum et al., (2009) suggested a high training volume to be more effective at stimulating adaptations in muscular strength than a low training volume, with a high-volume programme potentially involving 3 sets of 10–15 repetitions per exercise at a moderate load, 2–3 sessions per week, for 8–14 weeks.

> **Key point**
>
> Resistance training improves the muscular strength (10–40% increase) of pre-pubertal children through neuromuscular adaptations.

High-intensity training

Repeated sprint training, or maximal efforts against resistance (Wingate anaerobic test, isokinetic dynamometry, plyometrics), are effective in improving muscular power in pre- and early-pubertal children. The extent of muscle power increase in response to high-intensity training is much lower (2–12%) than the muscular strength adaptations to resistance training. Sprint running training by pre-pubescent boys and girls for 6–8 weeks improves leg peak power (4–10%) as measured by the Wingate Anaerobic Test (Grodjinovsky et al., 1980; McManus et al., 1997). Sprint speed of highly trained elite athletes over 100 metres has been shown to continue increasing from childhood to young adulthood, over and above the natural changes expected due to growth and maturation.

In addition to direct speed, many sports of an intermittent nature involve sudden changes of direction, change of speed, kicking, tackling or jumping, all of which require explosive power. Although the resistance-training-induced strength gains play a major role in the development of explosive actions, explosive high-velocity training, such as plyometrics, leads to greater improvements in explosive power (Hakkinen et al., 1985; Wilson et al., 1993). Indeed, it has recently been suggested that both resistance training and plyometrics should be included in an adolescent's training programme to maximise the benefits of strength, power, and motor skill in sports performance (Faigenbaum et al., 2009). Plyometrics involves exercises that utilise the stretch-shortening cycle (SSC) of skeletal muscle, such as jumping, hurdling, bouncing and skipping. The ability of the neural and musculotendinous systems to produce maximal force within the shortest amount of time possible (i.e. power) is enhanced by the SSC. This is why plyometric exercises are commonly integrated into training programmes where the development of explosive activities is important. Due to the nature of plyometrics, however, concern used to exist regarding its suitability for the growing child as it was thought they would be more susceptible to joint and soft tissue injuries resulting from the bounding-type activities. These concerns, however, were dismissed by the American College of Sports Medicine in 2001 and it is now advised that the participation of children in plyometrics should be closely supervised,

correct techniques must be learnt and training intensity and volume should be individualised.

Plyometric training, in isolation or in combination with resistance training, for 6–14 weeks duration, has been shown to improve anaerobic power and the performance of explosive actions (e.g. sprinting, jumping, and throwing) in pre- and early-pubescent children (Bishop et al., 2009; Diallo et al., 2001); Ingle et al., 2006; Meylan & Malatesta, 2009; Potdevin et al., 2011; Rubley et al., 2011; Wong et al., 2010). These findings have been demonstrated in both athletes and non-athletes, with a similar small relative increase (2–6%) in anaerobic power compared to the improvement with sprint training (4–10%).

> **Key points**
>
> Muscular power can be increased (2–12%) during childhood with high-intensity training, such as repeated sprints.
>
> The combination of resistance training with plyometrics maximises the strength and power gains and improves motor skill and sport performance.

Physiological mechanisms for anaerobic trainability

Muscular strength, an important component of muscular power, is improved with resistance training of pre-pubescent children with minimal change in muscle size (Faigenbaum et al., 2009; Lillegard et al., 1997; Ozmun et al., 1994; Ramsay et al., 1990; Sailors & Berg, 1987; Weltman et al., 1986). Strength gains in this population have, therefore, been primarily attributed to neural mechanisms. An improvement in neuromuscular activation has been associated with strength gains with the majority of adaptation occurring within the first 10 weeks of a 20-week programme. The relative increase in strength following resistance training, however, is greater than the changes in neuromuscular activation (Ozmun et al., 1994; Ramsay et al., 1990). Improvements in motor coordination and motor skill performance may be partially responsible for the improvement in strength, with the impact likely greater in more complex movements (e.g. arm curl, leg press) than stationary, isometric contractions. Elevated testosterone secretion in males during puberty is associated with large increases in muscle mass, hence the training-induced strength gains during adolescence and adulthood are primarily the result of muscle hypertrophy. The lower levels of testosterone in females may explain the limited increase in muscle hypertrophy and resultant strength gain following the onset of puberty.

Biochemical changes of the muscle accompany anaerobic training. Resting muscle ATP and PCr levels are elevated following training, providing a greater potential source of energy from anaerobic means for the performance of short-duration, high-intensity activities. In addition, the activity of several glycolytic enzymes is elevated and resting muscle glycogen content is increased, alongside a greater glycogen utilisation during exercise. Together, these biochemical changes are indicative of an enhanced anaerobic capacity and hence may be partially responsible for the improved anaerobic performance following resistance and/or high-intensity training.

Response to endurance training

Peak oxygen uptake

The effect of endurance training on the aerobic fitness of children is determined by the comparison of $\dot{V}O_{2peak}$ between trained and untrained individuals. As with adults, endurance training in children and adolescents elevates $\dot{V}O_{2peak}$. Trained boys and girls are commonly observed to utilise $> 60\ mL \cdot kg^{-1} \cdot min^{-1}$ and $> 50\ mL \cdot kg^{-1} \cdot min^{-1}$ of oxygen, respectively (Armstrong & Barker, 2011). An improved $\dot{V}O_{2peak}$ with training has been observed in a variety of trained individuals, including runners, cyclists, swimmers and cross-country skiers (Baltaci & Ergun, 1997; Bénéfice et al., 1990; Nottin et al., 2002; Rowland et al., 2000; Wells et al., 1973). The response of $\dot{V}O_{2peak}$ to endurance training appears to be independent of gender, with average increases of 6.7% and 5.9% in males and females, respectively (Armstrong & Barker, 2011). This increase in $\dot{V}O_{2peak}$ is smaller than that reported for adults. However, the direct comparison of children and adults has shown a similar training-induced increase in $\dot{V}O_{2peak}$ in both males and females (Eisenman et al., 1975; Savage et al., 1986).

Key points

Endurance training in children and adolescents can:

➤ Improve $\dot{V}O_{2peak}$ independent of gender

➤ Delay the lactate threshold point, i.e. it occurs at a higher percentage of $\dot{V}O_{2peak}$

➤ Improve endurance performance

As you may have experienced, either personally or as a coach/teacher, there is a wide range in the responsiveness of individuals to endurance training. Almost half of the $\dot{V}O_{2peak}$ change following training has been estimated to be the result of genetic influences in both adults and children

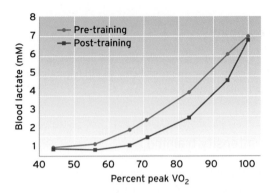

Figure 7.26 Blood lactate response to exercise and training. (*Source*: Adapted from Armstrong & Barker (2010))

(Bouchard & Rankinen, 2001; Danis et al., 2003). The relative importance of training for the change in relative $\dot{V}O_{2peak}$ in children has been estimated to be 35% (Danis et al., 2003).

Lactate threshold

As mentioned previously, LT is a physiological measurement commonly used as an indication of aerobic fitness. Similar to adults, the lactate curve in children and adolescents shifts to the right following endurance training (Figure 7.26), that is, blood lactate concentration at the same relative sub-maximal exercise intensity is lower post-training. As with adults, an increase in $\dot{V}O_{2peak}$ is not always observed following endurance training; however, an improved aerobic fitness may still have occurred as identified by the occurrence of LT at a higher percentage of $\dot{V}O_{2peak}$. In reality, therefore, an individual will be able to run at a faster speed before the same level of blood lactate is reached, and hence improve endurance performance time.

Physiological mechanisms for the training-induced increase in aerobic fitness

Physiologically, the greater $\dot{V}O_{2peak}$ found in trained versus untrained children is due to the greater level of oxygen delivered to the exercising muscle as a function of increased maximal SV, independent of gender. The adaptation in maximal stroke volume is dependent on factors influencing SV at rest (Nottin et al., 2002; Obert et al., 2003; Rowland et al., 2000), such as left ventricular dimension or expanded blood volume.

At the muscle level, the main training-induced changes in adults is an increase in the number and volume of mitochondria; however, due to methodological constraints, the adaptation of children's mitochondria following endurance training is unknown. Training-induced adaptations in the capacity for aerobic metabolism in children is demonstrated by an increased glycogen storage and elevated activity of oxidative enzymes. An increased oxidative capacity of the exercising muscles, and hence a reduced contribution of anaerobic glycolysis to energy production, may be responsible for the faster primary time constant and lower submaximal exercise lactate level following training.

Key points

Training-induced improvement in aerobic fitness is due to several factors:

➤ A greater maximal SV improves the delivery of oxygen to the exercising muscles

➤ Muscle glycogen stores are increased and oxidative enzyme activity enhanced

Check your recall
Fill in the missing words.

➤ Growth to adulthood follows a _____ curve shape indicating changes in the pace of growth during childhood.

➤ The science of _____ involves measurement of the human body and its individual parts.

➤ The period of maximal height gain is known as _____ _____ _____.

➤ The most accurate way to measure body composition is to measure the fat free mass and the _____ _____.

➤ Healthy bone has a unique balance of strength and _____ along with _____ and flexibility.

➤ The increase in bone size during growth sees increases in bone mass and _____ _____.

➤ _____ is essential for the development of healthy bones.

➤ Before birth muscles grow by hypertrophy and _____. After birth it is thought they grow by _____ only.

➤ Muscular _____ represents the maximal amount of force that can be generated during a contraction.

➤ Muscular _____ requires muscles to be able to complete repeated sub-maximal contractions.

➤ Gaseous exchange occurs at the _____ in unborn children.

➤ Basal HR at birth is around _____ beats·min^{-1}.

➤ The most common measures of anaerobic fitness include peak power output, mean power output and _____ _____.

➤ The differences in aerobic fitness observed between males and females increase from _____.

➤ In children a maximal aerobic test is likely to result in _____ being achieved rather than $\dot{V}O_{2\,max}$.

➤ In the formation of new bone, osteoblasts become trapped within the bone matrix and become known as _____.

➤ The epiphyseal plate, the cartilaginous region between the diaphysis and epiphyses, is the site of longitudinal bone _____.

➤ This plate becomes known as the epiphyseal _____ when the diaphysis fuses with the epiphyses on completion of bone growth.

Review questions

1. When does the peak height velocity occur for males and females during maturation?

2. What is the peak weight velocity for males and females?

3. Name three ways of assessing body composition.

4. In percentage terms what is the lean body mass difference between adult males and females?

5. What can help to increase the thickness and density of bones?

6. Name the three types of bone cell. What role does each of these play in the maintenance and functioning of the skeletal system?

7. In a long bone, what is the difference between the epiphyseal plate and the epiphyseal line?

8. Hypertrophy refers to what change in a muscle?

9. At what stage in development does muscular strength increase at its greatest rate?

10. Describe the changes in flexibility that occur for males and females during development.

11. What are the foramen ovale, the ductus arteriosus and ductus venosus?

12. How does average HR change during development?

Teach it!
In groups of three, choose one topic and teach it to the rest of the study group.

You are coaching a netball session for a group of 11–12 year old girls.

1. What would you expect in terms of growth and development differences within the group of girls?

2. What would the effect on skill performance be?

3. How could you plan a training session to cater for all abilities?

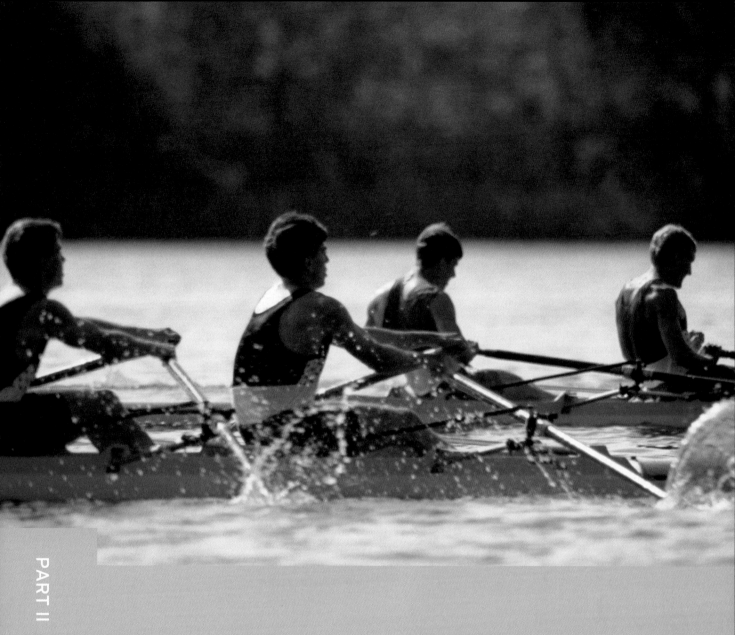

PART II

Applied exercise physiology

Part Two of this textbook contains the applied exercise physiology chapters. Aspects of sports performance and health, within the applied exercise physiology section of this textbook, are covered in chapters that relate to the predominant energy generation mechanisms. An overview of the mechanisms by which cells generate the energy required for their activities, including bringing about human movement for sports and exercise, follows this section. The intensity and duration of a sport or exercise session determine the predominant energy generation pathways. The first five chapters that make up Part II of *Exercise Physiology for Health and Sports Performance* are based around these mechanisms or pathways. Each of these chapters focuses on groups of sports aspects that relate to different intensities

and durations of exercise. While competing in a kayak marathon might appear to be fundamentally different to running a marathon, from a physiological perspective they have much in common. The energy demands of a marathon are similar, regardless whether it is a race completed on land or on water. By taking such a perspective, it is possible for an exercise physiologist to apply knowledge of the physiological demands of a sport to develop a sport-specific training programme. Similarly, in a health context, if an individual has a goal to improve their aerobic or cardiovascular fitness, regardless of the type of exercise that person would prefer to be involved in, by applying such an approach it is possible for a physiologist to design an appropriate exercise intervention or prescription. The final two chapters in Part II consider health and environmental physiology within an applied exercise physiology context.

Chapters 9-13 in Part II move along a continuum of intensity and duration from anaerobic to aerobic predominant sports and activities and also examine the special case of the physiology of games and intermittent sports.

As can be seen from Figure 1, maximal intensity of exercise can only be maintained for a short duration. In longer-duration activities the relative intensity falls dramatically. Interestingly, if Jamaican sprinter Usain Bolt, could maintain the pace of his 100m world record (9.58 s, at 37.58 km·hr^{-1}) he would complete a marathon (42.195 km) in around 1 hr 8 min. Despite the dramatic drop in power with increasing exercise duration male and female elite marathon runners can still complete the distance in just over 2 hr and 2 hr 15 min respectively. This achievement alone highlights the amazing adaptability of human energy generation mechanisms.

In the next chapter (Chapter 9), the focus is on sports performance and health aspects of power and power endurance sports such as athletic throwing events, weight-lifting and 100 m sprints. The focus is on explosive and speed activities of very high intensity and short duration, those up to a maximum of 10 seconds. Chapter 10 continues the anaerobic theme, focusing on the glycolytic pathway and sports and activities that rely on fast-rate glycolysis. This chapter includes high-intensity sports and types of exercise lasting between 10 and 90 s, which often place significant demands on glycolysis, as a source of ATP, and result in significant increases in lactate and H$^+$ concentrations. Chapters 11 and 12 examine the physiology of aerobic endurance sports but are split between those of a relatively high intensity, such as rowing and marathon running (Chapter 11), and lower-intensity activities such as the recreational activities of hill walking or walking or canoeing (Chapter 12). The nature of intermittent sports and games form a special case with regard to intensity and duration, and therefore the predominant energy generation mechanisms. Playing games such as rugby, basketball or field hockey, or sports such as boxing, wrestling or judo, along with many types of training session, places demands upon both aerobic and anaerobic metabolism. The special case of the physiology of games and intermittent sports is covered in Chapter 13. Chapter 14 covers a number of aspects of health that can be important considerations for physical education teachers and coaches, while Chapter 15, examines the physiological challenge created through exercise in different environmental conditions.

Table 1 provides an overview of chapters in Part II of *Exercise Physiology for Health and Sports Performance* and examples of sports relevant to each predominant energy generation mechanism. The placing of a sport in a particular category should be viewed as indicative only, as the intensity and duration of any sport can be manipulated by an athlete.

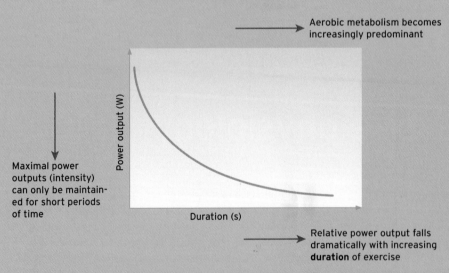

Figure 1 Decrease in power output with increasing duration exercise.

Table 1 Summary of the energy-system-based chapters in Part II and overview of the predominant energy generation pathways.

Chapter	Intensity	Duration	Energy pathways	Example sports
Chapter 9 Power and power endurance: the explosive sports	Maximal	≤ 10 s	ATP stores ATP-PCr AKR-ADR	**Power**: shot putt, discus, hammer, power lifts **Power endurance**: clean and jerk, 100 m run, flying 200m cycling
Chapter 10 Anaerobic endurance: the speed endurance sports	Very high	10 - 90 s	Glycolysis Aerobic metabolism	**Shorter duration:** 200 m kayak, 50 m swim, 400 m run, 1 km time trial cycling **Longer duration**: 500 m kayak, 200 m swim, 800 m run
Chapter 11 Aerobic endurance I: The high-intensity aerobic sports	High	≥ 90 s	Glycolysis Aerobic metabolism or pathway	**Short duration high intensity**: 1,500 m run, 400 m swim, rowing **Longer duration high intensity**: distance running, triathlon, 1,500 m swim
Chapter 12 Aerobic endurance II: The lower-intensity endurance sports	Lower	≥ 90 s	Aerobic metabolism or pathway	Mountaineering, hill walking, golf-walking between holes
Chapter 13 *A special case*: Intermittent sports and games	Varied	Game or session dependent	ATP-PCr, AKR-ADR Glycolysis Aerobic metabolism or pathway	**Games**: Football (various), netball, basketball, baseball, cricket, water polo **Intermittent sports**: judo, tennis, badminton **Training sessions**: interval training, fartlek training

ATP stands for adenosine triphosphate, ATP-PCr refers to the creatine kinase reaction in which phosphocreatine provides the energy and phosphoryl group to phosphorylate ADP to create further ATP, AKR stands for the adenylate kinase reaction, and ADR for the adenylate deaminase reaction, all of which are described in more detail in Chapter 9.

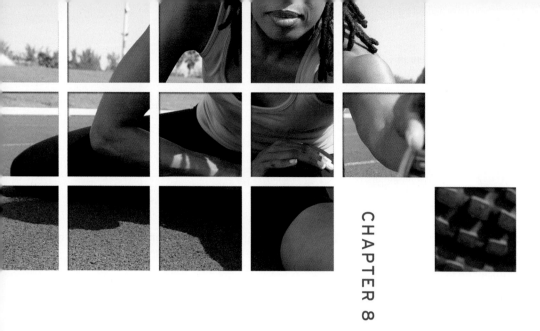

General concepts for applied exercise physiology

Learning objectives

After reading, considering and discussing with a study partner the material in this chapter you should be able to:

➤ summarise the energy generation pathways

➤ teach others about the predominant energy system for a range of sports

➤ explain enthalpy and entropy and their role in determining the free energy potential of a reaction

➤ describe in detail the functioning of enzymes

➤ identify the components of fitness

➤ summarise the key principles of training

➤ discuss the advantages of a periodised training programme

➤ highlight the key considerations for conducting valid and reliable fitness assessments

➤ explain strength and conditioning training

➤ critically analyse the role of warm-up and cool-down in any training programme

➤ discuss when flexibility training should occur in a training session

➤ identify different methods of flexibility training

This chapter provides an overview of key concepts that are essential to understanding applied exercise physiology. In the next section an overview of the energy generation mechanisms is provided, prior to examining bioenergetics and enzymology in more detail. Following this, we examine key concepts in training for sports and health, including an introduction to training methodology, exercise testing and the principles of training.

8.1 Energy generation for exercise

An overview: The metabolic pathways and their interaction

Every cell within the body requires *energy* to perform its functions. The energy required comes from the food that we eat and is essential for the maintenance of homeostasis. Cells are constantly catabolising and anabolising nutrients from our diet for growth, maintenance, repair, storage and cellular activity. The sum of all these reactions is our **metabolism**, taken from the Greek word *metabolismós*, meaning *change*. Even at rest the body uses large amounts of energy to maintain homeostasis, but when taking part in sport the energy demands multiply with the duration and intensity of the exercise. The sodium-potassium

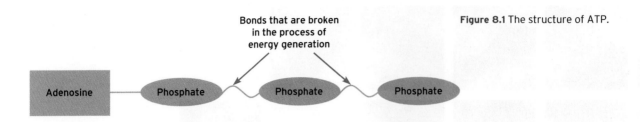

Figure 8.1 The structure of ATP.

pump, essential to the excitable muscular and nervous tissues, requires energy for its active transport mechanism, as do the muscles in order to bring about contraction for movement. The energy for sodium-potassium pump activation, muscular contraction and indeed most cellular activity comes from the high-energy compound **adenosine triphosphate** (ATP).

The basic structure of ATP, comprised of an adenosine molecule attached to three phosphoryl groups, is shown in Figure 8.1 and is described in more depth in Chapter 9. As can be seen from Figure 8.1, the final two phosphoryl groups of ATP are attached to each adenosine molecule by what are commonly referred to as high-energy bonds. When ATP is converted to ADP, energy becomes available which can be harnessed by cells to drive the activities they perform to maintain homeostasis. While cells maintain stores of ATP, the cellular demand for energy is such that the each cell must constantly synthesise ATP. Through the process of evolution, cells, such as muscle fibres, have developed a number of metabolic pathways through which ATP can be formed, dependent on the rate at which energy is required. In order to hunt or outrun predators humans needed pathways through which to synthesise ATP very quickly. For maintaining life during rest or lower-intensity activities such as planting and gathering food, more sustainable (longer-term, endurance) pathways for ATP synthesis were required. Alternative human metabolic pathways have evolved to serve these differing needs. In a modern sporting context, evolution has provided the body with several ATP generation pathways with different ones predominating in a 100 m sprint, a 400 m sprint or a marathon.

Adenosine triphosphate as an energy source

Adenosine triphosphate synthesis begins with the digestion of our food. The process of digestion can be thought of as the mining or drilling for crude oil from which the fuel for our bodies, ATP can be refined (synthesised). As described in Chapter 2, the 'crude' forms of fuel catabolised through digestion are glucose, fatty acids and amino acids. These crude fuels are transported (via the blood) to cells throughout the body where they are converted into the refined fuel ATP, the 'petrol' for our bodies.

ATP is most commonly catabolised such that one phosphoryl group (also referred to as a phosphate group in some textbooks) is removed and, in the process, energy is released which can be used to perform work. This reaction converts ATP to adenosine diphosphate (ADP) and a separate phosphoryl group (Pi). A simplified illustration of this reaction is shown in Figure 8.2, with a more complete illustration of this reaction found in Chapter 9. Adenosine diphosphate is also a high-energy compound, but only in sustained high-intensity exercise situations is this compound broken down further. More commonly, ADP is phosphorylated (Pi is bonded to ADP) to synthesise ATP. The pathway through which ADP is converted to ATP depends on the rate at which ATP is required by the body.

Key points

ATP, the body's energy supply, is formed from the carbohydrate, fat and protein in our diet.

Energy, released from the catabolism of ATP, is vital for all cellular activity, including muscle contraction.

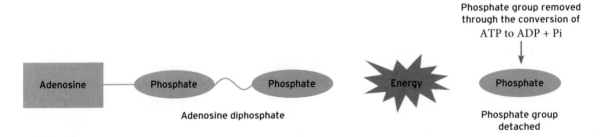

Figure 8.2 The hydrolysis of ATP to ADP + Pi which releases energy for cellular activity.

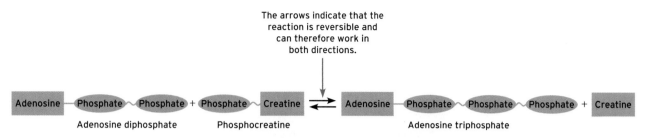

The arrows indicate that the reaction is reversible and can therefore work in both directions.

Figure 8.3 Illustration of the synthesis of ATP via the catabolism of phosphocreatine. The energy released by the removal of phosphate from phosphocreatine is used to synthesise ATP through the phosphorylation (bonding of a phosphate) of ADP.

Metabolic pathways

Cells have a number of metabolic pathways through which to synthesise ATP. There are two main anaerobic pathways and several aerobic pathways. Each of these pathways requires a number of chemical reactions to create ATP. *Aerobic* ATP generation refers to the necessity of oxygen within the metabolic pathway. *Anaerobic*, by contrast, indicates oxygen is not required for the chemical reactions within the pathway.

Anaerobic and aerobic pathways are essential for every cell in the body to function. Often, as exercise physiologists, we are primarily concerned with ATP synthesis in relation to the energy requirements for a sport or activity. The energy requirements, and therefore the predominant metabolic pathway, depend on the intensity and duration of the sport. The availability of different pathways and their predominance for different sports, by way of analogy, can be likened to the gears in a car engine. Just as a car has gears, so the body has a variety of pathways for ATP synthesis. Two low gears (1st and 2nd) for power and speed along with a top gear (3rd)– overdrive–for efficiency and long journeys. The 1st and 2nd gears, the phosphagen system and glycolysis, of the human 'car' represent the anaerobic pathways while the aerobic system comprises the 3rd gear.

Knowledge integration question

Explain why thinking of ATP as a cellular rechargeable battery might be a useful analogy.

Anaerobic system pathways

The phosphagen system

The simplest and fastest pathway for ATP synthesis is via the phosphagen system. The phosphagen system has more than one pathway for ATP synthesis and these are the focus of Chapter 9. However, in this overview we will highlight the primary pathway which is the adenosine triphophate-phosphocreatine (ATP-PCr) pathway.

Cells store phosphocreatine (PCr) within the cytosol and these stores can be used to synthesise ATP, as shown in Figure 8.3. The simple nature of the chemical reaction and the limited stores of PCr mean that this system is a rapidly available short-term energy system. The energy released from this reaction enables the phosphorylation of ADP. The arrows in Figure 8.3 indicate the reaction is reversible and at times of rest PCr will be synthesised to replenish cytosolic stores. In power sports ATP stores in the active muscles provide the energy for these explosive efforts, while for power endurance sports of 2–10 s duration, or where a sudden high-intensity burst is required, the ATP-PCr reaction provides the predominant pathway for ATP synthesis.

Key point

The phosphagen system (ATP-PCr pathway) is responsible for the fastest synthesis of ATP and is, therefore, the predominant energy system in short duration (up to 10 s) maximal intensity activities.

Glycolysis

The second anaerobic ATP synthesis pathway is via glycolysis. In sports requiring maximal effort lasting between 10 and 90 s, or for a sprint finish, such as in a cycling road race or rowing race, glycolysis represents the main pathway for ATP synthesis. Glycolysis enables the catabolism of either glucose or the storage form glycogen to synthesise ATP. Figure 8.4 provides an overview of glycolysis which takes place within the cytoplasm of the cell, all necessary substrates and enzymes being available within the

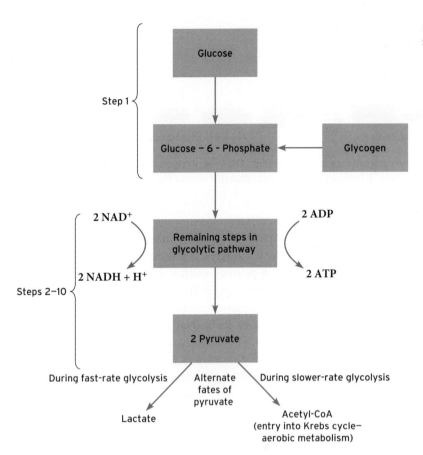

Figure 8.4 The glycolytic pathway and ATP synthesis.

intracellular fluid. The glycolytic pathway involves 10 reactions or steps to metabolise glucose and produce ATP and pyruvate. The 10 steps of glycolysis are described in more detail in Chapter 10. An important concept to note at this time, is that a greater number of steps or reactions are necessary to synthesise ATP than is required for the ATP-PCr reaction. It is for this reason that glycolysis takes a number of seconds to become the predominant ATP generation mechanism, taking over from the phosphagen system in maximal-intensity exercise.

Glycolysis does not require oxygen for any of the reactions in its 10 steps and is therefore an anaerobic pathway. The end of this pathway is the production of pyruvate during which a small amount of energy is produced, i.e. 2 or 3 molecules of ATP. The rate of glycolysis and the fate of pyruvate depend upon the intensity of exercise and hence the demand for energy. When exercising at a low intensity the rate of glycolysis is slower and the pyruvate produced is further catabolised via aerobic metabolism, in processes that require oxygen (see the Krebs cycle and electron transport chain later), to produce large amounts of energy in the form of ATP. Thus during *slower-rate glycolysis* pyruvate enters the mitochondria where it is finally broken down to carbon dioxide and water.

Knowledge integration question

Explain the difference between fast- and slower-rate glycolysis.

As the intensity of exercise increases so does the rate of glycolysis. During high-intensity exercise, such as a sprint finish in a race, the rate of H atom release (a by-product of glycolysis) is so great that it outstrips the rate at which it can be transferred to the mitochondria (by the carrier molecule nicotine adenine dinucleotide–NAD^+). Thus, during *fast-rate glycolysis* the H atoms bond with pyruvate in a further reaction to produce lactate (often referred to as lactic acid in a sports setting). This prevents the cellular pH falling, and so preserves enzyme activity.

Some textbooks refer to 'fast-rate glycolysis' as 'anaerobic glycolysis', and to 'slower-rate glycolysis' as 'aerobic glycolysis'. These terms can be confusing, however, as glycolysis is always an **anaerobic** process. It is the fate of pyruvate at the end of glycolysis that can be aerobic (oxidative metabolism) or anaerobic (conversion to lactate). It is for this reason that the terms fast-rate and slower-rate glycolysis have been adopted in this text. The glycolytic pathway is discussed in full detail in Chapter 10.

Key points

Glycolysis

➤ involves 10 reactions to produce ATP and pyruvate

➤ exercise intensity alters the fate of pyruvate, the glycolytic pathway remains unchanged

➤ low-intensity exercise–pyruvate enters aerobic pathway

➤ high-intensity exercise–pyruvate is converted to lactate

Aerobic system pathways

Carbohydrate, in the form of glucose or glycogen, is the only macronutrient that can be metabolised through glycolysis to synthesise ATP. Through the aerobic pathways, however, lipids, proteins and carbohydrates can all be catabolised to synthesise ATP due to the presence of carbon, hydrogen and oxygen in all three macronutrients. All the reactions to synthesise ATP via anaerobic pathways occur within the cytoplasm. Aerobic pathways include substrates that are found within the cytoplasm and mitochondria, where the reactions also take place. Depending on their development and role within the body, cells can have anywhere from none to several thousand mitochondria within the cytoplasm. The greater the numbers of mitochondria present

within a cell, the greater its adaptation towards aerobic metabolism.

In aerobic metabolism, each of the macronutrients has a specific pathway through which it is initially catabolised, prior to entry into the common pathways of the **Krebs cycle** (also known as the *citric acid cycle* or *tricarboxylic acid cycle*) and the **electron transport chain** (ETC). An overview of the pathways within the aerobic system is provided in Figure 8.5. Although up to 10% of ATP synthesis may be from protein sources, lipids and carbohydrates form the most important macronutrients for aerobic ATP synthesis.

The initial metabolic pathway for the catabolism of free fatty acids (lipids) is β-oxidation (pronounced beta-oxidation), while for carbohydrates (glucose and glycogen) it is glycolysis and for proteins (amino acids) the first pathway is deamination. The first common substrate in the catabolism of each macronutrient is acetyl coenzyme A (acetyl CoA). When free fatty acids, glucose and several amino acids have reached this stage in metabolism they enter the Krebs cycle. Due to their more complex structure, as illustrated by arrows (a) and (b) in Figure 8.5, amino acids can enter the Krebs cycle at a number of different points. Through the Krebs cycle, which takes place within the mitochondria, the three nutrients are further metabolised and additional hydrogen atoms removed for transfer to the ETC. While the ETC provides the most plentiful source of ATP, both the Krebs cycle and the ETC synthesise ATP for cellular activity.

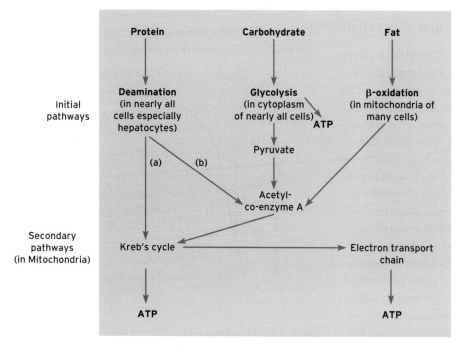

Figure 8.5 Pathways within aerobic metabolism and sources of ATP.

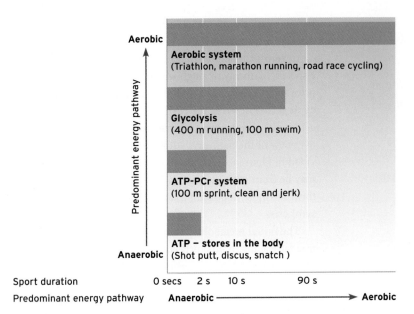

Figure 8.6 The predominant energy pathway for sports of different intensity and duration.

Key points

Initial pathways for the metabolism of the macronutrients are:

➤ Carbohydrate–glycolysis

➤ Lipid–β-oxidation

➤ Protein–deamination

Secondary pathways are the Krebs cycle and the ETC during which ATP is synthesized.

Aerobic metabolism is slower in the synthesis of ATP than anaerobic pathways, but produces a higher net yield.

Energy system predominance and interaction

The aim of the above brief overview of ATP and the cellular mechanisms for ATP generation, is to set in context the following chapters in Part II of this textbook. As mentioned at the start of this chapter each subsequent chapter is based around sports of different intensities and durations and the predominant energy generation mechanisms for those sports. The decision to divide Part II of the textbook into chapters on this basis was taken because the intensity and duration of a sport are critical to the physiological demands they place upon an athlete. This in turn will determine the predominant metabolic pathway(s). Figure 8.6 provides a theoretical model of the relationship between time duration (and by inference, intensity) and predominant energy sources for a variety of sports.

While this model is helpful in explaining the predominant pathway during sports of differing durations and intensities, a number of important concepts need to be kept in mind when adopting such an approach. As can be seen from Figure 8.7,

when we start to exercise all energy pathways contribute to total ATP synthesis. The concept of transitioning between metabolic pathways is an important aspect of ATP synthesis. Cells do not flick a switch to move from one pathway to another, although it might seem as such, given the necessity within a textbook to describe one pathway after another. In reality all pathways operate to synthesise ATP from the start of exercise. It is just that a particular pathway might provide the predominant energy source, dependent on the intensity and duration of exercise. This point is made particularly poignant by recent research that, as is illustrated in Figure 8.7, suggests glycolysis and the aerobic system respond more quickly to the demands of exercise than previously thought.

While current techniques lack the desired sophistication to examine the interaction in energy system contribution in as much detail as exercise physiologists would like,

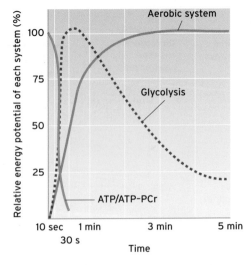

Figure 8.7 Energy system transitions during exercise.

recent data suggest that, even for sports of under 10 s duration, glycolysis plays a more significant role in ATP synthesis than first believed. Similarly, for sports or events under 60 s duration, the aerobic system provides a more significant contribution to total ATP synthesis than previously thought. This needs to be kept in mind when reading Chapters 9–13, and highlights the necessity for keeping current with research in the field. As techniques develop it may become possible for researchers to examine more closely the contribution of energy systems during exercise. In this way researchers may be able to confirm that the glycolytic and aerobic pathways provide a more significant contribution to total ATP synthesis at the start of exercise than previously believed. As a consequence, the timing of transitions between metabolic pathways suggested in this textbook should be seen as indicative rather than definitive. Future research will help to clarify further the interactions between cellular pathways in response to exercise of differing intensity and duration.

An overview of the cellular metabolic pathways and their interactions is provided in Figure 8.8. The figure is

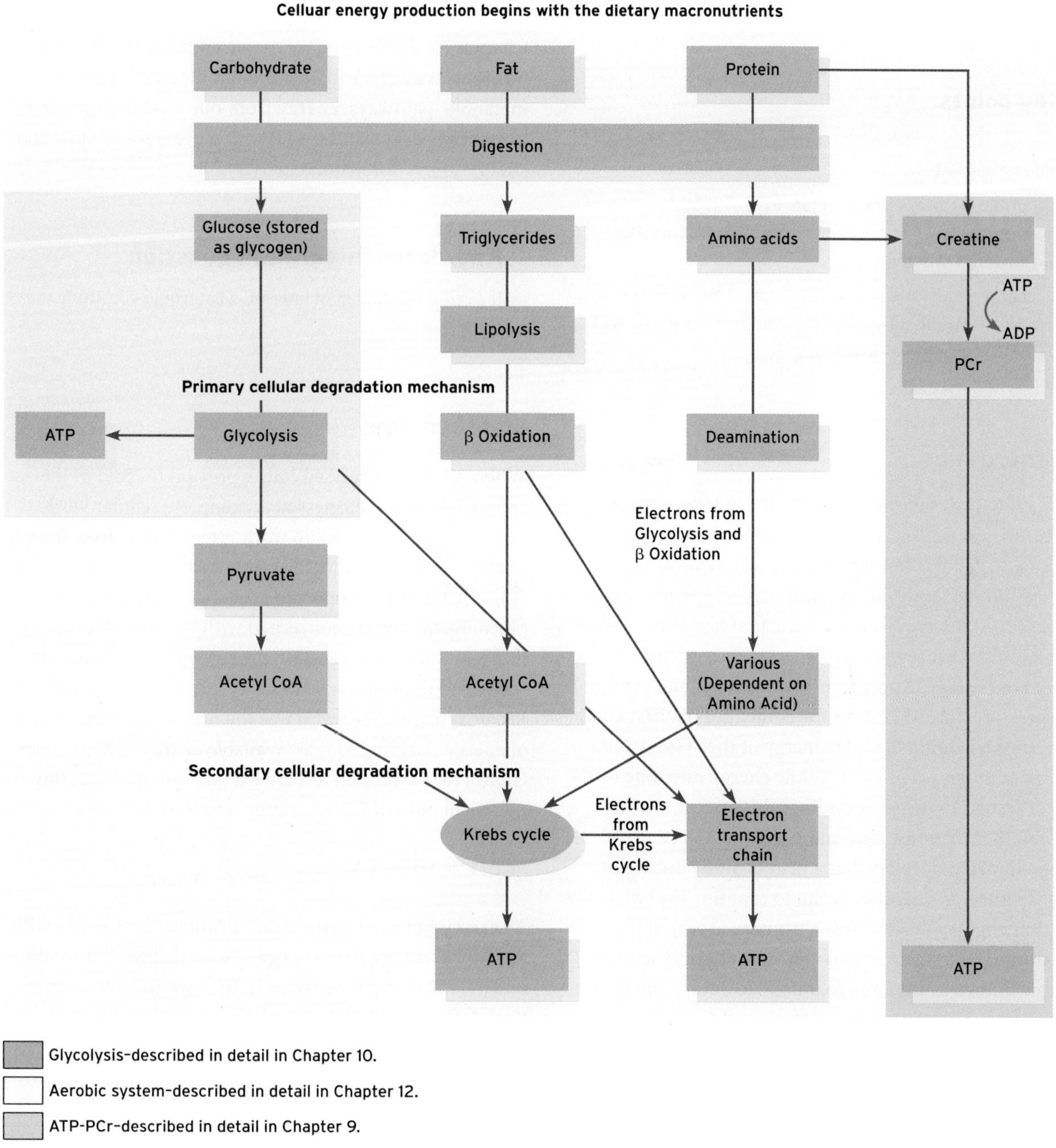

Celluar energy production begins with the dietary macronutrients

Figure 8.8 Primary cellular operation mechanisms – sources of ATP.

colour-coded to highlight the energy source that is the focus of each of the following chapters within this text-book. In Chapter 9 the phosphagen system is described in more detail, while in Chapter 10 the focus is upon gly-colysis as it relates to high-intensity anaerobic endurance performance. The interaction between glycolysis and aero-bic metabolism (the aerobic-anaerobic transition) is high-lighted in Chapter 11 prior to a more detailed examination of aerobic metabolism in Chapter 12. Finally, in Chapter 13 the interaction between energy generation mechanisms is a central aspect of the special case that is presented by inter-mittent sports and games.

Key points

There are three pathways for ATP synthesis: two anaerobic and one aerobic.

Anaerobic pathways: predominate in high-intensity, short-duration activity. Aerobic pathway: predominates in longer-duration activity.

All energy generation pathways operate at the start of exercise, while the subsequent demands placed on the ATP synthesis pathways are sport-specific.

Bioenergetics

In Chapter 2 energy and the forms it can take, such as chemical, heat or kinetic, were introduced. Energy is essential to cellular functioning and all chemical reac-tions within the body either require or release energy as they proceed. Also in Chapter 2 the first law of thermo-dynamics, the conservation of energy (energy cannot be created or destroyed only transformed from one form to another), was introduced. In the context of the first law of thermodynamics, the total energy of the system and its surroundings is constant. While energy might be lost from a system to the surroundings this energy is trans-ferred rather than lost. Thermodynamics, the study of energy transfer, developed as a field of study during the 19th Century, as scientists began to examine the efficiency of steam engines. As heat was a primary aspect of the functioning of a steam engine this new physical science became known as thermodynamics. However, this field of study is now more commonly referred to as **energet-ics** because scientists are concerned with the dynamics of all forms of energy, not just heat. The study of energy dynamics in living organisms is called **bioenergetics**. In an exercise physiology context, a basic knowledge of the principles of bioenergetics is helpful for gaining a deeper

understanding of energy transfer within anaerobic and aerobic metabolism.

When studying energetics, the matter within a struc-ture we wish to study is known as the *system* and every-thing else in the universe represents the *surroundings*. In bioenergetics terms, a cell or muscle, or the human body could represent a system of interest, in which case all other matter would represent the surroundings. As described in Chapter 3, cells require a continuous supply of energy to perform their specialised functions which include growth, repair and maintenance. For example, muscle fibres (cells) require energy to bring about movement (refer to Chapter 5). As humans we derive energy from the macro-nutrients within our diet. Through digestion and the metabolic pathways, energy from our food is converted to stored energy within ATP which provides the primary energy source for cellular activity.

Knowledge integration question

If a cell is the system of interest, what would constitute the surroundings?

Gibbs' energy

When ATP is hydrolysed only a portion (~25%) of the energy released is harnessed to complete cellular work. The energy available to do work is termed the **free energy** which is represented by the symbol ΔG (pronounced 'delta G'). The symbol 'Δ' refers to a 'change in' energy, as in bioenergetics we are concerned with the change in energy that takes place as a reaction proceeds and reactants are converted to products. The 'G' of free energy is a tribute to Josiah Willard Gibbs who was the first to describe this form of energy referring to it as 'available energy' (1870). Later, Gibbs (1878) went on to derive a fundamental equation for the calculation of Gibbs' energy which is:

$$\Delta G = \Delta H - T\Delta S$$

As exercise physiologists we are primarily concerned with the Gibbs' energy (free energy). Nevertheless, it is useful to understand each of the terms in the formula, for, as men-tioned above, not all the energy contained within ATP, or within the reactants of any chemical reaction, is available to do work. Table 8.1 provides an overview of all the terms in this equation, and also combinations of ΔH and ΔS that can lead to a negative ΔG, providing free energy for cellular activity.

Table 8.1 The relationship between enthalpy and entropy and the change in free energy (ΔG).

Gibbs' fundamental equation:

$\Delta G = \Delta H - T\Delta S$
Change in free energy = change in heat energy (enthalpy) − absolute temperature × change in energy dispersal (entropy)

Summary of enthalpy and entropy:

$+\Delta S$ a change in the system moving towards disorder − energy dispersing − catabolic
$-\Delta S$ a change in the system moving towards order− anabolic
$+\Delta H$ the reactants have lower heat energy than the products − endothermic − requires heat energy
$-\Delta H$ the reactants have higher heat energy than the products − exothermic − liberates heat energy

ΔG is negative (at a constant temperature):

always when reaction is exothermic ($-\Delta H$) and leads to dispersal of energy ($+T\Delta S$) − catabolic
if reaction is exothermic ($-\Delta H$) but leads to increased order ($-T\Delta S$) as long as $-T\Delta S < -\Delta H$
if reaction is endothermic ($-\Delta H$) but leads to dispersal of energy ($+T\Delta S$) as long as $+T\Delta S > +\Delta H$

Conversely ΔG is always positive:

if reaction is endothermic ($+\Delta H$) and leads to increased order ($-T\Delta S$) − anabolic

The role of enthalpy

The change in energy between the reactants and the products is known as change in **enthalpy** and written in Gibbs' fundamental equation as ΔH. If the reactants for a chemical reaction have greater energy than the products, the reaction releases heat energy to the surroundings and is said to be exothermic and the reaction will have a negative ΔH. The reason that ΔH is negative is because the reactants within the system lose heat energy to the surroundings. Conversely, if heat energy is taken from the surroundings as a reaction proceeds, the reaction is said to be endothermic and it will have a positive ΔH, i.e. the products will have more energy than the reactants ($+\Delta H$). Examples of an exothermic ($-\Delta H$) and an endothermic ($+\Delta H$) reaction are shown in Figure 8.9.

Within the body, endothermic reactions are coupled with exothermic reactions which provide the free energy necessary for the endothermic reaction to proceed. An example of paired $-\Delta H$ and $+\Delta H$ reactions can be seen from PCr catabolism and ATP synthesis. The energy from

the catabolism of PCr to creatine is harnessed within the cell to synthesise ATP. The catabolism of PCr can be thought of as a downhill reaction (Figure 8.9a), while the synthesis of ATP from ADP which requires energy represents an uphill reaction (Figure 8.9b). In this context, an analogy can be made to a ball on top of a hill. If a ball is given a little push to start it off, it will roll downhill spontaneously, whereas a ball at the bottom of a hill will require the input of energy to roll uphill. The little push at the top, or the large push from the bottom of the hill, synonymous to an exothermic or endothermic reaction, respectively, is required to start the reaction and is therefore referred to as the **energy of activation** (E_a). The E_a for the chemical reaction that occurs when a match is lit, is provided by the striking of the match on the side of the box. Within the body, enzymes act as catalysts to lower the E_a required for many chemical reactions to take place.

The role of entropy

The term ΔS, referred to as the change in entropy, relates to the second law of thermodynamics which states that

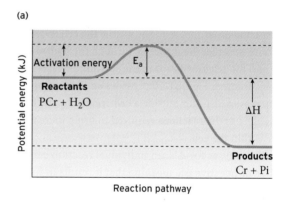

(a)

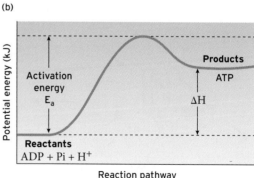

(b)

Figure 8.9 Examples of $-\Delta H$ and $+\Delta H$ reactions, (a) provides an illustration of an exothermic reaction, in this case the hydrolysis of PCr, and (b) provides an illustration of an endothermic reaction, the synthesis of ATP. In this example the energy from hydrolysis of PCr (a) provides the energy for the synthesis of ATP(b).

the dispersal or disorder of energy in the universe is constant or increasing. An example of dispersal can be seen through the diffusion of a solute from high concentration on one side of a permeable membrane to the lower concentration on the other side, such that after a given period of time the concentration of the solute would be the same on either side of the membrane. Energy attempts to disperse in this fashion. A piece of metal that has been heated will transfer heat energy to the atmosphere until it is the same temperature as its surroundings. In a similar way chemical reactions can result in a dispersal of energy from a concentrated form in reactants to a less concentrated form in products. A reaction involving the catabolism of a substance provides an example of taking something that is ordered and disordering it by breaking it into smaller products.

Biological organisms, such as cells, have the capability to facilitate reactions that decrease entropy within the cell. However, such reactions must be accompanied by another process so that overall there is an increase in the entropy of the universe. For example, cellular growth and repair increase order in a cell. The energy for this cellular activity comes largely from the hydrolysis of ATP. Large volumes of ATP have to be hydrolysed (disordered) to increase the order in a cell. Thus while the cell is becoming more ordered, the universe, through the hydrolysis of ATP and the release of heat to the surroundings, is becoming less ordered. Figure 8.10 provides an illustration of the increased disorder outside a cell created by the heat released from the reactions required to bring increased order within the cell.

In this way, as for ΔH, an individual reaction can have a positive or negative ΔS, meaning that it results in increased

or decreased order for a system, such as a cell. For instance, the hydrolysis of ATP to ADP and Pi would result in less order and would therefore have a positive ΔS (+ΔS), whereas the converse reaction would bring more order and would have a negative ΔS (−ΔS). It is important to note that the contribution of the ΔS term to ΔG is temperature-dependent. Changes in temperature affect the size of ΔS and may as a consequence alter the outcome of ΔG. The energy lost to disorder within Gibbs' fundamental equation is therefore represented by the term TΔS, as the temperature multiplies the change in entropy (ΔS).

Key points

Only a fraction of the energy released following ATP hydrolysis is available to do work–*free energy* (ΔG).

Enthalpy (ΔH) is the change in energy between reactants and products.

Entropy (ΔS) is a measure of disorder–energy unavailable for work.

Enthalpy, entropy and the change in free energy

Through these four possibilities (+ΔH, −ΔH, +ΔS, −ΔS), which are highlighted in Table 8.1, the possible combinations of enthalpy and entropy result in reactions having one of three possible outcomes:

- the ΔG is positive (+ΔG non-spontaneous reaction), meaning that the free energy of the products is higher than the free energy of the reactants.

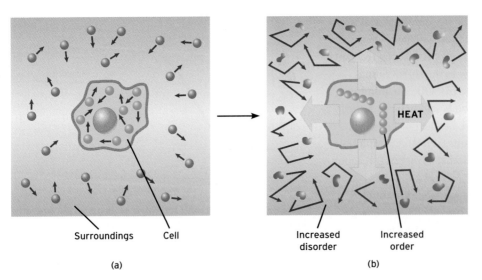

Figure 8.10 Illustration of increasing entropy. The reactions required to bring increased order to a cell (moving from a to b) results in the release of heat from the cell increasing the disorder in the surrounding (universe).

Surroundings   Cell   (a)   Increased disorder   Increased order   (b)   HEAT

- the ΔG is negative (−ΔG spontaneous reaction), meaning that the free energy of the products is less than that of the reactants.
- the ΔG = 0, meaning that the reaction has reached equilibrium–there is no free energy change.

Knowledge integration question

Explain enthalpy and entropy and how they relate to free energy.

The change in free energy, ΔG, is of particular interest to exercise physiologists and is very helpful in understanding how and why reactions within the energy generation pathways proceed. A −ΔG indicates that a reaction is spontaneous, while a +ΔG indicates a reaction is non-spontaneous. A spontaneous, −ΔG reaction can also be referred to as an **exergonic** reaction because it provides free energy that can be used to perform cellular work. Conversely, a non-spontaneous, +ΔG reaction requires energy and is therefore **endergonic**. Figure 8.11 provides examples of a number of high- and low-energy compounds that are found within the ATP-PCr reaction and the glycolytic pathways. In this context, ATP is a high-energy intermediary phosphate compound and will transfer energy through phosphorylation to lower-energy compounds such as Glucose 6-phosphate. Through this process ATP is hydrolysed to ADP, but can then be phosphorylated to ATP once more by the high-energy phosphate compounds such as phosphocreatine. It would be useful when reading about the phosphagen system in Chapter 9 and glycolysis in Chapter 10 to refer back to Figure 8.11 as this is helpful in explaining the bioenergetics involved in the relevant reactions and steps.

Key points

The meaning of changes in free energy (ΔG):

− ΔG: reaction is spontaneous and is referred to as exergonic (provides free energy for work).

+ ΔG: reaction is non-spontaneous and is referred to as endergonic (reaction requires energy).

Enzymology

In Chapter 2 we outlined the importance of enzymes as catalysts for the chemical reactions that take place within the body. In this section, which links with and leads on from bioenergetics, we examine in more detail the role of enzymes within the body. The branch of science that covers the structure and functioning of enzymes is called enzymology. An understanding of some further concepts relating to enzymes and their role within the body is beneficial in an exercise physiology context, prior to examining in detail the chemical reactions that take place within cellular metabolic pathways.

Enzymes are, with the exception of RNA ribozymes (a specialised type of enzyme), proteins that accelerate (catalyse) biochemical reactions without being altered by the process. They catalyse nearly all reactions within the body, increasing the speed of reaction. For instance, during maximal exercise ATP is required at a rate that would be impossible to supply without the action of enzymes.

In a laboratory, chemical reactions can be accelerated without enzymes through the use of external heat. By heating reactants the rate of reaction increases with rising temperature. The problem for humans is that we are homeotherms and sensitive to even small changes in temperature. A core body temperature over 42°C can be fatal, although muscle temperatures during high-intensity

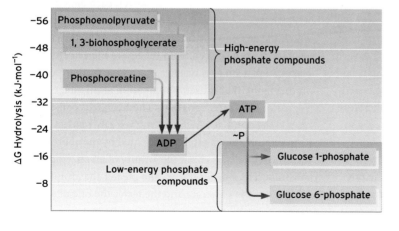

Figure 8.11 ATP as the high energy intermediate. Higher energy substrates such as phosphocreatine are able to phosphorylate ADP while ATP liberates sufficient energy to phosphorylate glucose.

exercise can reach this level without ill effect. Enzymes enable biochemical reactions to proceed at 10^5–10^7 times faster than they would otherwise, but within the temperature range tolerable for human life (30–42°C).

Enzymes are highly specialised and typically each will catalyse only a specific reaction, recognising only the substrates necessary for that particular reaction (the reactants in enzyme-catalysed reactions are known as substrates). As catalysts, enzymes lower the energy of activation required for a reaction by forming an enzyme-substrate complex which alters the shape of the substrate or brings substrates closer together to increase the likelihood of the reaction occurring. Each enzyme has a small active site which attracts the specific substrate(s) for the reaction it catalyses. Research suggests that substrates combine with enzymes either in a lock-and-key mechanism or by the enzyme altering its shape to incorporate the substrate(s).

> ### Knowledge integration question
>
> Why are enzymes important for cellular reactions?

Enzyme velocity

The velocity or rate at which an enzyme catalyses a reaction is dependent on a number of factors including temperature (as already mentioned), substrate concentration, enzyme concentration, cellular pH and ionic strength of the aqueous medium. Figure 8.12 provides an illustration of the effect of increasing temperature, substrate concentration and pH on enzyme activity. Enzymes cease to catalyse reactions at temperatures close to 0, but for each 10°C increase in temperature up to around 45–50°C, enzyme activity doubles. This is known as the Q_{10} quotient. The increase in enzymatic activity, which increases the reaction rate, occurs because the increase in temperature leads to an increase in the number of collisions between the substrate and the enzyme. Beyond 45–50°C, however, enzymes denature, which changes the shape of the protein and sharply decreases catalytic activity. This means that enzymes are ideally suited to catalysing biochemical reactions. This is one of the reasons why warm-ups are beneficial for sports performance. Enzyme activity and therefore ATP synthesis are enhanced by the increased muscle temperatures associated with a thorough warm-up.

The concentration or availability of a substrate will affect enzyme activity as shown in Figure 8.12b. The rate of the reaction initially increases linearly with increasing substrate concentration as more substrate molecules react

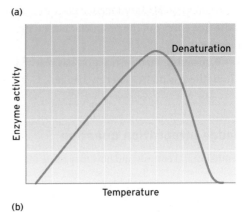
(a)

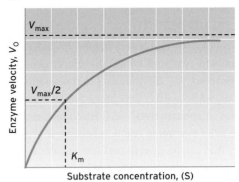
(b)

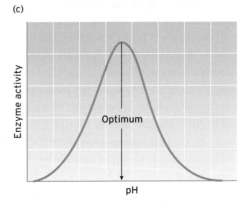
(c)

Figure 8.12 Effect of temperature, increasing substrate concentration and pH on enzyme activity.

with the enzyme. Ultimately, however, each enzyme has a V_{max}, that is, a maximal rate of enzyme activity, a point at which the enzyme is saturated and cannot further increase velocity. As can be seen from the figure the velocity line reaches a plateau as it reaches V_{max}. One further point on this figure that is useful to mention at this stage is the $V_{max}/2$ or **Michaelis constant**. The Michaelis constant represents the point at which enzyme velocity reaches half of its maximum and is often represented by the abbreviation K_m. The K_m tells us about the affinity of an enzyme for its substrate. The smaller the K_m the greater the affinity of the enzyme for the substrate and the faster the rate at which the reaction will proceed.

The catalytic activity of an enzyme is also dependent on the pH within its environment. As shown in Figure 8.12c all enzymes have an optimal pH range for most effective function; however, this is dependent on the location and reactions that they catalyse. Muscular enzymes operate most effectively within a pH range of 6.5–7.1, while in the stomach pepsin operates optimally at a pH of 2.0. Beyond their optimal range, just as for extremes of temperature, enzymes will start to denature.

Cellular regulation of enzyme activity

While the rate of an enzyme-catalysed reaction can be affected by substrate and enzyme concentration, temperature and pH, cellular regulation of enzyme activity, and therefore control of metabolic reactions, is brought about primarily through allostery, covalent modification and nervous-endocrine control. The fastest-acting regulation of enzyme activity, which occurs in milliseconds, is through **allostery**. Many enzymes, particularly those in the metabolic pathways, where control over speed of ATP synthesis is required, have multiple active sites. Enzymes have active sites which are available for substrate bonding (to form the enzyme-substrate complex which has been described). However, allosteric enzymes have additional active sites to which enzyme activators or inhibitors can bond. Indeed, it was in reference to these additional sites that the term allosteric was coined, from the Greek word 'allos' meaning 'other'. Allosteric activators and inhibitors, together refered to as allosteric effectors, bond to the additional active sites in order to regulate the activity of an enzyme. Various substrates, or molecules within the cellular environment, can serve as allosteric effectors and their role is particularly important for the control of metabolic pathways. For instance, as we will discuss in more detail in Chapter 10, the enzyme phosphofructokinase (PFK) plays an important role in controlling the rate of glycolysis, and the activity of PFK is in turn controlled by allosteric effectors. During exercise when the demand for ATP increases, PFK activator concentration rises, while the concentration of PFK inhibitors decreases. The net result of this allosteric effector change is a substantial increase in PFK activity and consequently a dramatic increase in the rate of glycolysis to meet the demands of exercise. Conversely, at times of rest the concentration of inhibitors rises and activators decreases resulting in a consequential fall in carbohydrate catabolism.

While allosteric regulation quickly moderates the rate of enzymatic activity, **covalent modification** can, within seconds, switch enzyme activity on or off. This regulatory modification occurs through the usually reversible bonding of a substrate to specific amino acids within the enzyme such as serine, histidine, tyrosine and threonine. One of the most common modifiers is inorganic phosphate which is attached to an enzyme through ATP hydrolysis. Interestingly, this enzyme phosphorylation, to regulate its activity, requires an enzyme itself, known as a *protein kinase*, to catalyse the reaction. The reverse process, dephosphorylation, is catalysed by another set of enzymes known as *protein phosphatases*. Covalent modification serves to activate some enzymes while it can inactivate other enzymes. By reversing the process, where possible, an enzyme can return to its pre-modified state. Enzymatic phosphorylation provides an important mechanism for controlling the rate of metabolism and is closely linked with the third regulatory mechanism, **nervous-endocrine control**. As was described in Chapter 3, hormones such as adrenaline are released during exercise to increase metabolism. The release of adrenaline serves to stimulate an increase in glycogen catabolism within muscle fibres (cells). This increase is brought about through the covalent modification of glycogen phosphorylase, the enzyme that catalyses the reaction to remove glucose, in the form of glucose-1-phosphate, from glycogen.

Classification of enzymes

Enzymes are classified in a number of ways and these reveal much about the function of the enzyme. Generally the first part of the name of an enzyme refers to the substrate with which it is associated, for instance creatine kinase catalyses the reversible reaction to form phosphocreatine from creatine and Pi. The second part of an enzyme name relates to the type of reaction it catalyses while the 'ase' indicates that the protein-based structure is an enzyme. **Kinases**, as with the term kinetics, are associated with work, for example the transfer of a phosphoryl group to or from a substrate. **Isomerases** and **mutases**, however, change the structure of the substrate, for example glucose phosphate isomerase, (discussed in the section on glycolysis in Chapter 10) changes the structure of the substrate in its reaction but does not alter the chemical composition. Another important enzyme category, within the cellular metabolic pathways, are the **dehydrogenases** which catalyse a specialised group of oxidation and reduction (redox) reactions (the loss or gaining of electrons). Dehydrogenases, such as lactate dehydrogenase, catalyse reactions that lead to the removal or addition of hydrogen atoms from or to a substrate.

Enzymes and cofactors

Enzymes are often associated with co-factors, which through participation in the reaction assist catalysis of the reaction. The B vitamins and many minerals such as zinc, magnesium and manganese serve as co-factors. Common examples within the metabolic pathways include riboflavin (vitamin B2) which forms the co-enzyme flavin adenine dinucleotide (FAD), Niacin (vitamin B3) which forms nicotinamide adenine dinucleotide (NAD^+), and pan-tothenic acid which forms Co-enzyme A (CoA). The links between enzymes and co-enzymes can be seen through the transfer of hydrogen atoms that occurs between NAD^+ and lactate dehydrogenase which is vital to fast-rate glycolysis.

Key points

The rate of enzyme activity is dependent on substrate and enzyme concentrations, as well as cellular temperature and pH.

Cells can regulate enzyme activity via allosteric effectors (bind to specific enzyme sites, can inhibit or activate enzyme), covalent modification (binding of substrate to amino acids within enzyme) or nervous-endocrine control.

8.2 Introduction to training methodology

Through study of exercise physiology, we examine the body's response to exercise and adaptations to training that occurs due to individual or multiple physiological stresses. This can relate to how we train to improve our own, our athlete's, or our team's sports performance, but equally it can relate to how exercise can contribute to improved health and well-being. Knowledge of the different aspects of fitness, as well as the principles that apply to developing training programmes, can help physical education teachers, coaches and health professionals.

The influence of well-being on sports performance and health

Our well-being, as an individual or an athlete, for health or sports performance, is affected by the interaction of the physiological, psychological, social-emotional, skill-related and spiritual factors that are depicted in Figure 8.13. While the primary focus of this textbook is upon the physiological factors that can affect health and performance, it should be

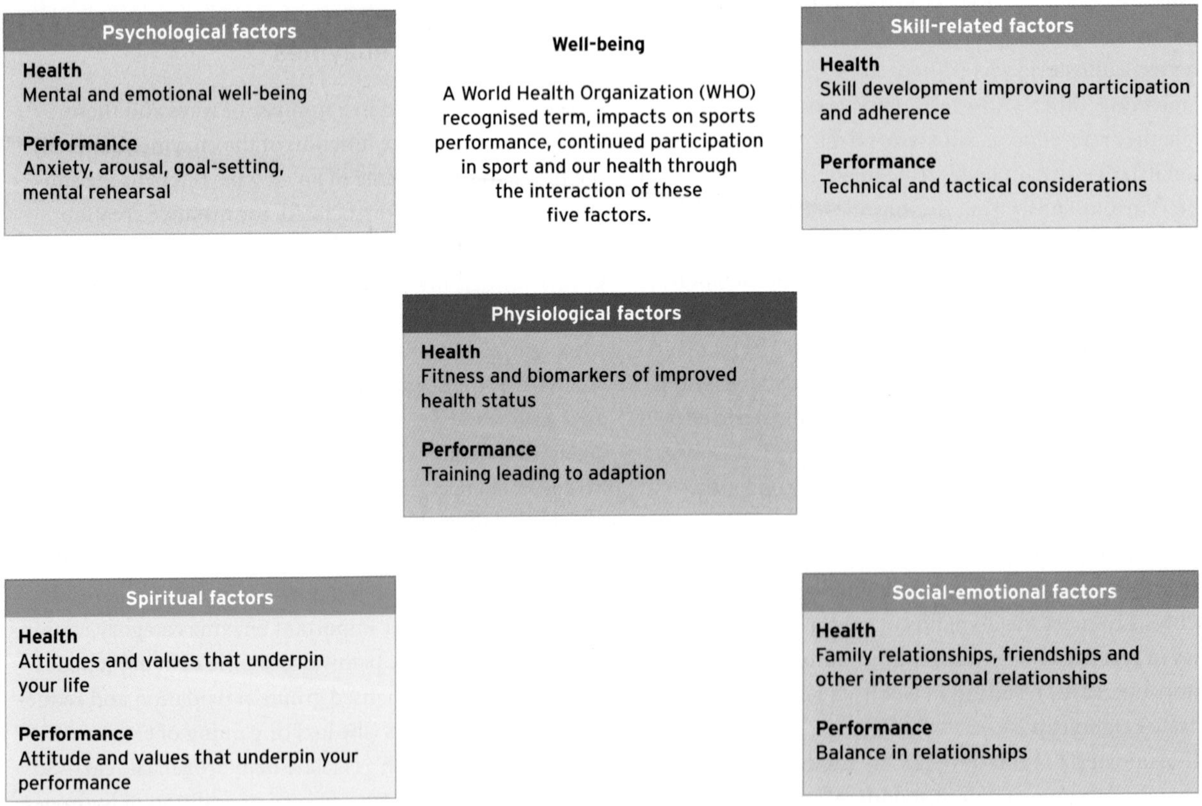

Psychological factors

Health
Mental and emotional well-being

Performance
Anxiety, arousal, goal-setting, mental rehearsal

Well-being

A World Health Organization (WHO) recognised term, impacts on sports performance, continued participation in sport and our health through the interaction of these five factors.

Skill-related factors

Health
Skill development improving participation and adherence

Performance
Technical and tactical considerations

Physiological factors

Health
Fitness and biomarkers of improved health status

Performance
Training leading to adaption

Spiritual factors

Health
Attitudes and values that underpin your life

Performance
Attitude and values that underpin your performance

Social-emotional factors

Health
Family relationships, friendships and other interpersonal relationships

Performance
Balance in relationships

Figure 8.13 The well-being model of sports performance and health.

kept in mind that actually all these factors interact to determine the well-being of an athlete or individual.

The relationship between, and the relative importance of, the individual components within the well-being model varies between individuals and across the lifespan. From a health perspective a large number of psychological factors can affect participation in sport and adherence to a training programme. Factors such as self-image and psychological readiness can impact upon an individual's decisions to participate in sport and physical activity. While many physical education coaching programmes advocate providing children with a variety of sports so that they can develop a range of motor skills and find a sport they like, there is evidence to suggest that adherence in sport is linked with the development of skills. With more technical and tactical knowledge, and skill in the sport, it appears that individuals develop more connection to that sport and are therefore more likely to continue long-term participation. Research clearly indicates that involvement in sport and physical activity improves fitness and a wide-range of biomedical markers, such as blood profiles, all of which can improve well-being. The attitudes and values a person holds determine the way they live their lives and can impact upon their health and wellbeing. While spirituality can relate to a particular religious belief, this is not the case for everyone and spiritual well-being is broader than a possible connection to a particular religion. It relates to the person's sense of self and how they bring meaning to the world and their purpose in life. Social factors, such as the relationship a person has with their family and team mates, can impact upon continued involvement in sport and upon well-being.

From a sports performance perspective, each of the factors in Figure 8.13 can impact upon well-being and therefore upon an athlete's performance in training and competition. Firstly, the psychological, skill-related and physiological components of a particular sport will vary according to the type of sport, such that the relative importance of each to golf, marathon running and rock climbing will differ. The interaction and relationship between the factors must be viewed as dynamic. At any one time an athlete's performance can be limited by any of the factors or their interaction. The relative importance of these components will change over time, between sports and individuals. The trick for us as athletes, coaches or physical educators seeking to improve performance, is to identify which of the components is the 'rate-limiter' at any particular stage in development. For example, in the sport of downriver kayaking, the inability to cross an eddy line to enter the downstream current could be due to variety of factors. The kayaker might not be able to cross the eddy line

due to technical (skill-related) errors, such as a not having the whole blade in the water, not being physically powerful enough (physiological) to punch through the eddy line, not having a good relationship with the instructor (social-emotional) and therefore not believing the teaching points provided, or having high anxiety levels (psychological) created by the thought of capsize. A good teacher or coach can spot the correct rate-limiter and alter the session or activity to address this issue and improve success.

Key points

Well-being for an athlete or someone wishing to improve their health is determined by the interaction of the following five factors:

1. physiological
2. skill-related
3. psychological
4. social-emotional
5. spiritual

As performers we need to identify which factor is the rate-limiter at any stage in our development.

Fitness for health and performance

A major part of the physiological aspects of sport, for health and performance, concerns fitness. To develop any sort of training programme for a sport or to generally improve health, we must ask some fundamental questions about the nature of the activity. One of the key questions has to do with fitness and how it can help improve health-related or performance-related fitness. From a sports performance perspective, a greater fitness level can help to improve performance, whether this is seen through quicker times, improved technical quality or improved decision making due to lower overall stress on the body. From a health perspective, being fitter can improve an individual's overall well-being and lower the risk of disease. It may also impact on other components such as psychological feelings of self-worth and social feelings of belonging.

At its most basic level, to be fit is to be healthy or in good athletic condition. From a health perspective, for instance, an individual could engage in a wide variety of sports to improve their cardiovascular fitness. Fitness for sports performance, however, has been shown to be highly sport-specific. Fitness for marathon running means something very different to that required for rugby or shot putt. As an athlete, teacher or coach, you must be able to identify the components of fitness that are the most important to a particular sport. The next section outlines the major components of fitness that will impact to a greater or lesser extent on a performer, depending on their sport. Each fitness component is described in more detail in this or one of the subsequent chapters. In developing a training programme it is important to identify which of these components are fundamental to improving performance.

> ### Key point
>
> Fitness is specific to each sport – an athlete, their teacher or coach must be able to identify the key components of fitness for that particular sport.

The components of fitness

The components of fitness, as illustrated in Table 8.2, can be divided into those that are broadly physiologically trainable and those that are highly skill-related and therefore perhaps most closely linked to the technique and tactics of a particular sport. For instance, aerobic endurance is an important component of fitness for distance running, many swimming disciplines and cycling; as a consequence, there would be similarities in the types of training undertaken by athletes in each sport. However, due to the highly specific nature of fitness, the training would employ the same exercise mode as the sport, i.e. running, swimming or cycling. It is for this reason that triathletes have to train in all three disciplines to maximise their performance. The key concern from a health perspective would be the physiologically trainable factors rather than the skill-related factors. While the mode of exercise for improvement in aerobic endurance or cardiovascular fitness for sports performance would be important, from a health perspective this would be less of a concern than the fact that training was undertaken and was being enjoyed.

Many of the trainable components of fitness are closely linked with the energy generation mechanisms.

As a consequence, the components of fitness, as shown in Table 8.2, are described in the energy-specific context and chapter within the text. Flexibility, however, because of its importance to so many sports regardless of the energy demands, is discussed in this chapter. In addition, because of the high skill-related dimension to agility, balance, co-ordination and reaction time, these components of fitness are also covered in this chapter.

Flexibility

The terms flexibility and mobility are often used interchangeably to refer to the range of motion about the joints of the body. *Mobility* does indeed refer to the range of motion about a joint. *Flexibility*, however, is more than this and also includes the stretch in the soft tissues that surround the joint. There are two forms of flexibility that can be identified–active and passive flexibility. *Active flexibility* refers to the ability of the muscles around a joint moving a limb through a range of motion. For example in the sport of rock climbing the ability to raise a foot high to reach a higher foothold requires active flexibility. The greater a climber's active flexibility the higher the hold he or she would be able to utilise. *Passive flexibility* refers to the range of motion through which a muscle can be placed with the aid of other muscles or gravity: simply put – stretching. Sitting and stretching to touch your toes would be an example of static stretching when the arms and the weight of the body (gravity) can be used to increase the range of motion.

Often included in warm-up and cool-down routines, flexibility is a significant component of fitness for sports performance and health. For example, a high level of flexibility in the shoulders, trunk and hips are essential for gymnasts. For the hips alone, gymnasts must have a high degree of flexion, extension, abduction and adduction to be able to perform a basic move such as splits to the front or side (box splits). A lack of flexibility can easily become

Table 8.2 The components of fitness and the chapter where each is covered.

Physiologically trainable components of fitness	Skill-related fitness components
Flexibility (this chapter) Anaerobic power (Chapter 9) Speed (Chapter 9) Strength (Chapter 9) Anaerobic endurance (Chapter 10) Muscular endurance (Chapter 10) Aerobic power (Chapter 11) Aerobic endurance (Chapter 12) Body composition (Chapter 13)	Agility } Coordination } Dynamic balance Balance Reaction time (The skill-related components of fitness are described in this chapter)

a rate-limiter for improvements in many sports including gymnastics and dancing. However, hyper-mobility is also a concern for gymnasts where too much shoulder flexibility can lead to shoulder dislocations. A balance, therefore, between flexibility and strength training must be maintained to protect joints along with maintaining an appropriate range of motion.

Dynamic balance

Physiologists describe three distinct components of fitness that most readily relate to the skilful aspects of a sport and these are balance, agility and coordination. In a sports performance context, these motor control aspects are perhaps more meaningfully combined and described as *dynamic balance*. In a health context, these three aspects are less often monitored as, in general, they have less relevance to the activities of daily life than components such as aerobic endurance and body composition. Balance is the ability to hold a static position such as a handstand for a length of time under control, while agility relates to a moving form of balance such that an agile athlete is able to make a series of movements but remain in balance. Coordination is the ability to effect efficient movements to achieve a goal. As individual components, they have a varying relationship to all sports depending upon the activity, but are perhaps more meaningful when combined as 'dynamic balance'. In a sporting context this refers to the ability to use skilful co-ordinated movement to maintain position or make progress on land, on or in water, or in the air. Balance and agility, as part of this movement are fundamental to the skilful aspects of any particular sport. There are similarities between the dynamic balance demands of some sports such as boxing, karate and taekwondo; or surfing, skiing and snowboarding; or football, rugby and field hockey. As a skill-related component of fitness, dynamic balance retains a uniqueness to it that requires practice of that specific activity to improve coordination, balance and agility.

Reaction time

Reaction time is the interval between the introduction of a stimulus and the beginning of a response, for example, how quickly a sprinter reacts, after the gun, to break from the starting blocks. It is a key aspect of sports performance and as such is defined by physiologists as one of the components of fitness. However, reaction time is less trainable in a physiological context than components such as strength or aerobic endurance and is best developed as part of skills training for any sport. Reaction time training for sprinters

is different when compared to tennis players or judo players, and so training for this component of fitness should be developed on a sport-specific basis. In a health context, as for dynamic balance, reaction time training would seldom be included in a planned exercise intervention.

Key points

As a teacher or coach, it is important to identify the fitness components of a particular sport, along with an individual's goals, to devise an appropriate training programme.

The identified fitness components should also form the basis for fitness testing.

Knowledge integration question

Which of the components of fitness could be classified as most important for health and which relate most to sports performance?

Assessing physiological fitness and the success of a training programme

There is a wide variety of tests that can be administered to assess fitness and training adaptations for any individual component of fitness. The tests commonly used are described in the following chapters and relate to the chapter-specific components of fitness. After identifying the components of fitness fundamental to a sport, it is necessary to decide upon the most appropriate battery of tests to assess an athlete's fitness for that sport, or to monitor the success of an ongoing training programme.

There are three main reasons for assessing fitness, and why regular fitness assessment might be important to an athlete, a coach, or a health professional. Firstly, by testing an individual's level of fitness prior to prescribing a training programme, the intensity and duration of the programme can be matched to his or her test results. Secondly, by carrying out tests before and after a training programme, they provide you, and the athlete, with valuable feedback about the success of the programme. It is important for all involved to know whether a training programme is bringing about the desired results.

A positive improvement in fitness can serve to reinforce to the athlete that the hard work in training is worthwhile (assisting motivation). Results from tests conducted at the end of a first training phase can also provide excellent information for programme development for the next phase of training. Thirdly, conducting regular fitness assessments helps to provide a more complete picture or profile of the athlete. In addition to fitness testing the following parameters are important to help the athlete and their coach assess progress towards agreed training and competition goals. Video analysis of technique can be an important part of skill development and psychological profiling and intervention strategies. Success is also dependent on good communication between the athlete and their coach. For health professionals prescribing exercise to improve an individual's health, each of these three factors could be applied to monitoring the progress of that individual. By testing regularly, we obtain more knowledge about the success of any training intervention.

Building up a physiological profile

For all athletes, especially those still growing, it is useful to keep a record of height and weight. A record of the health history of an athlete can help with monitoring their general well-being, along with monitoring evidence of possible over-training. Monitoring dietary intake can help an individual to modify their diet where necessary, and an athlete to monitor nutrition for repair and recovery from training and competition. Keeping previous race, performance and test records is a really useful way of monitoring development for an athlete. Although most often used as a coaching tool, a video clip diary, kept over time, can additionally provide an excellent record of performance development in skill-based tests. Records of physical changes, health history, diet, performance and test results, together build a more complete long-term picture of an athlete (physiological profile).

Key point

Keeping race results, video clips, height, weight, nutrition and health history records for a performer can form the basis of monitoring long-term athlete development.

Physiological fitness tests

The battery of tests selected for any individual or sport should be based on the key components of fitness for their sport or goals. The key components of fitness will be different for each sport or individual and the exact schedule of tests selected should reflect such differences. When designing a battery of tests, be inventive. The tests described in the following chapters are examples that could be adapted for a particular sport dependent on the demands of that particular sport.

There are many sports where all of the components of fitness are relevant to successful performance, or where a person wants to improve all aspects of fitness. This is where the skill of the coach or health professional is important. The battery of tests and subsequent training programme developed should be based on the most important aspects of fitness at any specific stage. If an exercise physiologist tried to test all possible components of fitness in a battery of tests and devise a training programme for each there would be no time for other aspects of training for an athlete or enough time in the day for an individual trying to improve their fitness. The coach, or health professional has to prioritise the key aspects of fitness for each intervention or phase of training. As flexibility is an important component of fitness for many sports, regardless of the energy demands, a number of tests for assessing flexibility are described in the following section.

Key point

Fitness tests should be specific to the sport and its components of fitness. They should be conducted before and after each phase of training.

Flexibility tests

There is a variety of generic measurements that can be used to assess flexibility. One of the most commonly used, as a measure of generalised flexibility, is the sit and reach test, shown in Figure 8.14. The sit and reach test assesses low back and hip flexibility and must be conducted after a participant has thoroughly warmed up and is ready to make a maximal stretch. The participant removes shoes and socks and places their heels against the box. In one slow, smooth movement they reach forward as far as possible, keeping their legs flat against the floor. The best of three trials (cm) is recorded. The advantage with this test is that it is simple to administer and relatively quick to complete. As a result it has proved a popular estimate of overall body flexibility. However, when compared with direct measurements, research indicates that it does not have a good correlation with hamstring flexibility and has a poor agreement with low back flexibility. In addition, it lacks sport specificity so might be best used as a measure of flexibility in a health context. Flexibility for sports performance is perhaps best measured using specific tests developed for a particular sport and based on the demands of the sport.

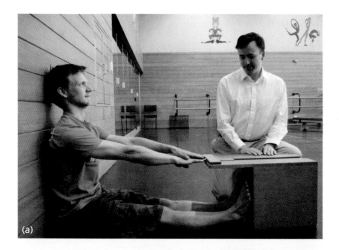

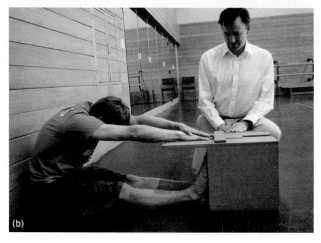

Figure 8.14 The Sit and Reach Test: the measurement box (a) starting position and (b) a participant completing an assessment (finishing position). Notice the participant has bare feet and straight legs. (*Source*: Simon Fryer)

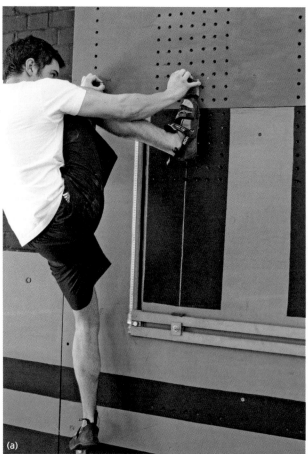

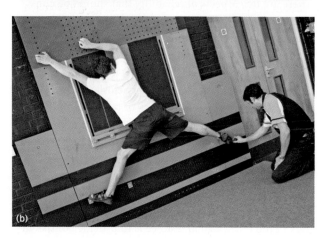

Figure 8.15 Sport-specific flexibility assessment for rock-climbing, (a) the high step test and (b) the lateral reach test (*Source*: Nicky Norris)

Figure 8.15 provides an illustration of two flexibility tests that were developed for the sport of rock climbing, where hip flexion and abduction is required to move between footholds during the ascent of a route. Both tests, called the high step test (HST) and lateral reach test (LRT) have been validated and checked for reliability for use with climbers of all ability levels. The two tests examine a climber's limits for a high step and abduction movement as illustrated. After a thorough warm-up, participants complete three trials on each test using their preferred leg for the high step or abduction movement. Both tests are conducted with the participant wearing climbing shoes. For the HST, the foot must be raised and placed on the wall between the shoulder and midline. The distance from the ground to the bottom of the climbing shoe is recorded in cm. For the LRT, the hand hold, a campus board rung is placed at shoulder height centrally to a 2.44 m-wide wall. The distance from the stationary foothold to the outside of the abducted climbing shoe is recorded in cm. In both tests the movement should be made in a smooth, continuous movement, and held stationary for 3 s during marking.

Guidelines for administration of testing

There are a number of useful guidelines that can be followed to assist with selecting existing tests, designing new ones and deciding upon the order for a battery of tests.

Test validity

A number of questions should be asked when considering the validity of a test. Does the test measure what it really should? For example, do the intensity and duration selected assess the aerobic system, the anaerobic system or a combination of both? How does the test match the physiological requirements of the sport for which it has been selected? Is it sufficiently specific to the sport? There are many tests that can be employed for each component of fitness and the most valid are the ones that should be selected for a battery of tests. An important consideration is whether the test has been statistically validated for use with that sport, and whether there are any results from other groups for validation and comparative purposes.

Test reliability

There are two aspects of reliability that should be considered when selecting a fitness test. These are the intra-tester (test-retest) reliability and inter-tester reliability. If a test is reliable, then when performed on two separate occasions (with no change in fitness), the results of the two tests should be the same or very close. If scores are different this may be due to a lack of test-retest reliability or due to an inconsistent measuring technique of the tester. In a similar way, there may be situations where two people carry out the testing for an athlete. In a reliable test the performer would achieve their score regardless of who was testing, in which case the test can be said to have inter-tester reliability. It should not matter who is carrying out the test – a good test needs to provide consistent results.

> ### Key point
>
> Tests need to be valid and reliable measures of performance. An analogy for this can be drawn from archery. The validity of a test refers to the ability of the arrow to hit the target and the reliability refers to the consistency (close grouping) of the arrows.

Test order

The order in which a battery of tests is organised will impact on an athlete's performance in each test. Ideally the tests should be ordered so as to minimise the effect on subsequent tests. For example, scores for strength tests will be negatively influenced by any maximal aerobic test carried out before the strength test, whereas aerobic results, after an appropriate rest, are not detrimentally affected by strength assessment. The following assessment schedule is therefore proposed:

- Collection of subject characteristic data (age, height, weight, body composition)
- Maximal strength tests
- Flexibility and agility tests
- Sprint tests
- Maximal aerobic or anaerobic tests
- Muscular endurance tests

If concerned about the influence of one test upon the score achieved on the later tests, testing could be completed over two days rather than one.

It is useful to keep a note of the order of testing as when conducting a repeat testing session, the battery of tests should be completed in the same order, with the same recovery time between tests, as for the previous assessment. This is to ensure that changes in results are related to changes in fitness rather than a change in the order of testing. Similarly if testing is conducted in the field, as opposed to in the laboratory with controlled environmental conditions, the weather and equipment used by an athlete should be taken in to account. That is not to say testing should be abandoned if there is a change in environmental factors, but they should certainly be recorded and taken into account when evaluating results. The period before testing can also have an influence on results. For instance, a heavy training session the night before testing can influence test performance the next day. When administering a battery of tests, a coach or health professional should try to mimic as closely as possible the lead in to the previous tests and, where possible, allow participants to take tests in a rested state.

Developing sport-specific tests

Generic tests can be used successfully to assess fitness for many sports. However, the performance demands of some sports make the development of sport-specific fitness tests highly desirable. With knowledge of the sport, the structure of generic tests, and the guidelines for administering tests, it is possible to develop tests that apply uniquely to a specific sporting context. A well designed test will be able to differentiate athletes of different performance levels and reveal training-related improvements in performance.

The duration, intensity or nature of the test should reflect the sport for which the assessment is being devised. For example, match racing in sailing requires some of the crew to perform 'coffee-grinding' to raise and lower the sails. A test for such crew members would be better designed according to the duration and intermittent nature of coffee-grinding during a race and performed on sport-specific apparatus rather than using a cycle ergometer. Tests such as the basketball sprint test (refer to Chapter 10 and Figure 10.12 for details) could be readily adapted to meet the needs of other specific sports. The structure of the basketball sprint test could be adapted to match the demands of another sport although the distances, intervals, number of repetitions and recoveries would have to be modified accordingly.

Key point

A variety of tests can be used to assess a training programme. Choose or develop ones that are the most specific to your sport and the type of training being undertaken.

Developing and designing training programmes

To improve fitness for a sport or for health purposes, a coach or health professional should develop individualised training programmes. Ideally such a programme would be based on the results of a sport- or goal-specific fitness assessment carried out prior to programme planning. This section covers the key components to be considered in the development of a training programme, from principles to guide the training to the general aspects of strength and conditioning training.

Principles of training

A number of robust principles of training have been identified by exercise physiologists and should be considered by a coach or health professional involved in the development of a training programme. The transfer of these theoretical principles to coaching practice, however, is not always simple, as highlighted by John Hellemans, the Dutch National Triathlon Coach (Sport in Action, p. 261).

Overload principle

In order to effect an improvement in fitness, a training programme must present an overload to the systems of the body. An overload is a training stimulus that is over and above that normally encountered. For example, if a previously sedentary person began an exercise programme, all training undertaken would represent an overload. Training for a period of time with an overload will bring about physiological adaptations for that individual, or in other words, will result in improvements in their fitness. This training principle must be adhered to during the design and implementation of any training programme. To improve fitness we must train with loads that are above those we would normally experience. To do this we can adjust the frequency, intensity or time (FIT) for which we train. Frequency is the number of times per week that we train, intensity is the level at which we work (for example at what percentage of our maximum heart rate we work) and time is the duration of each training session. Each of these parameters can be manipulated in programme design to create a training overload through which to achieve an improvement in fitness.

Progression principle

The principle of progression is very closely linked with that of overload. As physiological adaptations take and the participant becomes fitter, a training intensity that was previously an overload will decrease in its difficulty, and its effectiveness in stimulating training adaptations will decrease. *To continue to progress in training the FIT of training needs to be adjusted to cater for improvements in fitness.* The training overload must be progressively increased. A clear example of this can be related to weight training. A coach decides that a resistance (weight) training programme would improve an athlete's performance, and based on results from a fitness test, designs a training programme involving three sessions per week at a local gym. The load for each exercise in the initial weeks will represent an overload, however, as the athlete gets fitter, the weight lifted will need to be increased to maintain the overload and progress. A simple way to do this is to use the 2-for-2 rule. If the athlete can complete two repetitions more than planned in the last set of an exercise over two consecutive sessions, the training weight needs to be increased. For example, if 3 sets of 10 repetitions of bicep curls were included in the programme, and in the last set, for two sessions in a row, the athlete could complete

12 repetitions it would be time to increase the weight or resistance. By adjusting the FIT you can manipulate any aspect of your training to maintain a progressive overload.

Key point

A progressive overload must be applied during training to continue making fitness gains.

In weight training the 2-for-2 principle can be used to ensure a training overload is maintained.

Specificity principle

The specificity principle refers to the concept that improvements in fitness are directly related to the type of training undertaken. While there might be minor cardiovascular benefits for running having followed a swim training programme, the major improvements would be seen in swim performance. There are three important aspects of specificity that apply to training programmes.

Strength training specificity

Strength training (also referred to as resistance or weight training) is commonly employed by athletes from many sports to help improve performance. This form of training can help improve strength, power, speed and muscular endurance. Coaches and health professionals can tailor a training programme to develop some or all of these aspects of fitness depending on their relevance to a specific sport or training goal. Firstly, the exercises selected should be specific to the activity chosen. For example lower-body exercises for a cyclist should take priority over upper-body exercises, and movements made with weights should match as closely as possible movements made in the activity. Secondly, strength gains have been found to match the speed at which training was carried out. Therefore, if training was carried out at slow speed to develop strength, the maximal expression of strength would be found moving at that slow speed. If an athlete is training for an explosive event that requires power, then training speeds should reflect this to maximise possible gains. The importance of strength training specificity, optimising the transfer of training gains to a specific sport, is highlighted in the Sport in Action articles by Sasissa de Vries (p. 260), a Dutch triathlete, and her coach John Hellemans (p. 261). (See also 'Classic research summary' on p. 263).

Conditioning training specificity

Training results are specific to the muscles trained and there is often little transfer to other muscles even between events like running and swimming. A classic illustration (featured as the classic research summary on page 263) of this involved 15 healthy but sedentary subjects who completed swim training for one hour per day, three days per week, for 10 weeks. All subjects carried out swimming and running tests at the start and end of the study. Not surprisingly, the results found an 11% improvement in the swimming test scores for the group, but only a 1.5% change in the running test results. When training for a specific sport, be it cycling, swimming, running or any other requiring conditioning training, the overload should engage the specific muscles and include aspects of training that match the intensity and duration of the sport. In other words, if you wish to get fit for rowing you need to train in your boat as a regular part of your programme. In a similar fashion to the speed aspect of resistance training, the conditioning aspects of training should match the activity for which you are training – sprint training for anaerobic sprint events, primarily endurance-based training for aerobic events and a mix of intensities for intermittent sports such as rugby, tennis and water polo.

Programme specificity

There are a number of aspects with regard to programme design where specificity needs to be addressed. It is important for the programme planner to understand the relative contribution of aerobic and anaerobic pathways to ATP generation for a specific sport. The key aspect is for the training to relate to the intensity and duration of the sport. Training should mimic or 'model' the relative contributions.

In developing a training programme the focus of training should move from more generalised to more specific training at the start of a competition season or as an important event draws nearer. Periodisation, a specific form of training programme planning, which is described in more detail in the next section, breaks a programme into phases which increase in specialisation as an important competition approaches. The time at which training is carried out, at least for some sessions, should match competition times as closely as possible. Research indicates that adaptations to training are specific to the time of day during which the training took place. If training for an event which will take place in the morning it is better if at least some of the training is completed at the same time of day. In a similar way research has found that modelling competition in training can help make adaptations specific to the event.

Regression principle

When an athlete stops training they will lose any fitness gains they have made relatively rapidly. The effects of detraining can be seen very clearly in anyone who has broken a leg or arm and had it kept in plaster for six weeks. When the plaster is removed the resulting atrophy (loss in muscle size) is due to detraining or regression. The regression principle states that ceasing training, dependent upon the period and degree of detraining (ranging from normal active life but no training to complete bed rest), will result in a loss of fitness gains made through previous training. This has clear implications for breaks in training or off-season phases and the need to maintain some level of fitness. It is for this reason that many top athletes have maintenance programmes to retain a basic level of fitness before pre-season training. The same principle can guide the planning of a training programme for any level of athlete or for someone training to improve their fitness for health reasons.

Individualisation principle

If two rugby centres commenced the same training programme, the response of each would vary for each aspect of training. The individualisation principle is a sound coaching principle as well as a physiological one. Just as skill development sessions should be developed on an individual basis, training programmes should be developed in response to each performer's fitness assessment results and their training goals. Optimal training benefits are obtained through individually developed programmes. This does not, however, mean that all training should be carried out individually. During training, athletes will benefit from having sessions conducted individually, in pairs, small groups and larger groups throughout the programme.

Variation principle

Adding variety, such as by changing the number of athletes training at a particular session, the groups, the type of session, the warm-up or other aspect of the training programme can help with motivation and alleviate boredom with training. Dependent upon the level of competition, the training volume for an athlete can be over 1,000 hours per year, so the athlete or their coach needs to add variety to the programme to maintain motivation and enthusiasm. Variation in training loads can help not only with motivation, but can also assist in avoiding overtraining illnesses. Training close to your maximum in every session can overstress the body. Planning a combination of hard and easy training days into a training programme can help an athlete mentally and physically cope with the required volume of training and help to avoid illnesses or injuries.

This can be achieved by manipulating the FIT in a training programme, a central aspect of the next section which discusses periodisation, the long-term planning of a training programme.

Periodisation

Periodisation is based upon the General Adaptation Syndrome (GAS) – the body responds to a situation of stress by first showing *alarm reaction* (shock to the body and muscle soreness), then *resistance (adaptation)* which leads to improvement of performance, and finally *exhaustion* if the stimulus is maintained over too long a period of time. In response to strength and conditioning, the stress arises from the different forms of exercise encountered during training. However, in its broadest sense, stress is the reaction of the body to any demand. Figure 8.16 provides an illustration of

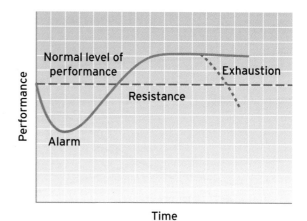

Figure 8.16 General adaptation syndrome (GAS) adapted from Selye (1956)

the GAS. Periodisation is a system of training programme design through which a performer can best develop their training over time, to peak for a major event or for a competition season, without going into the exhaustion phase.

Since the original model of periodisation was proposed by Matveyev in 1966, a number of variations in such planning have been created to suit athletes from different sports. Athletes from any sport and level of performance now have a wide range of periodisation options from which to develop an appropriate training programme. In addition to avoiding overtraining, periodising training can help avoid boredom, and allow an athlete to mentally break a whole year of training into manageable blocks. Having a phased programme, and knowledge of what is coming next in preparation for an event, helps an athlete cope with the training volumes to be completed. The athlete can see clearly where a specific session fits into the whole programme and can keep track of his or her progress.

The concept behind periodisation is to divide the training year into distinct phases. These phases build upon one another to prepare an athlete for a specific event or season of competition. Programmes can be designed over a short or long period of time and developed individually for an athlete. The possible phases within a periodised programme are shown in Table 8.3. The most common length

of time for a periodised programme would be a one-year plan; this is dependent on the level of performance and age of the athlete(s). The phases in a periodised programme have specific names. A macrocycle is the largest unit of a programme such as a training year. Macrocycles are subdivided into a number of mesocycles which last for one to several months. Mesocycles are comprised of a number of microcycles which are typically one week long. By structuring a programme in this way, it is possible for an athlete to put the next training session in context with the whole week's training, and to visualise how that week links to the next mesocycle and how the full programme leads to the event for which they are training.

Key point

Periodisation, dividing the training year into manageable and progressive phases, is an excellent way to set realistic goals for an athlete and to enable him or her to identify exactly where they are in the progress towards a main event or competition season.

Programme design

The basis of the success of periodised training is the variation in the volume (quantity) and intensity (quality) of training. Figure 8.17 provides a generalised model of periodisation and the relationship between the volume and intensity of training. The coach of an athlete needs to manage the volume and intensity of training through a programme so as to avoid overtraining and injury. During the early stages, the volume of training is emphasised over the intensity. As an athlete progresses through a programme, the emphasis would shift towards increased intensity and reduced training volume. As can be seen, the model training programme (macrocycle) is divided into four mesocycles. The mesocycles would be divided into a series of microcycles, but these are not shown on the generalised

Table 8.3 Phases within a periodised training programme.

Period of Training	
Long-term – lifetime programme Four-year–Olympic cycle	Marcocycles
One-year programme One-month programme	Mesocycle
One-week's training One-day or one training session	Microcycles

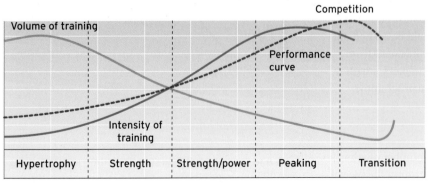

Figure 8.17 General model of periodisation

model. The hypertrophy phase of the model represents a preparatory phase and is designed to 'get the body ready to train' concentrating on increasing muscle mass and endurance. This is followed by a strength phase, towards the end of which one is likely see the cross-over between intensity and volume of training, with the quantity decreasing to allow a greater focus on the quality of the sessions. The strength and the strength/power phases represent the key phases of training, when the hard work is completed by the performer, ready for the final peaking phase that tapers training for the competition.

Key point

A periodised training programme is divided into four stages:

➤ Hypertrophy phase – preparation of body for hard training to follow; high volume, low intensity
➤ Strength phase – provides strength base; volume of training reduced, intensity increased
➤ Strength/power phase – great focus on session quality; continued volume reduction and intensity increase
➤ Peaking phase – final preparation for competition; low-quantity but high-quality training

An example programme

It is perhaps useful in understanding periodisation, to be able to examine a sample programme that was developed for a real athlete. The example included is one prepared for a judo player preparing for the 2001 World Championships, at which the player won a silver medal. The training year ran from September to September and included a number of preparation competitions through which the athlete continued to train and two competitions (European and World Championships) for which the athlete peaked. The programme included all strength and conditioning sessions for the competitive year, along with time allowed for travelling and competing in events. The information for the athlete included an overview of the entire macrocycle and details of each mesocycle, including re-assessment dates. Each microcycle lasted for one week and the programme included the training for each day of that week. The in-depth aspects of the programme provide details of the training programme for the athlete in the last preparation phase before the World Championships. A detailed World Champion preparation spreadsheet is available to download from the Companion Website.

As can be seen from the programme, at the end of the second and third phases there is an unloading week, which is designed to provide a drop in volume and intensity of training in order to avoid overtraining and to provide a psychological motivation by adding variety in the training programme.

Periodisation and fitness assessment

Fitness testing is included for any training programme to monitor whether a devised programme is working. Specificity, an important principle of training also applies to the choice of test battery. At the start of a macrocycle, for instance at the start of a training year, a complete battery of testing might be carried out to assess baseline fitness levels. From these results, the training programme can be developed with re-testing phases being linked with the completion of each specific mesocycle. For instance, the emphasis at the end of a strength phase could usefully be placed upon strength tests. It is important to know whether strength gains have been made as a result of the programme. If strength has not improved, the programme might not have included the correct exercises, repetitions and sets to bring about an improvement and may need alteration for future events.

Strength and conditioning

From a physiological perspective, sport- or goal-specific strength and conditioning form the cornerstones of any training programme or exercise prescription. Strength and conditioning programmes for a sport should be designed specifically around that sport, while for improved health the focus should be upon the individual's own training goals. Strength training involves the use of free and machine weights primarily to improve strength or power. As strength training is so closely linked with power, which is the focus of Chapter 9, this aspect of training is considered in more detail in that chapter. Conditioning training applies primarily to improvements in cardiovascular and muscular functioning, leading to improved aerobic and/or anaerobic performance. Conditioning training within a training programme should be closely linked to the energy demands of the sport or the health goal. As a consequence, energy-system-specific conditioning is considered within each of the subsequent chapters. There are a number of general concepts that apply to most forms of conditioning training that can usefully be covered at this point.

Conditioning training

This aspect of a training programme involves anaerobic and aerobic training specific to the intensity and duration of a sport. Table 8.4 provides an overview of the various

Table 8.4 Anaerobic and aerobic conditioning training methods.

Type of training	System trained	Covered in	Intensity	Repetition	Sets	Duration of repetitions
Sprint training	Anaerobic	Chapter 9	90-100% of maximum effort	5 - 10	1 - 5	5 - 30 s
Anaerobic intervals	Anaerobic	Chapters 10	85-100% of maximum effort	3 - 10	1 - 3	10 - 90 s
Medium-paced intervals	Aerobic	Chapter 11	70-80% of maximum heart rate	1 - 3	1	3 - 10 min
Fast-paced intervals	Aerobic	Chapter 11	80-90% of maximum heart rate	1 - 3	1	1 - 5 min
Fartlek* or speedplay	Aerobic	Chapter 11	70-85% of maximum heart rate	1	1	40 - 60 min
Long slow distance training	Aerobic	Chapter 11	50-70% of maximum heart rate	1	1	40 - 60 min

*Fartlek is a Swedish word meaning speedplay and refers to a form of training where the intensity is varied from easy to medium- to high-paced throughout the session.

forms of conditioning that can be undertaken as part of a training programme, which allow for a great deal of variety within a programme. One of the most versatile conditioning modes is interval training. In this type of training the repetitions, sets, interval lengths and recovery can be altered to match the intensity and duration requirements for a specific sport or training goal. For sprint training and short-duration interval training, the method for measuring each of the efforts is how close the athlete is to his or her maximum. As can be seen from Table 8.4, the recommended intensity for all other conditioning sessions is provided relative to maximal heart rate. As a consequence, it is beneficial to use heart rate as an indicator of effort during these training sessions. The development of heart rate monitors has made it relatively easy and inexpensive to monitor training effort which holds a great advantage in terms of accuracy of training intensity.

The more exact a coach or athlete is in monitoring training, the more accurately he or she can evaluate the success of the programme. Prescribing exercise based on a percentage of HR maximum (HR_{max}) is a very useful way to ensure that an athlete is training within the prescribed training zone. The most accurate way to calculate HR_{max} is for the athlete to complete a $\dot{V}O_{2max}$ or to design a test to take the subject to their maximum effort over a period of 8 to 12 minutes. Ideally the test should be sport and training specific, i.e. running based for distance runners. The HR_{max} recorded can subsequently be used to calculate the individual training zones (e.g. 50–70% HR_{max}) for conditioning training. A very common and simple method through which to estimate HR_{max} can be to use the 220–age formula which was first suggested by Fox et al. (1971). For example, if a performer was aged 23 years their predicted HR_{max} would be 197 beats per minute (beat·min^{-1}). This formula is based upon the principle that at birth maximal heart rate is around 220 beat·min^{-1} and decreases with age, at a rate of approximately one beat per year of life. Since this formula for estimation of HR_{max} was first proposed there have been many subsequent studies suggesting alternatives. One of the most useful for males and

CALCULATION

Estimation of maximal heart rate – the Tanaka et al. (2001) method

For a participant aged 23

$HR_{max} = 208 - (0.7 \times age)$

$HR_{max} = 208 - (0.7 \times 23)$

$HR_{max} = 208 - 16.1$

$HR_{max} = 191.9$

$HR_{max} = 192$ beat·min^{-1}

Table 8.5 Example target heart rate zones using results from a HR_{max} test as well as the 220-age and Tanaka et al. formulas.

Type of aerobic training	Intensity	Target HR zones – Max test	Target HR zones – 220-age	Target HR zones – Tanaka
Medium-paced continuous Training	70-80% of maximum HR	132-150	138-158	164-154
Fast-paced continuous training	80-90% of maximum HR	150-169	158-177	154-173
Fartlek* or speedplay	70-85% of maximum HR	132-160	158-167	134-163
Long slow distance training	50-70% of maximum HR	94-132	99-138	96-134

Note: Heart rate zones are calculated for a 23-year-old participant with a HR_{max} of 188 as directly measured, 197 using 220-age, and 192 using the Tanaka et al. (2001) formula.

females across all age groups was proposed by Tanaka et al. (2001) after testing over 18,000 participants. If estimating HR_{max} it appears best to use the Tanaka et al. method.

Table 8.5 provides an illustration of the range in determination of HR_{max} that can occur through the use of differing methodologies. Through a maximal running test a 23-year-old athlete's HR_{max} was determined as 188 beat·min^{-1}. The comparable maximal heart rates using the 220–age and Tanaka et al. formulas were 197 and 192 beat·min^{-1}, respectively. The differences in the target HR zones based on these maximums are also shown in Table 8.5. These results highlight the need to determine accurately rather than estimate HR_{max} whenever possible. As measured with a $\dot{V}O_{2max}$ test, HR_{max} varies with the mode of exercise such that higher values are obtained during a running test than a cycling test. This specificity of HR_{max} relative to the exercise mode should, therefore, be taken into account for exercise prescription. For a multi-sport athlete or a triathlete it is appropriate to determine HR_{max} for all disciplines involved.

Knowledge integration question

Explain what strength and conditioning are and why they should form part of an athlete's training programme.

Due to the consequences of the specificity principle, the majority of conditioning training, as well as HR_{max} determination, should match the movement within the sport as closely as possible. For instance, training for off-road runners such as fell or mountain runners should be ideally conducted on natural terrain or a treadmill for indoor sessions. Conditioning training for rowers should ideally be conducted in a boat, however, training on rowing ergometers is popular with coaches and athletes because the movements required closely match the demands of rowing on water.

Key points

The form of conditioning included in a programme should reflect the exercise mode, intensity, and duration of the specific sport or goal.

Prescription of training intensities commonly utilises the maximal HR for the calculation of HR training zones.

In addition to strength and conditioning, sufficient time must be available for skill development and other aspects of training – do not lose focus on the most important aspects of the sport or training goal.

Warm-up and cool-down

An appropriate warm-up and cool-down should feature in every training session and competition routine, but these components are sometimes neglected by athletes or coaches. This is especially true for those who train and compete outdoors during winter months. Cool-downs in particular can be neglected when it is cold and getting dark at the end of a tiring training session. In these conditions everyone wants to pack up, get changed and get warm, rather than thinking about completing a cool-down. An appropriate warm-up and cool-down, however, can improve performance, help avoid injury and promote recovery.

The benefits of a warm-up

An appropriate warm-up can improve performance and to some extent help with injury avoidance. Warm-ups should typically include a pulse raiser, followed by a variety of stretches or mobilising exercises and a more intense pulse raiser. The warm-up can also comprise general and sport-specific exercises, becoming more specific to the sport through the progression of the warm-up. The benefits of completing a warm-up include improvements in the following performance-related aspects:

- Increased blood flow. Sudden bouts of strenuous exercise without warm-up have been shown to lead to abnormal heart responses through inadequate oxygen supply to the cardiac muscle. Increased blood flow to the muscles reduces lactic acid build-up.
- Muscle temperature elevation increases the speed of reactions involved in metabolism, improving oxygen utilisation and the functioning of the energy systems.
- Nerve transmission and reaction time have been shown to improve in the early stages of exercise as a result of a warm-up.
- Strength and power at the start of exercise have been shown to increase as a result of the pulse-raising aspects of a warm-up.
- Flexibility is improved through a warm-up which may well serve to assist in injury avoidance.
- Improved psychological readiness for the training session or competition. The warm-up serves to focus the mind and body on the activity ahead. It enables an athlete to be mentally and physically ready for the sport, through increased arousal levels.
- All of the above have been shown to result in improved performance during the first minutes of strenuous exercise.

The benefits of a cool-down

How an athlete finishes a training session or competition routine has implications for their recovery from the exercise. Many athletes, coaches and health professionals are aware of the benefits and importance of a warm-up. However, fewer tend to focus on cool-downs to the same extent. In the rush to get packed away and changed at the end of a training session or competition, a cool-down can be neglected. Cool-down promotes the removal of metabolites that have accumulated during exercise, thereby assisting the body to decrease the effects of delayed onset of muscle soreness (DOMS – which is described in Chapter 9). It is also the optimal time to complete flexibility exercises. The frequent nature of training for many sports makes attention to a cool-down an important aspect for all taking part in exercise, be it for performance or health reasons. Completing a cool-down at the end of each training session or competition will improve recovery before the following day's activity.

The benefits of employing a cool-down strategy at the end of a training session include:

- Reducing the impact of DOMS that is often felt 1–2 days after strenuous training sessions through the gradual lowering of pulse rate and stretching exercises.
- Assisting the body with the removal of metabolites produced during exercise that might otherwise tend to pool in the legs.
- Stretching to improve flexibility has been shown to be most effective for warm muscles and is therefore best carried out during cool-down.

Knowledge integration question

Describe the mechanism through which cool-downs can help reduce the effects of DOMS.

Format for warm-ups and cool-downs

There a number of general principles that can be followed in the development of warm-up or cool-down sessions:

- Warm-ups should be specific, or become more specific as they progress, to the activity to be undertaken. For example, warm-ups should include boat activities for rowers and kayakers or increasing levels of physical contact and impact for sports such as rugby, wrestling or judo.
- The warm-up should include a pulse raising activity and a variety of mobilising exercises centered on the key joints involved in the exercise. Stretching exercises can be included where necessary for a sport or the needs of the individual (when recovering from injury). The muscles, however, will not be as warm at this stage, consequently flexibility training is often best completed at the end of a session.
- A cool-down included at the end of a session should include exercise to gradually lower heart rate to assist with the removal of exercise metabolites and flexibility exercises to promote recovery and improved flexibility.

Key points

The importance of warm-ups and cool-downs is now clear, hence they commonly feature as part of a training session, match or race.

Warm-ups prepare the body for the exercise to follow and should become progressively more specific.

Cool-downs have a positive impact upon recovery from training and competition.

Flexibility training

An essential component of any cool-down session relates to the inclusion of a range of sport-specific flexibility exercises. Developing an optimal level of flexibility specific to a sport can help to improve performance. This optimal level of flexibility relates to the fact that a lack of flexibility (hypomobility) could cause soft tissue injury during performance and become a rate limiter for skill development. Conversely, too much flexibility (hypermobility) can result in joint and soft tissue injury. Hypermobility of the shoulder joint of a kayaker or gymnast, for example, may in part be responsible for shoulder dislocation during training or performance. A balance needs to be maintained between flexibility training and muscle development (through strength training). There are three forms of flexibility training commonly used to improve flexibility: static stretching, ballistic stretching and proprioceptive neuromuscular facilitation (PNF).

Static stretches

This form of stretching involves the performer holding a position, usually for 10–30 seconds, in order to apply a stretch to the soft tissues surrounding a particular joint. The movement is made slowly and held in position for the length of the stretch. Static stretches have the advantage that they need only the athlete to perform them, they are simple to complete, are least likely to result in injury, and relative to other methods of stretching feel the least painful during execution.

Ballistic stretches

As the name suggests, ballistic stretches require motion and momentum to induce the stretch. This movement is most often completed in a bouncing, rhythmic fashion. Ballistic stretches often use the same exercises or positions as static stretches but are completed with movement to 'push' the stretch further. Martial arts exponents and hurdlers as athletes, who often make very dynamic movements in extreme ranges of motion, have traditionally used these stretches in their warm-ups and cool-downs. The disadvantages with this form of stretching result from the motion and momentum generated during the stretch. With the bouncing motion there is an increased risk of injury and a resistance to the stretch from the antagonistic muscle. Unless employed for a sport-specific reason static stretching has the same benefits as ballistic stretching with a lower risk of soft tissue injury.

Proprioceptive neuromuscular facilitation

This form of stretching requires an experienced partner to assist in each movement. There is a variety of PNF forms, the most commonly used of which involves an isometric contraction of the muscle to be stretched just prior to the stretch (contract–relax–contract method). Proprioceptive neuromuscular facilitation takes advantage of the fact that there is an increase in muscle relaxation after a muscle contraction. This is thought to occur due to a decrease in the muscle's protective contraction against the stretch, in response to the isometric contraction. As a natural protection against injury, the Golgi tendon organs, proprioceptors and muscle spindles together inhibit the stretch of a muscle as it reaches its limits of range of motion. The isometric contraction of the muscle prior to each stretch appears to inhibit the protection response, allowing further stretching of the muscle.

Figure 8.18 shows a contract–relax–contract PNF stretch for the hamstrings. This involves the partner kneeling next to the athlete and moving their leg (hamstring) muscle to its lengthened position. The performer then isometrically contracts the hamstrings against the resistance of the partner. The contraction is held by the performer for 5–6 seconds and then relaxed. During the post-contraction relaxation the partner moves the limb further into the stretch, lengthening the muscle further. This process is repeated three to four times for each stretch. This form of stretching has been shown to result in greater improvements in flexibility than for either ballistic or static stretching. It is very important, however, that the partner and the performer are trained in using this form of stretching, as due to the additional stretch applied there is an increased injury potential. The exercises on the website provide examples of a range of general flexibility exercises for adventure sports performers.

Key point

Flexibility training can most usefully be performed during a cool-down when muscles are warmest.

Static, ballistic or PNF stretches can be used to improve flexibility.

Due to injury risks, static stretching is the safest, yet, when performed correctly, PNF stretching is the most effective.

Introduction to ergogenic aids

There are a sufficient number of ergogenic aids available for performance enhancement that it would be possible

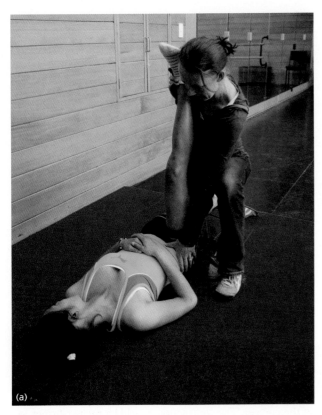 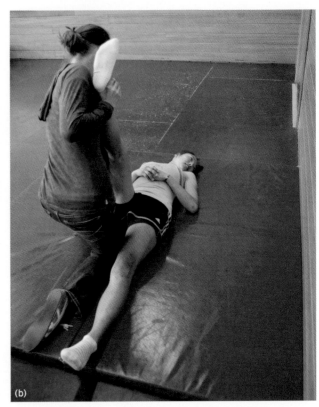

Figure 8.18 (a) and (b) Contract-relax-contract PNF exercise for the hamstrings. (*Source*: Simon Fryer)

to write a book with several volumes on the subject. As a consequence, in each subsequent chapter we will highlight a number of the most widely used (and abused) and well-researched legal and illegal aids. In its broadest sense an ergogenic aid describes any substance, material or technique that serves to improve work capacity or sports performance. Ergogenic aids include mechanical, pharmacological, nutritional, physiological and psychological performance enhancements.

Perhaps the broadest range of ergogenic aids can be found within mechanical aids for performance enhancement. Mechanical aids include equipment as diverse as video cameras, hypoxic tents, nasal strips, tyres for towing, elastic cords, weighted vests, compression suits, body suits and weight training equipment all of which can serve to enhance performance in a sporting context. Pharmacological and nutritional aids include legal substances such as vitamin supplements, energy drinks, protein supplements and creatine, as well as illegal substances such as anabolic steroids, amphetamines and diuretics. Physiological aids refer to substances or methods used to enhance physiological functioning and include legal methods such as acupuncture and massage, and illegal aspects such as blood doping with the use of erythropoietin (EPO).

There is a variety of psychological aids that can serve to enhance performance and these include, but are not limited to, music, crowd effect (cheering), imaging, hypnosis, meditation and tai chi.

The margins of victory in many sports are so small that ergogenic aids can make a significant difference to an athlete's performance. In a sporting context, this has led individuals to take supplements or use methods that are illegal and sometimes, despite short-term performance benefits, damaging to long-term health and in the worst case lead to death during training or an event. Any athlete or coach should consider carefully the ramifications of any particular ergogenic aid prior to introducing it into a training programme.

A central consideration, in terms of performance enhancement should be his or her diet. The basic nutritional strategy for performance in any sport, regardless of the intensity and duration of the activity, or when training towards a health goal, should be to follow a healthy balanced diet. Details of the components of a healthy diet were included in Chapter 2. The key aspect, where possible, is to plan your diet to maximise the *naturalness* of your food (minimising processed foods and cooking as much as possible), have *variety* and eat with *moderation*. With a balanced healthy diet it should be possible to supply all the required nutrients, vitamins and minerals within your normal meals.

There are many thousands of aids that are reportedly ergogenic which athletes from any sport can include to improve performance. Some of these work; however, very few have good quality research behind them to justify the claims made by the manufacturers. For instance, the nutritional supplement industry is worth billions of dollars worldwide, yet in most cases improvements in our basic diet can outstrip any manufactured supplement. There are some ergogenic aids, referred to in each following chapter, that do appear to work and through carefully controlled research have been shown to improve performance.

Check your recall
Fill in the missing words.

➤ The energy for muscular contraction comes from the compound _____.

➤ The energy required during explosive power activities, such as the shot putt, is provided by the muscle stores of _____.

➤ The fastest, and most simple pathway for ATP synthesis is the _____ system.

➤ A sprint finish in a rowing race is predominantly fuelled by the _____ pathway.

➤ The common pathways of aerobic metabolism are the _____ cycle and the electron transport chain.

➤ The initial steps in the catabolism of fatty acids (lipids) and proteins are _____ and _____, respectively.

➤ The interaction of the energy systems is dependent on the _____ and _____ of exercise.

➤ The portion of energy released from the hydrolysis of ATP that is available to do work is called _____ _____.

➤ The energy available for cellular activity is dependent on both enthalpy and _____.

➤ Enzymes act as _____ for all reactions that take place in the body.

➤ Five physiologically trainable components of fitness are aerobic endurance, strength, anaerobic power, flexibility and _____.

➤ Dynamic balance, a skill-related component of fitness, includes the three skills of balance, _____ and coordination.

➤ A common field test used for the generic measurement of flexibility is the _____ and _____ test.

➤ When choosing a test to measure a particular component of fitness, the validity and _____ of the test must be considered.

➤ The _____ principle of training states that for training to be effective, a stimulus must be greater than that normally encountered.

➤ Strength and conditioning training should be sport, or training goal, _____.

➤ Adding _____ to training can help avoid overtraining, improve motivation and alleviate boredom.

➤ Dividing the training year into manageable and progressive phases is called _____.

➤ Heart rate zones are often used as a guide for training intensity. These zones are calculated from the determination or estimation of _____ _____ _____.

➤ A warm-up increases blood flow and muscle _____.

➤ It is most useful to perform flexibility training during a cooldown when the muscles are _____.

➤ The function of an _____ aid is to improve sports performance.

Review questions

1. Name the two anaerobic pathways that synthesise ATP and give examples of sports in which the two pathways predominate.

2. Explain what the term 'slower-rate glycolysis' refers to?

3. What are the differing fates of pyruvate, the end product of glycolysis, during high-intensity and low-intensity exercise?

4. What are the initial steps in the catabolism of free fatty acids (lipids) and proteins, and at which stage do they then enter the aerobic pathway?

5. Does anaerobic or aerobic metabolism result in the higher net gain in ATP? Why, therefore, is this system not predominant all the time during life?

6. What is the portion of energy called that is released from the hydrolysis of ATP and is available to cells to complete work, and what factors influence the amount of energy available?

7. Name three variables that affect the rate at which an enzyme is able to catalyse a reaction and describe the relationship.

8. Name four of the five factors that inter-relate to determine an individual's wellbeing, and describe the importance of wellbeing within sport.

9. What is the specificity principle of training and how does it relate to aerobic conditioning?

10. What are the functions of warm-ups and cool-downs?

Teach it!

In groups of three, choose one topic and teach it to the rest of the study group.

1. Give an overview of the energy generation pathways. Describe the interaction of the pathways and provide examples of sports in which each system predominates.

2. Choose a particular sport and outline the contribution of the different energy generation pathways. Determine the most important components of fitness, how these could be tested, and what training sessions could be implemented to improve the fitness of these components.

3. Discuss how you, as a teacher or coach, may assess your athletes' physiological fitness and how you would monitor the progress of a training programme.

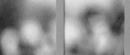
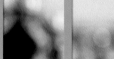

SPORT IN ACTION

Biography: Sarissa de Vries
Sport: Triathlon
(The Netherlands)

As a child, Sarissa began her love of sport as a gymnast. She then started swimming when she was 12 and competed in her first triathlon at the age of 16 years. Now at 22 years old, Sarissa has been seriously involved in Olympic distance triathlon for four years. With the appointment of a new Dutch head coach in 2010, Sarissa has improved her world ranking from 120 to 60 within one year. She is currently aiming for Olympic qualification.

Training to be an Olympic triathlete

Triathletes need to be competent in three disciplines, swimming, cycling and running, which means a lot of training hours. Normally I train 6–9 hours per discipline per week (i.e. a total of 18–27 hours per week) which

means training 2–3 times each day. I also do core stability training 2–3 times a week. I spend relatively more hours running during base training then other triathletes as that is my weak discipline. Closer to the race season the training gets more specific and is adjusted for the particular characteristics of the race I am working towards. Races can be in hot climates, involve sea swims and the terrain can vary between flat, technical and hilly. This requires very specific preparation in the weeks prior to the race.

John Hellemans became the new Dutch head coach in 2010. In addition to being a coach, John is a sports doctor so he has a lot of knowledge about how the human body works. He has guided some New Zealand athletes towards previous Olympic games, so he is a very experienced coach. Also, because he has raced himself for many years, he knows what it takes to be a successful triathlete. First we worked out that I had a lactose intolerance which was causing significant health issues.

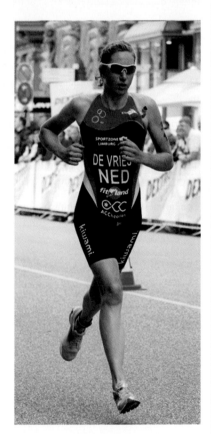

(*Source*: Mariska Lagerweij and Carin Willemsen)

These were resolved when I went on a lactose free diet. During my career I had also found that my weight fluctuated significantly which influenced my training and racing performance. With the help of the sport dietician and regular monitoring of my body composition (sum of 7 skinfolds and weight) I was able to manage this much better. Since John became my coach in 2010 I have made some significant changes to my training. I used to spend about 4 hours per week in the gym doing strength training. In contrast, John likes to involve strength training into the hours we already spend swimming, biking and running so it is more triathlon-specific. This means no more lifting weights, but activities like biking and running up hill and swimming with

hand paddles or arms only. These training methods result in very specific strength gains which translate directly to the movement patterns of swimming, biking and running. I also do more coupled ('brick') training sessions, such as running straight off the bike, and at least once a week we do a continuous swim-bike-run session. This way the body adapts to the changes in muscle activity required during competition. We perform these sessions at a controlled intensity, so I don't get as fatigued as in a real race, but it results in excellent sport-specific training adaptations.

I have learned how important recovery is. Without a proper recovery it becomes much harder to maintain training quality which subsequently affects the process of

adaptation. Eating the right foods in the right amounts and getting enough sleep are the most important components of recovery. Another thing I have learned is not to compete with my training partners during training sessions so I stay in control of the intensities which work for me. Although John has only been with us for a year I have already noticed big improvements. I am much stronger in all three disciplines. Where I got dropped earlier on hilly bike courses I can now ride uphill with the faster girls. I can stay on the feet in front of me during the swim when there are accelerations after turning the buoys and I am more capable of running a fast 10 km after already racing hard in the swim and bike.

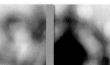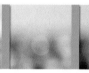

SPORT IN ACTION

Biography:
John Hellemans
Sport: Triathlon (national Dutch coach)

John Hellemans is a well-known New Zealand-based triathlon coach and sports medicine practitioner. He is currently the national coach for the Dutch Olympic triathlon team.

Coaching philosophy

My coaching philosophy has gradually developed from doing everything I could to assist the athletes in reaching their potential to a more holistic approach based on the notion: 'Better athletes, better people.' Sport, especially at the elite level, brings the best (sacrifice, courage, kindness) and the worst (cheating, abuse) out

of people. In this respect it is a very contained and relatively benign mirror of life. In my opinion, athletes who are at peace with the self and the world around them (acceptance) are more likely to compete consistently to their potential than athletes who are continuously fearful and/or at war. Toughness, courage, pride and honour can thus happily co-exist with tolerance, compassion, honesty and sacrifice. The pursuit of excellence in sport is enhanced by maintaining respect for others, including the competition.

Coach-directed, athlete-centred, team-supported

Today the coach needs to be able to work with a multidisciplinary team to maximise the outcome of the training

and racing. Doctors, physiotherapists, dieticians, psychologists and other health professionals, physiologists, biomechanists and engineers can potentially all add value. It is the task

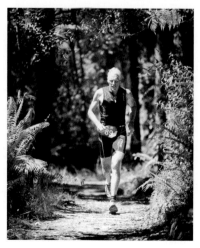

(*Source*: Dave Beeche)

➤

➤ of the coach to lead and direct this team. Information from these specialists needs to filter back to the athlete through the coach. It is the challenge of the coach to make sure that the team speaks with one voice so the athlete does not become confused.

The issue of control: attitude, training and nutrition

'If you are not prepared to do the work you might as well play cricket!' is a quote from well-known Finnish endurance coach Seppo Nuutilla. Although it is not altogether fair on the sport of cricket, it does sum up the basic requirement for participation in any type of endurance sport. Doing the work does not only relate to consistency and contents of physical training sessions but it also applies to two additional crucial areas which influence the long-term outcome of any training programme: nutrition and mental attitude. Nutrition relates to recovery and to balancing energy expenditure with energy input as well as exposing the body to the right balance of food groups and specific nutrients. Contrary to popular belief, mental attitude can also be trained and manipulated as much as physical training and nutrition. One of the aims of the mental conditioning process is to develop the skills to stay on task, especially when distracted and/or under pressure.

Stages of development

From a coaching perspective there are three distinct stages of development in a triathlete's career:

1. *The developing athlete* is the athlete young in training years and relatively new to the sport. They generally require instruction to which they will over time respond with feedback to the coach. The coach is clearly the teacher and instructor.

2. *The mature athlete* is the athlete who is more experienced in training and racing. They are able to make decisions for themselves and give input in planning, periodisation, training and racing. This is the stage where the coach and athlete work as a team. For me, as the coach, this is generally always the more interesting, enjoyable and challenging time of an athlete's career and often also the most satisfying.

3. *The champion athlete* generally has the confidence to lead their own programme. The coach takes a step back and acts as an advisor and trouble shooter.

It is true that some champion athletes never get beyond stage 1. They like to be told what to do and function well that way but in my experience this is rare. Most are somewhere between stages 2 and 3 depending on their personality and their relationship with their coach. During the first two stages the athletes learn how to train first, then how to compete and thirdly how to win. Learning to train, compete and win is first applied at club and regional level before the whole process is repeated at national level and then internationally. An added component is to learn to train, compete and win under pressure and/or with distractions. This is how most of the professional athletes serve an extensive apprenticeship before graduating to the more glamorous stage of their career. It is during these formative years of an athlete's career that the coach usually has the biggest impact.

Training

The principles of training pertain to frequency (how often), duration (how long), intensity (how hard), and periodisation (how to balance the components of training over shorter and longer time periods). This is something most textbooks agree on. What you do not find is how to optimise the execution of the training principles for the individual athlete. As no one athlete will respond in the same way as another, the nuances in individual training can make a huge difference for the development of the athlete over time. This is called the art of coaching. It is done not only by careful filtering of information acquired through monitoring, observation and feedback over time, but also by instinct. It is not uncommon that the data and feedback from monitoring and observation are unclear. In these instances the coach needs to rely on experience and instinct. This is often particularly the case in pressure situations.

Training intensity is the most controversial of the different components of training. A variety of sport science methods is available to assess training intensity zones which confirm that there is no one foolproof method available as yet. In our programme we have settled on lactate testing for running (lactate and heart rate at a certain pace), power testing for biking (power output and heart rate) and a critical speed test for swimming (time trials over 400 and 50 metres).

Monitoring

The use of monitoring has become common practice in endurance sport especially at the elite level. In our programme we use rates of subjective perception on a scale of 1 (very good) to 5 (very poor) for stress, nutrition, sleep, training performance and muscle soreness. Additionally, we monitor resting and training heart rate and more recently also heart rate variability. Measuring power output on the bike has also become common practice. The frequency of the monitoring varies during the year but is daily during periods of hard training. Body composition (sum of 7 skinfolds and weight) is done at monthly intervals. At altitude camps we also measure oxygen saturation (SpO$_2$) in the blood (an accurate measure for hypoxic stress) with the use of an

oximeter. Over time a picture develops regarding the athlete's individual response rate to training and related stress and how the monitoring data compare to race results.

Sarissa de Vries

When I inherited the national coaching job in the Netherlands, Sarissa de Vries was already a member of the national A squad. I noticed a very motivated athlete with some health issues and a lack of triathlon-specific strength, especially in the disciplines of biking and running.

Within a relatively short time we developed a good coach athlete relationship. With the help of the sports medicine doctor and nutritionist, Sarissa addressed her health problems and she set to work with lots of specific resistance training for her biking and running. She has been compliant with the monitoring protocols which has made me more effective as her coach. She has improved her world ranking from 120 to 60 within a year and she is now aiming for Olympic qualification, not an unrealistic goal.

CLASSIC RESEARCH SUMMARY

The specificity of swim training in relation to aerobic fitness by Magel (1975)

The research data available to Magel in the 1970s suggested that the maximal oxygen uptake of world class swimmers, as identified during running or cycling tests, was similarly achievable during swimming. In contrast, recreational swimmers demonstrated a lower VO2max for swimming as compared to running and cycling. It was suggested that the training state and prior sport-specific experience of an athlete may account for these variations in aerobic power. In 1975, Magel embraced this knowledge and conducted a very simple, yet effective, study on the specificity of the physiological adaptations to swim training.

In this study, Magel recruited 30 male participants (college aged recreational swimmers) who were split into two groups: an interval swim training group and a control group. The swim training consisted of a 10-week interval programme which was conducted for 1 h per day on 3 days of each week. In

contrast, the control group undertook no form of exercise training or organised physical activity for the same time period. Participants completed a running and a tethered swimming $\dot{V}O_{2max}$ test both prior to and immediately following the 10-week training phase. Gas analysis was conducted using the Douglas bag method.

The swim training involved maximal intensity repeat (50, 100 and 200 yards) and longer distance (300, 400 and 500 yards) swims utilising the front crawl. The participants repeated the designated swims when their heart rate (as measured from the carotid pulse) had returned to 70% of their maximum swimming heart rate. During the first two training weeks, swimmers completed one set of 10 × 50 yards and 5 × 100 yards repeat swims. Maximal swims of 200 and 300 yards were then included in the programme from week three, with the final five weeks of training involving a combination of all repeat and longer-distance swims. In the final two weeks of training participants covered 1,500–2,000 yards, increasing from an

average of 750 yards at the start of the programme.

Following the 10-week intense swim training programme, the recreational swimmers improved their swimming $\dot{V}O_{2max}$ but not their treadmill scores, clearly demonstrating the specificity of the cardiorespiratory adaptations to swim training. Additionally, the repeat swim times were reduced and exercise heart rates lowered, indicating an improved circulatory efficiency and endurance capacity. The difference between running and swimming $\dot{V}O_{2max}$ remained essentially unchanged in the control subjects. Following the findings of this early paper, and many more since, the importance of training specificity is now widely accepted. Refer to the text for more information on the specificity principle of training, or to the 'Sport in action' piece for an applied perspective.

Reference: Magel, J.R., Foglia, G.F., McArdle, W.D., Gutin, B., Pechar, G.S. and Katch, F.I. (1975). Specificity of swim training on maximum oxygen uptake. *Journal of Applied Physiology*, 38(1): 151–5.

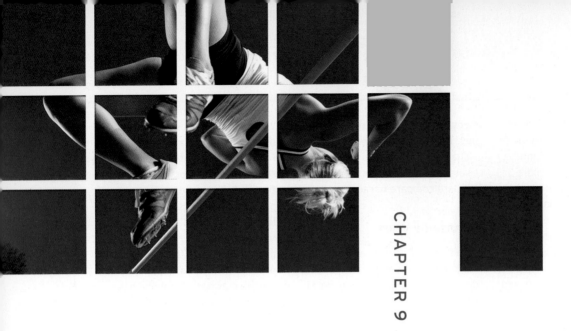

CHAPTER 9

Power and power endurance:
the explosive sports

Learning objectives

After reading, considering and discussing with a study partner the material in this chapter you should be able to:

➤ explain bond energies and the nature of bond forming and bond breaking

➤ describe the structure of adenosine triphosphate (ATP) and other nucleotides

➤ teach others about the apparent contradiction between bond energies and the amount of free energy available when ATP is hydrolysed

➤ teach others about the phosphagen system

➤ discuss the different forms of strength or resistance training

➤ describe the range of physiological tests for power and power endurance sports

➤ explain how speed can be measured

➤ discuss conditioning as it relates to power and power endurance sports

➤ outline the likely mechanisms of fatigue in power endurance sports

➤ explain the placebo effect

➤ teach others about the dangers of using steroids

➤ discuss the potential ergogenic effects of creatine

This chapter concerns the physiology of explosive sports. Some examples of sports that fall into this category are athletic throws and jumps, weight-lifting and sprinting which are shown in Figure 9.1. The time duration for sustaining such efforts is relatively short, up to around 10 s, but these represent the highest power outputs humans can achieve in a sporting context. As such, the intensity of these sports is maximal, within the confines of skilful performance.

These sports can be divided into those which are power-based (shortest duration) and those which require power endurance. Power endurance requires the expression of maximal effort through a number of movements, sustained for a longer, but still very short (under 10 s), time. The single explosive effort within the 2 s of a shot putt, is a good example of power while the 8–11 s for the clean and jerk in weight-lifting, requires power endurance for the two phases of the lift.

Adenosine triphosphate serves as the energy source for our bodies. To understand how cells derive the energy for cellular work from ATP, this chapter starts with an examination of *bond energy*. With this knowledge it is possible to have a deeper understanding of the metabolic significance of ATP and the hydrolysis reaction that enables the liberation of energy for cellular activity. After this, we examine the fastest mechanism available for ATP synthesis; the phosphagen system. ATP stores in the muscles

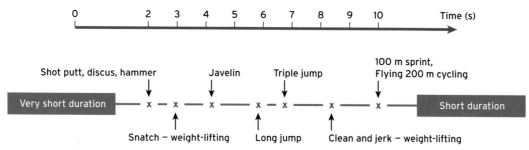

Figure 9.1 Duration continuum for a number of power and power endurance sports.

and the phosphagen system provide the energy for explosive sports. Following this, we discuss the physiology of power and power endurance sports. Within this section we examine the components of fitness and tests that relate to these types of sport, fatigue in power endurance sports and adaptations (chronic response) to power and power endurance training. Following this, because of the links between power and strength, a review of strength training, and suggested exercises, is included, along with suggestions for power and power endurance conditioning training. The final section on ergogenic aids focuses particularly on the use of creatine as a legal nutritional aid.

9.1 Energy supply for explosive sports

Bond energy

As was described in Chapter 2, atoms form chemical bonds which are held together by the forces of attraction between the atoms (the protons and electrons of the bonding atoms) forming the bond. Chemical reactions generally lead to the formation or breaking of chemical bonds. Typically, diagrams of the hydrolysis of ATP show the removal of a phosphoryl group leading to the release of free energy to complete cellular work. This is misleading, because it is not the breaking of the phosphoanhydride bonds between the outer phosphoryl groups that leads to the release of energy for cellular work, but the overall changes in bonds through the formation of the products (remember that H_2O is involved in the reaction to catabolise [hydrolyse] ATP). The hydrolysis of ATP is explained in more detail in the next section. However, prior to explaining the nature of this reaction, it is important to describe in more detail the general principles of bond formation, bond breaking and bond energy.

Chemical bonds are formed as a result of the forces of attraction between atoms. The attraction between atoms is such that energy is *released* during bond formation. In other words, chemical bonding is an **exothermic** process. Conversely, the forces of attraction between two bonded atoms must be overcome to break a chemical bond, hence energy is *required* and consequently, bond breaking is an **endothermic** process. If ATP hydrolysis simply involved the breaking of the final phosphoanhydride bond in ATP it would be an endothermic process and therefore require energy. Given this situation, that energy is required to break the phosphoanhydride bond (forming ADP and Pi), how is it that ATP can provide free energy for cellular activity? The answer to this question lies in the fact that the hydrolysis of ATP involves a combination of bond breaking and bond forming. The energy that we know is released from ATP is in actuality liberated because the bonds that are formed in the products of this reaction more than offset the initial breaking of the phosphoanhydride bond.

Key points

Breaking a chemical bond requires energy = endothermic.

Chemical bond formation releases energy = exothermic.

Energy is released from ATP when product bonds are formed, not when reactant bonds are broken.

In order to understand the change in energy between the reactants and products of reactions, chemists have created tables of bond energies, that is, the energy required to break a specific bond between two atoms. Table 9.1 provides an illustration of the bond energy required to break the bonds between a number of important atoms commonly found within cells. By way of example, the following calculation of the formation of H_2O can be used as an illustration of bond energies and energy transfer.

Table 9.1 Bond energies of some common cellular chemical bonds. Bond energy here refers to the average enthalpy required to dissociate the bond.

Bonded atoms	Bond energy (kJ/mol)*	Bonded atoms	Bond energy (kJ/mol)*
H—H	436	O—P	351
H—O	464	O—O	142
C—H	414	C=C	620
C—C	347	C=N	615
C—N	293	O=P	460
C—O	351	O=O	498

* Bond energy is an average for the dissociation of the bond (the energy required to break the bond). — represents a single bond and = represents a double bond.

As can be seen from the calculation box below, when water is formed from hydrogen and oxygen a substantial amount of energy (-486 kJ) of energy is released. For the formation of water from $2H_2$ and O_2 three bonds are broken and 4 new bonds are formed. In this reaction the bonds between the hydrogen atoms and oxygen atoms are broken which requires a total of $+1370$ kJ of energy. However, the formation of water results in the release of -1856 kJ and consequently a net gain of -486 kJ of energy. This example provides a useful example of the fact that if bond-breaking is accompanied by bond formation such a reaction can in overall effect be exothermic. This provides part of the explanation as to how we gain energy from the breaking of the bond between the final phosphoanhydride bond in ATP.

Adenosine triphosphate

The main energy source in the human body, and indeed that required for muscular contraction during everyday movements and sporting performance, is adenosine tri-phosphate (ATP). There are, however, other high-energy molecules which are used in the body for specific functions. The structures of the body's energy molecules are initially

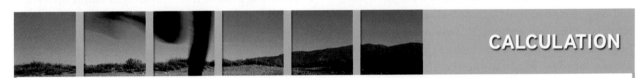

CALCULATION

Example of bond energies in the formation of water from the gases oxygen and hydrogen

$$2H_2 + O_2 \longrightarrow 2H_2O$$

$$H—H + H—H + O{=}O \longrightarrow O \quad + \quad O$$
$$\qquad\qquad\qquad\qquad\qquad /\backslash \qquad\quad /\backslash$$
$$\qquad\qquad\qquad\qquad\quad H\ \ H \quad\ \ H\ \ H$$

1 hydrogen molecule + 1 hydrogen molecule + 1 oxygen molecule $\longrightarrow$ 2 water molecules

Bond energies

Bonds broken	Bond energy (kJ/mol)	Total energy required (kJ/mol)
2 H—H	436	872
O=O	498	<u>498</u>
		$+1370$

Bonds formed	Bond energy	Total energy released
4 O—H	464	-1856

Energy change (ΔH) in the formation of water		-2486

The energy change between the reactants and the products in a reaction is referred to as the ΔH (the change in enthalpy, as was described in Chapter 8).

This reaction is exothermic as the energy required to break the H—H and O=O bonds is less than the energy released in the formation of water.

described, followed by a detailed examination of how ATP is broken down with the resultant release of free energy.

The structure of energy molecules

Cells require energy to perform their functions within the body, and the main energy currency is ATP. As can be seen from Figure 9.2, ATP is comprised of an adenosine moiety bonded to three phosphoryl groups. Each adenosine molecule is comprised of a *base* (adenine) and a *sugar* (ribose) which together form a **nucleoside**. Adenosine is just one of five nucleosides, the other four being guanosine, cytidine, thymidine and uridine. Each of these nucleosides can bond with up to three phosphoryl groups in the same way as illustrated for adenosine (Figure 9.2). When a nucleoside bonds with phosphoryl groups a **nucleotide** is created.

Adenine is one of five nucleic acid bases, illustrated in Figure 9.3, which are fundamental to cell structure and functioning. Nucleotides and nucleic acids are the other major class of nitrogen containing metabolites alongside amino acids and proteins (the nitrogen component in amino acids was described in more detail in Chapter 2). These five bases are common to every cell in the body and form essential components of deoxyribonucleic acid (DNA – our genetic coding) and ribonucleic acid (RNA – formed from DNA during transcription) which are found in the nucleus of every cell and used as the blueprint for its creation, development and functioning. If you have read anything about, or seen any illustrations of, DNA or RNA you may have seen the letters ACGT in DNA coding and ACGU in RNA coding, with these letters representing the five bases. Adenine, cytosine, guanine, thymine and uracil form the basis for the structure of DNA and RNA.

Each of the five bases bonds with a sugar, either deoxyribose or ribose, to form a nucleoside. As already mentioned, adenine bonds with ribose to form adenosine, the basic unit for ATP, which is an example of a nucleoside. Just as adenosine bonds with phosphoryl groups to form AMP (adenosine monophosphate), ADP and ATP, so each of the other four nucleosides can bond with phosphoryl groups to create a nucleotide. As with ATP, the addition of the final two phosphates to a nucleoside provides an energy store that can be used to fuel cellular activity. If ATP is the petrol for our bodies, then the other nucleotides represent diesel or liquefied petroleum gas (LPG), alternative fuels for the cells of the body. For example, guanosine triphosphate (GTP) is used as an energy source for protein synthesis and one molecule of GTP is produced during the Krebs cycle (which is discussed further in Chapter 12). Uridine triphosphate (UTP), by way of a further example, is used by the liver and muscles to provide the energy necessary for the synthesis of glycogen. Adenosine triphosphate, however, is the main source of energy for the cellular activity within the body including the muscular contractions that are necessary for sports performance.

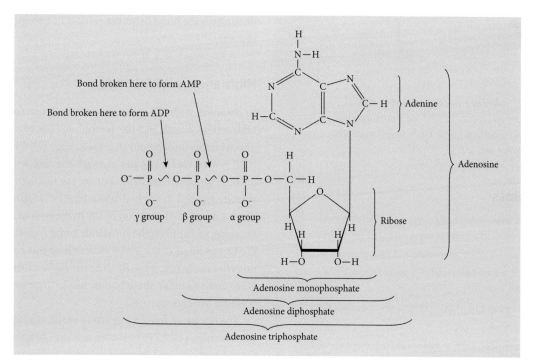

Figure 9.2 The chemical structure of ATP.

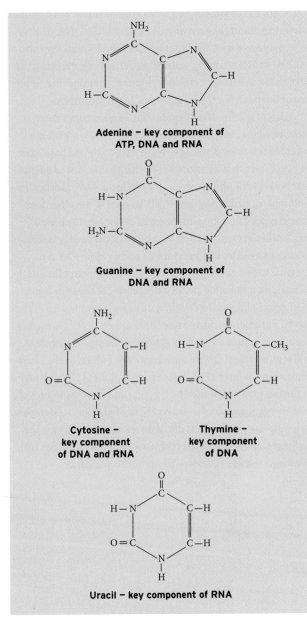

Figure 9.3 The structure of the five bases: adenine, guanine, cytosine, thymine and uracil.

Key points

ATP is the main source of energy for cellular activity, including muscular contractions essential for sport.

The structure of ATP: adenosine + 3 phosphoryl groups

Adenosine : a base (adenine) + a sugar (ribose) = a nucleoside

Nucleoside + up to 3 phosphoryl groups = nucleotide, e.g. ATP

Other nucleotides, such as guanosine triphosphate and uridine triphosphate, can also be used to fuel cellular activity.

Hydrolysis of ATP and the release of free energy

The energy released through the hydrolysis of ATP provides the energy required for exercise of any intensity or duration. This free energy enables the operation of the Na^+-K^+ pump, the powerstroke in muscular contraction and the release of the myosin head from its binding site on actin. To understand ATP hydrolysis more fully, it is important to understand both the bond energies within its chemical bonds (refer to Table 9.1) and the high-energy bonds depicted in Figure 9.2 by the symbol $\sim$. In addition, an appreciation of the complexity in the structure of ATP and its interactions with molecules around it in the aqueous environment of the cell is important.

The squiggles used to denote high energy in Figure 9.2 are common to many exercise physiology textbooks. They were introduced by Fritz Lipmann, who was the first to describe the complete structure of ATP. Lipmann intended the symbol to indicate that ATP was a high energy store. The use of the $\sim$ symbol has created two possible problems in the teaching of exercise physiology and biochemistry. Firstly, it has created a widespread misunderstanding of Lipmann's shorthand and established a notion of there being something different and special about these P—O—P bonds when compared with other chemical bonds. Secondly, it has led to a subsequent misinterpretation regarding the breaking of these phosphoanhydride bonds and the release of energy for cellular activity.

High-energy ATP bonds

In common with other textbooks we will use the term high-energy bonds and the symbol $\sim$. However, it is important to understand that the energy released from ATP is made available, not through the simple breaking of these phosphoanhydride bonds, but through the bonds that are formed in the hydrolysis of ATP. Figure 9.4 provides a detailed illustration of the hydrolysis of ATP. The breaking of the phosphoanhydride bond ($\sim$) and indeed the O—H bond in the water molecule in this reaction, does not release energy. As with all chemical reactions, energy is required to break these bonds, hence these aspects of the reaction are endothermic.

The release of free energy (ΔG), made available through the hydrolysis of ATP, however, is more complex than the simple breaking and forming of bonds as illustrated in the previous section for the exothermic formation of water.

This example was provided as an illustration of the general principles of bond energies. The structure of ATP and its electrochemical interaction with ions and water molecules within the aqueous intracellular environment, make the release of free energy through the hydrolysis of ATP, a more complex process.

Key point

Energy released from ATP hydrolysis is due to the bonds that are formed *not* the bonds that are broken.

Factors influencing free energy release from ATP

If we were to simply calculate the bond energies for the bonds broken and formed as shown in Figure 9.4, in a process similar to that conducted for the formation of water (previous section), we would find that the hydrolysis of ATP appears to be an endothermic reaction. However, as long ago as 1955, Podolsky and Sturtevant, following on from Fritz Lipmann's work, demonstrated through practical experimentation that the hydrolysis of ATP is in fact an exothermic reaction resulting in an enthalpy change (ΔH) of ~ -5.3 kcal·mol^{-1} (22.2 kJ·mol^{-1}). Furthermore, subsequent research has shown that the entropy (ΔS) change increases the energy available such that the ΔG (the free energy resulting from the hydrolysis of ATP) is ~ -7.3 kcal·mol^{-1}

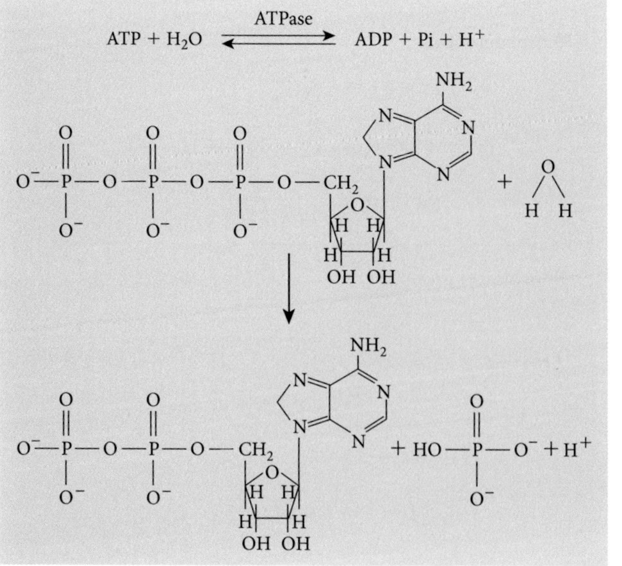

Figure 9.4 The hydrolysis of adenosine triphosphate.

(30.5 kJ·mol^{-1}). Refer to Chapter 8 for more details about enthalpy, entropy and free energy.

This begs the question as to what is so special about the chemical structure of ATP that makes it the high-energy intermediary for human cells? The answer relates to its electrochemical structure and its interaction with the chemicals that surround it. Firstly, as is described and illustrated in Chapter 10, the negatively charged oxygen ions shown in Figure 9.4 interact with Mg^{2+} within the cellular environment. Secondly, although shown as either negative or chemically neutral in Figure 9.4, the oxygen atoms associated with each phosphorus atom in reality share their electrons with other atoms. This makes the chemical bonds and the associated energies of the oxygen and phosphorus atoms more complex than is illustrated in Table 9.1 for an oxygen-phosphorus bond. In other words, the sharing of electrons between oxygen atoms means that the bond energy of each phosphate group is more complex than that shown in Table 9.1.

Thirdly, due to the negative charge on the oxygen atoms, as shown below each phosphorus atom (Figures 9.2 and 9.4), they repel each other and this affects the stability of an ATP molecule, making it more likely to release a phosphoryl group. Fourthly, the complexity of the exothermic nature of the hydrolysis of ATP is also affected by the water molecules that surround ATP within the aqueous environment of a cell. The protons associated with water molecules are attracted to the negatively charged oxygen molecules and this too affects the bonds within ATP and the amount of energy released through the hydrolysis of ATP. Finally, the hydrolysis of ATP as shown in Figure 9.4 provides an illustration of how ATP is catabolised during metabolism. In reality, however, the hydrolysis of ATP does not occur as an individual spontaneous reaction. The removal of a phosphoryl group from ATP only occurs when energy is required by a cell to do work, and as such, the catabolism of ATP is always associated with another cellular reaction. For example, when muscles are signalled to contract for movement, the hydrolysis of ATP only occurs during the movement, that is, it does *not* occur in advance to generate a store of free energy.

Key point

The electrochemical structure of ATP, and its interaction with surrounding chemicals, makes ATP a unique high-energy molecule for cellular energy supply.

The transfer of phosphoryl groups

The key features of ATP that makes it uniquely suitable as an energy store for all life forms, not just humans, relate to:

1. the special chemical structure of phosphorus as an element
2. the bonding potential of phosphorus
3. the ability of ATP to transfer phosphoryl groups

In all the reactions involving ATP, it is not the bond-breaking that is important, but the ability of ATP to transfer phosphoryl groups that makes it uniquely suited to being the high-energy intermediary for all living organisms.

When detached from ATP, the phosphoryl groups are often referred to as inorganic phosphates, and by the symbol Pi, because when removed from the carbon-based (organic) ATP molecule, what remains is an inorganic phosphate ion attached to four oxygen and one hydrogen atom, together known as a phosphoryl, or phosphate, group. In Figure 9.4, Pi is shown as HPO_4^{2-}, hydrogen phosphate; however, within a cell, Pi can exist as either hydrogen phosphate or dihydrogen phosphate (HPO_4^{2-} or H_2PO_4, respectively).

While either of the high-energy bonds (between the γ and β or the β and α phosphate groups – see Figure 9.2) can be broken during the catabolism of ATP, it is more common for the bond between the γ and β phosphoryl groups to be hydrolysed. In some situations, such as during intense exercise, the second high energy bond, between the β and α phosphoryl groups can also been catabolised to release further energy for cellular activity. This results in the adenosine molecule being bonded to only one phosphate group which is called, not surprisingly, adenosine monophosphate (AMP). The direct hydrolysis of ATP between the β and α phosphoryl groups occurs in the synthesis of proteins from amino acids. The bond at which this hydrolysis reaction occurs, resulting in the formation of AMP and pyrophosphate (PPi) can be seen in Figure 9.2. During such reactions ATP is hydrolysed at this bond to trap the newly synthesised protein (to stop the reverse reaction occurring). However, PPi is normally then quickly hydrolysed to provide further energy for the protein synthesis.

Knowledge integration question

During exercise, the energy required for muscular contraction is provided by ATP. In terms of its structure, what is unique about ATP that allows us to harness free energy from its hydrolysis?

The energy-generating pathways for explosive sports

Adenosine triphosphate stores within the muscles provide the energy necessary for power sports, such as a hammer throw, or the initial 2 seconds (s) of longer-duration exercise. For subsequent movement after the throw of a hammer, or for exercise of longer duration, ATP stores must be replenished. The phosphagen system has three mechanisms which serve in different ways to maintain maximal intensity effort beyond the 2 s provided by muscle ATP stores. The most important of these for immediate ATP re-synthesis, the ATP-PCr reaction, was introduced in Chapter 8 and will be covered further in the following section.

The phosphagen system

While the ATP for power sports, such as discus, is provided by stores within the muscles, the phosphagen system provides the predominant ATP synthesis pathway in response to the energy demands for power endurance sports such as the flying 200 m cycle race or a 100 m sprint. This section provides a more detailed explanation of the pathways within the phosphagen system. The phosphagen system, sometimes called the ATP-Phosphocreatine (ATP-PCr), alactic acid or immediate energy system, is the key mechanism for ATP regeneration during the first 10 s of exercise and is vital to power endurance sports.

Phosphocreatine and the ATP-PCr reaction

The structure of phosphocreatine (PCr), sometimes referred to as creatine phosphate, is shown in Figure 9.5. At

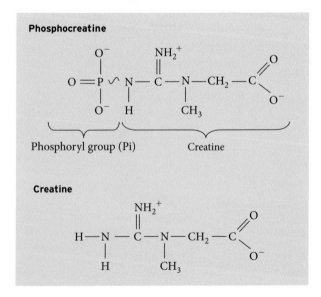

Figure 9.5 Structure of phosphocreatine and creatine.

$$\text{PCr} + \text{ADP} + \text{H}^+ \; \underset{\longleftarrow}{\overset{\text{creatine}}{\overset{\text{kinase}}{\longrightarrow}}} \; \text{Cr} + \text{ATP}$$

Figure 9.6 The creatine kinase reaction.

rest the muscular concentration of PCr is between 18–20 mmol kg^{-1}, about three to four times greater than the muscle stores of ATP. During maximal exercise ATP stores in the working muscle would be exhausted, as already mentioned, in 2 s of effort. However, the ATP is maintained through the breakdown of the PCr stores in a reaction catalysed by creatine kinase (CK).

The ATP-PCr reaction, sometimes called the creatine kinase reaction, is shown in Figure 9.6. As with other enzymes within the body there are different forms of CK. The most common form of CK found in skeletal muscle is structurally different from that found in the heart, smooth muscle and the brain. Within skeletal muscle CK3 (also known as CK-MM) is the most common form and is found close to the sarcomere M-lines because of its attraction to myosin protein filaments that form part of the M-line structure (see Chapter 5). The stores of ATP, ATPase and PCr are likewise maintained within the sarcoplasm, close to the muscular contractile units, the sarcomeres. The close proximity of the metabolites enables firstly, the rapid hydrolysis of ATP for muscular contraction and subsequently, the catabolism of PCr to maintain ATP concentrations (ATP-PCr reaction).

From the onset of exercise, muscle ATP stores are catabolised to supply the energy for muscular contraction. This reaction causes an increase in ADP and inorganic phosphate (Pi) concentration. The immediate proximity of PCr to the newly created ADP molecules, along with the presence of creatine kinase, enables the ATP-PCr reaction to proceed at a fast rate and maintain ATP supplies for muscular contraction. During exercise the reversible ATP-PCr reaction favours the formation of ATP, whereas at rest aerobic metabolism enables the regeneration of PCr stores within the muscle.

As can be seen from Figure 9.5, PCr is created from the bonding of creatine and Pi molecules. The bond created stores energy which is released when PCr is broken down during exercise, enabling the formation of ATP from ADP. Creatine is consumed within the diet as a constituent of meat or can be synthesised in the liver from the amino acids glycine, arginine and methionine. The supplementation of dietary creatine has been suggested as an ergogenic aid for power-based sports and is widely sold commercially. The role of creatine in improvement of performance

in explosive activities is discussed later in this chapter in the nutrition and ergogenic aids section and is the subject of the classic research summary on pages 292–3.

Key points

Muscle ATP stores supply the energy required during the first 2 s of exercise.

Power sports: energy exclusively supplied by ATP stores, e.g. shot putt or hammer throw.

Power endurance sports: following depletion of ATP stores, the phosphagen system is the key pathway for ATP regeneration (2–10 s).

The ATP-PCr reaction:

$$\text{PCr} + \text{ADP} + \text{H}^+ \; \rightleftharpoons \; \text{Cr} + \text{ATP}$$

The main reaction of the phosphagen systems

The predominant power endurance pathway (2–6 s)

The adenylate kinase and adenylate deaminase reactions

As exercise duration approaches 6 s of maximal effort for a power endurance sport, PCr stores would be substantially diminished when compared with resting concentrations. At the same time, as a consequence of the continued demand for ATP, muscular ADP concentrations would have risen. Data for elite 100 m sprinters, with a drop from maximal running speeds occurring from around 60 m, appear to support this notion. However, recent times by Usain Bolt, who has been able to sustain maximal running speeds through to 75–90 m, might challenge this notion. The PCr concentration begins to fall as muscular stores are limited and PCr cannot be resynthesised during high-intensity exercise. The rise in ADP concentration triggers two reactions that serve to maintain all out effort and to stimulate glycolysis activation. The first reaction, the adenylate kinase reaction, is a supplementary phosphagen energy system that results in the formation of additional ATP to maintain maximal effort. The second reaction, the adenylate deaminase reaction is also described here because, although not a reaction that creates additional ATP, it is triggered by rises in AMP concentration, a product of the adenylate kinase reaction, and serves to activate glycolysis, the next key metabolic pathway beyond the phosphagen systems.

Adenylate kinase reaction (AKR)

As the name suggests, this reaction, shown in Figure 9.7, is catalysed by the enzyme adenylate kinase (sometimes called *myokinase* or when referring to the reaction in cells other

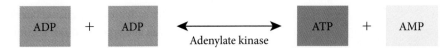

Figure 9.7 The adenylate kinase reaction.

than muscle tissue as *AMP kinase*). As muscular ADP concentrations rise during high-intensity exercise, adenylate kinase catalyses a reaction that breaks the phosphoanhydride bond of one ADP releasing sufficient energy to bond a Pi to another ADP to create an ATP and an AMP moiety (Figure 9.7). The ATP synthesised serves to maintain ATP concentration, while the rise in AMP concentration plays an important role in the activation of glycolytic enzymes. In other words, increased muscular AMP concentrations, the result of the adenylate kinase reaction, stimulate the rate of glycolysis to sustain maximal power output beyond 6 s.

The adenylate deaminase reaction (ADR)

In the section on protein metabolism in Chapter 2 the process of amino acid deamination was described. As a result of deamination the amine, or nitrogen component of an amino acid, is removed. This process enables the remaining part of an amino acid, the α-keto acid, to be metabolised to produce an alternative supply of ATP. In the adenylate deaminase reaction (ADR), with the addition of water, the amine component of AMP is removed to leave inosine monophosphate (IMP) and the amine group which forms ammonia (NH_3) (Figure 9.8). The ADR reaction occurs during high-intensity exercise to reduce the build-up of AMP within the sarcoplasm. A high level of AMP would inhibit the adenylate kinase reaction and interfere with sustained ATP production.

During recovery, much of the IMP can be converted back to AMP through a two-step process that involves GTP. The remaining IMP is further catabolised to inosine, by the removal of the Pi, and then to hypoxanthine, through the removal of the ribose sugar. At this point of catabolism the AMP remnant, hypoxanthine, can be removed from the muscle fibre. The other product of the ADR, the base ammonia (NH_3), quickly accepts an H^+ to become an NH_4^+ which serves as a further activator of glycolysis. Hydrogen ions are widely available for this reaction as high-intensity exercise results in an increased acidity of the blood. Ammonia and hypoxanthine are actively transported from the muscle fibre and subsequently excreted from the body via the urea cycle. The effect of acidosis, rising H^+ concentrations, during sustained high-intensity exercise is discussed in more detail in Chapter 10.

The degradation of ATP to IMP only normally occurs when a maximal effort moves beyond 10 s towards 45 to 60 s duration, such as during an elite athlete's 400 m sprint, 100 m swim or 1 km track cycling time trial. Figure 9.9 provides an overview of ATP hydrolysis and the reactions within the phosphagen system that can lead to the degradation of ATP to IMP.

Key points

As maximal effort continues towards 6 s, PCr stores begin to decline and ADP begins to accumulate, stimulating the adenylate kinase reaction.

The adenylate kinase reaction:

$$ADP + ADP \rightleftharpoons ATP + AMP$$

serves to maintain ATP concentration.

AMP activates glycolytic enzymes.

In situations where maximal effort continues beyond 6 s, AMP is further degraded to IMP in the deaminase kinase reaction.

Key points

In situations where maximal effort continues beyond 10 s, AMP is further degraded to IMP in the adenylate deaminase reaction.

The adenylate deaminase reaction:

$$AMP + H_2O \rightleftharpoons IMP + NH_3$$

Prevents AMP build up which would inhibit AKR and interfere with sustained ATP production.

$$NH_3 + H^+ \rightleftharpoons NH_4 \text{ (an activator of glycolysis)}$$

During recovery IMP is either converted back to AMP or further degraded to hypoxanthine which is, alongside ammonia, removed from the body via the urea cycle.

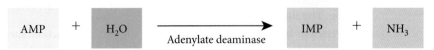

Figure 9.8 The adenylate deaminase reaction.

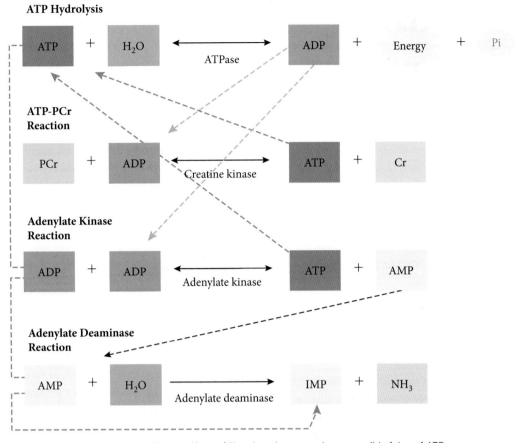

ATP Hydrolysis

ATP-PCr Reaction

Adenylate Kinase Reaction

Adenylate Deaminase Reaction

Figure 9.9 ATP hydrolysis and the reactions of the phosphagen system – possible fates of ATP.

The reactions within the phosphagen system, the immediate source of energy for muscular contraction can be thought of in two phases. The hydrolysis of stored ATP provides the explosive energy for the first 2 s of exercise. Beyond the first 2 s of exercise the ATP-PCr reaction, supported increasingly by the AKR from around 6 s (when muscular ADP concentration begins to rise) provide the predominant pathways for ATP synthesis for the 10 s of power endurance sports. Beyond 10 s the second anaerobic pathway, glycolysis, increasingly becomes the predominant metabolic pathway for ATP synthesis. The role of glycolysis as the predominant ATP synthesis pathway for maximal performance in sports of a longer duration than 10 s, can be thought of as **anaerobic endurance** and is the focus for the next chapter, Chapter 10.

Key points

The predominant energy production mechanisms during power and power endurance sports are:

Power sports: muscle ATP stores (0–2 s)
Power endurance sports: phosphagen system (ATP-PCr reaction, 2–10 s; adenylate kinase reaction, 6–10 s)

Metabolic pathways and maximal power output

Absolute peak power output is attained by human effort within the first 2–4 seconds of exercise, somewhere between power and the very start of power endurance activities.

Beyond this, power output drops so that the attainment of peak power during power endurance, anaerobic endurance and aerobic endurance activities is relative to the rate of ATP re-synthesis. Maximal effort, however, is a key component across the energy systems for many sports. The phosphagen system is responsible for maximal power output for very short and short duration, power and power endurance, activities. Maximal power output through glycolysis (anaerobic endurance) and through the aerobic system (aerobic power) are covered in the relevant chapters to follow.

Knowledge integration question

What energy systems and reactions provide energy for an elite athlete during a 100 m sprint? Can a legal ergogenic aid help in the performance of power endurance sports, and, if so, how does it function?

9.2 The physiology of power and power endurance sports

As was introduced in Chapter 8, *anaerobic* relates to metabolic pathways that do not require oxygen to synthesise ATP. The body has two main mechanisms through which to regenerate energy anaerobically: the phosphagen system and fast-rate glycolysis. Anaerobic mechanisms provide the 1st and 2nd gears for energy production. The 1st gear (muscle ATP stores and the phosphagen system) provides the energy required for *power* and *power endurance* sports like shot putt, 100m sprints, as well as power lifting and Olympic weight-lifting. *Power* represents an expression of strength at speed (strength/speed = power) and involves very short explosive movements such as those in the throwing events in athletics. *Power endurance* involves the use of a maximal expression of force over a more sustained period, up to 10 s, such as seen during an elite runner's 100m sprint.

Power and power endurance components of fitness

In addition to anaerobic power, power and power endurance sports are closely related to two further components of fitness, strength and speed. These components, shown in Chapter 8, Table 8.3, are normally described as separate aspects of fitness, and can be individually defined. In a sports performance context, however, strength and speed are related and integral to power and power endurance. **Strength** represents the maximum force a muscle or group of muscles can generate. It is most often associated with strength training, and is commonly measured by a one repetition maximum (1RM). In isolation, strength is of less immediate importance to sport; however, as a component of power, it is of great importance. **Speed** represents moving from one point to another as quickly as possible and is calculated by the formula distance/time, for example, metres per second ($m \cdot s^{-1}$). **Power**, the resultant of strength and speed (calculated by the formula, force (strength)/speed, e.g. watts per second ($W \cdot s^{-1}$)) is an essential component of fitness for many sports. Shot putt, the take-off in long jump, a slam-dunk in basketball, shoulder throws in judo and the Olympic lifts all rely on power. Power represents the functional application of strength at speed.

Key points

The fitness components for explosive sports are strength, speed and power.

Power represents the ability to generate strength at speed.

The maximal expression of strength or force in strength training can only be maintained for a matter of seconds. In a similar way, maximal speed, as demonstrated in the 100 m sprint, is achieved in the first few seconds and can be maintained for a relatively short period of time. As such, the time duration for the expression of maximal strength and speed, along with their clear link with power, make these aspects of fitness vital to anaerobic *power* and *power endurance*. Figure 9.10 illustrates shot putt as an example of power performance. The photo shows Jacko Gill (New Zealand), World Youth Champion (2011) who won that title immediately after releasing the shot. The athlete takes their throw from inside a circle (2.135 m diameter) with a 10 cm high stop board at the front edge. There are two main styles of putting; the glide and the spin. Currently there is a fairly even split between gliders and spinners at international level. In senior competitions the men's shot weighs 7.26 kg, with the women's weighing 4 kg. It is clear therefore that strength and power are key components of shot putting. The power which an athlete imparts on the shot putt, along with technical factors such as angle of release (optimal angle around 40° for gliders and about 35% for rotary/spin throwers), is vital to the distance travelled by the shot. The strength of the arm and the velocity at which the arm can move combine to form the resultant power, crucial components to the performance of a shot putter. An inspiring performance story from Jacko Gill's earlier years in the sport is told in the Sport in Action piece on p. 291.

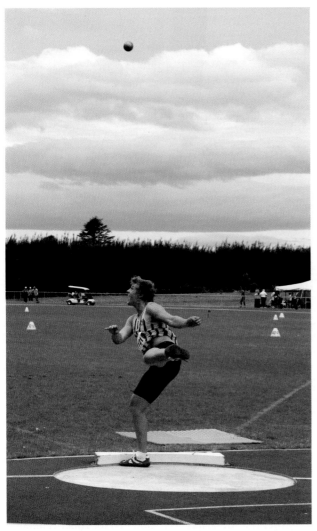

Figure 9.10 Anaerobic performance: shot putt. (*Source*: Dean Flyger)

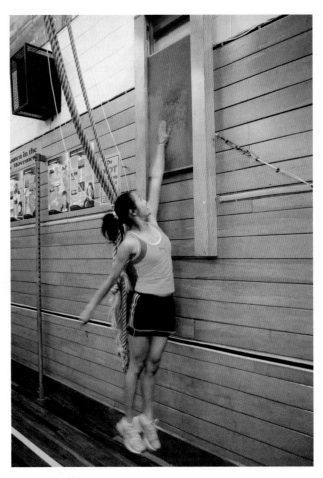

Figure 9.11 Athlete performing vertical jump using a jump board. (*Source*: Simon Fryer)

Tests of anaerobic power and endurance

Anaerobic power – the application of strength at speed – is an explosive aspect of sport, and tests to examine this aspect of fitness should reflect this. If possible these should be sport-related; however, there are a number of generic anaerobic power tests that could be completed as described, or adapted to a specific sport, as part of a monitoring programme.

Field tests

Vertical jump

The vertical jump test provides a measure of anaerobic power. To complete the test, having chalked their nearest hand fingertips, the participant stands sideways to the measuring board (see Figure 9.11), 15 cm from the board. They raise their arm and stretch to the highest point they can reach, making a mark on the board. The performer then re-chalks their fingertips and performs a counter-movement jump to touch as high as possible with their fingertips on the measuring board.

The best of three trials is recorded. The vertical jump height is determined by taking the standing height away from the jump height:

$$\text{vertical jump} = \text{jump height} - \text{standing height (cm)}$$

Standing broad jump test

The standing broad jump provides an alternative to the vertical jump for assessment of leg power. Interestingly, the standing long jump as it was known then, was an Olympic event between 1900 and 1912, and during that time American athlete Ray Ewry set the world record with a standing long jump of 3.47 m. The current world record, which was set in 1968 by Norwegian Arne Tvervaag, stands at 3.71 m. This test requires very little equipment and can be completed in a laboratory, gymnasium or other suitable venue with a non-slip floor. The test can also be conducted into a long-jump pit to provide a softer landing for athletes. From a comfortable standing position, legs slightly apart and behind the take-off line, the athlete jumps two-footed and lands (also two-footed) as far away from the take-off line as possible. The distance from the take-off line to the back of the heels is recorded. The athlete's score is taken as the best of three trials.

Upper-body power tests

There are a number of upper-body tests that can be used to assess power for athletes where upper-limb power is important for performance purposes. Medicine balls, which typically can be purchased in weights ranging from 1 kg to 12 kg, provide opportunities for a variety of upper-body power assessments to suit a specific sport. Examples include seated or standing overhead throws, reverse or backwards overhead throws, chest passes and underarm passes. In addition, within some sports there are specific tests of upper-body power such as the power slap test which was developed for use within the sport of rock climbing.

Margaria-Kalamen power test

The Margaria-Kalamen power test, a well-established measure of the anaerobic power production of the lower extremities, provides an alternative test, although it requires a very accurate timing device and a staircase (with at least 9 steps of a height of 17.5 cm) with a flat 6 m lead up area. The illustrations in Figure 9.12 show (a) the set-up of equipment for testing and (b) a participant completing the Margaria step test. Starting 6 m from the stairs, the performer sprints to and up the flight of steps as quickly as possible. The steps are ascended three at a time: contacting the 3rd, 6th and 9th steps. The timing device is triggered upon contact with the 3rd step and stopped when the 9th step is reached.

The time is recorded as the best of three trials. The formula can then be used to calculate power:

power (watts) = (body mss (kg) × 9.807 (m·s^{-2}) × vertical height (m) ÷ time (s)

Vertical height is that from step 3 to step 9, the normal acceleration due to gravity is represented by 9.807, and

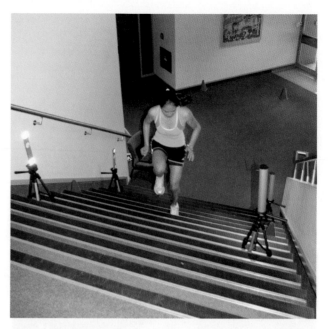

Figure 9.12 Participant completing the Margaria Step Test. Notice the timing gates placed on the 3rd and 9th steps. Participants start 6 m from the bottom of the flight of steps (indicated by the orange cones). However, the test time for each participant is determined from the time taken to pass between the two timing gates. (*Source*: Simon Fryer)

time is the time taken to complete the climb from the 3rd to the 9th step.

A good example of adapting available fitness tests for a specific sport is found with the Margaria-Kalamen anaerobic power test which has been modified for American football athletes (Hetzler et al., 2010). The football stair climb test (FST) increased the vertical height to be covered (20 steps, 3.12 m), ascending 4 steps at a time so that the average best test time was 2.05 s, and was found to be reliable for the measurement of peak anaerobic power in collegiate football players.

Sprint and acceleration tests

Although not a direct measure of power, a measure of running velocity is generally accepted to be related to power. In order to capture the duration of power endurance activities, short sprints (30–50 m) may be more appropriate than longer sprints (e.g. 100 m). The distance selected, however, will be dependent on the goal, age and anaerobic fitness of the individual. Acceleration in sprint running is heavily dependent on the power of the legs and as such, the time taken to run 10 m from a standing start can be used as a test of power.

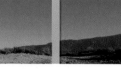

CALCULATION

Margaria-Kalamen power test Example

A 19-year-old (body mass = 73 kg) climbed a vertical height of 1.05 m (the distance from the 3rd to the 9th step) in a time of 0.826 seconds. Their power output is calculated as follows:

Power = (body mass × 9.807 × vertical height) ÷ time

Power = (73 × 9.807 × 1.05) ÷ 0.826

Power = (751.70655) ÷ 0.826

Power = 910 Watts

Laboratory tests

In addition to the numerous field tests, anaerobic power and power endurance can be measured through laboratory testing. The validity of the vertical jump test can be improved in the laboratory with the use of a force platform and computer analysis. From the recording of the ground reaction forces and the acceleration of the body's centre of mass, peak power output can be calculated.

More commonly, however, cycle tests are utilised in the laboratory for the measurement of power output. The two main cycling tests are the Wingate Anaerobic Test (WAnT) and the Force-Velocity Test (FVT).

The WAnT is used to determine leg peak power and mean power. As the test is primarily used for the determination of anaerobic endurance, through the calculation of mean power and fatigue index, it generally lasts either 30 or 60 seconds. The detail of the WAnT is therefore discussed in Chapter 10, primarily as a test of anaerobic endurance. The FVT involves a series of short (5–8 s) maximal sprints against increasing resistance, aiming to reach maximal pedalling rate as quickly as possible. With an increase in the applied resistance, peak pedalling velocity falls in a linear fashion. As power is a measure of the rate at which work is performed, power output can be calculated from this test by multiplying the force by the velocity.

Isokinetic dynamometry, in addition to the assessment of muscular strength, can be used for the accurate measurement of peak power output. Additionally it can calculate mean power output and the decline in power output during fatiguing exercise, as an assessment of anaerobic endurance. As a common measure of muscular strength, more information on isokinetic dynamometry is provided in the following section.

Key points

Tests for the measurement of power and power endurance:

Field tests:

➤ Generic: vertical jump, standing broad jump, Margaria-Kalamen power test,

➤ Sport-specific: Power slap test (rock climbing), football stair climb test (FST; American football)

➤ Laboratory tests: Wingate anaerobic test (WAnT), force-velocity test, vertical jump test, dynamometry

Tests of strength and speed

Strength tests

Assessment of *strength* development needs to be based around the most appropriate exercises for the specific sport. There are several methods for monitoring strength changes, including the use of free weights, resistance exercise machines, or dynamometers. The 'gold standard' for evaluating strength is the 1RM (one repetition maximum) effort; however, as this test is not suitable for all, a variety of strength tests is used.

Free weights

Free weights are perhaps the most common equipment used for the assessment of strength. They are readily available and of a low cost which makes them appropriate for repeated testing during a training programme. The options of muscles and movements to be tested is extremely varied, from focusing on a single muscle to whole body strength, as assessed with multiple joint movements such as the squat or the power clean. These options allow for the strength testing of a particular movement pattern specific to a sport. In addition, due to the balance factor involved, a test that closely simulates athletic activities should be adopted. An example of a sport-specific strength test using free weights is the prone bench pull, as performed by rowers.

As mentioned above, the 1RM is the 'gold standard' of strength testing and is a test of the maximum weight that can be lifted for one repetition. Repeated lifts (e.g. 5–10 repetition maximum), however, can also be used as a measure of strength. The number of repetitions should be based upon the sport and the age and experience of the athlete. Later in this chapter, a selection of weight training exercises appropriate for a number of sports are described, and these could easily form the basis for a strength assessment.

Fixed weights

Due to the nature of resistance exercise machines, movement only occurs in one plane of motion, hence there is no balance control involved (an advantage for the testing of inexperienced individuals). Similar to free weights, the external resistance applied by the machines is constant. The use of resistance machines for strength testing will likely be preferred over free weights in younger, and less experienced, individuals. A disadvantage of fixed weights is that the movement possible is limited by the machine and hence may not be as sport-specific as those that can be performed using free weights.

Dynamometry

In addition to the use of free or fixed weights to assess strength, dynamometry can be utilised in the laboratory. The movements on a dynamometer, however, are restricted and will therefore be less specific to the sport of interest. Despite this, it allows for the assessment of both upper- and lower-limb strength, isometric and isokinetic (contraction at a constant velocity) strength, and can also examine the strength of both concentric and eccentric contractions. This is very useful to determine whether the strength of agonistic muscle pairs are balanced, an important aspect in the sporting world for the prevention of injury. Isokinetic dynamometers are commonly used for strength testing, although the cost and lack of accessibility can be major disadvantages in the use of these protocols.

Key points

Strength testing:

➤ One repetition maximum (1RM) is the 'gold standard'

➤ Can use free weights, fixed weights or dynamometry

Dynamometry:

➤ Allows for the testing of isometric and isokinetic strength

➤ Can determine the strength of both concentric and eccentric contractions

Speed tests

An athlete's *speed* could be assessed very simply as a land-based or water-based assessment of time taken to cover a specific distance. Example distances for land-based tests could be 10 m, 20 m or 30 m etc. up to a maximum of around 100 m depending on the ability of the individual athlete. A sprint training session with the New Zealand All Blacks rugby team is illustrated in Figure 9.13. Similarly, water-based speed tests could be performed for swimmers, kayakers or similar. The accuracy of timing is very important for speed tests. Where possible, the use of timing devices with electronic sensors should be used to increase accuracy. With such sensors an infra-red beam is cut off as the athlete passes each sensor, starting and stopping the timer.

Strength training for power and power endurance sports

While strength training can be beneficial and applied to all sports, not exclusively power and power endurance sports, this topic is covered in detail in this chapter because of the close relationship between strength and power, as described above. To improve fitness a training programme may often include a carefully planned strength programme based around the FIT principle to manipulate the duration and intensity of the sessions. A strength programme designed to improve sports performance should be designed specifically for that sport, while for improved health the focus should be upon the individual's own training goals.

In its simplest form strength training involves adding resistance to a muscular contraction so that an overload is created. Exercises conducted with an overload will result in increases of strength. Many towns and cities around the world have gyms and health clubs where it is possible to undertake a strength training programme. A strength training programme can be manipulated to focus

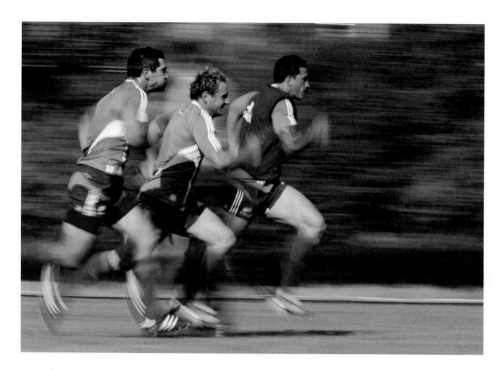

Figure 9.13 Members of the New Zealand All Blacks rugby team sprinting during a fitness session. (*Source*: Georgie/ RugbyImages)

on hypertrophy strength, power or muscular endurance improvements. Individual exercises within a strength training programme can be designed using bodyweight, free weights, machine weights, elastic cords or a combination of these. The wide range of training equipment now available means that many exercises can be designed for each muscle, either in isolation or as part of a functional group for a compound lift. Carrying out a preacher curl would be an example of a muscle (the biceps) being trained in isolation, whereas a power clean, a very important exercise for athletes, works a large number of muscles in a coordinated movement pattern. Time for weight training may be limited, and as a consequence compound exercises could form the basis for a strength programme. A further benefit of compound exercises is that the contraction of muscles in coordinated groups is more akin to the movements required in many sports. When recovering from an injury, an athete's rehabilitation programme might include more single muscle group exercises, but generally compound lifts are more appropriate for sport-related strength improvement. Therefore, in accordance with the specificity principle, a strength training programme should ideally be comprised of exercises that match the movements within the sport, with the FIT adjusted to meet strength, power or muscular endurance outcomes.

Strength training programmes can be manipulated to achieve a variety of outcomes by adjusting the exercises, weight, repetitions (reps), sets and recovery. Table 9.2 provides details of the variation in reps and sets that would

be required depending on the desired outcome; strength/ power, strength, hypertrophy or endurance. The weight for each exercise can be determined using the knowledge of the teacher, coach or athlete, or by experimentation, such that in the last set the athlete can only just complete the required repetitions. For safety reasons is better for an athlete to start using a lower weight and build this up over time. This helps the athlete to avoid sacrificing technique for extra weight.

As an athlete adapts to training, the 2- for-2 rule could be applied to make decisions about when to increase training load. Unless already heavily involved in strength training, teachers, coaches and health professionals should ideally attend an accredited strength training course prior to assisting with strength training programmes.

Table 9.2 Repetitions, sets and recovery times for each strength training outcome.

Outcome	Strength/ power	Strength	Hypertrophy	Muscular endurance
Repetition range	1 – 3	5 – 8	8 – 12	15+
Sets	3 – 5	4	2 – 4	3
Rest between sets	3 – 5 mins	3 –5 mins	1 – 3 mins	1 min

Alternatively, contact could be made with an accredited strength training coach at a local gym who would have knowledge and experience of a wide range of exercises and techniques.

Key points

Strength training programmes can be designed to develop a range of muscular goals: strength, power and muscle size.

Manipulation of exercise repetitions, sets and resistance brings about the desired results.

With adaptation, an increase in training load should be applied, e.g. the 2- for-2 rule.

Strength training exercises

Table 9.3 provides a range of strength training exercises from which the most appropriate for a particular sport or training goal can be selected. Illustrations can be found on the National Strength and Conditioning Association website. When using free weights, particularly for the compound lifts, an athlete should take additional care with technique. The use of wooden discs provides an excellent way to learn the technique for compound lifts before increasing the load. Once learned correctly, compound lifts are highly specific to sports performance and represent a very efficient form of strength training. When very high loads are being lifted using free weights, such as the 1–3 reps for the development of strength/power, the use of an experienced spotter is essential to minimise the risk of injury.

The number of exercises in a session would typically range from 8 to 12, and those selected should be the ones that are the most specific for an athlete's sport or a training goal. For example, in terms of specificity for rowing, it is clear that the major requirement relates to upper-body and leg strength. However, the lower back and abdominals are important as assistor muscles and weaknesses in these aspects of a rower's development would negatively impact on his or her performance. A strength training programme for rowers, therefore, should include exercises for the development of upper body, leg, lower back and abdominal strength.

Key points

Strength training: 8–12 sport-specific exercises per session

Free weight exercises, particularly the compound lifts, require good technique for safe and correct execution – a strength training coach can help develop the correct technique.

Table 9.3 General exercises that could be included in a strength training programme.

Body part	Exercise	Equipment
Shoulders	Lateral raise	Dumbells or machine
	Shoulder press	Barbell, dumbells or machine
	Shrugs	Dumbells
	Upright row	Barbell
Legs	Leg press	Machine
	Leg extension	Machine
	Leg curl	Machine
	Lunge	Dumbells
	Calf raise	Dumbell
Upper back	Seated row	Cable pulley
	Lat pulldown	Machine
	Bent-arm pullover	Dumbell
	One-arm dumbell row	Dumbell
	Chin-ups	Chin bar or beam
Lower back	Back extension	Machine or floor exercise
	Prone cobra	Dumbells
Chest	Dumbell flys	Dumbells
	Press-ups	Floor
	Bench press	Barbell or machine
	Incline bench press	Barbell or machine
Arms	Tricep press	Machine
	Tricep extension	Machine
	Bicep curl	Ez bar, barbell or dumbell
	Reverse curl	Ez bar, barbell or dumbell
Abdominals	Abdominal curls	Machine, floor or Swiss ball
	V-sits	Floor
	Hanging leg raise	Hanging from pull-up bar
Compound lifts	Power clean	Olympic bar
	Deadlift	Olympic bar
	High pull	Olympic bar
	Squat (front)	Olympic bar
	Squat (back)	Olympic bar
	Military press	Olympic bar

Note: Some useful training video clips of a range of these weight training exercises can be found at National Strength and Conditioning Association website http://www.nsca-lift.org/ under 'For the public' and 'Free training videos'.

Programme order

Having selected the exercises for a weight training programme there are a number of ways they can be ordered depending upon the outcomes desired. For maximal strength and power gain, where maximising rest between sets is important, exercises can be carried out from largest to smallest muscle groups (for example bench press before tricep extension or pressdown). Alternatively, the exercises could be ordered by switching between upper-body and lower-body exercises (for example Lat Pulldown to Squat). For hypertrophy and muscular endurance training you could consider moving from small to large muscle groups (triceps extension before bench press) or completing all exercises for one body part before moving on to the next.

By altering the order of exercises, or splitting routines into separate body part sessions, it would be possible for an athlete to train in the gym up to six days per week. However, this degree of weight training specialisation would be more appropriate to sports where strength or muscle size were major aspects of the sport. This is not the case for many sports, consequently, a typical training programme would include three strength sessions per week.

In addition to weight training, there are a number of alternative forms of resistance training that might prove beneficial for athletes in many sports. One of the most important of these is *plyometric training* which is often developed in conjunction, or within, a strength training programme. This form of strength training, referred to as 'complex' training, can be adopted to impact upon the power or endurance capacity of muscles. An example of this type of training would be bench press matched with clap press-ups – a strength exercise to pre-load the system followed by a plyometric power exercise. Plyometric exercises use pre-tensioning of muscles to increase force generation which can be harnessed in the gym for training purposes and within the technique for sports such as basketball, and athletic events like high jump and long jump.

Key points

Plyometrics:

➤ By pre-tensing a muscle, force generation is improved

➤ Important training for power development

➤ Often developed alongside, or within, a weight training programme – known as *complex training*

Yoga and *functional stability training* both offer forms of exercise that can help with core strength and flexibility for sport and could be considered as part of a strength and conditioning programme. Finally, *circuit training*, a combination of strength and conditioning work, can provide an efficient form of training for many sports.

A carefully planned and balanced resistance training programme can be a central part of injury prevention or rehabilitation for any athlete or individual wishing to improve their health and well-being. A key part of injury prevention is about keeping a balance between muscle groups around the main joints of the activity. For instance in rowing and kayaking where 'pulling from the shoulder activities' make up a large part of the demands of the sport, strength training programmes should include 'pushing' exercises as well as pulling exercises to avoid muscle imbalances. A further example would be to ensure a balance in the strength of the quadriceps and hamstrings in sports such as soccer and rugby where a great deal of kicking is involved. Having suitable rest and recovery periods between training sessions, a good basic diet, as well as including a warm-up and cool-down before and after training, can assist with avoiding overtraining illnesses and injuries.

For rehabilitation purposes the use of a physiotherapist or similar medical professional can be very helpful in planning and supporting injury recovery strategies. In addition, they can provide specific resistance training exercises that can be used during the later stages of injury recovery to assist with strengthening the muscles around joints.

Knowledge integration question

What is the relationship between power, strength and speed? What field tests can be used to estimate power and how can this power be improved through training?

Conditioning training for power and power endurance sports

As a result of the association of power with speed and strength, much of the conditioning training for power and power endurance sports has close links with strength training as described above. The key for power and power endurance sports, as for developing conditioning programmes for any sport, is to match the training to the duration and intensity of the event and the key movements involved. In this way, the training for a shot putter, while sharing some similarities, will also have major differences to the training for a 100 m sprinter. Training should be related to sports performance and the predominant metabolic pathways.

Conditioning training for power sports should therefore be linked with improvements in both the speed and strength aspects of performance. As such, the strength and conditioning programmes for power athletes will overlap greatly. Strength training exercises, coupled with plyometric exercises based around the sport-specific movements, would form the key components for a training programme. For example, in shot putt, in addition to whole body weight training exercises, throwing sessions with over and under-weight shots along with medicine ball throws would provide the bulk of strength and conditioning training to complement skill-based components. The speed aspects for the shot putter would depend on whether the athlete was a glider or rotator in the circle, and would focus on speed of movement or rotation, weight transfer and coordination of movement.

A key aspect of conditioning training for power endurance athletes would be adaptation of the phosphagen system as the predominant energy source for these events (which is discussed in more detail in the following section). Research in the field provides a number of helpful points that should be kept in mind when training for power endurance events. Around 6 s of maximal exercise is sufficient to deplete 50–60% of PCr stores within the working muscles and this rises to 90% depletion by around 25–30 s. During recovery, the half-life for PCr resynthesis is around 30 s, so it takes between 3 and 4 minutes, to approach 100 % replenishment of PCr. These figures can help with setting both the duration of exercise and the required recovery time for ATP-PCr training. When planning training for the ATP-PCr system, the recovery between repetitions is especially important, for if insufficient time is allowed the training would be based on the glycolytic metabolic pathway improvement rather than the ATP-PCr pathway.

Depending on the sport, there are a wide number of types of training that can be undertaken to improve power endurance performance. Hills have been used for many years to improve both speed and strength. Uphill sprints can be used to improve leg strength and downhill sprints in different sessions to improve speed. The choice of hill for the type of session is vitally important to provide an appropriate incline and length for the duration of the repetition. In sprint training, tyre and parachute towing, attached to the runner by a harness, have become popular techniques for improving athlete power endurance. This type of sprint training is illustrated in Figure 9.14 where New Zealand rugby player Hosea Gear is parachute running. These methods have been less closely examined through research, however, than more traditional forms of training such as hill running.

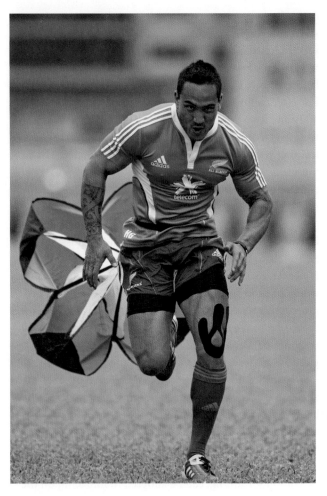

Figure 9.14 Parachute running: a form of resistance sprint training. (*Source*: Georgie/RugbyImages)

Key points

Focus on adaptation of the phosphagen system:
➤ Strength and speed raining
➤ 100% replenishment of PCr stores takes 3–4 min; allow sufficient recovery between repetitions

Sprint training for power endurance sports:
➤ Uphill and downhill sprints to improve strength and speed
➤ Tyre and parachute towing

Fatigue in power and power endurance sports

Fatigue, as it relates to sports performance, is an important concept for athletes and exercise physiologists. In straightforward terms fatigue relates to a temporary inability of muscles to perform at a required work rate. As a physiological concept, fatigue has provided a complex challenge for exercise physiologists and biochemists, and to date, a widely accepted answer remains elusive. The complexity exists because of the number of potential metabolites that might provide the explanation for fatigue, the likelihood is that the answer differs according to the exercise duration and muscle fibre type, as well as the difficulties of *in vivo* examination of fatigue by fibre type.

Research findings to date support the concept of fatigue being specific to the predominant ATP synthesis pathway and to the muscle fibre type. The cause of fatigue therefore is different in power endurance sports, which are the focus of this chapter, compared to anaerobic endurance sports (Chapter 10) and aerobic sports (Chapter 11 and 12). In recent years, however, a number of *in vitro* studies on mammalian muscle fibres have presented a challenge to the most widely accepted theories of fatigue. A concern with such studies is that they present findings of research primarily conducted on frog and rat muscle tissue rather than human fibres, although there are strong functional similarities between them. However researchers in the field are left with little alternative, because the techniques used at present are too invasive to be conducted with human participants and the currently available *in vivo* techniques do not allow examination of individual fibres. It is possible that current in vivo techniques mask, rather than reveal, the causes of fatigue because changes in metabolite concentrations in response to exercise relate to whole muscle response instead of differentiated fibre dynamics. Consequently, taking these difficulties into account, we examine the most widely supported models of fatigue as they relate to the exercise intensity and duration that is the focus of each chapter.

Key points

Fatigue is the temporary inability of a muscle to perform the required work.

The cause of fatigue is specific to the predominant ATP synthesis pathway and muscle fibre type.

In power endurance activities the exercise intensity necessitates a high rate of ATP hydrolysis and re-synthesis primarily through the ATP-PCr reaction, but also through the adenylate kinase reaction which was described previously. As the duration of maximal exercise moves towards 6 s,

the PCr stores begin to diminish, Pi begin to accumulate and, despite the positive contribution of the adenylate kinase reaction, muscular ADP concentrations increase. In addition, it is believed that the high intensity of exercise during power endurance sports leads to a breakdown of intracellular Ca^{2+} transport within the muscle fibre. The accumulation of Pi and breakdown of Ca^{2+} transport have been linked with a disruption in the excitation of muscle fibres required for muscular contraction. Accumulation of ADP within a muscle fibre has been shown to inhibit ATP hydrolysis and the decrease in PCr stores associated with maximal activity results in a drop in the rate of ATP re-synthesis. The presence of these potentially fatiguing metabolites within the muscle fibre makes it difficult to pin-point the exact mechanisms behind fatigue.

Returning to the definition of fatigue, specifically we are talking about a reversible drop in performance (power output) during muscular activity. Within the confines of the muscular protective mechanisms, power sports, fuelled by ATP stores, provide a peak power output at around 2–4 s of exercise. Beyond this, the fast rate of ATP synthesis through the ATP-PCr reaction enables high intensity to be maintained in power endurance sports. When we examine the drop in power output associated with power endurance sports this will occur at a point that is specific to a particular sport, but by way of example, appears to occur at around 6 s in the 100 m sprint. The decline in PCr concentrations associated with power endurance sports is thought to provide a primary mechanism for fatigue in power endurance activities. In addition, recent research indicates that the accumulation of Pi also plays a significant role in power endurance fatigue, one that, over time may prove to be the major determinant of fatigue.

To examine the role of Pi in fatigue it would be useful to revisit the structure and function of the sacroplasmic reticulum (SR), muscles fibres and the sodium potassium pump (Na^+-K^+ pump). Each of these aspects of cellular physiology was examined in Part I of this textbook and it is worthwhile reading these again, but from a functional perspective. While each of these aspects was examined in a specific chapter, in reality they are structurally located close together and represent the largest consumers of ATP during exercise. Within a muscle fibre approximately 50% of the Na^+-K^+ pumps are located within the T-tubule network which invaginates each muscle fibre, and to function these pumps require ATP. The T-tubules along with the SR form the triad junctions which assist in coordinated muscular contraction. As the wave of depolarisation sweeps along the T-tubules this stimulates the terminal cisternae of the SR to release calcium (Ca^{2+}) which enables muscular contraction to take place. The re-sequestering of Ca^{2+} to the SR takes place via Ca^{2+} pumps located on the terminal cisternae and ATP is required for this process. Calcium released from the SR into the sarcoplasm is free to bond with troponin C and facilitate movement of tropomyosin away from the myosin binding sites, enabling crossbridges to form. The formation of crossbridges and the sliding of filaments, being the mechanism through which muscular contraction takes place, require ATP to detach the myosin heads from the actin filaments. The SR triads are located close to the sarcomeres to facilitate muscular contraction. Through this structure the three heaviest users of ATP during exercise are located in close proximity to facilitate muscular contraction during exercise. As a consequence ATP consumption and Pi accumulation will be significantly higher at the localised sites.

In recent *in vitro* studies Pi accumulation has been associated with a decrease in Ca^{2+} sensitivity and Ca^{2+} release from the SR. Both of these factors have been demonstrated to lead to a decrease in myofibrillar force production, which by definition relates to an increase in fatigue. The decrease in Ca^{2+} sensitivity relates to myofibrillar crossbridge formation, with an accumulation of Pi being found to decrease the sensitivity of troponin C to free Ca^{2+} within the sarcoplasm. This situation may be exacerbated by a Pi-induced inhibition of SR Ca^{2+} release, reducing the available Ca^{2+} within the sarcoplasm during muscular contraction. Both factors lead to a reduction in crossbridge formation and a concomitant decrease in force generation.

In summary, it appears that the decline in PCr and the deleterious effects of Pi accumulation provide the most likely sources of fatigue, reversible power output decline, associated with power endurance performance. It is likely that in type II fibres, particularly type IIx which are recruited most heavily for power endurance sports, such concentration differences are most marked. In contrast, type I fibres appear to be relatively fatigue-resistant.

Key points

As the duration of maximal exercise duration approaches 6 s:

PCr stores ↓   Pi ↑   ADP ↑

ADP accumulation inhibits ATP hydrolysis.

Pi accumulation is associated with reduced Ca^{2+} sensitivity and release from the SR.

The most likely mechanisms of fatigue in power endurance activities are the fall in muscle PCr and the negative effects of Pi accumulation on myofibrillar force production.

Knowledge integration question

During power endurance sports, the ability to produce maximal muscular contractions falls over time. What is this situation referred to, and what factors are responsible for bringing about this fall in power output?

Physiological adaptations to power training

Training to improve power and power endurance requires a combination of sprint – high-intensity, very short duration activity – and strength training. Research findings clearly indicate that these forms of training result in improvements in performance, as shown through increases in speed, power or strength following this type of training. There is a general agreement between exercise physiologists as to the adaptations to aerobic endurance training. However, research findings in the less-studied field of anaerobic (including power and power endurance activities) metabolism are more equivocal. The physiological adaptations in response to sprint and strength training described in this section represent those that are more widely supported in the literature. As with other aspects of anaerobic physiology, there is a greater divergence in views as to the mechanisms behind anaerobic adaptations to training. The reasons behind these differing views relate to several factors:

- The smaller body of knowledge compared to aerobic endurance training
- The reliance on animal studies – making inferences from animals to humans
- A greater variation in the types of training and assessment equipment used compared to that employed for aerobic-based research

An example of this can be found in the uncertainty that exists regarding the notion of human muscle fibre *hyperplasia*. Research with animals has identified incidences of both hypertrophy (increase in muscle fibre size) and hyperplasia in response to training. The application of this finding to humans is yet to find common acceptance among exercise physiologists for whom muscle hypertrophy is the most widely accepted consequence of sprint and resistance training.

The more commonly agreed adaptations to sprint and resistance training include increases in:

- muscular strength and size
- ATP, PCr and creatine stores

- ATP-PCr enzyme activity
- neuromuscular functioning
- efficiency of movement
- ligament and tendon strength
- bone mineral content
- fat-free mass along with an associated decrease in body fat percentage

Sprint and resistance exercise leads to a greater recruitment of type II muscle fibres than aerobic exercise and as a consequence this type of training results in an increase in the cross-sectional area of type II muscle fibres. Type I fibres also increase in size through power and power endurance training but to a lesser extent. It is thought that the increases in muscle fibre cross-sectional area relate to increases in the size and number of myofibrils along with associated increases in the number of myosin and actin filaments within each sarcomere. In addition, research suggests there is a gradual shift of some type I fibres to the structural composition of type II fibres, which serves to improve power and power endurance performance.

There appears to be a general agreement as to the increase in activity of the phosphagen system enzymes, creatine kinase and adenylate kinase, in response to sprint and strength training. As was described earlier in this chapter, CK catalyses the reaction to synthesise ATP from the breakdown of PCr and adenylate kinase (sometimes referred to as myokinase) catalyses ATP synthesis from two ADP. These mechanisms serve to maintain the supply of ATP during power endurance activities. Sprint training particularly has been found to enhance creatine kinase and adenylate kinase activity resulting in improved power endurance performance. Results regarding increased ATP and PCr stores in response to training, however, remain equivocal, although research identifying differences between endurance and power athletes revealed higher resting muscle stores of these substrates in power sports performers.

Knowledge integration question

What are the most effective types of training for the improvement of power and power endurance activities? What factors need to be considered in the development and execution of a power training programme?

Strength gains through resistance training can be up to 25% or more, dependent upon the training status of the individual and the type of programme followed. With regard to strength training the use of low repetitions and higher relative loads is associated with greater gains in strength, while higher repetitions and lower relative loads results in greater incidences of muscle fibre hypertrophy. In the early stages of a strength training programme research indicates that gains are more related to improvements in neuromuscular functioning – coordination of movement – than to hypertrophy. Beyond 8–12 weeks, subsequent strength gains appear to result from improvements in contractile force and muscle fibre size. The neuromuscular adaptations associated with sprint and resistance training result from an improvement in muscle fibre recruitment and improved efficiency of movement. They occur more quickly for simple one-limb movements, such as that encountered in a bicep curl, than for more complex and technical movements, such as a power clean, sprint action or shot putt.

Key points

Anaerobic training for power and power endurance sports is primarily sprint and resistance training.

Training adaptations mainly concern muscle and energy system alterations:

➤ Muscle – increased strength and muscle fibre size (mainly type II fibres)

➤ Metabolism – increased resting stores of ATP, PCr and creatine, improved phosphagen system enzyme activity

Ergogenic aids for power for power endurance performance

After a brief introduction outlining the range of ergogenic aids available for power and power endurance athletes, we will highlight the use of anabolic steroids and creatine as examples of illegal and legal performance enhancement supplements.

There is a variety of mechanical aids that can assist power and power endurance performance and these include free weights, video analysis, tyre towing, parachute running and the use of elastic cords for speed and strength improvement. The use of the crowd to clap a rhythm for athletes in the jumping events provides an excellent example of a psychological aid for power endurance athletes. Another example can be found from the sport of Olympic weight-lifting where each athlete chooses his or her own motivational music to play as he or she enters the stage for their lift. For power and power endurance sports performers it is also beneficial to monitor protein intake and increase this above the levels for the normal population. Nutritionally, as was described in Chapter 2, protein intake for any athlete should be increased to between 1.0–2.0 g per kg of bodyweight. For those involved in the power and power endurance sports, or for those wishing to develop their power for performance, daily intake should be at least 2.0 g per kg of bodyweight per day.

Androgenic anabolic steroids

Androgenic anabolic steroids (referred to as 'anabolic steroids' in this text) began their usage as medical treatments for patients with muscle wastage and hormonal deficiencies in the early 1950s. Immediately, the potential benefits for sports performance, particularly for power and power endurance events, was recognised by medics involved in sport, coaches and athletes themselves. The 1952 Helsinki Olympics, which saw Soviet Union women athletes dominate in the throwing events, were perhaps the first time that the effect of steroid usage to enhance sports performance was seen on a world stage. Anabolic steroids, amongst a wide number of substances or techniques, are banned for use in sports, originally by the International Olympic Committee and now by the World Anti-Doping Agency (WADA). National governing bodies for sport, working in conjunction with WADA now have extensive in- and out-of-season programmes to test for the illegal use of anabolic steroids for improved sports performance. The legality of anabolic steroids varies by country. Most commonly the possession of steroids is treated less seriously than procurement for onward supply, and this is adopted in countries such as Canada and the UK. In other countries such as the USA and Australia, possession, buying or selling of steroids is illegal, while in complete contrast anabolic steroids are legal in Mexico, Panama and Thailand.

Evidence from the throwing events in athletics, with regard to when world records were set, and results from more recent Olympic Games, suggests the prevalence of anabolic steroid use is declining in some sports, perhaps due to the increased risk of getting caught. At the 2008 Beijing Olympic Games the gold medal winning performances for shot-putt and discus were 7–16%

lower than their respective world records for males and females, all of which were set over 20 years ago (between 1986 and 1990). When we normally consider the differences between winning and losing at Olympic level to be between 1% and 2%, these declines in performance would appear to be significant. Outside the Olympic Games there are, however, a number of sports where anabolic steroid use is still implicated. It is suspected that steroid use is widespread within American football, baseball and bodybuilding.

The structure and function of anabolic steroids

Anabolic steroids include the male hormone testosterone, and the synthetic derivatives of testosterone. The structure of testosterone is illustrated in Figure 2.13 in Chapter 2. Testosterone is produced primarily in the testes (95%) but also in the adrenal cortex (5%) and is derived from cholesterol. Testosterone is the most important anabolic and androgenic hormone in the body. Anabolic, as was discussed in Chapter 2, refers to reactions that synthesise larger products. Testosterone, through its anabolic effect, leads to growth of bone, muscle and other tissues within the body. The androgenic effects of testosterone, referring to changes in primary and secondary sexual characteristics, include enlargement of the penis and testes, the growth of hair on the face and genital area, along with changes in the voice and an increase in aggressiveness. There are a wide range of anabolic steroids designed to mimic the anabolic effects, but minimise the androgenic effects. While synthetic steroid users seek to harness the anabolic effects, it is the androgenic effects, which can be reduced but not eliminated, that provide the major side effects. Table 9.4 provides examples of some common anabolic steroids and their possible side effects.

Anabolic steroids can be taken orally, through the wearing of a patch or by injection into a muscle. Within the body, like natural hormones, they are transported within the blood to cells around the body. As steroid-based synthesised hormones, anabolic steroids are transported into the cell and bind with specialised androgen receptors. The combined receptor and steroid unit is then translocated to the nucleus of the cell where it stimulates a change in cellular functioning. Specifically, at the nucleus the receptor-steroid unit causes the synthesis of messenger RNA molecules which in turn stimulate an anabolic effect across the cell. In muscle fibres, the specific target cell for steroid

Table 9.4 Common androgenic anabolic steroids and possible side effects of steroid use for males and females.

Common steroids	Side effects (males)	Side effects (females)
Methenolone (Primabolan)	Gynecomastia	Facial hair development
Stanozolol (Winstrol)	Testicular atrophy	Clitoral hypertrophy
Methandrostenolone (Dianabol)	Reduced sperm count	Reduced breast tissue
Oxandrolone (Anavar)	Reduced testosterone production	Menstrual abnormalities
Nandrolone (Deca Durabolin)		
Testosterone enanthate (Delatestryl)	Reduced HDL levels/increased LDL levels	
Testosterone cypionate (Depo-testosterone)	Liver damage/jaundice	
Boldenone (Equipoise)	Increased aggression and psychiatric disorders	

users, anabolic steroids stimulate a dual effect. Firstly, they promote protein synthesis, and secondly, they appear to slow down catabolism of the muscle which normally follows training (especially heavy weight training). These steroid-induced effects, when accompanied by a strength training programme can result in increases in muscle fibre size, strength, speed and power.

Key points

Anabolic steroids:

➤ A banned substance for use in sports (IOC and WADA)

➤ Mimic the effects of testosterone: anabolic and androgenic effects

➤ Promote muscle protein synthesis and slow down muscle catabolism

➤ When accompanied by strength training, can increase muscle fibre size, strength, speed and power – ultimately improving performance

The effectiveness of anabolic steroids

Studies of the effectiveness of anabolic steroids have, however, been inconclusive with regard to the extent to which such adaptations can be brought about through steroid use. The positive findings from early studies in the field were called into question because of a lack of *experimental control*. Without appropriate control in the design of an experiment, extraneous variables (outside influences) might just as easily explain the difference between pre- and post-test scores. For example, without appropriate experimental control a placebo effect could explain differences in strength gains at the start and end of an anabolic steroid study. A classic example of the placebo effect occurred in a steroid experiment conducted by Ariel and Saville (1972), the results of which are described in more detail below.

In several later, more controlled studies, researchers were unable to replicate earlier findings with regard to reported strength improvements and muscle hypertrophy. This led to speculation as to whether anabolic steroids actually worked, although anecdotal evidence from users strongly supported their effect. It is now believed that the lack of evidence supporting the effect of steroids on muscular strength and size in controlled studies relates to the size of dose and method for administration. In a research context, participants have been administered far smaller doses of steroid than are reported for user levels in sports settings. In addition, *stacking*, *cycling* and *pyramiding* of drug doses have been adopted by users to multiply the effects of steroid dosages. Stacking involves a practice of using more than one steroid at a time, while cycling provides phases of use and non-use to minimise side effects. Pyramiding involves gradually increasing and decreasing the dose of steroid. These real-world regimes have not been used in a research setting and steroid users suggest this was why increases in muscle size and strength remain equivocal.

It was not until a tightly controlled set of studies conducted by Bhasin et al. (1996–2001), where larger steroid doses were administered, that clear evidence of the strength and muscle size benefits of anabolic steroids were found. In the first of these studies, 40 participants were administered either 600 mg of testosterone enanthate or a placebo (injected intramuscularly) once a week for each of the 10 weeks of the study. Results indicated that when accompanied with strength exercises, steroid use resulted in significant improvements in muscle size, fat-free mass and strength.

Key points

If taken in large enough doses, anabolic steroids are effective in increasing muscle size and muscle strength

but anabolic steroids are an illegal substance with negative side effects and large penalties are enforced when an athlete is caught using this ergogenic aid.

The placebo effect and steroid use

While steroids have been found to improve strength and muscle size it is also very interesting to realise the effects of the mind on performance improvement, as seen through the placebo effect. A *placebo effect* occurs when the body's response to a substance is determined by the individual's expectation of effect rather than by any physiological effect of the substance. As mentioned above, a placebo is often given during blind drug trials and represents an inert substance that to the eye looks identical to the substance under test. In this way, the individual cannot tell whether the substance they are taking is the trial drug or a placebo. This type of control, which should ideally be double blind, is essential when investigating the ergogenic effects of a new supplement. Double blind refers to the fact that neither the participant nor the researcher is aware of which substance is being administered, ensuring the researcher does not present any subliminal expectations to the participants. It is perhaps because of a lack of this type of control that some products, originally released as ergogenic aids, were later unable to be found to have the same performance benefits in controlled double blind studies.

A classic study that revealed the effect a placebo can have on performance was conducted by Ariel and Saville (1972). In this cleverly conceived study, the researchers recruited experienced weight-lifters to take part in an anabolic steroid study. From a pool of 15 volunteers, who they had told would be selected based on their performance during a four month pre-study period, eight participants were randomly selected (improvements during the four-month pre-study period were in reality ignored) to enter the study. To further emphasise the reality of the study for the participants, two of the eight volunteers were then rejected during a sham medical screening. The remaining six participants were then given a placebo, but were told it was in fact the anabolic steroid dianabol. The participants took the dianabol placebo for a period of four weeks. The volunteers continued their normal weight-training schedules during the duration of the four months of the

pre-test and the four weeks of the study. Strength assessments were conducted during the final seven weeks of the pre-treatment and during the study. The competitive nature of the pre-treatment period meant that even though the volunteers were experienced weightlifters they made improvements during this phase of the experiment. The group improved their lifts by 11 kg during the final seven weeks of this phase, but during the treatment phase, when they thought they were taking an anabolic steroid, they improved their lifts by a further 45 kg. This represented a great improvement for experienced weight-lifters and clearly demonstrated the placebo effect.

Risks of steroid use

While more recent controlled evidence suggests that anabolic steroid usage, in conjunction with strength training, can increase muscle size and improve strength, their side-effects, illegality, and contravention of the rules of sport make their use highly questionable. There are high risks involved in their procurement and usage. The illegal nature of steroids, other than by prescription, means it is impossible to know the true origin and content of a purchased product and as such self-administration is highly questionable. As an athlete, the risks of getting caught through the development of new testing procedures, and the seriousness with which steroid use is looked upon by most governing bodies of sport, regardless of the morality of taking steroids to enhance sports performance, make steroid use a potentially career-ending, if not life-threatening, decision.

Clenbuterol – an illegal ergogenic aid

Prior to examining the ergogenic effects of creatine monohydrate, a legal nutritional supplement, it is worth highlighting the case of *clenbuterol* which is associated with increased muscle mass and decreased fat mass. Clenbuterol is associated with anabolic steroids, because, in the past, athletes took it in place of steroids in the final weeks before competition to maintain the anabolic effects, but avoid the risks of a positive steroid test. It is also interesting to examine the case of clenbuterol, as it is one of the β_2 adrenergic-agonists that can be used in the treatment of asthma, which is one of the focuses of Chapter 14.

Clenbuterol first came to light as an ergogenic aid in the early 1990s, while more recently 2010 Tour de France winner Alberto Contador tested positive for the drug during a rest day urine test. As a β_2 adrenergic-agonist, clenbuterol is a sympathomimetic amine, meaning that its effect mimics those of adrenaline and noradrenaline leading to stimulation of the nervous system. It is thought through this action that clenbuterol stimulates enhanced protein synthesis and fat metabolism. In some European countries clenbuterol is licensed, like salbutamol in the UK, USA, Australia and New Zealand, as a bronchodilator to treat and prevent exercise induced asthma. In 1992, however, it became a banned anabolic agent by the IOC and continues to remain on the list of prohibited substances compiled by WADA. In contrast, salbutamol, by medical exemption, is a permitted β_2 adrenergic-agonist for the treatment of asthma. Potential side effects of clenbuterol are linked to its stimulant effect and include insomnia, anxiety, heart arrhythmias and heart failure.

Creatine monohydrate

The now popular nutritional supplement *creatine monohydrate* appears to have a legal ergogenic effect, not only for power and power endurance sports, but also for lactate tolerance in anaerobic endurance sports, which are described in Chapter 10, and in intermittent sports (the focus of Chapter 13). Creatine is a naturally occurring compound contained in meat and fish or synthesised within the body. The majority (over 90%) of the body's stores of creatine are held within muscle fibres. The body has a natural turnover rate of about 2 grams per day – ~2 g are provided in the diet and ~2 g are excreted from the body within the urine. Thus, during normal conditions, the body's levels of creatine remain constant. Vegans and vegetarians take in much smaller volumes of creatine in their diet, so rely on endogenous synthesis of creatine and, perhaps as a consequence of their reduced intake, also excrete less creatine in their urine.

Creatine monohydrate - the ergogenic effect

Once inside the muscle fibre, creatine readily combines with phosphate to create PCr. The importance of PCr, as the body's immediate source for ATP re-synthesis during high-intensity exercise, was described in detail in the section on the phosphagen system, earlier in this chapter. Consequently, increased stores of PCr have been linked with improvements in the performance of strength, power, power endurance, anaerobic endurance and intermittent sports. Research by Harris and colleagues (1992) revealed that PCr and creatine stores within the muscle can be increased through supplementation of dietary creatine. A loading dose of 20 grams per day for six days resulted in an increase of 20% in total muscle creatine, of which one third was converted to PCr. The consequent rise in muscular PCr concentration is thought to increase the capacity of the ATP-PCr pathway, thereby delaying fatigue for power endurance activities.

Creatine monohydrate and performance

Since these findings were published, and in light of the success of British athletes such as Sally Gunnell and Linford Christie at the 1992 Olympic Barcelona Games, who reportedly trained using creatine, the supplement has been the focus of numerous subsequent studies. Research findings have indicated improvements in tests relating to strength, power, anaerobic endurance and repeat sprint laboratory test performance. Studies by Balsom and colleagues (1993) and Casey and co-workers (1996) found creatine supplementation improved sprint performance by delaying the effects of fatigue, increasing peak power and also increasing total work. Although some studies have found no effect of creatine supplementation, the majority report improvements during laboratory-based tests. Less clear-cut results have been found in performance-based-tests. It appears that the closer the required power output is to an individual's maximum, or when high-intensity repeat activity is required, the better the impact on performance. In swimming, for instance (even in short (25 m) sprints), perhaps due to the highly technical nature of the sport, results remain equivocal with a number of studies reporting no improvement in performance through creatine supplementation. In contrast, during repeat sprint swimming (10×50 m), creatine supplementation was found to result in an improvement in performance as measured through swimming time.

Dosing strategies

In terms of creatine monohydrate loading doses, research indicates that either a sustained low dose, or an initial high loading followed by a lower maintenance dose, can result in equal success. A loading regime of 20 grams per day for six days followed by 2 grams per day for the remaining 22 days resulted in a very similar increase in total muscle creatine stores when compared to a 3-grams-per-day regimen.

More recent research suggests that with prolonged creatine use the response of muscle to the supplementation decreases over time, resulting in a lower muscle concentration and, with this, a drop in performance benefits. To combat the loss in ergogenic effect, it has been suggested that interruptions in supplementation protocols enhance subsequent muscular uptake and maintain ergogenic benefits. Results of research indicate that a 4-week washout following a 12-week creatine supplementation phase is beneficial for maintaining creatine stores above baseline. The effects of such a regimen, along with the ergogenic effect of creatine for sports performance, do, however, require further research.

The moral dilemma

Creatine monohydrate is a legal supplement that appears to improve performance in power, power endurance and anaerobic endurance. There is, however, an ethical or moral decision an athlete must make when choosing to supplement with creatine monohydrate. Depending on the views of the individual athlete, creatine monohydrate supplementation goes against the spirit of the WADA policy as a substance that is taken in abnormal quantities with the aim of improving performance. The choices an athlete has to make with regard to any supplementation are very personal and can be illustrated by the case of one British athlete who won a bronze medal in the 1999 Judo World Championships. After discussion with the athlete about creatine supplementation the athlete made the decision not to take creatine monohydrate, despite its ergogenic effects, because of their own ethical standpoint. For them, in a competitive sport context, the use of creatine monohydrate was cheating. Each athlete has to make up their own mind about the use of creatine monohydrate or any other ergogenic aid. Research appears to suggest that there are no long-term health effects of taking creatine. To date, however, there has not been a longitudinal study regarding the long-term effects and it is worth bearing this in mind when making a decision to use creatine monohydrate as a supplement. The use of a wash-out phase, as was described above, would appear to lessen any potentially harmful effects.

Key points

Ergogenic aids for power and power endurance sports:

➤ illegal: anabolic steroids and clenbuterol

➤ legal: creatine monophosphate

Creatine monophosphate:

➤ Combines with phosphate in the muscle to form PCr (crucial for ATP re-synthesis)

➤ Improves strength, power and power endurance

➤ To maintain muscle concentration and ergogenic effect, a wash-out period may be beneficial

Check your recall
Fill in the missing words.

➤ ATP stores within the _____ fuel power sports and the first two seconds of power endurance activities.

➤ The main energy source for power endurance sports is the _____ system.

➤ Adenosine is a nucleoside composed of the base _____ and the sugar _____ .

➤ The bonding of adenosine with three _____ forms the energy storing molecule essential for muscle contraction.

➤ Energy is released for cellular metabolism through the _____ of ATP.

➤ The catabolism of ATP is presented in the following reaction:

$$ATP + H_2O \longrightarrow \text{_____} + Pi$$

➤ ATP can be replenished very quickly from the breakdown of phosphocreatine (PCr) in a reaction catalysed by the enzyme – _____ _____ .

➤ The ATP-PCr reaction is the predominant energy pathway during the initial _____ seconds of maximal intensity exercise.

➤ Creatine supplementation is common among _____ athletes.

➤ In addition to the ATP-PCr reaction, ATP can be re-synthesised from two ADP molecules through the _____ _____ reaction.

➤ A build-up of AMP following this reaction stimulates an increase in the rate of _____.

➤ The build-up of _____ is reduced through the adenylate deaminase reaction.

➤ Fatigue occurs during exercise when a drop in expected _____ occurs.

➤ Training for power and power endurance sports involves a combination of high-intensity, short-duration activities and _____ training.

➤ Sprint and strength training results in a variety of muscle adaptations, including:

1. _____

2. _____ and

3. _____ .

Review questions

1. How would you define power and power endurance? Describe a sporting example of each of these.

2. Describe the mechanisms responsible for energy production in activities of up to 10 seconds duration.

3. What do the terms exothermic and endothermic mean?

4. Why is the symbol ~ possibly misleading when used to represent the bonds between the phosphoryl groups in ATP?

5. Why is the breakdown of ATP to ADP very different from the breakdown of AMP to IMP?

6. What is the relationship between power, strength and speed?

7. Give three examples of field tests for the assessment of power. Describe one of these tests in detail.

8. What variations in sprint training are currently included in the training programmes of power athletes?

9. Describe the muscular adaptations to sprint and resistance training. What is meant by hypertrophy and hyperplasia?

10. What are the most likely explanations for fatigue of the muscle fibres during power endurance activity?

Teach it!
In groups of three, choose one topic and teach it to the rest of the study group.

1. Give an overview of the energy sources for power and power endurance sports. Include both phosphagen system reactions involved in the re-synthesis of ATP in your discussion.

2. Explain how the hydrolysis of ATP results in the release of free energy for cellular work.

3. Discuss various forms of resistance training appropriate for the development of muscular power.

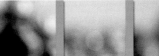

SPORT IN ACTION

Biography:
Jacko Gill
Sport: Athletics, shot putt

Jacko joined the shot putt discipline of athletics at the age of nine years, and competed at the Auckland Children's Championships only three weeks later. In 2010 Jacko won the World Junior Athletics (under 20s) title at the age of 15 years. He followed this up with the World Youth (under 18s) title in 2011, with a new world record throw of 24.35 m. At the age of 16 years, Jacko became the youngest person ever to throw the Olympic shot over 20.00 m, beating the previous youngest athlete (18 yrs 10 months) by two- and-a-half years. Jacko holds 12 different world age records from the age of 13–18 years.

Jacko's rise to the top!

I joined athletics at the age of nine years, and three weeks later competed at the Auckland Children's Champs. Even back then, my inclusion wasn't to simply make up the field. I finished fourth in the shot putt, beaten by three large Samoan

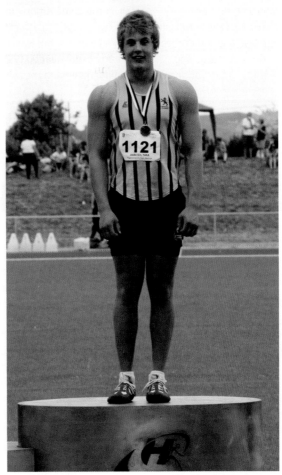

(*Source*: Didier Poppe)

➤

➤

athletes, and I remember thinking to myself 'I am fourth in ALL of Auckland and only in three weeks!' Auckland was pretty big to me then, probably my whole world! So I asked my Dad what would it take to win, and the candle was lit. One year later I won my first Auckland record re-writing the distance in the process. At age 11 years I met my Dad's friend, Graham May, who became my mentor. He was always getting me to push the boundaries and to think hard about how I would keep ahead of my competitors each year. I also began weight-lifting at this stage, dispelling many of the old wives' tales about the strength training of children that abound in sport. Nigel Avery taught me how to 'snatch' and 'clean and jerk' which enhanced the speed of the gift I already had. I chose to train alone, only with Dad and sometimes Mum, as I found I could focus and work harder without interruptions.

I believe this training at a young age prepared my body for my teenage years, when I began to grow and big gains in strength were made.

At the age of fifteen I was selected to compete for the New Zealand team at the World Junior (under 20s) Athletic Championships held in Canada. I remember being late for qualifying and had to report to the call-in tent where everyone waited before they competed. As I walked in, the lady at the desk yelled to me that the 1,500 m call-in tent was next door, to a chorus of laughter from those I was hoping to impress. I was 87 kg and 1.88 m tall, but I had never seen such a collection of huge men. Most were 19 years of age, weighing over 130 kg and were 1.95–2.15 m tall. In the competition I fouled my first two qualifying attempts and, with only one to go, was headed for an early exit. I needed 19.22 m from my final qualifying throw to remain

in the competition – I responded with a throw of 19.27 m. I had made the final by a mere whisker. No one had noticed me with the top throw being 20.10 m. After injuring my finger during warm-up for the final, I lay down in the call room and had to devise a plan B. I knew I had maybe two throws in me at best so it would be 110% first off. My competitors started slowly, with the first seven only just breaking the 18.0 m line. This was my chance to shock, and I took it. My first throw was 20.24 m (I had never thrown over 20.00 m before). Nobody would look at me as I walked from the circle and I knew they were on the run. Round two extinguished any hope the field had of reining me in with my gold-medal-winning, and world-under-18 record, throw of 20.76 m. I was always confident I would take a medal. However, there is always an element of 'best man on the day'.

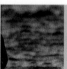

CLASSIC RESEARCH SUMMARY

Long-term creatine intake by Vandenberghe and colleagues (1997)

Creatine appears to provide a nutritional supplement that has an ergogenic effect for power and power endurance sports. In addition, creatine has been indicated as leading to increases in fat-free mass. Vandenberghe and colleagues' study investigated the effects of long-term creatine supplementation on resistance (strength) training and intermittent exercise. The study was conducted with 19 female sedentary

volunteers, to examine the effects of long-term creatine usage on performance and body composition.

The study had three phases, an initial four-day loading phase where only creatine was supplemented, a ten-week training phase where strength training was conducted in addition to low-dose creatine supplementation and finally a 10-week detraining phase where the participants continued to take creatine after ceasing strength training. The study was double-blind and the participants were randomly assigned to either creatine or placebo group. In the

loading phase, participants in the creatine group took 5 g creatine four times per day (20 g per day) for four days. The placebo group followed the same regime, but took maltodextrine tablets in place of creatine. The doses were taken in tablet form and were designed to look and taste the same. During the ten-week training phase the dosage for both groups was dropped to a lower dose of 2.5 g twice a day (5 g per day) for the course of the study. During this phase all participants followed a strength training programme that involved six exercises: leg press, bench press, leg curl, leg extension, squat and shoulder press. The load for each session was 70% 1RM values, with 1RM re-assessments after five and ten weeks of this phase. In the detraining phase the participants (of which there were 13 who continued in the study, 7 creatine and 6 placebo) stopped training but continued taking the lower dose of creatine (or placebo) for the additional ten weeks of detraining. Creatine and ATP concentrations were determined by use of nuclear magnetic resonance (NMR) spectroscopy of the right gastrocnemius muscle. The intermittent exercise protocol involved five sets of 30 arm flexions with a two-minute rest period between each set. The torque during each repetition was recorded. Body composition was assessed using underwater (hydrostatic) weighing at the start of the study, post five weeks and 10 weeks of training.

The participants reported no side-effects and felt they could not guess whether they were taking creatine or the placebo. The four-day loading phase led to a 6% (from 22.5 to 24.2 mmol·kg wet wt^{-1}) increase in

PCr stores which remained elevated to a similar level across the training and detraining phases. The 1RM lifts total for the placebo group was 465 kg at the start of the study and rose to 553 kg at week five and 606 kg by the end of the training phase (10 weeks). This represented an initial increase (from start to week five) of 88 kg and a total increase (from start to week 10) of 141 kg, representing a 30% increase. The total lifts for the creatine group rose from 481 to 612 and finally 711 during the same time phases, representing a 48% increase over baseline levels. In response to the intermittent exercise testing the ten-week creatine and exercise programme led to 11, 18, 20, 21 and 25% higher scores for the five sets of lifts when compared with the placebo group. The fat-free mass of the participants rose for both groups but was higher for the creatine group. At five weeks there was a 2.5% increase in fat-free mass for the placebo group whereas there was a 4.5% rise for the creatine supplement participants. At ten weeks these values were 3.7 and 5.8% respectively.

These results indicate that long-term low-dose creatine supplementation maintained PCr levels about 6% above baseline levels after being established by a higher-dose loading phase. The low-dose and training phase led to improvement in performance (1RM value and intermittent arm-flexion torque) for both creatine and placebo groups; however, the rise was significantly higher for the creatine group. The detraining phase led to similar losses in strength, however, the PCr levels remained elevated for the creatine supplementation group. The higher PCr levels returned to baseline within four weeks of cessation of creatine supplementation. The study presented evidence that creatine supplementation in sedentary females enhanced muscle strength development during strength training.

Full reference: Vandenberghe, K., Goris, M., van Hecke, P., van Leemputte, M., Vangerven, L. and Hespel, P. (1997). Long-term creatine intake is beneficial to muscle performance during resistance training. *Journal Applied Physiology*, 83(6), 2055-63.

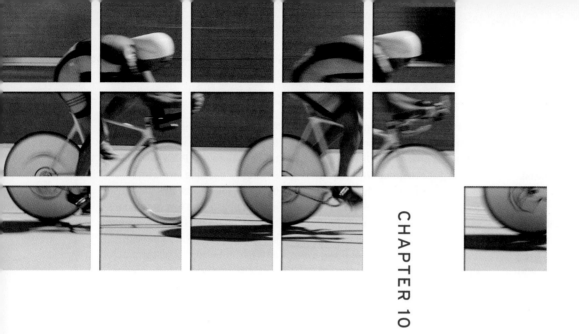

CHAPTER 10

Anaerobic endurance:
the speed endurance sports

Learning objectives

After reading, considering and discussing with a study partner the material in this chapter you should be able to:

➤ explain the pathway and reactions in glycolysis

➤ teach other about fast- and slower-rate glycolysis

➤ discuss the role of lactate, H^+ and phosphate in fatigue for anaerobic endurance sports

➤ describe tests of anaerobic endurance such as the Wingate and maximal accumulated oxygen deficit tests

➤ summarise different methods of conditioning training for anaerobic endurance sports

➤ define muscular endurance

➤ identify a number of egrogenic aids with the potential to improve anaerobic endurance performance

In this chapter the focus is upon sports that place significant demands on the glycolytic pathway, the second anaerobic energy generation mechanism. Examples of a range of shorter- and longer-duration speed endurance sports are illustrated on the duration continuum in Figure 10.1. As a result of the high intensity associated with such sports, athletes accumulate high concentrations of lactate and H^+ during performance. While not responsible for fatigue in anaerobic endurance sports, blood lactate concentration, which can be easily measured in laboratory and field settings, provides a useful indication of the exercise intensity. There are linear relationships between exercise intensity, lactate concentration and perception of fatigue. The level of lactate in the blood is indicative of the rate of glycolysis and hence the work rate of the individual. In maximal efforts that continue beyond 10 s, tolerance of fatigue, and the pain encountered, is a key concern for athletes in terms of optimal performance. The duration of the anaerobic sports (10–90 s) means the tactics for athletes involved in the shorter-duration sports will differ compared to those in sports approaching or just passing 90 s duration. In shorter speed endurance sports the focus is on how hard an athlete can push themselves to maintain relative intensity: how much pain can they tolerate: Due to the duration of the longer speed endurance events, an element of pacing is involved. Push too hard, too early and performance is detrimentally affected. An optimal level of exercise intensity must be achieved, one that will result in high lactate and H^+ concentrations but enable successful completion of the event. It is important to note, however, that lactate accumulation is not the culprit of fatigue, but it is indicative of the intensity of exercise and is a relatively simple measure of anaerobic performance. Further discussion of lactate as a substrate within anaerobic performance appears in the following sections.

When an athlete exercises at maximal level the initial source of energy comes from ATP stores and then from

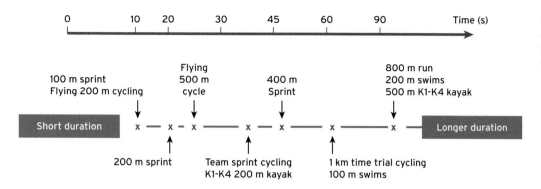

Figure 10.1 Duration continuum for a number of anaerobic endurance sports.

ATP synthesised via the phosphagen system, as described in Chapter 9. If the phosphagen system represents the 1st gear for ATP resynthesis, then glycolysis comprises the 2nd gear: the second anaerobic pathway for ATP synthesis during maximal exercise. The glycolytic pathway is activated from the start of exercise and after 6–10 s becomes the predominant mechanism for ATP replenishment in activities that last between 60–90 s. The relatively large variance here (60–90 s) relates to recent research findings regarding the transition to predominantly aerobic metabolism. Just as recent research suggests the activation of glycolysis, and hence realisation of ATP, occurs more rapidly during maximal exercise than exercise physiologists had previously thought, the same appears to occur in the transition to aerobic system predominance. It was previously thought that the aerobic system was sluggish and took from 1.5 to 3 min before it provided the predominant contribution to ATP synthesis during maximal exercise. It is now believed that this transition occurs earlier, somewhere between 60 and 90 s from the start of exercise. Nevertheless, anaerobic pathways, and predominantly glycolysis provide the highest contribution to ~60 s and remain to contribute around 45% of energy by 90 s of all-out efforts. As a consequence, for sports or events lasting from 10 to 90 s, glycolysis

provides a vital role in ATP synthesis. An illustration of the transition in the relative contribution of ATP-PCr, glycolysis and aerobic metabolism to total work or energy output is shown in Figure 10.2.

The role of glycolysis is not, however, limited to the first 60–90 s of high-intensity activity as an anaerobic pathway. As was introduced in Chapter 8, while fast-rate glycolysis and the accumulation of lactate is associated with anaerobic endurance sports, slower-rate glycolysis provides an important pathway within aerobic metabolism. Beyond an exercise duration of 90 s, slower-rate glycolysis provides an important pathway for carbohydrate metabolism for high-intensity aerobic sports, while fast-rate glycolysis makes a significant contribution to certain aspects, such as the finishing kick in a race. The contribution of glycolysis to aerobic metabolism is covered in detail in the next chapter, Chapter 11.

This chapter begins with a more detailed description of the glycolytic pathway along with discussion of the possible fates of pyruvate, the end-product of glycolysis. Following this, the physiology of speed endurance sports is covered and includes sections on components of fitness, appropriate fitness tests, conditioning, mechanisms of fatigue and adaptation to training in anaerobic sports. The final

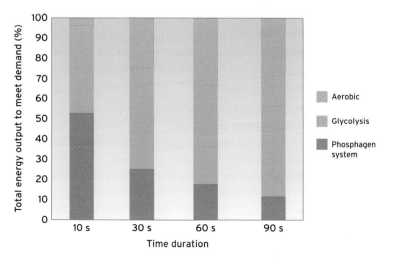

Figure 10.2 Relative contribution of phosphagen system, glycolysis and aerobic metabolism to total energy output during all-out effort up to 90 seconds' duration.

section of the chapter examines ergogenic aids for anaerobic endurance activities including sodium bicarbonate and beta-alanine.

10.1 Energy supply for speed endurance events

Glycolysis

Taking over from the phosphagen system in explosive sports (2–10 s exercise duration), fast-rate glycolysis becomes the predominant fuel source for the speed endurance events (10–90 s exercise duration). Glycolysis forms the second of the body's anaerobic pathways, meaning that it does not require oxygen for any of the reactions that take place during the catabolism of glucose or glycogen. At a cellular level, glycolysis serves two main functions; to synthesise **pyruvate**, a substrate for further catabolism in the Krebs cycle, and **ATP**, the energy source for cellular activity. These functions are demonstrated in Figure 10.3 which provides an overview of the reactions or steps in glycolysis.

As a simple consequence of the greater number of reactions involved, glycolysis takes longer than the phosphagen system to become the predominant energy system during high-intensity activity. Adenosine triphosphate synthesis via glycolysis increases from the start of exercise such that after 6–10 s glycolysis becomes the predominant energy generation mechanism. The glycolytic pathway was first described by Gustav Embden and subsequently demonstrated by Otto Meyerhof, two German physiologists (further detail of their work can be found in Chapter 1). Consequently, glycolysis is also referred to as the Embden-Meyerhof pathway. Glycolysis describes the degradation of carbohydrate (in the form of *glucose* or *glycogen*) to pyruvate through a series of 10 steps or reactions (11 for glycogen) to produce a net gain of two ATP molecules for each glucose molecule (Figure 10.3). As glycogen enters the pathway at glucose-6-phosphate, however, the expense of one ATP during step 1 is avoided resulting in a net gain of three ATP molecules for each glycogen molecule. Glycolysis and glycogenolysis (discussed in the following section), take place within the cytosol, the gel-like mass that surrounds the organelles within the cytoplasm. All the substrates and enzymes necessary for these reactions are found within the cytosol of the cell.

In Chapter 8 an overview of cellular energy generation mechanisms was presented. Two forms of glycolysis were referred to – *fast-rate* and *slower-rate* glycolysis – the rate being dependent upon the intensity of exercise. These differential rates of glycolysis are also referred to as *anaerobic* and *aerobic* glycolysis in some textbooks. However, by employing these terms there is a possibility of misinterpretation. Glycolysis is an anaerobic process, it does not require oxygen for any of the ten steps within the pathway. The reference to anaerobic and aerobic refers to the fate of pyruvate, the end product of glycolysis, which is determined by the intensity of exercise. During high-intensity or fast-rate glycolysis, pyruvate is converted to lactate, a process that does not require oxygen and is therefore *anaerobic* – hence *anaerobic* glycolysis. During lower-intensity exercise, when slower-rate glycolysis is preferred, pyruvate provides a metabolite for *aerobic* metabolism, specifically the Krebs cycle, and consequently this is sometimes termed *aerobic* glycolysis. The type of muscle fibre will also affect the fate of pyruvate. In Chapter 5 the structure and functioning of type I, type IIa and type IIx fibres was described. In type I and type IIa fibres the greater mitochondrial density and capillarisation, particularly in type I fibres, favours the transport of pyruvate to the mitochondria where it is further catabolised in aerobic metabolism. In type IIx fibres, which have a lower mitochondrial density and capillarisation (and which are more heavily recruited during high-intensity exercise) pyruvate is reduced to form lactate. As a unique case, glycolysis in erythrocytes always results in the formation of lactate as their mitochondria are removed during development to maximise their oxygen carrying capacity. As a result of the glycolytic activity of red blood cells, capillary blood samples maintain a lactate concentration of 1 mM, even at rest . The possible fates of pyruvate are shown in Figure 10.3. As mentioned in Chapter 8, to avoid the possible confusion of the terms aerobic and anaerobic glycolysis, the terms slower-rate and fast-rate glycolysis will be used throughout this textbook.

Key points

Glycolysis:
- The *anaerobic* process of CHO degradation to form *pyruvate* and *ATP* takes place in the cytoplasm
- Involves 10 reactions
- Results in the net gain of two (glucose) or three (glycogen) ATP molecules

The fate of pyruvate is dependent upon the intensity of the exercise:
- High-intensity exercise: pyruvate converted to lactate (anaerobic process)
- Lower-intensity exercise: pyruvate utilised as a substrate for aerobic metabolism (the Krebs cycle)

Glycogenolysis

As was introduced in Chapter 2, glucose is stored in long highly branched molecule chains called glycogen. Glycogen is formed through the process of *glycogenesis* and ~400 g of glycogen are typically stored in the body at rest, ~350 g in the muscles and the remainder in the liver. During exercise, and specifically for glycolysis, glycogen has to be catabolised to release the stored glucose molecules. The process of glycogen breakdown is called *glycogenolysis* and involves two reactions to convert glycogen to glucose-6-phosphate which can enter at step 2 of the glycolytic pathway. The reactions within glycogenolysis are shown in Figure 10.3. In the first step, glycogen is converted to glucose-1-phosphate through

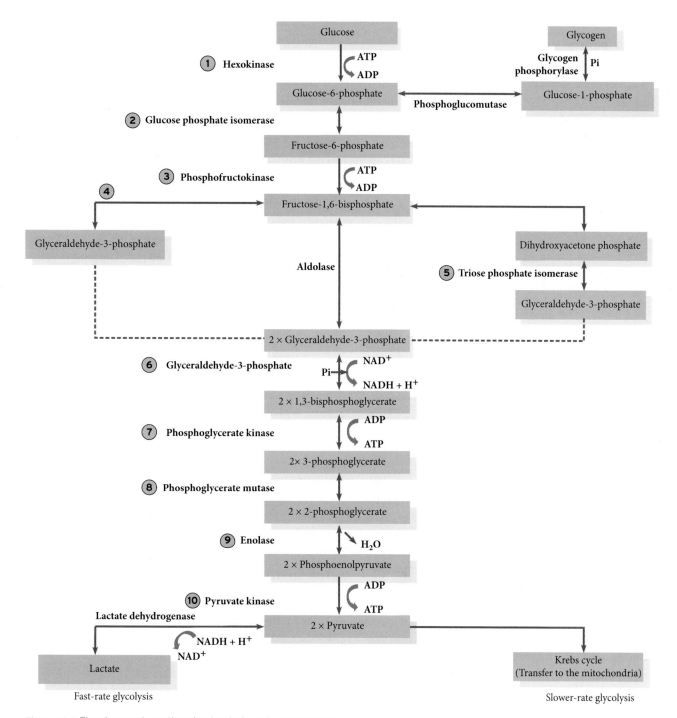

Figure 10.3 The steps and reactions in glycolysis and glycogenolysis.

a reaction catalysed by glycogen phosphorylase during which a glucose molecule is detached from the glycogen chain and a phosphate added. In the second step, catalysed by the enzyme phosphoglucomutase, the phosphate is moved from the first carbon to the sixth carbon resulting in the formation of glucose-6-phosphate which then enters the glycolytic pathway.

Key points

Glycogen, the storage form of glucose, must be catabolised into single carbohydrate units (glucose-6-phosphate) before it can enter the glycolytic pathway.

This process is known as glycogenolysis.

Knowledge integration question

In relation to the food that we eat, how is energy produced during the final sprint of an 800 m race?

The glycolytic pathway

The ten steps of the glycolytic pathway begin with a single molecule of glucose and end with the formation of two pyruvate molecules, along with a net gain of two ATP molecules. Although not as rapid as the phosphagen system, glycolysis provides the predominant pathway for ATP synthesis as PCr stores begin to diminish. An overview of the reactions or steps within glycolysis is provided in Figure 10.3.

In Figure 10.4 a more in-depth analysis of each step is provided including details of the changes in the chemical structure of the metabolites. To understand fully and identify the changes at each step in glycolysis, it is worthwhile using the written descriptions in conjunction with Figures 10.3 and 10.4. At first, the language used to describe the substrates and enzymes within each step can seem off-putting; however, by making reference between the text and the figures the names are in actuality quite logical and helpful to the reader. For instance, the first step in glycolysis involves the addition of a phosphate group to the sixth carbon of glucose, hence the product is called glucose-6-phosphate. In addition, it is worth noting that enzymes with the words *mutase* or *isomerase* in their name catalyse reactions that change the structure of the substrate without further catabolism or anabolism. All other, enzymes add or remove chemicals from the structure. For instance, hexokinase catalyses the addition of a phosphate group to glucose

in the first step of glycolysis, i.e. anabolism. In contrast, phosphoglucomutase catalyses the movement of phosphate from carbon 1 to carbon 6 during the formation of glucose-6-phosphate in the second reaction of glycogenolysis, i.e. isomerism. With this knowledge, and reference between the text and Figures 10.3 and 10.4, it is possible to identify what happens in each of the steps in glycolysis.

Knowledge integration question

What are the substrates and products of glycolysis? How and why is lactate formed during high-intensity exercise and what does the accumulation of lactate represent?

The energy consuming steps (1–3) of glycolysis

The first step in glycolysis, the conversion of glucose to glucose-6-phosphate is catalysed by the enzyme *hexokinase*. Through the hydrolysis of ATP a phosphate is added to carbon 6 of glucose. This results in a net loss of ATP as a result of the first step (net ATP = -1). The second step in glycolysis re-arranges the chemical structure of glucose-6-phosphate to form the isomer (same chemical composition, different structure) fructose-6-phosphate, catalysed by the enzyme glucose phosphate isomerase. During the third reaction a second phosphate is added to the structure from the breakdown of a further molecule of ATP. Catalysed by the enzyme phosphofructokinase (PFK), the major rate-limiting enzyme of glycolysis, fructose-6-phosphate is phosphorylated to form fructose-1,6-bisphosphate which, as the names suggests, and as is shown in Figure 10.4, has a phosphate group bonded to carbon 1 and also to carbon 6. The further use of ATP in the phosphorylation of the original glucose molecule means that at this step the process of glycolysis results in a net loss of two ATP molecules (net ATP = -2). So far glycolysis has cost, not created energy.

The splitting of the hexose ring to form two 3 carbon chains (Steps 4 & 5)

At the fourth step of glycolysis the enzyme aldolase catalyses the splitting of fructose-1,6-bisphosphate (a hexose, 6 carbon ring) into two triose (three carbon chain) molecules, dihydroxyacetone phosphate and glyceraldehyde-3-phosphate (G3P), each of which contains one of the phosphate groups. Catalysed by triose phosphate isomerase, dihydroxyacetone phosphate is then restructured in

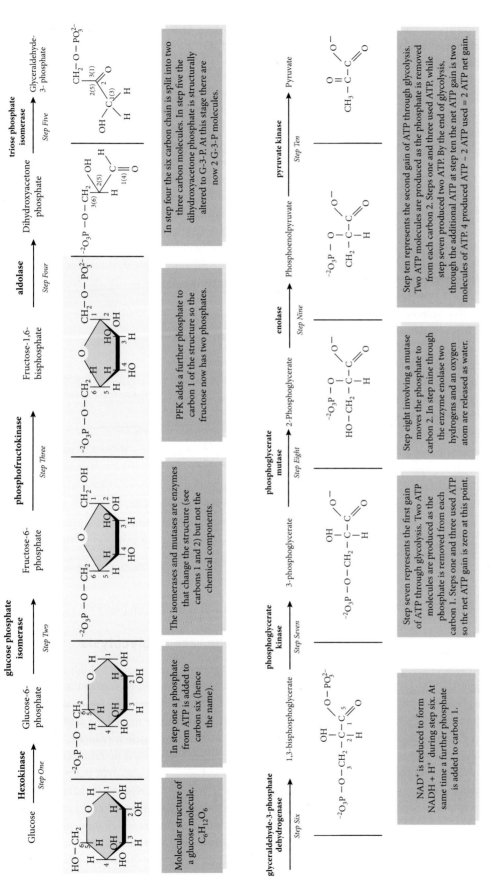

Figure 10.4 Detailed illustration of the 10 steps in the glycolytic pathway including the changes in the chemical composition and structure of the substrates.

the fifth step of glycolysis to form another glyceraldehyde-3-phosphate. This reaction is necessary because only glyceraldehyde-3-phosphate can participate in the subsequent reactions of glycolysis. At this point the newly created glyceraldehyde-3-phosphate molecule can pass, along with the original glyceraldehyde-3-phosphate molecule, to the sixth step of glycolysis. From this point on, therefore, there are two molecules of each metabolite, derived from the original single glucose molecule.

The phosphorylation of glyceraldehyde-3-phosphate (Step 6)

During the sixth step of glycolysis, catalysed by the enzyme glyceraldehyde 3-phosphate dehydrogenase, a further phosphate is bonded to the first carbon of each triose to form 1, 3-bisphosphoglycerate. In addition, two hydrogen atoms, one from G3P and one from Pi, reduce nicotinamide adenine dinucleotide (NAD^+) to $NADH + H^+$. As a co-enzyme carrier, NAD^+ facilitates H atom transport for the reduction of pyruvate to form lactate, or to the mitochondria for use within aerobic metabolism. NAD^+ will be described in more detail in the section on lactate below and in Chapter 12 where aerobic metabolism is discussed. In summary, step six involves the addition of a further phosphate and the removal of one hydrogen atom from each of the trioses, resulting in the formation of 1, 3-bisphosphoglycerate, a reaction that is catalysed by glyceraldehyde 3-phosphate dehydrogenase. Up to this point, the sixth step of glycolysis, there continues to be a net loss of two ATP (net ATP = −2).

Production of ATP and a structural change (Steps 7 and 8)

It is at step seven that the first synthesis of ATP occurs within the glycolytic pathway. Phosphoglycerate kinase catalyses the phosphorylation of ADP through the energy released by the removal of the phosphate group from carbon 1 from each 1, 3-bisphosphoglycerate molecule. This results in the creation of an ATP from each of the trioses. The energy balance for glycolysis after step seven is, therefore, a net ATP gain of 0 (two ATP consumed during steps one and three; two ATP produced at step 7). In step eight of glycolysis the remaining phosphate in 3-phosphoglycerate (the product of step seven) is transferred, in a reaction catalysed by phosphoglycerate mutase, from carbon 3 to carbon 2. The product of this reaction is named, not surprisingly, 2-phosphoglycerate.

Dehydration and the final production of ATP (Steps 9 and 10)

In the ninth reaction, 2-phosphoglycerate is dehydrated (an H_2O molecule is removed from each of the trioses) in a reaction catalysed by enolase to form phosphoenolpyruvate. In the tenth, and final, step of glycolysis, pyruvate kinase catalyses the phosphorylation of a further ADP for each of the trioses, resulting in the production of two further ATP and two pyruvate molecules. At the end of glycolysis, therefore, there is a gain of two ATP (net ATP gain = +2). As mentioned previously, the fate of pyruvate at the end of glycolysis is determined by the exercise intensity. During fast-rate glycolysis, pyruvate is converted to lactate and during slower-rate glycolysis, pyruvate becomes a substrate for aerobic metabolism.

Key points

The glycolytic pathway:

➤ Involves the degradation of one glucose molecule to two pyruvate molecules with a net gain of two ATP molecules

➤ Involves 10 steps, or reactions

➤ Steps one and three consume a single ATP molecule each (net ATP = −2)

➤ Steps seven and ten produce two ATP molecules each (one for each triose at each step) (net ATP = 4 − 2)

Pyruvate is either used as a substrate for aerobic metabolism or is converted to lactate, depending on exercise intensity.

See 'Classic research summary' on pages 321–2.

Control of the rate of glycolysis

It is now clear that upon the initiation of high-intensity exercise glycolytic rate increases, becoming the predominant energy source after 6–10 seconds. In situations where exercise intensity is lowered, or indeed the activity ceased, the demand for ATP by the muscle is reduced. Tight control over the rate of glycolysis is therefore essential to ensure ATP production via the glycolytic pathway meets the needs of the active muscle cells. What changes occur within the muscle during exercise to alter the rate of glycolysis: There are two main factors which influence the rate of glycolysis: substrate levels and the activation of glycolytic enzymes. These factors are discussed in the following sections.

Increased reaction substrates

During exercise the muscle can utilise either blood glucose or muscle glycogen as carbohydrate fuel sources. Blood glucose is carried across the sarcolemma by glucose transporters, particularly GLUT4. The increase in both GLUT4 availability and blood flow during exercise function to enhance the muscle uptake of blood glucose, where it enters the glycolytic pathway. A further factor influencing the involvement of glucose is the activity of hexokinase, the enzyme responsible for catalysing its phosphorylation to glucose-6-phosphate. Glycogenolysis also results in the formation of glucose-6-phosphate, which, as an inhibitor of hexokinase, reduces the uptake of glucose into the cell and hence the contribution of glucose to glycolysis. This is particularly prudent during high-intensity exercise as muscle glycogen is the main substrate for glycolysis, with blood glucose making a minor contribution. An elevated level of glucose-6-phosphate, independent of its source (glucose or glycogen), is one factor that increases the rate of glycolysis. As a substrate for steps 7 and 10 of glycolysis, increased ADP concentration also plays a small role in the activation of glycolysis.

Enzyme activity

The main control of glycolysis is brought about through the functioning of key enzymes within the pathway. As one of the first steps in glycolysis, glycogenolysis, controlled by the activity of glycogen phosphorylase, will be considered first. Phosphofructokinase (PFK) is the main rate-limiting enzyme which catalyses the third reaction of glycolysis, and the control of its activity will subsequently be discussed. The activation of pyruvate kinase is under similar control to that of PFK, hence the activity of this enzyme is also touched on in the final section.

Glycogen phosphorylase

During exercise, an increase in the proportion of active glycogen phosphorylase occurs, resulting in an increased rate of glycogenolysis, elevated levels of glucose-6-phosphate, and a faster glycolytic rate. The change from inactive to active glycogen phosphorylase is partly stimulated by the hormone adrenaline, which is released under conditions of stress. This can occur prior to an event, when feeling anxious and aroused, or during general exercise. Adrenaline binds to its cell membrane receptor initiating the formation of a second messenger (cyclic AMP), which subsequently activates glycogen phophorylase. The

active form of glycogen phosphorylase, however, can only catalyse the breakdown of glycogen when Ca^{2+} increases above a certain level, as when muscle is stimulated to contract. This ensures that glycolytic energy production is initiated rapidly following the onset of exercise to meet the metabolic demands of the muscle, but also conserves the glycogen stores during periods of low energy demand. During low-intensity exercise, however, adrenaline concentration remains constant. In this situation, it is the release of Ca^{2+} from the sarcoplasmic reticulum that activates glycogen phosphorylase via the activation of the protein calmodulin. In addition to the roles of adrenaline and calcium, the accumulation of ADP during high-intensity exercise increases the net activity of glycogen phosphorylase. Following the cessation of exercise, when ATP stores are replenished, glycogen phosphorylase activity is inhibited.

Phosphofructokinase and pyruvate kinase

As the catalyst for the third step in the glycolytic pathway, phosphofructokinase activity is increased with the accumulation of its substrate, fructose-6-phosphate. In addition, a range of metabolites are involved in its control. At rest, skeletal muscle contains higher concentrations of ATP and PCr, while levels of ADP, AMP, Pi and NH_4^+ are low. In this situation, PFK activity is inhibited by the high ATP and PCr concentrations. Additionally, H^+ enhance the inhibition by ATP, and citrate, found in the cytoplasm when aerobic metabolism is meeting the energy demands (refer to Chapter 12 for further detail), acts as an inhibitor of PFK.

The initiation of high-intensity exercise, however, results in a fall in ATP and PCr, while ADP, Pi, AMP (product of adenylate kinase reaction) and NH_4^+ (product of adenylate deaminase reaction) increase. These changes function to increase the rate of glycolysis through the activation of PFK. An acidic pH, however, inhibits the activity of PFK. During high-intensity exercise, the pH of the muscle falls, due to an increased H^+ concentration, primarily the result of glycolysis. An *in vivo* reduction in PFK activity due to muscle acidity, however, has not been found. This is likely due to a greater stimulatory effect of the elevated ADP, AMP, Pi and NH_4^+.

In addition to the effects of these molecules on PFK activity, the activation of pyruvate kinase, the catalyst for the final glycolytic reaction, is similarly influenced. The fall in ATP and PCr, and the increase in ADP, with exercise are responsible for the stimulation of pyruvate kinase activity and hence acceleration of glycolysis.

Key points

Glycolytic rate is altered to ensure the energy needs of the cell are met during high-intensity exercise.

Two main factors influence the rate of glycolysis:

1. Substrate levels
   a. Increased muscle glucose, glycogen and glucose-6-phosphate increase the rate of glycolysis
2. The activation of glycolytic enzymes
   a. Glycogen phosphorylase is activated by adrenaline and Ca^{2+}, leading to an increase in glycogenolysis and the rate of glycolysis
   b. Phosphofructokinase (main rate-limiting enzyme) is activated by a fall in ATP and PCr, and increased ADP, AMP, Pi and $NH4^+$, and inhibited by high ATP, PCr and citrate

Lactate

Lactate or lactic acid?

The terms *lactate* and *lactic acid* are often used interchangeably, although when we refer to hydrogen atoms being transferred to pyruvate during high-intensity exercise, the more correct term would be lactate. Conversely, if referring to pyruvic acid the correct term would be lactic acid. Pyruvate and lactate are salts of their respective acids and at physiological pH, i.e. at the pH within human cells, pyruvic acid and lactic acid dissociate (lose a H^+ from their structure) to their salt forms. The chemical formula for lactic acid is $C_3H_6O_3$, and its corresponding salt lactate is $C_3H_5O_3$. As lactic acid appears as lactate at physiological pH, the correct term for the reduced form of pyruvate following fast-rate glycolysis is lactate, which will be used throughout the current text.

The purpose of lactate formation

Pyruvate, the product of glycolysis, is converted to lactate under conditions of high-intensity exercise, where the metabolic needs of the muscle are unable to be met by aerobic metabolism. As discussed later in this chapter, the H^+ associated with lactate formation is a contributing factor to the development of fatigue, so what is the purpose of the formation of lactate?

The structure and function of NAD

The conversion of pyruvate to lactate is catalysed by the enzyme lactate dehydrogenase and, in addition, requires the coenzyme nicotinamide adenine dinucleotide (NAD) (refer to Figure 10.3). As the name suggests, nicotinamide adenine dinucleotide, is formed from two nucleotides; adenine (as within the structure of ATP), and niacin (formed from vitamin B_3). Put simply, NAD is a carrier for hydrogen, and hence can exist in either an oxidised (NAD^+) or reduced (NADH) form (Figure 10.5). In step 6 of glycolysis, glyceraldehyde-3-phosphate (G3P) is converted to 1,3-bisphosphoglycerate with the addition of NAD^+ and Pi (see Figures 10.3 and 10.4). One hydrogen atom is removed from G3P and a further hydrogen is removed from Pi. NAD^+ accepts one of these hydrogens, becoming the reduced form NADH, while the other hydrogen remains free in solution: $NAD^+ + 2H = NADH + H^+$. As NAD^+ carries a positive charge, and hydrogen ions (H^+) are also positive, the reduction of NAD^+ occurs by the simultaneous addition of a single H^+ and two electrons (e^-), resulting in the formation of a neutral molecule, NADH (Figure 10.5b). As such, NADH can serve to shuttle H^+ and electrons to the mitochondria for use in the aerobic generation of ATP, or to pyruvate for its conversion to lactate within the cytoplasm. The fates of pyruvate following both fast-rate and slower-rate glycolysis, including the roles of NAD, are illustrated in Figure 10.6.

Key point

Nicotinamide adenine dinucleotide (NAD) is a co-enzyme which functions as a hydrogen carrier.

The role of NAD during exercise

A low concentration of NAD^+ exists within the cell, hence NADH must be oxidised back to NAD^+ at a sufficient rate to allow glycolysis to continue. During low-intensity exercise, slower-rate glycolysis allows NAD^+ to keep pace with the rate of hydrogen removal from glyceraldehyde-3-phosphate (Figure 10.6). The hydrogen ion and electrons from NADH are transferred to the mitochondria where they are utilised for metabolism within the electron transport chain (more detail is provided in Chapter 11). The oxidised NAD^+ is then available to continue to assist in glycolysis (picking up further H^+ and electrons). At lower intensities of exercise the pyruvate can be utilised in aerobic metabolism to form additional ATP molecules (Figure 10.6).

In contrast, the phosphorylation of ATP through glycolysis during high-intensity exercise, is required at a faster rate than which hydrogen atoms can be transferred to the

(a)

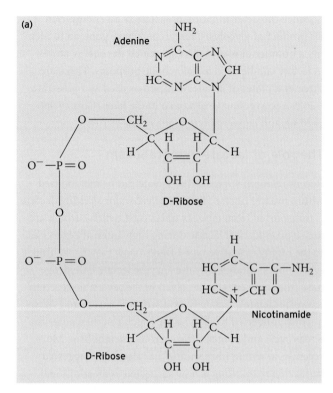

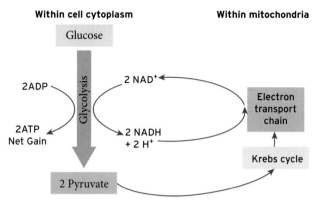

Fate of pyruvate during slower-rate glycolysis

Fate of pyruvate during fast-rate glycolysis:

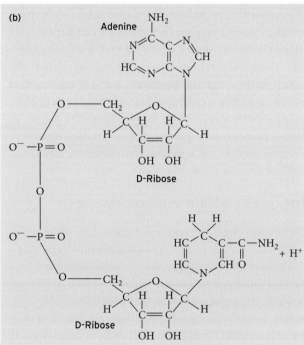

Figure 10.6 Fate of pyruvate during slower-rate and fast-rate glycolysis.

Figure 10.5 Structure of nicotinamide adenine dinucleotide in its (a) oxidised (NAD^+) and (b) reduced form ($NADH + H^+$).

mitochondria. As a consequence, the hydrogen atoms are transferred to pyruvate, in a reaction catalysed by lactate dehydrogenase, to form lactate (Figure 10.6). The formation of lactate during high-intensity exercise, therefore,

enables NAD^+ to continue to function as a shuttle for hydrogen atoms which enables glycolysis to continue synthesising ATP at the rate required. Although the formation of lactate, and the concomitant rise in H^+, results in a drop in cytoplasmic pH, which has been linked to fatigue during high-intensity exercise, glycolysis would be impaired faster without the regeneration of NAD^+.

As can be seen from Figure 10.5(a) the oxidised form of NAD^+ has an N^+ within the nicotinamide nucleotide. When two hydrogen atoms are transferred to NAD^+ during step 6 of the glycolytic pathway, one of the electrons is transferred to this N^+ leaving an H^+ and a hydrogen atom. The second hydrogen atom in the reduction of NAD^+ bonds with carbon 6 of nicotinamide as shown in Figure 10.5(b), leaving the remaining H^+ within the aqueous cytoplasm. When the formula for this reaction is written the reduced form of NAD^+ is expressed as $NADH + H^+$, when we refer to the movement of hydrogen and electrons it is the new molecule NADH that transfers them to the mitochondria.

Knowledge integration question

In terms of its function, why is NAD^+ such an important co-enzyme for metabolism?

Lactate concentration can be measured relatively simply in the laboratory and the field from a capillary blood sample. The processes for lactate sampling in the laboratory and field are illustrated in Figure 10.7. Research indicates that beyond a threshold point (this point, referred to as the lactate threshold, is described in detail in Chapter 11), lactate concentration levels rise linearly with increasing exercise intensity. The rises in lactate concentration can be used to indicate the glycolytic contribution to energy production. Information regarding lactate concentration levels can be useful for training and performance in sports where fast-rate and slower-rate glycolysis make a significant contribution to energy production. This is discussed further in Chapter 11.

Key points

Low-intensity exercise:

➤ NADH transfers H^+ and electrons to the mitochondria which regenerates NAD^+

High-intensity exercise:

➤ Glycolytic rate too fast for NAD^+ regeneration at the mitochondria

➤ The conversion of pyruvate to lactate regenerates NAD^+

Lactate formation is essential to maintain sufficient levels of NAD^+ to allow glycolysis, and hence ATP generation, to continue at the required rate during high-intensity exercise.

The fate of lactate

In 1907 Frederick Hopkins and Walter Fletcher identified the relationship between muscle activity and rises in lactate concentration within the working muscle. They also demonstrated that skeletal muscle itself is able to remove lactate produced by the muscle. Later, Carl and Gerty Cori, who worked with Otto Meyerhof to identify correctly the steps in glycolysis, demonstrated a pathway through which lactate can be transferred to the liver for glucose glycogen synthesis. This research revealed that lactate is not a waste product of fast-rate glycolysis, but an energy intermediate that can be utilised to synthesise glucose and glycogen.

Since the determination of lactate as an energy-rich by-product of glycolysis, researchers have gone on to identify a number of routes through which the energy stores in lactate can be used for metabolic purposes. There are three main fates of lactate: oxidised or used as a substrate (~70%), conversion to glycogen in the liver (Cori cycle) (~20%), and conversion to amino acids (~10%).

The role of lactate in metabolism

Recent research suggests that lactate can be metabolised within muscle fibres. Through *intercellular shuttling* lactate is transported from type IIx fibres (fast twitch), which are major producers of lactate during high-intensity exercise, to the highly oxidative type I fibres (slow twitch). Within type I fibres, catalysed by the enzyme lactate dehydrogenase (the same enzyme involved in the reversible reaction to create lactate), lactate is oxidised to pyruvate and subsequently converted to acetyl CoA which can then enter the Krebs cycle and contribute to aerobic metabolism. More recently, a 'within fibre shuttle' has also been suggested. *Intracellular shuttling* is now suspected as an additional fate of lactate as lactate dehydrogenase (LDH) has been observed within the mitochondria of skeletal and cardiac muscle. This fact suggests that muscles are in fact able to convert lactate to acetyl CoA within their own mitochondria. These two mechanisms establish the importance of muscle fibres as not only producers, but also consumers of lactate. In addition, *cardiac muscle* (the heart) can utilise lactate directly as a substrate for glycolysis. This mechanism is particularly important during sustained high-intensity exercise when glucose concentrations may fall through glycolytic consumption.

The role of lactate in gluconeogenesis

The process of glucose synthesis from lactate, described in the Cori cycle, is one form of **gluconeogenesis**, i.e. the synthesis of glucose and glycogen from indirect (non-dietary) carbohydrate sources. There a number of pathways through which glucose can be synthesised from non-dietary carbohydrate sources and these are described in the next section. Through the Cori cycle, as demonstrated in Figure 10.8, muscular lactate, and indeed pyruvate, can be transported to the liver and converted to glucose or glycogen. Research indicates that the Cori cycle provides a significant pathway for glycogen synthesis in the liver, second only to dietary sources. The uptake of lactate by the liver, and subsequent gluconeogenesis, is important during prolonged exercise as a mechanism to prevent the development of low blood-glucose levels (hypoglycaemia).

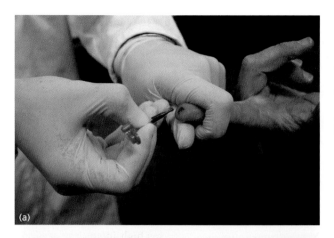

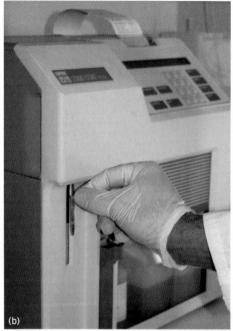

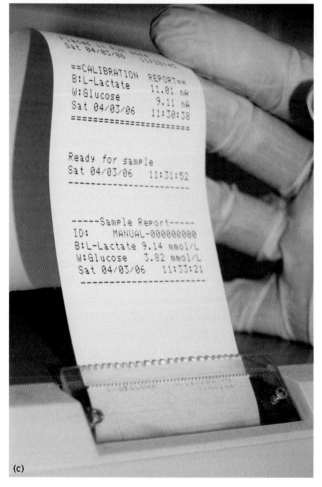

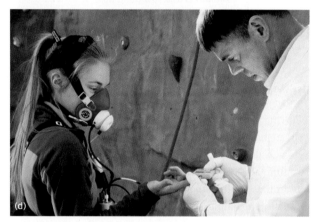

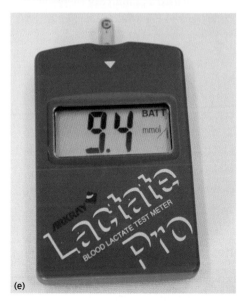

Figure 10.7 Laboratory and field measures of capillary lactate concentration: laboratory analysis depicting (a) blood sampling, (b) introduction of the sample for analysis, and (c) printout of result; field analysis showing (d) blood sample being taken from a climber and (e) readout obtained in the field. (*Sources*: (a, b, d, e) Simon Fryer, (c) Nicky Norris)

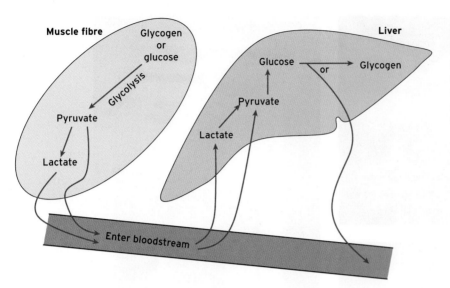

Figure 10.8 The Cori cycle. Pyruvate and lactate diffuse into the bloodstream and are transported to the liver. In the liver both lactate and pyruvate can be converted to glucose which can re-enter the bloodstream for uptake by other cells or be converted into glycogen and stored in the liver.

Knowledge integration question

What sporting situations lead to a build up in muscle and blood lactate? Why is the production of lactate so important and in what ways does it help and hinder the functioning of both the muscle and other organs in the body?

Conversion of lactate to amino acids

Following its production from the oxidation of lactate, pyruvate has several fates. Its role in the Cori cycle is discussed above. A further fate is its transamination to the amino acid alanine, catalysed by the enzyme alanine transaminase. This is the most common pathway for the production of alanine. Alanine has close links to the metabolic pathways and can be used as a source of energy via the glucose-alanine cycle (refer to Figure 2.20, Chapter 2).

Key points

Pyruvate, the final product of glycolysis, is converted to lactate during high-intensity exercise.

Lactate has three main fates:
1. Substrate for heart metabolism, oxidised by skeletal muscle
2. Converted to glucose in the liver (Cori cycle)
3. Converted to alanine, an amino acid linked to the metabolic pathways

Gluconeogenesis

Gluconeogenesis refers to the creation of glucose from non-dietary carbohydrate sources. There are a number of gluconeogenesis pathways for glucose synthesis which are activated particularly during longer-duration activities or when dietary carbohydrate intake is reduced. The *neo* in gluconeogenesis, meaning 'new', can be helpful in distinguishing between this and other similar terms covered in this chapter such as glycogenesis, glycogenolysis and indeed glycolysis (remember that *glycogenesis* involves the formation of glycogen from glucose, *glycogenolysis* refers to the breakdown of glycogen to glucose and *glycolysis* is the degradation of glucose (or glycogen) to produce pyruvate and ATP).

Non-dietary substrates for gluconeogenesis include: *lactate* and *pyruvate*, (the Cori cycle); *amino acids* (the glucose-alanine cycle (refer to Chapter 2, protein metabolism) and the glucose-glutamine cycle, which involves a similar deamination process of *glycerol* (the backbone of triglycerides). The liver plays a key role in gluconeogenesis and is the site for the Cori cycle, glucose-alanine cycle and conversion of glycerol to glucose. Additionally, a small proportion of total gluconeogenesis (e.g. the glucose-glutamine cycle) takes place within the kidneys (~10%). Gluconeogenesis is stimulated by the adrenal cortex hormone *cortisol*, the adrenal medulla hormones *adrenaline* and *noradrenaline*, and by the pancreatic hormone *glucagon*.

10.2 The physiology of anaerobic endurance sports

Lactate, given its appearance in fast-rate glycolysis, is a useful indicator of anaerobic effort and exercise duration. To understand the physiology of anaerobic endurance sports it is important to be clear that while lactate concentrations can rise dramatically in sports of these durations, it is not the lactate itself that is the cause of fatigue. There is no evidence to suggest that lactate is detrimental to performance and a cause of fatigue. While muscular fatigue is a complex phenomenon, it appears more justifiable that it is the H^+ associated with lactate, and the resultant change in acidosis within the muscle, that provides one of the most likely cause of fatigue in anaerobic endurance sports.

The scale for measuring the relative acidity or alkalinity of a solution is pH. The pH scale was established by the Danish biochemist Søren Sørensen (1868–1939) where the *p* relates to the power or concentration of *H* – hydrogen ions. The scale ranges from very acidic solutions such a hydrochloric acid (found in the gastric fluids of the stomach, see Chapter 2) which has a pH of 1.0 to highly alkaline solutions such as sodium hydroxide (found in drain cleaner) with a pH of 14.0. Figure 10.9 provides an illustration of the pH scale. The blood, with a normal resting pH of 7.35, has a narrow band of tolerable limits in pH from 6.9 to a maximum pH of 7.5. During maximal anaerobic exercise muscular pH can drop to 6.3 from a normal resting pH of around 7.0.

As discussed earlier, lactate is not a waste product of metabolism, but is an intermediary energy substrate that can be used directly by the heart (cardiac muscle) and may also provide an immediate energy source for the muscle fibre through the operation of an intracellular shuttle. In addition, lactate can be oxidised to synthesise glucose through the Cori cycle or within other muscle fibres (following intercellular shuttling). In contrast, the accumulation of H^+ associated with the synthesis of lactate has been implicated in fatigue. To protect against the deleterious effects of increasing acidosis, the body has a number of substrates that serve as buffers to the increasing H^+ concentrations. Intracellular and extracellular buffering

provides a temporary measure, protecting against the change in pH associated with fast-rate glycolysis. The operation of the buffering mechanisms is covered in 'fatigue in anaerobic sports' later in this section.

Components of fitness related to anaerobic endurance

In this section we will focus on two aspects that are linked to the duration of anaerobic endurance exercise (10–90 s). As the name suggests, one is anaerobic endurance, and the other, due to the time duration of training repetitions for this aspect of fitness, is muscular endurance.

Anaerobic endurance, also referred to as anaerobic capacity, relates to the ability to sustain high-intensity exercise. It is integrally linked with the body's 2nd gear – fast-rate glycolysis. In events lasting longer than 10 s, and up to around 90 s, glycolysis becomes the predominant pathway for energy production. The intensity of exercise during anaerobic endurance events is high, so energy production occurs through fast-rate glycolysis. As was introduced above, fast-rate glycolysis results in the production of lactate and H^+. It is the H^+ that have been implicated in fatigue in anaerobic endurance sports.

Muscular endurance relates to the ability of a certain muscle or muscle group to maintain repeated muscular contractions against a given resistance. This resistance could represent a small percentage of your maximal contraction or a higher percentage. The closer a load is to your maximum the shorter the time for which the effort can be maintained. There are many examples where muscular endurance can impact upon performance. This is clearly illustrated in the rock climbing Sport in Action piece by Katherine Schirrmacher on p. 320–1. The ability to perform the repeated contractions necessary to complete

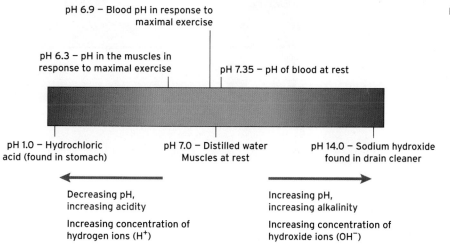

Figure 10.9 The pH scale.

pH 6.9 – Blood pH in response to maximal exercise

pH 6.3 – pH in the muscles in response to maximal exercise

pH 7.35 – pH of blood at rest

pH 1.0 – Hydrochloric acid (found in stomach)

pH 7.0 – Distilled water Muscles at rest

pH 14.0 – Sodium hydroxide found in drain cleaner

Decreasing pH, increasing acidity

Increasing concentration of hydrogen ions (H^+)

Increasing pH, increasing alkalinity

Increasing concentration of hydroxide ions (OH^-)

long-distance canoeing and kayaking races, or pumping the sail in windsurfing and poling in cross-country skiing all rely on muscular endurance. The load for each individual paddle stroke, sail pump or poling action would be small relative to maximum possible contraction, thus enabling the athlete to maintain the action for long periods of time. If an athlete fatigues before the end of a race or training session one aspect he or she might need to develop could be their muscular endurance. As the examples show, this component of fitness in a sports context is most closely linked to performance in aerobic events. In a health context, however, muscular endurance is typically developed in sessions such as circuit training, where there is dual strength and conditioning components. Typically, sessions last 30–60 minutes and include a range of exercises and sets, with individual repetitions lasting between 30–60 s duration. In this way, such sessions have a combined muscular strength and cardiovascular training effect.

Tests of anaerobic endurance

In past decades there was a smaller research concentration on anaerobic endurance when compared with aerobic performance. As a consequence, a smaller number of anaerobic performance tests were developed for laboratory and field testing. In the past twenty years, however, this situation has changed and there is now a wide variety of tests available to measure anaerobic endurance. In this section we will focus on those that have been more widely assessed for validity and reliability.

Wingate Anaerobic Test

The Wingate Anaerobic Test (WAnT) is a 30-second maximal sprint test performed on a cycle ergometer. Developed at the Wingate Institute and first proposed in 1974, the WAnT has been used to assess anaerobic fitness for a wide variety of sports. A cycle ergometer commonly used for the test can be seen in Figure 10.10. The height of the saddle needs to be adjusted to the correct height for the participant. This can be achieved by the participant placing either heel on one pedal at its lowest point. The saddle height is adjusted correctly when a slight bend in the leg remains.

The participant should complete a five-minute warm-up with a resistance (load) of 1 N for females and 1.5 N

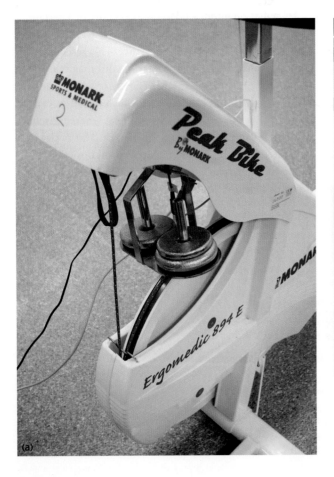

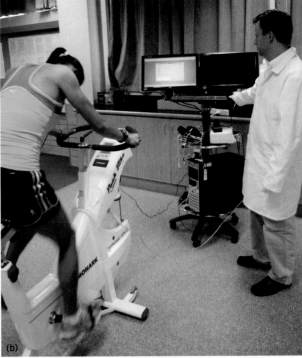

Figure 10.10 Set-up for the Wingate Anaerobic Test: a cycle ergometer showing the cradle to which the load is added (a) and a participant ready to complete the test (b). The photocell on the flywheel is connected to a computer program that calculates the power output during the WAnT test. (*Source*: Simon Fryer)

for males at a pedal rate of 60 rpm. Following this, the participant prepares for the test by setting the pedal on the lead leg at about '10 o'clock'. The load for the test is usually set at 7.5% of bodyweight, although this can be adjusted up or down to suit the individual, depending on their level of anaerobic fitness. A photocell on the flywheel is used to count flywheel revolutions and from this the power output for the test is automatically calculated by a computer. From the first strike on the pedals at the start of the test, the participant must cycle as hard as possible for the duration of the test, but remain seated throughout. Figure 10.11 provides an illustration of a typical power curve for a WAnT. The higher the peak power output, and the longer he or she can maintain close to this output, the better their anaerobic fitness. Another measure calculated at the end of the test, the fatigue index, can be used to provide further information on the athlete's anaerobic fitness. The peak power output reading from a test can be used as a measure of anaerobic power, whereas, the fatigue index is a gauge of anaerobic capacity.

The WAnT data used in the above example, found the participant to have a 45% fatigue index, indicating a 45% loss of their initial power output through the duration of the test. This loss of power is reflected in the downward trend of the power curve (Figure 10.11). For elite anaerobic athletes the decrease in power as shown by their fatigue index can be less than 10%, with a smaller decline in power seen in the power curve.

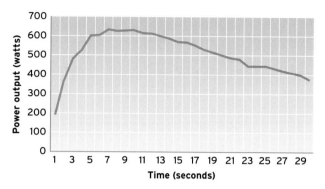

Figure 10.11 Power curve for WAnT.

Basketball sprint test

The basketball sprint test involves four sprints, out and back, of an increasing distance, the layout of which is shown in Figure 10.12. The athlete completes the test four times with a two-minute rest between each repetition. The time for each repetition is recorded to the nearest 0.1 s. The distance for each repetition varies according to the dimensions of the court, but typically the length of the court is between 22–28.65 m, although for some school gymnasiums the court might be smaller than this. This would make the total distance for each repetition around 110–143 m depending on the specific court dimensions. As long as all tests are conducted at the same venue, these differences are not important, unless trying to make a comparison to norm tables.

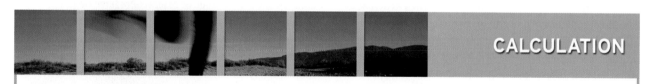

CALCULATION

Wingate anaerobic test example

The fatigue index associated with the power curve shown in Figure 10.11 can be calculated from the following information.

Peak power output (PPO) of 648 watts; minimum power output (MinPO) of 355 watts:

Fatigue Index (%) = (PPO − MinPO)/PPO × 100

= (648 − 355)/648 × 100

= (293/648) × 100

= (0.4522) × 100

= 45.22%

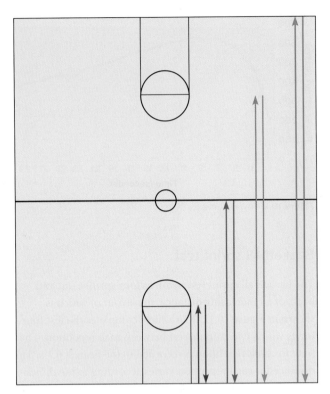

Figure 10.12 The participant sprints to (1) the freethrow line and back (9.14 m), (2) the halfway line and back (typically 22-28.65 m), (3) the far freethrow line and back (typically 35-48 m), and (4) the far baseline line and back (typically 44-57 m). (*Source*: Adapted from Semenick 1984.)

Anaerobic treadmill test

This treadmill test was developed by Cunningham and Faulkner and involves running to exhaustion at a speed of 12.9 km·hr^{-1}. To warm up for the test the participant should complete a 5-min run on the treadmill at a speed of 10.5 km·hr^{-1} with the gradient set at 0%. After stretching and mentally preparing for the test, the treadmill is adjusted to a 20% incline and a speed of 12.9 km·hr^{-1}. The participant then straddles the treadmill belt (one foot either side) and commences the test in their own time. The participant continues running until they reach volitional exhaustion, i.e. they cannot keep pace with the treadmill. The test time is recorded to the nearest 0.1 s, starting from the moment the participant ran unsupported on the treadmill until they touched the sides of the treadmill or stepped off at the end of the test.

Maximal accumulated oxygen deficit test

The maximal accumulated oxygen deficit (MAOD) test was developed in the 1980s as a method of assessing anaerobic endurance ability. More recently, the MAOD test has

been criticised as a test because of potential problems with primarily its validity, but also to some extent its reliability (Noordhof et al., 2010). The test though, presents an interesting conceptualisation of anaerobic contribution and is therefore worthwhile considering as a test for further development and one that might provide a basis for creating a sport-specific measure. The test is normally completed using a treadmill or an electromagnetically braked cycle ergometer and is well suited to the measurement of $\dot{V}O_2$ through online gas analysis.

Completion of an MAOD test requires a minimum of two testing sessions to complete the assessment. At the first session the participant completes a series of sub-maximal stages prior to running or cycling to exhaustion to provide an estimate of his or her $\dot{V}O_{2max}$. On a treadmill (10.5% incline) the speed is increased at the start of each stage, whereas, on a cycle ergometer the workloads are increased from a starting intensity of between 75–100 W. The intensity of exercise is increased to within a range of 30–90% of maximum during the sub-maximal stages.

The number of stages (4–10) has varied considerably between studies, but typically the length of each stage is 4 min to enable a steady state $\dot{V}O_2$ to be achieved at each stage. It is necessary to have sufficient stages to create an accurate linear regression. However, the inclusion of 10×4-min stages would mean that a participant would be required to complete at least 40 min of exercise prior to completing the maximal aspect of the test. A submaximal stage of the test lasting this long would negatively impact upon the $\dot{V}O_{2max}$ achieved. As a consequence, a number of researchers have begun to use 4×4-min stages prior to completing the $\dot{V}O_{2max}$. The $\dot{V}O_2$ during minutes 3 and 4 of each stage is averaged to provide the data point for linear regression modelling. After the sub-maximal stages the intensity of exercise would be increased at 1 min intervals until volitional exhaustion to provide an estimate of $\dot{V}O_{2peak}$ or $\dot{V}O_{2max}$.

The treadmill velocity or power output at each stage, and the $\dot{V}O_2$ (mL·kg^{-1}·min^{-1}) at the end of each stage, are recorded to calculate the supramaximal exercise load for the second test. A linear regression is calculated from this data to predict the exercise load.

During the second test the participant would then run or cycle to exhaustion based on a treadmill velocity or power output equivalent to 110–125% of their $\dot{V}O_{2max}$ (i.e. supramaximally). During the test the participants $\dot{V}O_2$ (mL·kg^{-1}·min^{-1}) is measured and recorded throughout to calculate the MAOD. Typically, the supramaximal

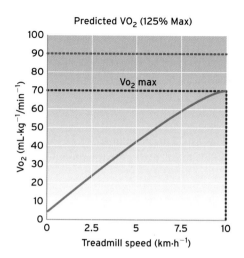

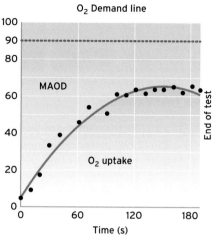

Figure 10.13 Method for determining MAOD. The participant ran at 12.5 km·h^{-1} for 2.5 min resulting in a MAOD of 88.5 mL O$_2$eq·kg^{-1}.

test lasts between 2 and 3 min. The MAOD is calculated from the difference between the oxygen demand (taken from the linear regression) and the $\dot{V}$ O$_2$ during the test. Data from breath-by-breath online gas analysis is then analysed to convert the oxygen consumption rate (mL·kg^{-1}·min^{-1}) relative to the time for each breath into an oxygen deficit (mL O$_2$ eq·kg^{-1}). Figure 10.13 provides an illustration of how the extrapolation line from the sub-maximal data creates the oxygen demand for the MAOD, the difference between the O$_2$ demand and the oxygen uptake providing MAOD which is recorded as a total in mL·kg^{-1}.

Repeat sprints

A variety of repeat sprint tests can be devised, related to the specifics of a sport, to assess anaerobic capacity. The sprint might be repeated a number of times with a recovery between repetitions, with the time for each sprint recorded. The lower the increase in sprint times, the better the athlete's anaerobic endurance. This test is easily adapted for a wide range of sports by changing the number of repetitions, sets and recovery time, dependent on the demands of the sport.

Running-based anaerobic sprint test

The running-based anaerobic sprint test (RAST) was developed in the late 1990s by Draper and Whyte and requires an athlete to complete 6 × 35 m sprints with a 10 s turnaround between each repetition. At the start of the test, before commencing the warm up, the athlete's mass is measured. The warm-up consists of 10 min increasing intensity exercise. After 3 min of light jogging the athlete completes 3 min of mobilising exercises prior to completing 10 increasing speed sprints, such that by the end of the

warm-up the athlete has completed one sprint at maximum speed. The athlete then recovers (walking and standing) for 3 min prior to starting the test.

Ideally, dual-beam bi-directional timing lights should be used for maximal accuracy, with a stopwatch used to time the 10 s turnarounds. If using timing lights the athlete starts just behind the light beam at the start gate. If using a stopwatch the athlete starts with his or her foot just behind the start line. Each sprint is made from a standing start. The athlete aims to sprint through the finishing line or gate as fast as possible (not slowing before the line). Between each sprint the athlete has 10 s to slow and return to the line for the next sprint, as a consequence the test is bi-directional, with 3 sprints in each direction.

The times of the athlete's 6 sprints can be recorded and kept for comparison with future test results. Additionally, it is possible to convert to an estimation of power and rate of fatigue using the formulas shown in the calculation box above.

6 × 150 m Rowing Test

Similar in format to the repeat sprints, the 6 × 150 m rowing anaerobic test on a rowing ergometer offers an alternative repeat anaerobic test that might be appropriate for athletes from a variety of sports. Ideally the rowing ergometer should be programmable such that it could be programmed for the 150 m intervals with 30 s recoveries. Each sprint takes approximately 25–40 s and the time and average power can be recorded for each sprint. A sample of test results for an athlete on the 6 × 150 m row is shown in Table 10.1. A power curve can be constructed using either the power outputs or time for the six sprints. Figure 10.14 illustrates a power curve based on the power output for the athlete whose results are shown in Table 10.1. The higher

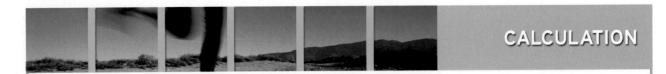

CALCULATION

Running-based anaerobic sprint test example

The following example is based on a 74 kg athlete who completed the first and fastest 35 m sprint in 4.79 s. Using the following formula, based on the Harman (1995) power calculation, it is possible to calculate an estimation of power output.

$$\text{Power} = \frac{\text{mass} \times \text{distance}^2}{\text{time}^3}$$

$$= \frac{74 \times 35^2}{4.79^3}$$

$$= \frac{74 \times 1225}{109.902239}$$

$$= \frac{90650}{109.902239}$$

$$= \underline{824.82 \text{ W}}$$

As for the WAnT, a fatigue index for a RAST can be calculated from the formula below, the example being based on a peak power output (PPO) of 825 W and an minimum power output (MinPO) of 376 W:

$$\text{Fatigue Index (\%)} = (\text{PPO} - \text{MinPO})/\text{PPO} \times 100$$

$$= (825 - 376)/825 \times 100$$

$$= (449/825) \times 100$$

$$= (0.5442) \times 100$$

$$= 54.42\%$$

the initial power output, the higher the athlete's anaerobic power, whereas the smaller the gradient of the trend line, the better the athlete's anaerobic endurance and performance on the test.

Table 10.1 An athlete's results for a 6 × 150 m rowing test.

Repetition no.	Time (sec)	Mean power (watts)	Heart rate (beats·min^{-1})
1	34.1	238	132
2	34.3	234	140
3	35.5	211	161
4	35	219	165
5	36.1	200	174
6	35.7	208	179

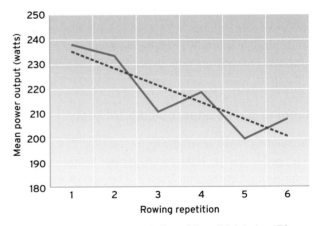

Figure 10.14 Graphic representation of the athlete's 6 × 150 m rowing results as shown in Table 10.1. The best fit line (red dotted line) indicates the general trend across the test. The higher the initial power output and the more horizontal the trend line, the better the performance.

Muscular endurance tests

A variety of bodyweight-resistance circuit-training-style exercises or sport-specific drills can be used to assess muscular endurance ability. The key with these exercises is to maintain the quality of the movements throughout the test time. Exercises can be carried out on a singular basis, such as how many sit-ups can be completed in a minute, or in a mini-circuit with, for example, press-ups, sit-ups, tricep dips and star jumps, with 30 s on each exercise. The type of exercises and organisation of the test could be designed specifically for a sport and could include sport-specific drills as well as generic exercises.

Knowledge integration question

What is the relationship between fatigue index and anaerobic endurance? What cycle test could be employed to determine fatigue index and how could this measure be improved through training?

Conditioning for anaerobic endurance sports

As for many sports, strength training should form an integral part of a training programme for any anaerobic endurance sport. Significant improvements in anaerobic performance will be brought about if a conditioning programme is designed in conjunction with a strength training programme. The conditioning programme for an anaerobic endurance sport athlete should be focused primarily on speed and speed endurance sessions, both of which can be developed through interval training.

Interval training provides an ideal form of training through which to improve anaerobic endurance. Through such training the timing of exercise and recovery periods can be closely monitored and altered to match those of the sport and the goals for training. Similarly, changes in exercise repetitions and recoveries can be made as training progresses. Typically, for anaerobic endurance performance improvement, high-intensity exercise bouts with short recovery periods are employed. The intensity and/or duration of exercise could be increased and the recovery duration decreased to maintain the training stress over time.

This form of training for anaerobic endurance sports is both physically and mentally demanding. The intensity of such training, which typically should be between 85–100% of maximum, brings with it a psychological and physiological challenge. The motivation of the athlete and the inventiveness of the teacher or coach will therefore be essential for maintaining the quality of training sessions. Variety in the location of sessions, types of training, providing short-term as well as long-term goals and groups working together, can all help with increasing motivation and thereby improving anaerobic fitness.

As well as matching the intensity for a given sport, which will naturally be high for anaerobic sports, the duration of conditioning training should also match the demands of the sport. Three forms of conditioning training would therefore be beneficial to athletes involved in sports that last between 10–90 s. *Speed training* over shorter distances or times would be beneficial for maximising intensity and improving neural transmission, (the speed of nerve impulse travel to the working muscles). In such efforts the typical time duration would be about 10 s. The recovery between repetitions would be around 3–5 mins. The second form of training, *speed progression* training, would be based around a time duration of 10–40 s and consequently the intensity would again be close to maximal throughout each effort. The basis behind such training would be to improve speed and to improve the functioning of the glycolytic pathway. The work/recovery ratio would have to be carefully planned to ensure the glycolytic pathway was predominant during each effort, without creating large rises in lactate and H^+. In these sessions, the intensity of the efforts would require recoveries of 5–10 minutes between repetitions. *Speed endurance* training would require efforts that were up to and slightly over the sport-specific distance, with repetitions typically lasting 40–90 s, and consequently, the intensity of training would be slightly lower than that for speed and speed progression training. As an example of over-distance training a 400 m runner might complete a session with 2 or 3 $\times$ 450 m repetitions. In this type of session, to ensure a high intensity is maintained, recoveries might be up to 10 min between repetitions.

Fatigue in anaerobic endurance sports

As was introduced in Chapter 9, the mechanisms behind muscular fatigue, because of their complexity, are not yet fully understood. The most popular model of fatigue in anaerobic endurance sports suggests that the reversible drop in performance is related to increases in muscular H^+ concentration. It appears that the increasing acidosis, associated with high-intensity anaerobic endurance sports, leads to an inhibition of glycolytic enzymatic activity and also interferes with the excitation–contraction coupling mechanism during muscular contraction.

Acids, bases and pH

Acids, such as lactic acid, dissociate in solution to release their H^+, increasing acidity. **Bases**, such as ammonia (NH_3) which is produced during the adenylate kinase reaction (described in Chapter 9), accept H^+ in solution to form hydroxide ions (OH^-) thereby increasing alkalinity. The acid-base balance of solution depends on the concentration of hydrogen and hydroxide ions present. Where $H^+ >$ than OH^- the solution is acidic, when $H^+ = OH^-$ the solution is neutral, and when $H^+ < OH^-$ the solution is alkaline. The maintenance of blood pH within tolerable limits is essential to life. Acidosis arising in diseases such as diabetes, and alkalosis in response to the low PO_2 at altitude, are potentially fatal if left untreated. The body's buffering mechanisms (discussed below), which operate within all the body's fluids (i.e. intracellular and extracellular fluid, and plasma within the blood), are responsible for maintaining pH at rest and importantly during exercise.

Knowledge integration question

Why does acidosis accompany anaerobic endurance activities? What negative effects does this have on the muscle and how can homeostasis be regained?

Buffering mechanisms

Carbonate - blood buffer

Lactate and H^+ produced in muscle fibres during fast-rate glycolysis can diffuse across the sarcolemma to the blood. This provides the primary mechanism through which the effect of increasing H^+ on cellular acidosis is delayed. Within the blood, where pH levels also require homeostatic control, carbonate (HCO_3^-) provides a buffer against H^+ diffusing from the working muscles. Through carbonate buffering, the H^+ binds with HCO_3^- to produce water and carbon dioxide. The equation for this reaction is:

$$HCO_3^- + H^+ \longrightarrow CO_2 + H_2O$$

The CO_2 produced during carbonate buffering is expelled from the body via the lungs during respiration. It is of interest to note that the additional CO_2 resulting from H^+ buffering within the blood during high-intensity exercise explains why Respiratory Exchange Ratio (RER) values rise to above 1.0 during maximal exercise, such as during a $\dot{V}O_{2max}$ test. The RER was introduced in Chapter 6 and provides a ratio of the carbon dioxide produced to the oxygen consumed during the catabolism of fat and carbohydrate. At rest and during low-intensity exercise, fat provides the main fuel for ATP generation. As exercise intensity increases towards maximum, carbohydrate, through glycolysis, becomes the predominant fuel for ATP re-synthesis. The RER value for metabolism of fat is 0.70, while the RER for glucose is 1.0, meaning that for every molecule of oxygen consumed, a molecule of carbon dioxide is produced. This represents the highest value RER can reach through aerobic metabolism. During a maximal aerobic test, however, when carbonate buffering is in operation to protect against the falling pH, the additional CO_2 produced results in RER rising above 1.0. Consequently, one indicator used by exercise physiologists to assess whether $\dot{V}O_{2max}$ has been reached is to examine whether the RER has risen to at least 1.15.

Kidneys - blood buffer

As has already been described, the maintenance of pH levels within tolerable ranges is vital to homeostasis. Consequently, the body has a number of additional mechanisms through which to protect against increasing acidosis. The kidneys play an important role in the maintenance of the acid-base balance within the body. They filter H^+ from the blood and either excrete them from the body via the urea cycle or use them to create further bicarbonate ions for blood buffering. It is the kidneys that are responsible for the regulation of bicarbonate levels within the blood.

Ammonia - cellular buffer

Blood proteins and haemoglobin provide alternative buffers for H^+ when increasing concentrations exceed carbonate buffering capacity. During high-intensity exercise, the adenylate deaminase reaction (refer to Chapter 9) catabolises AMP to form inosine monophosphate (IMP) and the base ammonia (NH_3). The ammonia created through this reaction accepts H^+, forming ammonium (NH_4+), prior to their removal from the body via the kidneys. The equation for this reaction is:

$$NH_3 + H^+ \longrightarrow NH_4^+$$

Muscular acidosis during maximal exercise

Despite the effects of the body's buffering mechanisms during maximal intensity exercise, the levels of lactate and consequently H^+ rise dramatically. Research indicates that enzymes function optimally within narrow pH bands. The increasing acidosis within the muscle fibre appears to inhibit the functioning of enzymes such as PFK (described earlier in this chapter) and therefore hinder the rate of glycolysis. In addition, the decreasing pH is thought to result in interruptions in the contraction of individual sarcomeres, thereby weakening muscular contraction. The feelings of fatigue that follow maximal anaerobic endurance exercise are also thought to result from the change in cellular pH. Chemoreceptors and nocioceptors within the muscle fibres detect the fall in pH and relay these as feelings of pain to the brain.

Although not responsible for fatigue in anaerobic endurance sports, the rise in blood lactate concentration is indicative of increases in H^+ concentration and the consequent fall in cellular pH. Physiologists have therefore commonly used capillary blood lactate concentrations as an indicator of exercise intensity and reliance on anaerobic metabolic processes, specifically fast-rate glycolysis. Resting blood lactate concentration is around 1.0 mM (produced by red blood cells whose only mechanism for energy production is through glycolysis). During maximal exercise lactate concentrations can reach as high as 25–30 mM in motivated athletes. A typical lactate concentration for a university student on the Wingate anaerobic test (30 seconds duration) is around 10–12 mM.

Inorganic phosphate – friend or foe?

The role of inorganic phosphate ions (Pi) in buffering and fatigue presents an interesting case study for anaerobic endurance sports. The possibly deleterious effect of Pi and its role in fatigue during power endurance sports was highlighted in Chapter 9. Previously, however, the most commonly held view was that Pi provided an important sarcoplasmic H^+ buffer. This buffering role, along with the forms of Pi found within muscle tissue, are described next, before an examination of the possible role of phosphate in fatigue during anaerobic sports.

Pi as a friend

It has been argued that within the sarcoplasm, Pi, resulting from the hydrolysis of ATP, serves as a buffer against the increased H^+ concentration associated with the formation of lactate during fast-rate glycolysis. The hydrolysis of ATP which provides the energy for muscular contraction during exercise liberates Pi in the form of HPO_4^{2-} which can accept an H^+ to form $H_2PO_4^-$ and buffer cellular pH levels. Research findings indicate that this reaction occurs within the sarcoplasm as both forms of Pi have been

isolated following high-intensity exercise. The equation for this reaction is:

$$HPO_4^{2-} + H^+ \longrightarrow H_2PO_4^-$$

Pi as a foe

More recent research, however, suggests that increases in the concentration of Pi, regardless of its form, are deleterious to performance. Firstly, just as was described in Chapter 9, it has now been suggested that increases in Pi result in a decrease in myofibrillar force production due to decreased Ca^{2+} sensitivity and SR Ca^{2+} release. Indeed, as exercise duration increases, this situation would be exacerbated. Research also suggests the effect is most evident in type II muscle fibres which are recruited most heavily in anaerobic endurance sports. Secondly, it has been demonstrated that Pi bonds with free Ca^{2+} during high-intensity exercise which serves to reduce further the available Ca^{2+} during muscular contraction. Thirdly, it has been speculated that the duration of anaerobic endurance sports might be such that as Pi accumulates it starts to move into the SR where it bonds with Ca^{2+}. This action of Pi passing from high concentration to low within the SR, serves to further decrease Ca^{2+} release into the sarcoplasm.

Pi – a friend and a foe?

Taking all these aspects together, while it might appear that Pi serves as a temporary buffer for H^+, as it starts to accumulate during high-intensity exercise it has a negative effect on performance, contributing significantly to fatigue. If the findings of more recent research translate to human muscle tissue during anaerobic performance, then it is perhaps likely that both the decreased pH originating from the increase in H^+, and the accumulation of Pi, contribute to fatigue in anaerobic endurance sports.

> ### Key points
>
> Fast-rate glycolysis:
>
> ➤ The predominant energy system during anaerobic endurance sports
>
> ➤ Results in accumulation of lactate and H^+ (leads to a fall in pH)
>
> Buffers:
>
> ➤ Help to maintain pH within a tolerable range
>
> ➤ Found in the blood (carbonate) or within cells (ammonia, phosphate)
>
> ➤ The kidney helps to maintain blood pH by filtering H^+ from the blood

The triad junction

To date, when asking the question whether Pi is friend or foe, the evidence currently suggests that the jury is still out. Further research in this interesting aspect of physiological fatigue is required to clarify the role of Pi in anaerobic performance. While considering the respective roles of Pi and H^+ accumulation as mechanisms of fatigue, it is also relevant and interesting to consider other proposed mechanisms that may also in part explain the power output drop. Researchers have speculated that the power drop associated with increasing fatigue in anaerobic sports might relate to a triad junction-led alteration in the rate of Ca^{2+} release from the SR. Upon sensing the decline in ATP concentrations, particularly in type II fibres, the triad junction might respond by reducing Ca^{2+} release as a safety mechanism to avoid complete cellular ATP depletion and potential muscle damage. An area of rapid growth with regard to fatigue is that of reactive oxygen species (ROS), such as superoxide and hydrogen peroxide. It is speculated that ROS, produced in active muscles, contribute to fatigue by their negative effect on SR Ca^{2+} release and myofibrillar force generation. Which of the ROS are important, and how they are produced remains to be clarified. Research with ROS scavengers has led to a reduction in fatigue in isolated muscle fibres, which supports the involvement of ROS in fatigue. Finally, in the section below we will briefly examine the role of magnesium as a potential contributor to fatigue.

The special case of magnesium and its role in fatigue

Whilst only representing around 0.1% of our body mass, magnesium (Mg^{2+}) represents the fourth most abundant cation (after Na^+, K^+ and Ca^{2+}) and is particularly prevalent in the bones and muscles. Within the body, magnesium ions (Mg^{2+}) serve a number of important functions including enzyme activation, calcium signaling and cell membrane functioning. Magnesium ions are also involved in the synthesis of DNA and RNA and are found within the structure of a number of proteins and nucleotides. As can be seen from Figure 10.15, ATP actually exists bonded to Mg^{2+} to form an ATP-Mg^{2+} complex, consequently, Mg^{2+} is involved in all the energy generation pathways. ATP has a strong affinity for Mg^{2+}; however, due to the lower affinity of ADP and AMP, Mg^{2+} concentration rises as ATP concentration falls. Recent research has led to speculation that the rise in Mg^{2+} might also serve to inhibit the Ca^{2+} release channels within the SR, thereby contributing to reduced Ca^{2+} release from the SR and impaired muscle contraction.

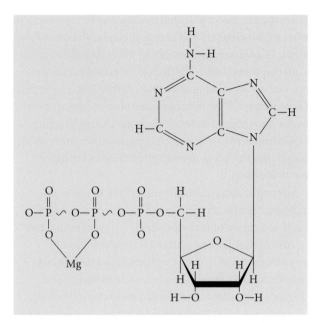

Figure 10.15 The attachment of Mg^{2+} to ATP.

Key points

Fatigue in anaerobic endurance sports is probably linked to a fall in muscle pH, which affects glycolytic enzymatic activity and excitation–contraction coupling.

Additionally, increases in reactive oxygen species and Mg^{2+} (forms complex with ATP) during high-intensity exercise, may reduce Ca^{2+} release from the SR and impair muscular contraction.

Physiological adaptations to anaerobic endurance training

Improved glycolytic capacity

Anaerobic endurance training leads to improvements in glycolytic metabolic functioning and fatigue resistance. It leads to greater glucose uptake during recovery and increased resting glycogen stores. As the primary fuel source for anaerobic activities, the increase in glycogen stores will result in an increased anaerobic ability during exercise. A key mechanism for the improvement in anaerobic endurance capacity relates to improved glycolytic enzyme activity. Just as sprint and strength training result in improvements in phosphagen enzyme activity, so anaerobic training, such as interval work, improves the activation of enzymes such as phosphofructokinase (PFK) and hexokinase (HK). As was described earlier in the chapter

HK catalyses the first reaction in glycolysis where glucose is converted to glucose-6-phosphate and PFK catalyses the third step in glycolysis (fructose-6-phosphate to fructose-1,6-bisphosphate). Both reactions involve the addition of Pi to the substrate. Research indicates that improvement in enzyme activity for PFK and HK can be as high as 50% above pre-training levels.

Some studies have found additional improvements in the functioning of glycogen phosphorylase and lactate dehydrogenase (LDH), but these findings are less consistent. Glycogen phosphorylase serves as the catalyst for the initial reaction in glycogen catabolism, through the process of glycogenolysis. Lactate dehydrogenase is the enzyme responsible for catalysing the conversion of pyruvate, the product of glycolysis, to lactate. Although the increases in glycolytic enzyme activity are not as substantial or as influential as those realised through aerobic training, the increased glycolytic enzyme activity still results in improved force generation and ability to sustain contractions during anaerobic endurance exercise. In addition, anaerobic training will also lead to a transition in the properties of type II fibres to favour glycolysis. More specifically, type IIa fibres will shift towards the structural properties of type IIx fibres. This shift will result in additional fibres favouring glycolysis which will, in conjunction with enhanced enzymatic activation, serve to improve further glycolytic ATP synthesis.

Buffering capacity

Anaerobic endurance ability is also improved after training through improved buffering capabilities within the blood and active muscles. Research indicates that buffering capabilities are improved by up to 25% in response to anaerobic training. The net effects of the increased buffering capacity will be to delay the on-set of fatigue, thereby, improving anaerobic performance. In addition, anaerobic training has been shown to lead to an increased H^+ tolerance, thought to be linked with an increased motivation or an improved ability to cope with the pain associated with decreasing pH.

Knowledge integration question

What physiological adaptations occur following anaerobic endurance training and what roles do they play in the improvement of 400 m running performance?

Aerobic metabolism

Lastly, anaerobic training has been shown to result in small improvements in aerobic metabolism which also serve

to delay the onset of fatigue. Anaerobic endurance training, such as interval sessions, has been shown to result in improved activity in Krebs cycle enzymes such as citrate synthase, succinate dehydrogenase, and malate dehydrogenase (refer to Chapter 11). Although these improvements are not as substantial as those realised through aerobic training, they still contribute to reducing the anaerobic load and increasing time to fatigue in anaerobic endurance sports. The effect of anaerobic training on aerobic enzymatic activity, whilst perhaps appearing counterintuitive, should not be surprising, given the significant contribution of the aerobic pathways to total energy (ATP) generation during anaerobic endurance sports. This contribution is shown clearly in Figure 10.2.

Key points

Adaptations to anaerobic endurance training:
➤ Improved glucose uptake and resultant glycogen storage during recovery
➤ Improved enzyme activity (glycolysis and Krebs cycle)
➤ Improved buffering capabilities

Combined, these adaptations delay fatigue and improve anaerobic endurance performance.

Ergogenic aids for anaerobic endurance sports

This section examines ergogenic aids that would be beneficial to performance in anaerobic endurance sports. Initially, nutritional ergogenic aids are discussed. As a consequence of the likely importance of H^+ to fatigue in these sports, the main focus in this section will be upon ergogenic aids that can serve to enhance buffering capability to delay the onset of fatigue. The ergogenic aids covered in this chapter are legal substances that an athlete can take to improve buffering capacity.

Nutritional ergogenic aids

In common with the explosive sports, the basic starting point prior to any performance enhancing dietary manipulation should be an athlete's normal diet. Where possible, an athlete should attempt to ensure his or her nutrition provides a *well balanced diet*. In addition, attention should be paid to the moderation, variety and naturalness of dietary choices which were described in more detail in Chapter 2. The main focus in the development of nutritional ergogenic aids has been around maintaining energy delivery and delaying fatigue. For example, in Chapter 9 the potential performance enhancement provided by creatine supplementation was discussed. As was described, research indicates that creatine supplementation leads to enhanced muscular creatine and phosphocreatine concentrations. Creatine is briefly mentioned here because research indicates that, as well as enhancing performance in power and power endurance sports, creatine appears to also have an ergogenic effect for anaerobic endurance sports. The improved PCr stores brought about through creatine supplementation will provide enhanced stores for immediate ATP synthesis, thereby having a glycolytic sparing effect, albeit for a very short period of time. Creatine supplementation would perhaps be more beneficial to an anaerobic endurance athlete in a training setting where an ergogenic effect has been identified in relation to strength training. The main focus in this chapter, however, is on substances that can act as buffering agents.

Buffers as ergogenic aids

Bicarbonate and, more recently, β-alanine have been studied in a variety of settings to assess their capacity to provide a buffer against the increasing acidosis arising in response to anaerobic endurance performance. As was described earlier in this chapter, carbonate buffering provides a short-term reprieve from the increasing acidosis associated with fast-rate glycolysis. Almost as soon as the buffering effect of carbonate was discovered, exercise physiologists began to experiment with ways to enhance concentrations in the blood. More recently, researchers have begun to examine the potential of β-alanine as a supplement to assist in pH buffering.

Bicarbonate

Bicarbonate ingestion, in the form of sodium bicarbonate (baking soda), appears to have an ergogenic effect for anaerobic endurance and high-intensity short-duration aerobic endurance sports. Rather than entering muscle fibres and increasing the pH there, sodium bicarbonate takes its effect by increasing blood alkalinity, which serves to stimulate an increase in the shuttling of lactate and H^+ from the active muscle fibres to the bloodstream. It appears that pH reactive transport proteins, originally identified by Roth and Brooks in 1990, respond to the rise in blood pH associated with bicarbonate supplementation, by increasing the rate of lactate and H^+ transport to the blood.

The dual action of extracellular buffering and increased rate of lactate and H^+ transfer to the blood is believed to assist in maintaining pH in muscle fibres and the blood, thereby delaying fatigue. The effects of bicarbonate buffering are also thought to lead to a decrease in central fatigue (feelings of fatigue) which also appears to delay the onset of fatigue during anaerobic endurance sports. Research indicates that the effects of bicarbonate buffering are most effective for high-intensity sports lasting from 1 to 7 minutes in duration, including intermittent exercise. As a consequence, bicarbonate has a potential ergogenic effect that has application to aerobic and intermittent sports (covered in Chapters 11 and 13) as well as those in this chapter.

It appears that the most effective loading dose for bicarbonate ingestion is 300 mg per kg body mass which should be ingested one to two hours before exercise, along with the consumption of 1 L of water. There have been incidences of gastrointestinal upset (bloating, abdominal pain, cramps and diarrhoea) reported in response to sodium bicarbonate ingestion, but these effects can be lessened by taking the dose in 10-minute intervals starting two hours before exercise. Used in this way sodium bicarbonate supplement should present no major health risks, and indeed, it is commonly used as a stomach antacid. Excessive or long-term use can present harmful effects including alkalosis, and muscle contraction interference and should therefore be avoided.

β-alanine

In recent years the buffering capacity of *carnosine*, a dipeptide derivative of the amino acids alanine and histidine, has been investigated. Carnosine, found in high concentration in muscle fibres, represents an effective H^+ buffer. More recently, it has been suggested that the role of carnosine might additionally, or possibly alternatively, serve to improve performance by increasing Ca^{2+} sensitivity, thereby offsetting one of the negative effects of Pi accumulation. The availability of carnosine within the muscle appears to be limited by the availability of β-*alanine*. As a consequence, research groups such as Harris and colleagues set out to investigate the effects of β-alanine supplementation on H^+ buffering and performance. In their research, β-alanine supplementation was found to increase carnosine stores within the muscle by 42–80%, dependent on the loading regimen. In a study of maximal isometric contraction endurance, increased carnosine stores resulted in 11–14% improvements in time to exhaustion. In a cycle ergometer study, designed to elicit exhaustion in 150 seconds, time to exhaustion was increased by 12% and 15%

after a 4- and 10-week supplementation period, respectively. It appears that β-alanine supplementation offers an ergogenic effect; however, the mechanism through which this works, increased Ca^{2+} sensitivity or as a buffer to H^+, requires further investigation. Nevertheless, β-alanine supplementation does appear to provide an effective supplement to delay fatigue and improve performance in anaerobic endurance and short-term high-intensity aerobic endurance exercise. Further research is required to ascertain the potential benefits to sports performance and the mechanism through which it takes effect.

Phosphorus

An interesting possible ergogenic aid that is also worth discussion in this section is that of phosphorus, in the form of sodium phosphate. Prior to recent research findings, as was described above, Pi was thought to serve primarily as a sarcoplasmic buffer to the rise in H^+ associated with anaerobic endurance sport. As a consequence, it was speculated that sodium phosphate supplementation might serve to reduce the effects of fatigue.

The mineral *phosphorus* is found in the body as the salt phosphate. Most of the body's phosphate is combined with calcium forming calcium phosphate which is the main constituent of our teeth and bones. Phosphate can exist in its inorganic form (Pi) or combined with organic matter to form the organic phosphates found in ATP, PCr, or the phospholipids that form the basis for cell membrane structure.

Sodium phosphate loading has been postulated as a mechanism for improving performance and decreasing fatigue through pH buffering. Results from studies have been far less convincing for phosphate than for bicarbonate or β-alanine supplementation. It is also suggested that increasing extracellular and intracellular phosphate concentration through supplementation increases the phosphagen available for PCr and ATP synthesis. There is, however, a lack of research evidence to support this theory and recent research findings regarding the potentially negative effects of Pi accumulation perhaps explain why no clear evidence of the benefits of sodium phosphate supplementation has been found.

Key point

Buffering supplements, such as sodium bicarbonate and β-alanine, may act as ergogenic aids, improving anaerobic performance.

Check your recall
Fill in the missing words.

➤ For sports of 10 to 90 seconds duration, _____ is the key mechanism for energy production.

➤ Glycolysis is the conversion of glucose or glycogen to _____.

➤ Additionally, _____ is produced to supply the active muscles with energy.

➤ For each molecule of glucose broken down through glycolysis there is a net gain of _____ ATP.

➤ _____ rate glycolysis occurs during high-intensity exercise.

➤ The conversion of lactate to glucose occurs through the _____ cycle which takes place in the liver.

➤ An important hydrogen carrier required for the process of glycolysis, and the conversion of pyruvate to lactate, is called _____ _____ _____.

➤ The two main components of fitness that are related to anaerobic endurance sports are anaerobic endurance and _____ _____.

➤ A common cycle test of anaerobic endurance is the _____.

➤ The most popular model of fatigue in anaerobic endurance sports is that increased muscle _____ concentration inhibits glycolytic _____ activity and interferes with excitation–contraction coupling.

➤ Increased Pi during high-intensity exercise may decrease muscle force production by impairing the release of _____ from the sarcoplasmic reticulum.

➤ The best training for anaerobic endurance is _____ training.

➤ Anaerobic training improves glycolytic enzyme activation, such as that of _____, an increase in resting _____ stores, and a shift from type IIa to type _____ muscle fibre type.

➤ Due to its capacity to provide a buffer against increasing acidosis, _____ is a common ergogenic aid in anaerobic endurance sports performers.

Review questions

1. Why does it take longer to gain energy from glycolysis than the phosphagen system? What are the fuels for glycolysis?

2. How is the rate of glycolysis controlled? Which enzymes are involved in this process?

3. At what point in glycolysis is the 6 carbon ring of glucose broken?

4. Explain why there is a build up of lactate with fast-rate glycolysis.

5. Explain the fates of lactate following fast-rate glycolysis?

6. What are the differing fates of pyruvate following fast-rate and slower-rate glycolysis?

7. With relation to the buffering of blood lactate, describe how Respiratory Exchange Ratios greater than 1.0 can occur during maximal exercise?

8. In relation to anaerobic endurance, what is meant by the term buffering? What is the difference between the buffering mechanisms of the muscle cell and the blood stream?

9. What are the potential dual roles of Pi in terms of muscular fatigue in anaerobic endurance sports?

10. Describe how buffers can function as ergogenic aids and how improving buffering capacity may help a rock climber improve their performance on a route.

Teach it!

In groups of three, choose one topic and teach it to the rest of the study group.

1. The rate of glycolysis must meet the cellular demands for energy. Discuss the factors involved in the control of glycolytic rate.

2. What is the best form of training for anaerobic endurance and what physiological adaptations occur as a result of this training?

3. Describe in detail two tests of anaerobic endurance, one generic test and one sport-specific test.

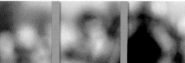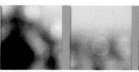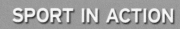

SPORT IN ACTION

Biography: Katherine Schirrmacher

Adventure sport: rock climbing

Katherine has been climbing for 20 years and during that time has

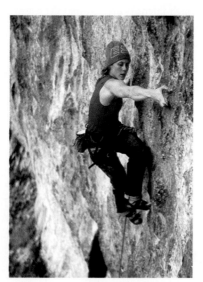

(*Source*: Alex Messenger)

climbed many different rock types and across disciplines including bouldering, sport climbing and trad climbing. She has climbed at crags all over the world but began her career on the Welsh sea cliffs, and Lake District crags along with trips to the Italian Dolomites. In the past four years Katherine has found herself drawn to the more physical nature of bouldering, sport climbing and competition climbing Katherine has climbed bouldering problems up to V9, led 8a on bolts and E7 6c on trad routes. Since entering climbing competitions she has made the finals in three World Cup bouldering events, with her best finish so far being 11th place. Last year she took time out from climbing to have her first child a girl named Vanessa. Katherine lives in Sheffield with her husband Nic and coaches climbing in her spare time.

Raindogs

Raindogs is like the 100 metre sprint but it's only 12 metres high, and takes 1 minute and 20 seconds to climb. Requiring a very specific type of fitness, almost only applicable to this route, Raindogs is the ultimate test of power endurance. There is no section of desperately hard moves but the climbing is relentless and resting is almost impossible. After all the difficulties below, the final move, needing one more burst of power, unusually is grabbing the lower-off chain at the top. People are known to spend days falling off here. A short bit of white rock at Malham Cove, it is swamped by the 100 metre sweep of cliff above it. This is one of Britain's classic bolted routes and at the magic grade of 8a, many people aspire to climb it. It's a benchmark which I wanted to test myself against.

The climbing is intricate and purposeful. Every hand movement seems to involve about three foot changes. There are many different and subtle possibilities depending on your body shape. In fact, despite high climbing standards today, it is so complicated no one has yet succeeded on the route on their first go with no prior knowledge. Once you get past the first bolt the movements are long, sometimes powerful and you have to climb fast. The clock starts ticking right away and it's a race against time before your arms drain and the route spits you off.

From the very first moment, I was drawn into the route. None of the moves seemed especially hard, it was simply a question of putting it all together. Simple? The journey began, both in the steps I had to take to get myself physically in shape and mentally as time and time again I fell and I wondered whether I would ever reach the top.

I spent a period of time on it trying 'links', climbing from the second bolt to the top, then first bolt to the top and finally ground to the top.

Within a matter of about three days I found myself climbing from the first bolt to the top so I tried from the ground. However hard I tried, nothing would get me to the top. Within a couple of metres of the chain and within a matter of seconds my arms would give out and gravity got the better of me.

Conditions were vital: too cold and I wouldn't be able to feel my fingers, too warm and my fingers would slip on warm rock, wet rock was a no go. I battled with hot weather and became obsessed with the forecast and the temp gauge in my car. At the bottom one of the pockets stays stubbornly damp even when the sun is shining hard and needs a rag stuffing in to dry it, in order to stop fingers slipping. Clutching at straws I stuffed newspaper cuttings of Kelly Holmes' Olympic success into the pocket, hoping that some of her success would rub off on me.

A re-think was needed and the following year I geared myself properly to the route convinced that nothing was going to get between me and the top. I practised circuits in my local

climbing wall lasting 1 minute and 20 seconds & kept up a dose of powerful climbing. Pull-ups, push ups and other core body exercises took over my normal 'having fun at the climbing wall'. It was time to get serious. Within a short time I was actually climbing the best I had ever climbed and when I went on the route I was already better than I had been the previous year.

I can clearly remember the day I did it. I smiled when I saw 12°C on the temperature gauge as parked my car. The previous day on the route, I had arrived within one hand movement of the top but for some reason my body seemed to fold in flat at the knees like an envelope bringing me downwards dangling again on the rope. However the moment I finally grabbed the chain, my whole body was working as one, strong from the toes to the knees, and up through my arms. The tip of my middle finger crept through the chain. For an instant my body wasn't sure if it could make it but my mind took over as the rest of my finger curled through. Letting out a cheer, the job was done.

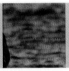

CLASSIC RESEARCH SUMMARY

Equilibrium constant of isomerase and phosphorylation of glyceraldehyde-3-phosphate by Meyerhof and Junowicz-Kocholaty (1943)

This is the first of three classic papers on the elucidation of the glycolytic pathway by Otto Meyerhof. It specifically involves steps 4, 5 and 6 of the glycolytic pathway. Two to four years prior to this paper it was identified

that during glycolysis the hexose ring, hexose diphosphate (known today as fructose-1,6-bisphosphate), was split into two triose phosphate isomers (glyceraldehyde-3-phosphate and dihydroxyacetone phosphate), catalysed by the enzyme zymohexase (now known as aldolase). In the presence of an isomerase, dihydroxyacetone phosphate is then converted to glyceraldehyde-3-phosphate, which is subsequently oxidised and phosphor-

ylated to form 1,3-diphosphoglycerate. Prior to this paper by Meyerhof and Junowicz-Kocholaty, it was proposed by Warburg and Christian (1939), that this final reaction occurred through an intermediate, 1,3-diphosphoglyceraldehyde, in the presence of an oxidising enzyme and cozymase.

With this knowledge, Meyerhof and Junowicz-Kocholaty aimed to determine the equilibrium constant of isomerase ([dihydroxyacetone

➤

phosphate]/[glyceraldehyde-3-phosphate]), and to identify whether the above intermediary step existed. To do this, they improved the technique used for the measurement of very small amounts of glyceraldehyde-3-phosphate, and adapted available methods for the preparation of a variety of enzymes. This research demonstrated that the equilibrium constant of isomerase was 20–25 (i.e. 95–96% dihydroxyacetone phosphate and 4–5% glyceraldehyde-3-phosphate). The quantities of the two triose phosphates was found to be unaffected by the presence of

inorganic phosphate (required for the phosphorylation of glyceraldehyde-3-phosphate) whether or not in the presence of the oxidising enzyme of Warburg. As the equilibrium constant remained stable in these altered conditions, Meyerhof and Junowicz-Kocholaty indicated that the previous suggestion of an intermediary step in the oxidation and phosphorylation of glyceraldehyde-3-phosphate was 'premature', in that the idea was circulated before research had fully verified their thinking. Now that the glycolytic pathway has been fully elucidated, it is clear that Meyerhof

and Junowicz-Kocholaty were indeed correct in saying that glyceraldehyde-3-phosphate is oxidised directly to 1,3-bisphosphoglycerate, as is described in the above section of the text and illustrated in Figures 10.3 and 10.4.

Reference: Meyerhof, O. and Junowicz-Kocholaty, R. (1943). The equilibria of isomerase and aldolase, and the problem of the phosphorylation of glyceraldehyde phosphate. *Journal of Biological Chemistry*, 149: 71–92.

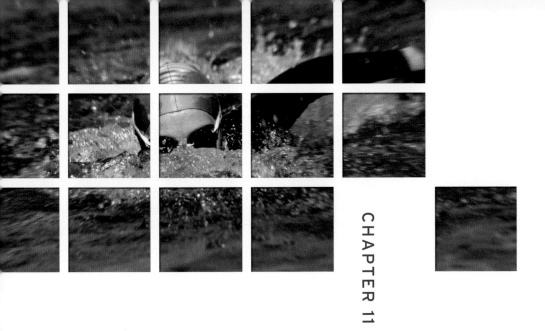

CHAPTER 11

High-intensity aerobic endurance sports

Learning objectives

After reading, considering and discussing with a study partner
the material in this chapter you should be able to:

➤ define the aerobic-anaerobic transition

➤ critically analyse the different methods for identifying the
aerobic-anaerobic transition

➤ explain the importance of the aerobic-anaerobic transition
to aerobic endurance athletes

➤ compare and contrast the lactate threshold, maximal
lactate steady state and critical power tests for use with
athletes

➤ describe what is meant by the term steady state

➤ summarise excess post-exercise oxygen consumption
(EPOC)

➤ discuss the concept of exercise economy

➤ describe the likely mechanisms of fatigue in high-intensity
aerobic endurance sports

➤ highlight the metabolic and cardiovascular adaptations to
aerobic endurance training

➤ teach athletes about the benefits and most beneficial regimen for carbohydrate loading

➤ explain the potential ergogenic effect of caffeine for
sports performance

As a result of the diversity of aerobic sports, both in
terms of the intensity and duration, two chapters have
been devoted to the aerobic endurance sports. The current chapter focuses on high-intensity aerobic endurance
sports, while Chapter 12 examines the physiology of lower-
intensity aerobic endurance sports. The relative intensity
of aerobic endurance sports is closely related to the duration of the event. By way of example, Figure 11.1 provides
an illustration of a velocity–distance curve for the world
records for a number of athletics events. As can be seen
from this figure, the highest velocities occur for the events
in the anaerobic zone.

Within the anaerobic zone, as a result of the maximal
intensity involved and the increasing duration of the effort,
the velocity curve falls sharply through this zone. We then
enter the aerobic high-intensity zone and we see the shape
of the curve begin to plateau. The lesser velocity decline in
this zone reflects the ability of the aerobic energy system,
as the main fuel source, to sustain high-intensity exercise
across a wide duration of activity from 1,500 m (~3.30 min)
to a full marathon (~2.00–2.15 h). As we enter the lower-
intensity aerobic zone we see a further drop in intensity for
marathon performance at the end of an ironman triathlon.
Given that the duration of a full ironman triathlon is in
excess of 8 hours for elite athletes, their times for the marathon (between 2 h 30 min and 2 h 48 min) are a further

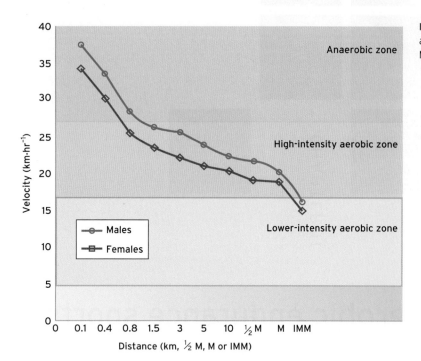

Figure 11.1 The velocity duration curve for athletics world records. ½ M = half marathon, M = marathon, IMM = Ironman marathon time.

reflection of the sustained performance ability of the aerobic system. In events of a duration longer than an elite full marathon (just over two hours), we begin to see a further decline in intensity and velocity, and these will form the focus of Chapter 12. The current chapter considers a range of sports that fit within the high-intensity aerobic endurance category, of which some can be seen in Figure 11.2.

As a consequence of their higher relative intensity, the duration of the activities in Chapter 9 (2–10 s) tended to be shorter than those covered in Chapter 10 (10–90 s). Despite this, the high-intensity endurance activities covered in this chapter still have a relatively wide range in duration, from events like the 1,000 m sprint kayak or canoe (3–4 min duration) to the marathon run (2–3 h duration). As can be seen from Figure 11.1, the duration of an individual aerobic endurance event has a direct impact upon the relative intensity of performance. Clearly, it would not be possible for an athlete to maintain the physiological intensity they achieve in a 1,500 m race over the distance required for a marathon. When planning training for an aerobic endurance sport the duration of the event should be central to decisions made about the preparation programme. A high degree of physiological specificity is required for training to improve performance in high-intensity aerobic endurance sports, as for all the sports covered in Part II of this book.

The pace judgement involved in aerobic endurance sports means that athletes will operate in a zone close to the transition between aerobic and anaerobic exercise. This transition point is often referred to as the anaerobic threshold. The anaerobic threshold and the related lactate threshold, have been shown to have significant correlation with race performance. It is likely that a delayed

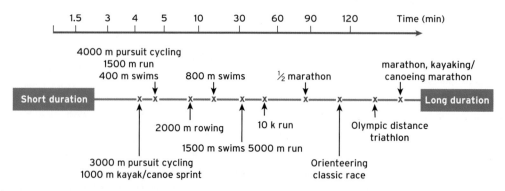

Figure 11.2 The duration continuum for high-intensity aerobic sports.

aerobic-anaerobic transition contributed to the bronze medal success of Tim Brabants in the Sydney Olympic Sprint Kayak race, as described in the Sport in Action piece on p. 347. As a consequence of the importance of the aerobic-anaerobic transition to high-intensity aerobic endurance, this chapter begins with a review of this aspect of physiology. In addition, we will examine the concept of critical power, a more recent concept, which has been found to be linked to race performance. Following this, we examine the physiology of high-intensity aerobic endurance sports, including specific concepts such as fatigue, adaptations to training and ergogenic aids to improve performance.

11.1 Aerobic endurance sports and the importance of the aerobic-anaerobic transition (AAT)

Aerobic endurance

Aerobic endurance refers to the ability of the body to produce energy for exercise involving the whole body during sustained exercise. There are a number of different terms, often used interchangeably, that have been used to refer to this aspect of fitness: these include aerobic capacity, aerobic power, cardiovascular fitness and cardiorespiratory fitness. The metabolic pathways within the aerobic system become the predominant energy source for sports or events that last for longer than 60–90 s. The aerobic system has specific pathways through which carbohydrates, lipids and proteins can be catabolised in the presence of oxygen to produce energy for exercise.

The functional capacity of the aerobic system has traditionally been assessed by conducting a test for maximal oxygen uptake ($\dot{V}O_{2max}$). An individual's $\dot{V}O_{2max}$ represents the maximum volume (V) of oxygen (O_2) he or she can consume per minute (dot above the V) to provide energy via aerobic metabolism during an exercise test of increasing intensity. There is a variety of ways this can be measured or estimated, such as through the multi-stage fitness test (Bleep or Beep test) or in a laboratory on a cycle ergometer, a treadmill or a rowing ergometer. In a physiology laboratory, gas analysis equipment can be used to measure the exact volumes of oxygen consumed and carbon dioxide produced during a maximal test. If such a precise measurement of aerobic endurance is not required, or for safety reasons is not advisable, there is a variety of sub-maximal methods that can provide an estimate of an individual's aerobic power. A number of these methods are described in Chapter 12.

More recently, the transition between aerobic and anaerobic systems has been measured as a way to assess the functional capacity of the aerobic system. This change has occurred because stronger correlations have been observed between the aerobic-anaerobic transition and race performance than between $\dot{V}O_{2max}$ and race performance. In other words, the point at which an athlete makes the transition to an increasingly anaerobic performance is a better predictor of race pace than his or her $\dot{V}O_{2max}$. Consequently, because the focus is on high-intensity aerobic endurance sports, we will examine the aerobic-anaerobic transition in this chapter and then in Chapter 12 move on to examine the concept of $\dot{V}O_{2max}$ in more detail.

Key points

'Aerobic' means requiring or using air (oxygen).

Aerobic endurance refers to the ability to sustain whole-body exercise.

High-intensity aerobic endurance sports:

➤ Duration ranges from 90 s to around 2 h

➤ The aerobic system provides the main energy pathway

The $\dot{V}O_{2max}$ or the aerobic-anaerobic transition can assess the aerobic capacity.

Aerobic-anaerobic transition

A clear understanding of the aerobic-anaerobic transition (AAT) is very important for those interested in high-intensity aerobic endurance performance. As a result of early research findings in the field, the AAT has become closely associated with the formation of lactate. Indeed, research concerning the existence of an aerobic-anaerobic transition developed from the early work regarding the nature and production of lactate.

The Swedish physiologist Carl Scheele, introduced in Chapter 1, first isolated lactic acid in samples of sour milk in 1780. It is through this link with milk, a product of lactation, that lactic acid and lactate gained their names. In 1807 another Swedish scientist, Jöns Berzelius, isolated lactic acid in muscle, calling it *sarcolactic acid*. Berzelius went on to determine that the concentration of sarcolactic acid in a muscle was associated with prior exercise. As the intensity of exercise increased, so the sarcolactic acid concentration increased. By 1833 the chemical composition and formula for lactic acid, $C_3H_6O_3$, had been determined. In 1907 Frederick Hopkins and Walter Fletcher studied exercise to fatigue in amphibian muscle, and discovered that lactic acid concentration increased during anoxic (low or no oxygen) conditions. Later, Hill and Lupton (1923) suggested the increase in lactic acid during exercise was the consequence of insufficient oxygen supply.

The terms *aerobic* and *anaerobic* glycolysis arose from the conclusions drawn by Lupton and Hill regarding the formation of lactic acid during exercise. 'Aerobic glycolysis' was used to describe slower-rate glycolysis where the presence of oxygen is sufficient to enable pyruvate to be completely oxidised. More correctly, it refers to a pattern of glycolysis where lactate removal is equal to lactate synthesis (resulting in no or only a small net gain in lactate during exercise). 'Anaerobic glycolysis' described the fate of pyruvate during fast-rate glycolysis where lactate synthesis exceeds lactate removal resulting in an accumulation of lactate within muscle fibres and the blood.

As described in Chapter 10, the use of these terms has led to some confusion in physiological pedagogy, due to the fact that glycolysis is an anaerobic (not requiring oxygen) metabolic process. It is the fate of pyruvate, the end-product of glycolysis, which is determined by the intensity of exercise and the supply of oxygen. This is why the terms *slower-rate* and *fast-rate glycolysis* have been used throughout this textbook.

Traditionally, the metabolic processes are described by starting with short-term high-intensity exercise and then moving on to consider endurance activities. In this way textbooks move from anaerobic to aerobic metabolism. For some activities this matches the transition in energy production from the onset of exercise. However, for the high-intensity aerobic endurance activities that are the focus of this chapter there are times when the reverse pattern of energy system contribution occurs. Sports such as 1,500 m running, 400 m swimming and rowing are predominantly aerobic sports but draw upon anaerobic metabolism for short in-race bursts or for the finishing 'kick'. An understanding of this conceptual difference is important when considering the transition from aerobic to anaerobic metabolism.

During an aerobic endurance race athletes attempt to maintain an exercise level that is as high as possible, thereby maximising aerobic metabolism, while avoiding substantial reliance on anaerobic (fast-rate glycolysis or phosphagen system) metabolic processes that would lead to early fatigue. This point of exercise intensity, maximising aerobic metabolism while remaining just below substantial reliance on anaerobic metabolism, represents the AAT.

The term AAT has been adopted for this textbook as an umbrella term encompassing the wide number of terms that have been used previously to describe this transition. For want of a better term, the anaerobic threshold has most

commonly been used to describe the transition from aerobic to increasingly anaerobic exercise. The term anaerobic threshold, however, has a specific meaning which, as was clearly argued by Brooks and Davis in the 1980s, precludes its use as an umbrella term. The AAT is an important physiological transition point for high-intensity aerobic endurance athletes. As a consequence, the various terms and concepts related to the AAT will be discussed in this section prior to describing a number of methods that can be used to identify this transition point.

Key point

The aerobic-anaerobic transition (AAT) represents the point during exercise at which maximal aerobic metabolism switches to rely mainly on anaerobic metabolism resulting in the subsequent accumulation of lactate.

Anaerobic threshold

Interest in the identification of an individual's AAT arose from a clinical rather than a sport-related concern for cardiac and cardiovascularly-compromised patients. It was thought that the AAT provided a sub-maximal method for the assessment of exercise capacity for cardiac patients. Since then, interest in the AAT has spread to a sports performance context. The AAT is traditionally identified using invasive blood lactate analysis techniques or through the use of non-invasive gas analysis. The gas analysis methods were originally developed in the 1960s for a clinical setting where non-invasive techniques for AAT might be preferred. The use of gas analysis to identify the AAT was originally termed the **anaerobic threshold** (*AnT*) by Wasserman and McIlroy (1964) but is sometimes referred to as the **ventilatory threshold**. Wasserman and McIlroy suggested that a breakaway in pulmonary ventilation equated with the rise in lactate accumulation associated with increasing anaerobic exercise. During exercise $\dot{V}_E$ initially rises linearly with increasing intensity; however, at a specific point for each individual a breakaway in ventilation occurs. This point was identified by Wasserman and McIlroy as the AnT and was said to coincide with the rise in CO_2 produced during blood lactate and H^+ buffering (introduced in Chapter 10). Thus, the AnT indicates non-invasively the point at which the body begins to accumulate lactate, i.e. the lactate threshold. Later research highlighted difficulties in the identification of the ventilatory breakpoint and consequently other aspects of gas kinetics were examined to assess their possibility as a more clearly defined marker of AnT. Currently, the most widely used non-invasive indicator of AnT is the combined

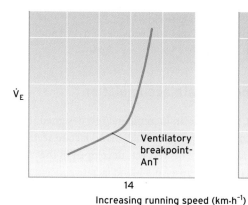
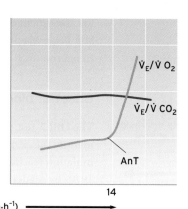

Figure 11.3 Markers of anaerobic threshold.

use of the ventilatory breakpoint and the ventilatory equivalents for oxygen and carbon dioxide ($\dot{V}_E/\dot{V}O_2$ and $\dot{V}_E/\dot{V}CO_2$, respectively). The $\dot{V}_E/\dot{V}O_2$ represents the ratio of air expired to oxygen consumed, while the $\dot{V}_E/\dot{V}CO_2$ is the ratio of expired air to carbon dioxide produced. Figure 11.3 provides an illustration of these AnT indicators, showing that the AnT occurs where there is an increase in $\dot{V}_E/\dot{V}O_2$ without a concomitant rise in $\dot{V}_E/\dot{V}CO_2$. In this example the AnT occurred at a treadmill running speed of 14 $km \cdot hr^{-1}$.

During assessment of the AAT for an athlete, the transition is now more commonly identified by the analysis of lactate kinetics due to a number of difficulties with the indirect assessment of AnT by gas exchange analysis. The ventilatory breakpoint, as already mentioned, is not always easy to identify which can make AnT detection problematic. Research has also indicated that patients with McArdle's disease (described in Chapter 14), who cannot produce lactate, still have a ventilatory breakpoint during incremental exercise, revealing a separation of LT and AnT. In addition, other research has shown a separation of AnT and lactate threshold (LT) which places limitations on the validity of non-invasive gas exchange assessment of the AAT. As a consequence, when a higher degree of accuracy is required for the assessment of AAT, the LT has more commonly been used to assess the transition from aerobic to increasingly anaerobic exercise.

The $\dot{V}O_{2max}$ test, which will be described in Chapter 12, has traditionally been the gold standard measure of aerobic endurance. It is now more common, however, for exercise physiologists to conduct an LT test and, more recently, critical power (CP) tests to assess aerobic endurance as it relates more closely to race performance. The point at which an athlete's LT or CP occurs is a more accurate predictor of race success than his or her $\dot{V}O_{2max}$ in aerobic endurance events such as 10 km running. In the next section we will move on to describe the LT, prior to introducing the concept of CP.

Lactate threshold

The assessment of LT is based on research that has shown that as an athlete increases their effort towards maximum, they make a transition towards increasingly anaerobic exercise, and lactate begins to accumulate in muscle fibres and blood. Lactate is produced continuously and removed during metabolism. At rest, and during lower-intensity exercise, lactate removal matches its synthesis and so blood lactate concentration remains relatively constant. As exercise intensity increases, such as during a $\dot{V}O_{2max}$ test or for the finish of a race, lactate is produced at a faster rate than it can be removed. As a consequence, lactate and H^+ begin to accumulate in the muscles and blood.

Key points

In aerobic endurance sports athletes attempt to race at an intensity level close to the point at which exercise shifts from being predominantly fueled by the aerobic system to being increasingly fueled by the anaerobic systems.

This point is known as the aerobic-anaerobic transition (AAT).

Key points

The concentration of lactate, which is constantly being produced within the body, is dependent upon the balance between its production and removal.

An increase in exercise intensity enhances fast-rate glycolysis, which results in a significant rise in lactate concentration as its removal is unable to match its production.

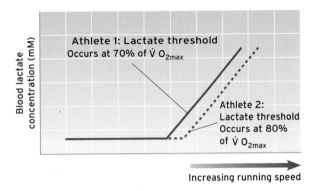

Figure 11.4 Lactate threshold occurring at different points for two athletes with the same $\dot{V}O_{2max}$.

The LT represents a level of work after which the body's lactate removal mechanisms cannot keep pace with the rate of lactate synthesis. When exercising at an intensity above the LT, lactate and H^+ accumulate in the blood and are, in part, thought to lead to fatigue. The higher the percentage of an athlete's $\dot{V}O_{2max}$ at which the lactate threshold occurs, the better for race performance. In other words, two 10 km runners with the same $\dot{V}O_{2max}$ but with differing LT (occurring at 80% and 70% of $\dot{V}O_{2max}$) would differ in race performance. The race winner would be the athlete who could run at the higher percentage of $\dot{V}O_{2max}$ before an increasingly heavy reliance on anaerobic metabolism. An illustration of this can be seen in Figure 11.4. Research indicates that an athlete's lactate threshold is a better predictor of his or her performance than $\dot{V}O_{2max}$ alone. In addition to exercise intensity, heart rate (HR) at the point at which LT occurs can be used as a basis for training programme development. The practical use of LT testing for the development of training programmes is discussed in a following section 'Practical use of AAT determination'.

Lactate-concentration-related measures of AAT

There is a wide variety of lactate-based measurements for the AAT including mathematical transformations of the data to identify the transition point more clearly. The assessments of AAT based on lactate analysis includes the onset of blood lactate accumulation (OBLA), lactate minimum speed, LT (as introduced in the previous section) and the maximal lactate steady state (MLSS). As the most common methods for lactate analysis of AAT are LT and MLSS, they are the focus of this section. However, a brief mention of OBLA is included as it is often linked with LT assessment. A more complete review of the variety of methods

for assessment of AAT was completed by Krista Svendahl and Brian MacIntosh in 2003 and provides a useful additional resource.

Onset of blood lactate accumulation

The OBLA test represents an incremental test designed to identify the exercise intensity at which blood lactate accumulation reaches 4 mM. This test was developed in the 1970s by Mader et al. because, at a blood lactate concentration of 4 mM, there appears to be a relationship between the lactate concentrations in the muscle and blood, which is not found as clearly above or below this concentration level. This test has been used quite widely; however, the assumption that a blood lactate concentration of 4 mM is synonymous with AAT ignores the wide individual variation in AAT. As a consequence, the use of LT or MLSS tests for AAT identification, and the monitoring of training induced changes, would be more beneficial for athlete populations.

Lactate threshold test protocol

The LT represents the point after which lactate begins to accumulate in the blood. The LT test, in common with OBLA and AnT, is conducted as an incremental test (most commonly 4-min stages). It can be conducted in the laboratory on a treadmill, cycle ergometer or rowing ergometer. In this situation, the starting intensity is dependent upon the athlete's current level of competition and training programme, that is, it is based on an estimation of the athlete's current fitness level. The increase in intensity during the test is easily achieved on the equipment in the laboratory. Blood lactate concentration, HR, and sometimes the rating of perceived exertion (RPE) (a psychological response to exercise), are measured at the end of each stage. The test is ended when a significant rise (> 4 mM) in lactate is observed.

The LT test can also be administered in the field. A set distance (rather than time), dependent upon the sport, is completed during each stage of the test. Suggested repetitions for the three major endurance sports are: swimming, 300 or 400 m; cycling, 3 or 4 km; running, 1 or 1.6 km (Hellemans, 2000). As with the starting intensity selected in the laboratory, the distance selected in the field is dependent on the athlete's fitness level. The more difficult aspect of lactate threshold testing in the field, compared with the laboratory, is the increase in intensity between test stages. A five-point subjective scale of exercise intensity is used by coaches of national athletes 1–easy, 2–steady, 3–moderately

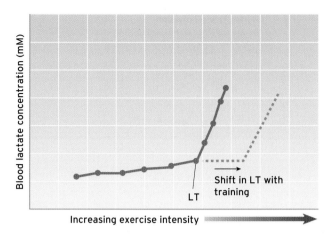

Figure 11.5 Lactate threshold curve and the rightwards shift following threshold training.

hard, 4–hard and 5–very hard. In relation to lactate threshold testing, the athlete would complete a repetition at each of these intensities, creating an incremental test. Similar to laboratory testing, blood lactate, HR and RPE are measured at the end of each stage.

> ## Key points
>
> Lactate threshold test:
>
> ➤ An incremental workload to identify AAT
> ➤ Can be performed in the laboratory or in the field

Figure 11.5 provides an illustration of a model lactate curve, along with representation of the effects of training on the lactate curve. Threshold training results in a shift of the lactate curve to the right, indicating that an athlete can, for example, run, cycle or row at a higher intensity before crossing the LT. This, in turn, leads to an improved performance in high-intensity endurance sports. Lactate samples are relatively easy to obtain, do not present great practical difficulties and represent an efficient method for AAT identification. The lactate threshold point appears to provide a valid and reliable marker of the AAT; however, this will be influenced by the quality of the protocol employed.

The identification of lactate threshold

A number of different protocols have been used to identify LT. These have included continuous and discontinuous test protocols with stages of varying duration and sampling periods. The duration of each increment, along with the increasing intensity of exercise, affects the identification of LT. Consequently, increments should be as small as

practically possible, with the duration for each step being around four minutes to enable blood lactate concentration to reflect the increment for that step. Sometimes it is beneficial during an initial athlete assessment to conduct the LT test twice, with smaller steps being made during the second test to identify more closely the exercise intensity at which LT occurs for that individual. An LT test should be conducted with specificity in mind, for example, on a treadmill for a runner.

The simplest way to identify the LT is by visual inspection of the lactate concentration data. As with the detection of AnT (ventilatory breakpoint) however, the LT can sometimes be hard to pinpoint by visual inspection. Because of this, a number of test protocols and mathematical approaches to LT identification have been developed to identify the LT more clearly. Three of these approaches are illustrated in Figure 11.6. Beaver and colleagues (1985) recommended the use of a logarithmic transformation of oxygen consumption and corresponding lactate data (*log-log transformation*). The *Dmax* method, developed by Cheng and co-workers (1992), involves the creation of a plot of oxygen consumption and lactate concentrations during an incremental test. As is illustrated in Figure 11.6, a general direction (GD) line is drawn between the first and last points on the plot. The LT represents the point at which the greatest distance (distance maximum or Dmax) occurs between the lactate- $\dot{V} O_2$ curve and the GD line. The *individual anaerobic threshold (IAT)* method involves a data collection period beyond the termination of exercise. The IAT test, proposed by Stegman and colleagues (1981), requires lactate samples to be collected post-exercise until, following the initial rise, blood lactate concentration returns to the level at maximal exercise (as can be seen in Figure 11.6). Having plotted the blood lactate data, the IAT is identified by drawing a tangent line from (a), the point at which lactate returned to the maximal exercise concentration to (b), the blood lactate curve. The tangent line is drawn as a straight line that just touches, but does not intersect, the lactate concentration data. The best LT method for the prediction of performance may depend on the sport and the duration of event.

> ## Key points
>
> Methods of lactate threshold identification:
>
> ➤ It can be identified visually or with mathematical transformation
> ➤ Mathematical approaches include: log-log transformation, the D-max method or the individual anaerobic threshold

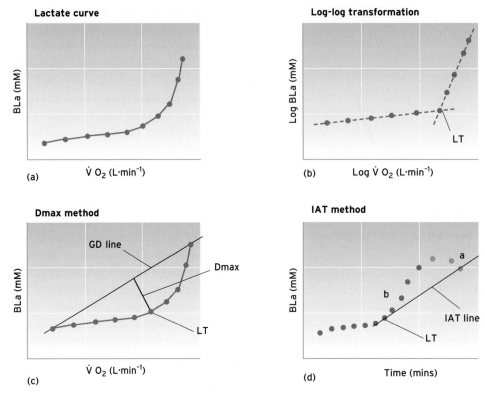

Figure 11.6 Illustration of the log-log transformation, Dmax and IAT methods for LT detection.

Maximal lactate steady state test (MLSS test)

An alternative approach to obtaining the AAT point through the use of lactate sampling is provided by the use of an MLSS test. The tests already described for ATT identification, AnT, OBLA and the various forms of LT, are based around the execution of an incremental test. The aerobic-anaerobic transition is identified through MLSS by use of a series of 30-minute constant-intensity tests. The MLSS exercise intensity is the maximum that can be maintained for a 30-minute period with a less than 1 mM change in lactate concentration during the last 20 minutes of the test. Although first developed in the 1980s, one of the most useful methods for the identification of MLSS was that proposed by Dekerle and colleagues (2003). The first stage in MLSS testing is for an athlete to complete a $\dot{V}O_{2max}$ test. The $\dot{V}O_{2max}$ test is required to calculate the work intensity for the MLSS which is completed on a different day. In the first MLSS assessment the athlete completes a T_{30} (MLSS 30 min) at an exercise intensity equivalent to 75% of $\dot{V}O_{2max}$. Blood lactate samples are collected at the start of testing and every five minutes until the last collection at the end of the 30th minute. On a separate day the athlete completes a second T_{30}, the intensity of which is determined by the result in the first test. If an

MLSS was reached or lactate concentration fell during the final 20 minutes of that test, the second test is completed at an exercise intensity 5% higher than in the first test. If the lactate concentration rose by more than 1 mM during the first test the exercise intensity is decreased by 5%. The T_{30} tests would need to be repeated, increasing or decreasing the exercise intensity until an MLSS was identified. The obvious disadvantage with this method relates to the time taken for testing, although this would probably decrease in future tests. Laplaud and colleagues (2006) developed a single incremental test to estimate MLSS. However, the mean 10 beats $\cdot$ min^{-1} HR differences between the incremental test and the constant-intensity test for MLSS determination may preclude its use with athletes. A 10 beats $\cdot$ min^{-1} difference in HR can represent a large difference when establishing training zones for athletes.

Practical use of AAT determination

As a high-intensity aerobic endurance athlete, whether a runner, cyclist, rower or cross-country skier, you aim to push yourself as hard as possible without straying too far into your anaerobic reserve. Knowledge of your AAT enables you to train at the most effective intensity to optimise training success and subsequent sporting performance.

The success behind using LT and MLSS as methods for the development of training programmes lies in their close correlation with performance in 30–60-minute races. Research indicates that both MLSS and LT can be used as better predictors of success in races over these durations than $\dot{V}O_{2max}$ test performance alone. It is not practical, nor desirable, for lactate samples to be collected regularly during training sessions. For this reason, the HR at which the AAT occurs is commonly used to maintain the correct exercise intensity when training just below, at, or just above the AAT. It may be that the AAT is identified at the start of a training phase, to help with programme design. Further AAT testing may then be used during, and upon completion of training, to monitor the success of, training and to identify the training-induced elevation in AAT.

Key points

The most commonly used methods to identify AAT are LT and MLSS.

A LT test is conducted using an incremental workload.

An MLSS test uses a constant workload through the duration of a test.

See 'Classic research summary on page 350.

Lactate threshold testing was the most commonly used method for the determination of training intensity in many endurance sports. Coaches of elite sport today, however, have adopted alternative methods to determine exercise training intensities. The main shift has been toward training with power or velocity, which is particularly relevant to the sports of cycling and swimming, respectively. The concept of critical power, and an overview of its measurement, is now discussed.

Critical power

The concept of critical power (CP) is not a new one, and dates back to the mid-1960s. At that time, the concept was suggested as a theoretical maximal exercise intensity that could be sustained for a period of time without fatigue. In the 1980s this concept was developed into a test that could be used in a sporting context. Conceptually, CP refers to an exercise intensity that is between the LT and $\dot{V}O_{2max}$, and approximately equivalent to MLSS. Exercise at an intensity that is at, or close to, an athlete's LT can be maintained for relatively long periods of time, e.g. for the completion of a marathon run. The maximal intensity required at the end of a $\dot{V}O_{2max}$ test, however, can be sustained for only a limited period of time. The exercise intensity for an MLSS tests can be sustained for 30 min and is consequently closely related to CP. Critical power was suggested as an exercise intensity above LT, but sustainable for a duration typically between 20–30 min. Figure 11.7 provides a representation of exercise intensity zones as they relate to the concepts of LT, MLSS and CP, such that LT and MLSS/CP represent the upper and lower limits of the heavy intensity exercise zone. The point at which MLSS and CP are achieved appears to represent a threshold above which exercise intensity becomes very heavy. It is important to note that while CP and MLSS have been shown here as occurring at the same time, research indicates that they are only approximately equal: in reality CP often occurs at an exercise intensity that is slightly above MLSS (approximately 5%).

Research has shown that CP is highly individual and generally occurs between 70–90% of $\dot{V}O_{2max}$. As a consequence, the power output or HR at CP for one person might represent the LT for another. Over time the concept

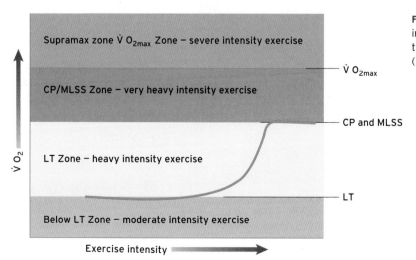

Figure 11.7 Conceptualisation of exercise intensity zones and their relation to lactate threshold (LT), maximal lactate steady state (MLSS) and critical power (CP).

of CP, and tests of CP, have been extended and applied to a wider number of sports including running, rowing and swimming. In running, CP has been found to have a correlation of r = −0.85 with 10 k running time and a r = −0.79 correlation with half marathon time. For cycling r = −0.71 and r = −0.91 correlations have been found between CP and 17 km and 40 km time trial performance. In swimming, where the concept has been converted to a critical velocity (CV), a correlation of r = 0.86 was found between CV and 400 m freestyle swim mean velocity. These findings show that, similar to LT and MLSS, CP is highly related to sports performance.

Figure 11.8 provides a theoretical example of results from a CP test displayed in three related panels which illustrate the relationship between power output, time to exhaustion (TTE) and work completed. When originally developed by Scherrer and Monod (1965), the authors

suggested that two key parameters could be calculated through critical power testing, both of which are illustrated in Figure 11.8. The first, CP, is the main focus of the test, while the second parameter is the anaerobic work capacity (AWC or W'). The anaerobic work capacity is illustrated in Figure 11.8a by the shaded area W'. While CP (also shown in Figure 11.8a) represents the maximal power attainable for a sustained period of time, the AWC represents a finite store of energy available at the start of exercise from anaerobic sources.

Critical power can be determined by anywhere between 2 and 10 exhaustive exercise trials depending on the protocol being used. Typically, the exercise intensity (power) for each trial is set such that exhaustion is reached between 1 and 30 min. In this example the exercise intensity was set at 450, 300, 250 and 225 W. The time to exhaustion for these examples was 90, 180, 300 and 420 s respectively which

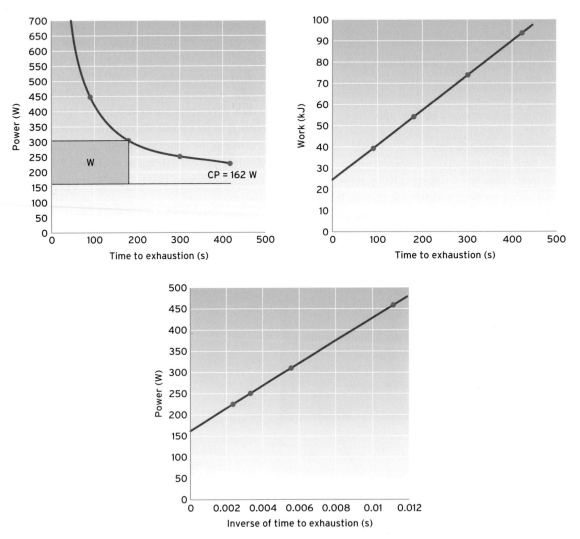

Figure 11.8 Figures depicting the nature of critical power in relation to power, work and time to exhaustion.

gave rise to the plot in Figure 11.8a. The CP for the athlete in this model was calculated at 162 W (details of how to calculate CP are provided below). As can be seen from Figure 11.8a, when the power output is plotted against the time to exhaustion we see the characteristic hyperbolic curve that is typical of the decline in power with increasing duration of exercise (refer to Figure 8.1 in Chapter 8). The higher the power output required the shorter the time period for which the output can be maintained. As shown in Figure 11.8a the line representing CP acts as an asymptote to the power curve, such that the distance between the power curve and CP approaches zero as the lines trend towards infinity. In this way, in line with the classical model developed by Scherrer and Monod (1965), CP represents an exercise intensity that can be sustained for a relatively long theoretically infinite period of time.

In the example (Figure 11.8), four exercise trials have been illustrated and when work completed (W') and power are plotted against time to exhaustion and the inverse of time to exhaustion, the linear relationship between these parameters is revealed. The longer the time to fatigue the greater work is completed (panel b) and the greater the power output required, the shorter the duration of time to exhaustion (remember that for mathematical reasons time is inversed in panel c). The work limit (W_{lim}) for a test is calculated by multiplying the power output (P) by the time limit (T_{lim} – the time for which work can be sustained before exhaustion) in the following equation:

$$W_{lim} = P \times T_{lim}$$

The simplicity of CP testing (very little equipment is required and the test does not require invasive techniques such as lactate sampling) and its relationship with MLSS and performance make this test a useful one for athletes. There are a number of sport-specific protocols that can be used to establish an athlete's CP. Such protocols vary but can be complex and time-consuming depending on the accuracy required; however, a straightforward laboratory method for calculating CP can be completed using a cycle ergometer equipped with power measurement and a stopwatch. Results are then generated with the use of statistical software.

A typical protocol involves three tests to exhaustion, ideally on separate days; however, these can be completed on the same day with suitable rest between each effort. After a 5-min warm-up the athlete should complete a constant cadence and intensity ride to exhaustion. Exhaustion would be defined as when the cadence cannot be maintained within 5 rev·min^{-1} for a period of over 5 s. The intensity for each of the tests should be set such that

Table 11.1 Suggested power outputs (W) for critical power testing using a cycle ergometer.

Fitness estimation	~10 min duration	~6 min	~1 min
Average level	170	195	220
Competitive sport player	230	265	300
Endurance athlete	300	345	390
Higher level endurance athlete	370	425	450

(*Source*: Adapted from School of Sport and Health Sciences, University of Exeter)

ideally, exhaustion is reached within 1, 6 and 10 min respectively for each test. Table 11.1 provides suggested power outputs to reach exhaustion within these timelines for individuals of differing fitness levels.

Table 11.2 provides an illustration of a dataset collected from a 13-year-old male where, due to his young age, the work intensities were set at 140, 147 and 170 W. Once the test was completed the power outputs and time to exhaustion (TTE) were used to display the results on a plot

Table 11.2 Example data for a CP test of a 13-year-old male participant.

P 1 (W)	140
P 2 (W)	147
P 3 (W)	170
TTE 1 (s)	429
TTE 2 (s)	332
TTE 3 (s)	159
1/t 1 (s)	0.002331
1/t 2 (s)	0.003012
1/t 3 (s)	0.006289
CP (W)	123.635
AWC (J)	7401.392
R^2	0.996

Note: When using Statistical Package for the Social Sciences (SPSS), after running the regression model, CP is found from the constant value which and AWC from the predictor constant. R^2 is provided here so that when using this data set as a test model the model can be checked for accuracy. R^2 relates to the meaningfulness of the relationship between the variables. An $R^2 = 0.996$ indicates that was a meaningful relationship between the variables TTE and Power – which is shown very clearly in the linear relationship revealed in Figure 11.9.

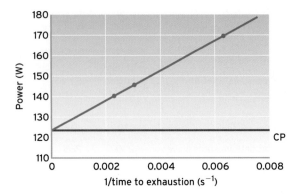

Figure 11.9 Example figure of CP using the data from Table 11.2.

(Figure 11.9) and then a statistical package such as Excel or Statistical Package for the Social Sciences (SPSS) could be used to calculate the participants CP. To complete the plot firstly the inverse of time would need to be calculated (1 – t [s]). From this data, a plot such as that shown in Figure 11.9 could be created. The CP was then calculated by running a regression equation, where power (W) was the dependent variable and inverse of time (1/t or 1–t as above) was the independent variable. As can be seen from Table 11.2, the calculated CP for the participant was 124 W and the AWC was 7401 J or 7.4 kJ.

Through determination of CP, an athlete or coach is provided with an individualised parameter that can be used to determine training intensities. Research indicates that CP can be used as a viable alternative to HR and lactate-designed programmes. Once CP intensity is known, for instance in (W) for a cyclist, this can be used to design training sessions that are at, above or below CP. There would be no need to measure lactate response to exercise or to wear a HR monitor during training, when a programme was designed from CP data.

Key points

Critical power:

➤ is commonly used for the determination of training zones for elite athletes

➤ is the maximal exercise intensity that can be sustained over a set period of time

➤ generally occurs between 70–90% $\dot{V}\,O_{2max}$

Knowledge integration question

What are the similarities and differences between the LT, MLSS and CP tests?

11.2 The physiology of high-intensity aerobic endurance sports

The physiology of high-intensity aerobic endurance sports is closely related to the transition between aerobic and anaerobic metabolism. As such, an understanding of the concepts of LT, AnT and CP is important when considering them. The primary macronutrient for energy supply in these sports is carbohydrate in the form of glucose or glycogen. This has implications for glycogen storage, the enhancement of which is discussed in the next section: ergogenic aids for high-intensity aerobic endurance sports.

Firstly, this section discusses steady-state exercise, cardiovascular drift, exercise economy and oxygen debt as they all are important physiological concepts that relate, in particular, to aerobic endurance exercise. Following this we move on to discuss conditioning training, probable causes of fatigue and adaptations to training.

Steady-state exercise

In Chapters 9 and 10 the focus was upon anaerobic sports of short duration and high intensity during which a steady-state exercise level would not be achieved. Many of the sports that are the focus of this chapter and Chapter 12 enable a steady state to be achieved due to their sub-maximal exercise levels and longer duration. A *steady-state* exercise level is illustrated in Figure 11.10, and occurs when the energy supply for exercise meets the energy demands. At the start of exercise, respiration, heart rate and oxygen consumption rise to meet the body's energy requirements. If an athlete exercises against a constant and sub-maximal workload, the heart rate and oxygen consumption will begin to plateau and after 3–4 minutes, a steady state will be reached (the nature of the steady-state plateau is an essential part of the Åstrand-Åstrand aerobic capacity test which is described in Chapter 12).

Figure 11.10 shows the plateau associated with steady state for three exercise intensities or workloads. As illustrated, the time to reach steady state increases as workload is increased and takes around 4 minutes in response to an initial workload. If the workload is subsequently increased the athlete will require a shorter time, of around 1–2 minutes to reach steady state for the second workload.

When exercise intensity or workload is increased above a critical level for any athlete he or she will not be able to attain a steady state for heart rate, oxygen consumption or respiration. This critical level is closely related to the concepts of MLSS and CP which were

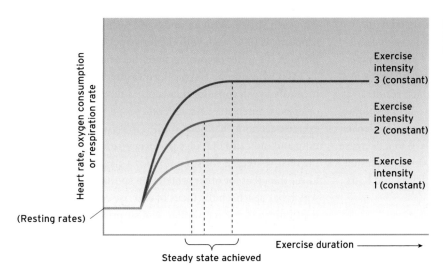

Figure 11.10 Steady-state exercise heart rate, respiration rate and oxygen consumption plateau.

described in the previous section. In effect, these concepts relate to a **steady-state$_{max}$** (SS$_{max}$), that is, a maximal intensity of exercise that can be sustained for a period of time. Although MLSS and CP were conceptualised as unique physiological measurements, research suggests the exercise intensities at which MLSS and CP are reached are similar. While during a CP test, given the exercise to exhaustion nature of the test, it is not appropriate to measure lactate concentration, the exercise intensity (power output) an athlete could maintain during an MLSS test would be closely related to his or her calculated CP or SS$_{max}$. Exercise intensity (demand) is related to physiological response (HR, lactate accumulation, etc.) and consequently, both CP and MLSS relate to a notion of a SS$_{max}$.

The research interest in the AAT and SS$_{max}$ should not be surprising, given that both constructs are important functional aspects of high-intensity aerobic endurance performance. Race performance is certainly correlated with MLSS, CP, the AAT and SS$_{max}$. Research also indicates that individuals who train for a specific aerobic endurance sport reach steady state for any given exercise intensity more quickly than sedentary individuals, and can exercise against heavier workloads before crossing the threshold above which steady state cannot be achieved. Improved aerobic capacity, demonstrated through increases in the number of mitochondria, development of capillaries and enzyme functioning, are responsible for the improved steady-state capacity.

Cardiovascular drift

An interesting response to prolonged, steady-state exercise is that of **cardiovascular drift**. This is associated with

long-duration exercise and/or exercise in a hot environment. Figure 11.11 provides an illustration of cardiovascular drift.

Recalling from Chapter 6, cardiac output ($\dot{Q}$) is the resultant of stroke volume (the blood volume ejected from the heart in one beat) and heart rate (the number of times per minute the heart beats). The rise in heart rate associated with cardiovascular drift is thought to be caused by a drop in stroke volume which is associated with prolonged exercise or exercise in the heat. To maintain $\dot{Q}$ for a particular steady-state exercise intensity, heart rate must rise if the stroke volume drops. The drop in stroke volume is thought to occur for a number of reasons, all or some of which could occur during exercise. The upright body position during most aerobic endurance sports, for example running, kayaking and cycling, means that venous return must compete against gravity. It is thought that during exercise at a constant workload there is a progressive decrease in venous return which in turn leads to a decrease in stroke volume and necessitates a rise in heart rate. The

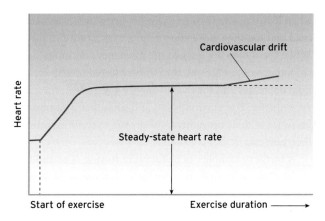

Figure 11.11 Illustration of cardiovascular drift.

rise in body temperature and sweating associated with exercise are also thought to contribute to a decrease in stroke volume during prolonged exercise. As body temperature rises during prolonged exercise or exercise in the heat blood is diverted to the skin for cooling, which results in a decreased venous return and, consequently, stroke volume. This situation can be further exacerbated by the incidence of water loss through sweating which can lead to a decrease in blood volume and hence venous return through plasma removal to help maintain tissue hydration levels and body core temperature during exercise.

Key points

Cardiovascular drift:

➤ rise in exercise HR that is not attributed to increased exercise intensity

➤ associated with long-duration exercise or exercise in a hot environment

➤ occurs when blood flow is diverted to the skin to aid heat loss resulting in decreased SV and increased HR to maintain $\dot{Q}$

Exercise economy

Exercise economy relates to the energy demands of a given workload for any individual athlete. The relative efficiency of an athlete will have a significant impact on his or her response to a given workload. Exercise economy provides the interaction point between physiology and the skilful aspects of performance in sport. An example of efficiency can be found in rock climbing. When comparing climbers of different abilities the more skilful climber tends to be more efficient and smoother in their movements. Each movement and grasp of a new hold requires less effort and fewer muscle fibres to grip the hold. In a similar way, when learning a new route a climber grips tighter to each hold and requires more effort to make each movement. When the moves are learned the movement becomes smoother, more efficient, the effort required to grip each hold decreases and the overall energy demands of the climb are reduced. The more efficient and smoother a climber becomes in their movement, the greater exercise economy they possess.

A further example can be found in rowing. The ability of the same individual to move through the water at a set speed is influenced not only by their physiological ability, but many other factors such as the angle of the blade entry and exit, the duration of the stroke, and body movement with each stroke. With an optimised technique, exercise economy is improved, with the movement of the boat through the water becoming smoother and more efficient.

Exercise economy is typically measured by the assessment of oxygen consumption across a range of workloads or exercise intensities. As with other aspects of physiology, exercise economy has been studied most with regard to running and indicates that race performance is improved when the relative oxygen consumption for a given workload is lower than that for other athletes. In sports like swimming, which has also been the focus of exercise economy research, the findings have been similar. Not surprisingly, higher level swimmers were more efficient than less skilful swimmers who spent more time and energy maintaining a horizontal body position in the water. The results from swimming have application to other more technical aerobic endurance sports such as rowing, kayaking and cross-country skiing for they stress the importance of the skilful aspects of the sport. In sprint kayaking for example the interaction between the paddler's physiology, their boat awareness, feel for the water and use of the blade are critical for performance. The development of technical aspects alongside improved physiological performance are essential for exercise economy. Research indicates that if you improve exercise economy you delay fatigue and improve performance.

Key point

The more economical you are the lower the relative energy demand at any given exercise intensity level.

Oxygen deficit and Excess Post-exercise Oxygen Consumption (EPOC)

When we start to exercise there is an immediate rise in the body's demand for oxygen, which results in an increase in heart rate and breathing frequency to match oxygen delivery to the exercise requirements. As has been described, it takes time for the supply of oxygen to the active muscles and aerobic metabolism to meet the demands of exercise and therefore to reach a steady state during sub-maximal exercise. This delay in the rise of aerobic metabolism and oxygen consumption at the start of exercise, first identified by Archibald Hill and Hartley Lupton in 1922, creates what they termed an **oxygen deficit**. The maximal accumulated oxygen deficit (MAOD) test described in Chapter 10 represents a measure of oxygen deficit. The higher the exercise intensity the longer it takes for the body to reach steady state and the larger the oxygen deficit incurred.

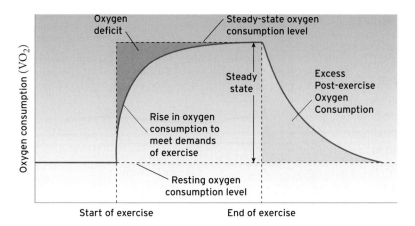

Figure 11.12 Oxygen deficit and excess post-excercise oxygen consumption.

Figure 11.12 demonstrates that oxygen consumption (shown in red) does not rise immediately to meet the demands of the steady-state exercise and as such a deficit (shown in yellow) is incurred. This deficit is repaid post-exercise.

When exercise ceases and the additional oxygen for exercise is no longer required, oxygen consumption should theoretically immediately return to resting levels. As can be seen from Figure 11.12 this is not the case. Oxygen consumption, and indeed heart rate and ventilation rate remain elevated post-exercise. George Brooks and colleagues (1971) termed the post-exercise elevation in oxygen consumption the **excess post-exercise oxygen consumption** (EPOC). The EPOC is also commonly referred to as the **oxygen debt**. The longer the duration and the higher the intensity of the exercise, the longer it takes for oxygen consumption to return to resting levels. The EPOC associated with completion of a 100 m race will be smaller that that after a 500 m kayak sprint or fell race and therefore will repaid in a shorter time.

The exact nature of the mechanisms behind the EPOC associated with exercise is not known; however, research has indicated that there are a number of likely reasons behind the slow return of oxygen consumption to resting levels. A major reason behind the elevated levels of oxygen consumption (above resting levels) is to repay the oxygen deficit incurred at the start of exercise. Oxygen stores in the blood and myoglobin are depleted during the start of exercise and the EPOC is thought, in part, to be associated with restoring oxygen stores. The longer the duration of exercise and the higher the intensity, the greater is the rise in body temperature associated with the increased metabolism. High-intensity aerobic endurance exercise, such as that encountered during a marathon, can raise the body temperature by around 3°C. This rise in body temperature post-exercise causes an increase in metabolic rate which in turns requires an increased level of oxygen consumption.

As the temperature drops over time, post-exercise oxygen consumption also drops. It is believed that a further part of EPOC is associated with the removal of CO_2 and the conversion of lactate to glycogen. As was described in Chapter 8, the onset of exercise causes the release of adrenaline and noradrenaline which serve to stimulate an increase in metabolism. These sympathetic nervous system hormones are not immediately removed from the blood and continue to stimulate metabolism, and consequently oxygen consumption, prior to their removal. It is likely that the EPOC is also related to tissue repair and the re-sequestering of Ca^{2+}, K^+ and Na^+ ions to their non-exercising compartments within muscle fibres. Further research is ongoing in this interesting area of physiology; however, it appears there are a number of mechanisms behind the continued elevation of oxygen consumption post-exercise.

Knowledge integration question

Upon cessation of exercise we can feel that HR and ventilation remain elevated. What are the likely reasons for this and how do exercise intensity and duration affect the rate of recovery?

Key points

The commencement of exercise results in:

➤ an immediate rise in muscle demand for oxygen = increased HR and V_E

➤ a time delay to match oxygen supply to demand (i.e. to reach steady-state exercise) is the oxygen deficit

Oxygen deficit is an important factor in the increased O_2 consumption after exercise – known as the excess post-exercise oxygen consumption (EPOC) or oxygen debt.

Conditioning for aerobic endurance sports

Due to the wide variation in intensity and duration that can be found in aerobic sports, the physiology of these sports is covered in two chapters (this chapter and Chapter 12). There would consequently be overlaps in the training methods covered if conditioning was considered in both chapters. To avoid such overlap, aspects of conditioning training for competitive aerobic sports are covered in this chapter, while in Chapter 14 we will consider exercise prescription for health.

In Chapter 8 a brief outline of general aspects for conditioning training was provided. Table 8.5 provides an overview of a number of different forms of training that could be considered for any athlete. An aerobic athlete might use all of these forms of training depending on the duration and intensity of the sport in which he or she takes part. There is, however, a much greater range of training methods that could be employed by a coach or an athlete which would be beneficial to aerobic endurance performance. Some of these are illustrated for marathon kayaking in Anna Hemmings' Sport in Action piece (p. 348). In this section we will consider a number of types of conditioning training that could form the basis for an aerobic endurance athlete's programme.

In making decisions about the types of training to include it is very important that attention is paid to the principle of sport specificity. Clearly, following this principle of training (which was outlined in Chapter 8), a conditioning programme for a runner should be based around running whereas that for a triathlete would need to include all three disciplines; swimming, cycling and running. Additionally, however, choices for a training programme should be specific to the intensity and duration of the sport.

Training intensity

Regular physiological testing can help with the design of a sport specific training programme. As was outlined in Chapter 8, HR monitors can be used to set and check the intensity of training for any particular session. Such intensities could be set from two possible starting points and careful consideration should be paid to which is more appropriate for use with a particular athlete. A test, such as a $\dot{V}O_{2max}$ (which will be described in more detail in Chapter 12), could be used to identify an athlete's HR_{max}. Once this is determined it is possible to specify the intensity of training session relative to his or her HR_{max}. This method was used to identify the intensity of training

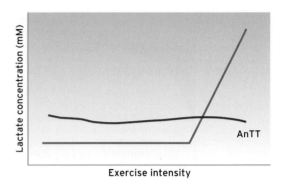

Figure 11.13 Illustration of Bompa's anaerobic threshold training, where lactate concentrations are likely to be between 4 mM and 6 mM.

for types of conditioning training shown in Table 8.5. Increasingly, however, the results of LT, MLSS and CP tests have been used to prescribe the intensity of training for aerobic endurance athletes. An athlete's HR response for one of these given measures can be used to prescribe the intensity of sessions, with sessions differentially designed to be below, at or above the HR at LT, MLSS or CP. The choice of which of these measures would be most beneficial for an athlete would be based upon the duration of the sport and the type of sport itself. Training based around the HR at LT has most commonly been used in running, whereas CP has been used as the basis for exercise prescription in cycling and swimming (where the parameter critical velocity is used). An illustration of training based around LT, using the terminology developed by Bompa, can be seen from Figure 11.13.

Anaerobic threshold/pace-tempo training

As can be seen from Figure 11.13, anaerobic threshold training (AnTT) refers to training that is just above LT. Very similar in concept to (race) pace-tempo training, the idea with such training is to increase the speed at which LT occurs and to improve running economy. Depending on the duration of the event or sport an athlete is training for, LT will be close to race pace for an athlete. Pace-tempo training, as the name suggests, is designed to improve race pace by working at a tempo just above normal race pace. Bompa suggested that repetitions for AnTT might vary between 90s –1 hr depending on the duration of the competition event, and the tempo is relative to race pace for the repetition or session. Research suggests that AnTT or pace-tempo training will enhance both aerobic and anaerobic metabolism, making this form of training particularly useful for high-intensity aerobic endurance sports.

Fartlek training

As for anaerobic endurance athletes, interval sessions provide an incredibly versatile form of training for aerobic endurance athletes. As is shown in Table 8.5, the intensity and duration of the work phases, along with the number of repetitions, sets and length of recoveries can be manipulated to meet specific training goals. As such, interval sessions should provide an integral part of any aerobic athlete's training programme. Additionally, fartlek and long slow distance (LSD) sessions, also illustrated in Table 8.5, are beneficial forms of training for aerobic endurance athletes.

The word *fartlek* is a Swedish word meaning *speedplay* and relates to a form of continuous training in which the intensity of exercise is varied throughout the effort. Fartlek training has mainly been associated with running; however, it can have application to other sports. In middle distance running, Kenyan athletes have become famous for changing the pace of a race throughout its duration such as applying a surge in race pace followed by a drop in pace. This race strategy has enhanced fatigue for athletes not used to this type of pace change; however, fartlek training can help to alleviate the fatiguing effects of race pace changes. An example of a 35-min fartlek session might include 3 exercise intensities (individually devised, but based around high-, moderate- and low-intensity efforts) with efforts at each intensity lasting for varying duration (1–5 min).

Long slow distance training

Long, slow, distance training, which should be carried out at an exercise intensity between 50–70% of HR_{max}, has a number of potential benefits for athletes. This form of training can lead to improved oxidative capacity and thermoregulation as well as facilitating a sparing of glycogen. It is worth noting that, because this form of training is by definition below race pace, there should not be an over-reliance on LSD as this might negatively affect exercise economy.

Strength training

An overview of strength training can be found in Chapter 9 and a well balanced training programme for an aerobic endurance athlete should include both strength and conditioning training. Although not always considered for aerobic endurance athletes, strength training has been shown to provide a number of benefits to performance. Strength training is thought to benefit aerobic endurance athletes by reducing muscle imbalances and assisting with recovery from injury. In addition, strength training can serve to improve hill climbing and the 'kick' during a race.

Key points

Conditioning for aerobic endurance events should include:

➤ anaerobic threshold training – to increase speed at which LT occurs and to improve exercise economy

➤ fartlek training – to increase ability to cope with changes in race pace

➤ long slow distance training – to improve oxidative capacity and thermoregulation

➤ strength training – to reduce muscle imbalances and aid recovery from injury

---

Fatigue in high-intensity aerobic endurance sports

Short-duration events

The mechanisms for fatigue in high-intensity aerobic endurance sports relate to the duration of the event. For endurance sports, those on the left of the duration continuum (Figure 11.2), a number of possible contributors to fatigue have been postulated. Fatigue in sports, such as rowing and cycling (3,000 and 4,000 m pursuit), is closely linked with anaerobic endurance fatigue. The most commonly reported mechanism for fatigue is the increasing acidosis, associated with increasing H^+, as a consequence of an extended reliance on fast-rate glycolysis due to the high intensity of effort. More recently, however, Pi and K^+ have been implicated as possible alternatives or contributory explanations of fatigue. The possible mechanisms, along with current thinking about the role of decreasing pH in fatigue, were described in Chapter 10, but have clear implications for performance in shorter-duration aerobic sports that are the focus of this chapter.

Long-duration events

As the duration of aerobic endurance sports increases the relative intensity falls (see Figure 11.1), with glycogen depletion increasingly becoming the major mechanism behind fatigue. Glycogen stores in the muscles and liver are the major substrate for ATP regeneration, particularly during high-intensity aerobic endurance sports. It is likely that the intensity and duration of these sports is such that, past a critical point, glycogen stores become depleting to fatigue. Research indicates that during running, glycogen stores are used 40 times faster than while walking. It is for this reason that glycogen stores can be sufficient to provide the energy for a day walking in the hills but can be depleted before the completion of a marathon. Glycogen depletion leads to an increased reliance on fat metabolism and a consequential decrease in race pace and has also been associated with an increase in central fatigue. Within fatigue research two aspects of this phenomenon have been identified: peripheral and central fatigue. In Chapters 9 and 10 the focus of discussion in relation to fatigue has been on the periphery, i.e. fatigue within the muscles. Central fatigue, most often associated with longer-duration sports, relates to the feelings of fatigue associated with high-intensity performance. Research indicates that athletes report increased perceptions of fatigue when continuing to exercise in a glycogen depleted state. The feeling of 'hitting the wall' in a marathon (often at around 18–22 miles) can largely be attributed to glycogen depletion. There are a number of studies that indicate that carbohydrate loading before exercise, and glucose intake during exercise, can decrease the likelihood of, or at least delay, glycogen depletion. Strategies of delaying or avoiding glycogen depletion are discussed in the section on ergogenic aids.

Key points

Fatigue during high-intensity aerobic endurance sports:

➤ short-duration events – associated with fall in pH, further potential contributing factors include increased Pi and K+

➤ longer-duration events – glycogen depletion becomes a major mechanism of fatigue

While discussing feelings of fatigue and ways of delaying it, it is also interesting to consider the effects of three hormones released during longer-duration exercise. During aerobic endurance sports (also covered in Chapter 12) the hormones **aldosterone** and **anti-diuretic hormone** are secreted by the adrenal cortex and the pituitary gland respectively, to stimulate Na^+ and water reabsorption from the kidneys and so help maintain hydration. As the duration of exercise progresses **endorphins** are released into the bloodstream which help to block the feelings of pain associated with exercise and to promote the feelings of well-being associated with exercise. Each of these endocrine responses serves to delay the effects of fatigue during high-intensity aerobic endurance sports.

Knowledge integration question

How does the duration of an aerobic endurance event relate to the mechanism of fatigue? How can fatigue be delayed in such sports?

Physiological adaptations to aerobic endurance training

The completion of an aerobic training programme, based on the conditioning training methods described above, will lead to a variety of physiological adaptations in response to the training stress. This section describes the key adaptations that occur in response to aerobic training and so provide the basis for improvement in performance for any of the sports in this chapter or the lower-intensity sports covered in Chapter 12. The adaptations to aerobic training include alterations in cardiac, respiratory, muscular and metabolic function.

Aerobic power adaptation

The most obvious response to aerobic training is an improvement in aerobic power ($\dot{V}O_{2max}$) which results in an increased ability to maintain a higher intensity and duration of exercise. The intensity, duration, type and specificity of training will all influence the extent of any physiological adaptation. The extent to which adaptation occurs will also be dependent upon the individual's previous training and their individual response to the training stimulus. For instance, improvements in $\dot{V}O_{2max}$ have been shown to occur primarily within the first 6–12 months of training. After this time, improvements in performance tend to be related to improvements in their LT and exercise economy. Consequently, if an individual is new to aerobic training their improvement in $\dot{V}O_{2max}$ will be significantly greater than that for an experienced athlete. Nevertheless, through training, experienced athletes can still continue to improve their performance. Individuals respond differently to any training stimulus and therefore coaches, or the athletes themselves, need to monitor the response to training and alter the programme if the desired results are not being realised.

Key point

Aerobic training improves aerobic power, primarily within the first 6–12 months of training.

Adaptations of skeletal muscle fibres

Muscle fibre size and type

In Chapter 6 the properties of different muscle fibre types were described in detail. During aerobic activities type I fibres are primarily recruited for exercise. In response to aerobic training type I fibres tend to decrease slightly in size. At first this might seem contrary to logic; however, during aerobic training type I fibres are not required to produce maximal forces, but to complete repeated lower-intensity contractions. As was described in Chapter 9, strength training is associated with hypertrophy (increase in muscle fibre size). Consequently, aerobic endurance athletes should undertake a strength training programme, to maintain muscle strength and size, in conjunction with aerobic training. By combining strength and aerobic training an athlete can maintain muscle size and strength, along with making aerobic gains.

The protein degradation within muscle fibres in response to aerobic training is thought to arise from changes in the production of the hormones cortisol and testosterone. In response to aerobic training, levels of cortisol tend to increase. Cortisol has been shown to be associated with protein degradation in type I muscle fibres. In contrast to this, plasma levels of testosterone, an anabolic hormone (stimulates protein synthesis) tend to fall in response to aerobic training. Together, these hormonal changes combine to create a predominantly catabolic environment within type I muscle fibres.

In addition to the reduced size of type I muscle fibres, research findings indicate there are also changes in the properties of type II fibres. In response to aerobic training, type IIx fibres alter their structure and functioning to that of type IIa fibres and, similarly, type IIa shift towards the properties of type I fibres. These adaptations of type II fibres enhance their oxidative capacity, particularly in response to high-intensity aerobic endurance exercise. Training-induced changes in the metabolism of type I muscle fibres are discussed below.

Key points

Muscle fibre type adaptations to aerobic endurance training:

➤ diameter of type I muscle fibres falls – increased cortisol and decreased testosterone promote a catabolic environment

➤ strength training should be included in programmes to maintain muscle strength and size

Muscle fibre structure and metabolism

Although aerobic training results in a decrease in the size of type I muscle fibres there are a number of structural changes within these fibres that promote increases in aerobic endurance performance. In response to aerobic training there is an increase in the oxidative capabilities of type I muscle fibres. Endurance training brings about increases in the capillary density, myoglobin concentration, mitochondrial size, number and function, which together serve to improve the aerobic capability of the trained fibres. The number of capillaries surrounding each muscle fibre can increase by 10–15% through training, thereby enhancing the amount of oxygen available for active muscle fibres. In addition, more oxygen can be stored due to an increase in myoglobin concentration within type I muscle fibres. Myoglobin concentration has been shown to increase by as much as 75–80% above pre-training levels.

Further to these improvements in oxygen delivery and storage, aerobic metabolism is also improved through changes in mitochondria. These are the site of oxidative phosphorylation within muscle fibres and have been shown to increase by up to 35% in size and 15% in number in response to aerobic training. Further to this, their increased efficiency has been demonstrated to be due to greater enzyme activity. As an example, the Krebs cycle enzymes *citrate synthase and succinate dehydrogenase* (SDH) increase their activity in response to endurance training (the Krebs cycle is described in detail in Chapter 12). Interestingly, the intensity of training appears to dictate the degree to which SDH activity is increased; higher-intensity training promotes a greater increase in SDH activity compared to lower-intensity aerobic training.

In addition to increases in enzyme activity within the Krebs cycle, the enzymes involved in β-oxidation (the start of lipid catabolism: refer to Chapter 12) respond to aerobic training. The resultant increases in enzyme activity for fatty acid metabolism can be as much as 25% (or even higher) and have a glycogen-sparing effect. In addition, the muscles can store greater amounts of triglyceride which creates an increased lipid pool immediately available for β oxidation and fatty acid oxidation. Training has been shown to more than double the resting muscle triglyceride stores. These changes result in a decrease in RER values for a given work intensity. A decrease in RER during aerobic endurance exercise provides evidence of the shift towards fat oxidation as a consequence of aerobic training. It is thought that the shift to fat oxidation is accompanied by a decreased response of the sympathetic nervous system (SNS) to exercise. At the start of exercise the SNS, through the release of the hormones adrenaline and noradrenaline, increases metabolism and the body's reliance on glycogen as a fuel source. As a result of training the SNS response to exercise is blunted, decreasing the emphasis on carbohydrate as the main fuel source.

As well as improvements in fatty acid storage and oxidation, aerobic training appears to result in increases in glycogen synthesis and storage. Aerobic training appears to trigger an improved insulin response, leading to an increased uptake of glucose by muscles. The enhancement in glycogen storage brought about through this mechanism has been demonstrated to lead to improved aerobic endurance performance and to result in a delayed onset of fatigue. Glycogen sparing also appears to be enhanced through a training-induced improvement in mitochondrial functioning which serves to slow glycogen oxidation and decrease lactate production.

Knowledge integration question

What training-induced adaptations contribute toward the increased reliance on fat oxidation by the muscles?

Key points

Type I muscle fibres show:

➤ increased capillary network – enhanced oxygen availability

➤ mitochondrial adaptations: increased, number, size, and function (increased aerobic enzyme activity) = improved oxygen storage and aerobic metabolism

➤ increased triglyceride storage

➤ increased metabolism of fat has a glycogen-sparing effect

➤ improved insulin response increases muscular glucose uptake and glycogen storage

Combined, these adaptations result in an improved aerobic endurance performance.

Cardiovascular changes with training

Aerobic training results in a lower resting heart rate and a decreased heart rate response to exercise (maximal HR is normally little altered in response to training). The mean resting heart rate for a sedentary individual is about $72 \text{ bts} \cdot \text{min}^{-1}$. As a result of aerobic training the resting heart rate can fall below $50 \text{ bts} \cdot \text{min}^{-1}$. Despite a lower resting and sub-maximal heart rate response, an athlete's $\dot{Q}$ (the resultant of heart rate and stroke volume) has been shown to increase in response to endurance training. The increase in $\dot{Q}$ is brought about through improvements in stroke volume. Aerobic training results in the heart increasing in size, causing an increase in the volume of blood ejected from the left ventricle with each contraction.

Training-induced LT adaptations

In sustained endurance training one of the key adaptations is an improvement in LT. In an AAT test, improvements in LT can be found by a shift to the right of the lactate curve as is illustrated in Figure 11.5. Aerobic training results in improvements in LT, conversely, research indicates that the most effective way to improve oxidative functioning is to train at or just above the exercise intensity at which LT or AAT occurs. Improvements in LT have been found to be specific to the exercise mode. Running training results in a greater shift in the point at which LT occurs in a treadmill test compared to a cycling test. Consequently, LT test apparatus should as far as possible match the demands of the sport.

Key points

Aerobic endurance training results in:

➤ variety of cardiovascular, respiratory and muscular (structural and metabolic) adaptations

➤ initially, $\dot{V}O_{2max}$ improved, subsequently LT and exercise economy improved

➤ all adaptations have a positive impact on aerobic endurance performance

11.3 Ergogenic aids for high-intensity aerobic endurance sports

Beyond a healthy balanced diet, the key legal manipulation that could be beneficial to high-intensity aerobic endurance performance is carbohydrate loading. Certainly for longer-duration sports such as marathon running, where glycogen depletion represents a significant possible cause of fatigue, the employment of a glycogen loading strategy and the use of in-race carbohydrate feeding can help to maintain performance. As a consequence, this section begins with a review of carbohydrate loading. Although aerobic metabolism is the predominant source of ATP, a significant energy contribution from fast-rate glycolysis continues in short-term aerobic endurance events. The use of bicarbonate and β-alanine supplements (as discussed in Chapter 10) may therefore also be beneficial as pH buffering agents in events such as a 1,500 m run or a 400 m swim. Following discussion of carbohydrate loading, we will consider the case of caffeine, as a widely available, legal supplement which has a wealth of research describing its possible ergogenic effects.

Carbohydrate loading

Carbohydrate loading (also referred to as carbo-loading, glycogen loading or glycogen super-compensation) involves the manipulation of diet to increase the muscle glycogen stores prior to an endurance event. As was discussed in the section on fatigue, glycogen depletion leads to feelings of 'hitting the wall' and has been shown to be detrimental to performance. Research indicates that for prolonged, high-intensity sports (over 60 min, $\geq 75\%$ of $\dot{V} O_{2max}$), carbohydrate loading can improve performance by increasing the time to exhaustion, or, in other words, delaying fatigue. The classic studies into glycogen depletion and carbohydrate loading took place in the 1960s and form the basis from which modern forms of carbohydrate manipulation were developed. Research by Bergström and colleagues, published in 1966 and 1967, provided a major breakthrough in the understanding of the effects of glycogen loading on performance. Bergström and Hultman (1966) carried out a one-legged cycle test to deplete muscle glycogen stores in the exercising leg. The participants exercised for several hours after which muscle biopsies were taken to record the levels of glycogen stored within the leg muscle. After a 3-day period, during which a high-carbohydrate diet was followed, the glycogen levels of the exercised muscle were nearly double those in the non-exercising leg. This study indicates that a bout of glycogen-depleting exercise prior to adopting a carbohydrate rich diet results in a higher storage of glycogen in muscle. In 1967, Bergström and colleagues published findings regarding the effect of diet on performance. In this study, nine participants followed a normal diet, then three days of a low-carbohydrate diet and finally three days of a high-carbohydrate diet. After each diet they completed a cycle ergometer ride to exhaustion (at 75% $\dot{V} O_{2max}$). The mean exercise time following a normal diet was 115 minutes, which decreased to 60 minutes after the low-carbohydrate diet. However, after three days of a high-carbohydrate diet the time to exhaustion increased to a mean of 170 minutes. These and subsequent studies have indicated that carbohydrate loading can increase muscle glycogen stores by 40–100%, depending upon the regimen followed.

A classic model for carbohydrate loading was developed from the results of these findings. This model involves an athlete altering their diet and exercise pattern in the final

week before a competition. After three days following a low-carbohydrate diet (i.e. a fat and protein based diet) an athlete performs an exhaustive exercise bout to deplete glycogen stores. In the remaining days before the event the athlete adopts a high-carbohydrate diet. Following this model glycogen stores are severely depleted before bouncing back above normal resting levels, hence the term glycogen super-compensation.

The use of this dietary manipulation undoubtedly led athletes to increase their pre-race glycogen stores, but a number of drawbacks meant this was not reflected in optimal performance, hence alternative strategies were developed. The three days following a low-carbohydrate diet and exhaustive exercise caused feelings of fatigue, dizziness and led to mood change, including decreased self-confidence and self-belief prior to competition. These changes appeared to have a detrimental effect on subsequent performance. Further to this, following the classic model also interfered with an athlete's final taper to the event. Identification of these drawbacks led to the development of a modified carbohydrate-loading regimen by Sherman and colleagues (1981, 1982). The Sherman model involved a decrease in exercise in the week prior to competition and an increase in carbohydrate consumption to represent 70% of the total calorific intake. Following the Sherman model, athletes were found to have very similar pre-race gains in muscle glycogen storage to the classic model, but without the side effects. This model not only provided a more straightforward method for increasing muscle glycogen storage, but also presented a regimen that matches the alterations in training associated with the taper for competition.

Research indicates that a typical glycogen loading diet should contain around 500–600 g of carbohydrate per day. Table 11.3 provides an example of a one-day menu where the carbohydrate contribution would be within this range. As indicated in the table, increases in total carbohydrate ingestion should come from complex carbohydrates as found in foods such as wholewheat pasta, bread and cereals, not through the consumption of simple sugars. Consuming a high-carbohydrate diet prior to competition can improve performance and delay fatigue. Athletes should consider one further aspect before the adoption of a pre-race carbohydrate loading regimen. The improvements in performance for cycling have been better than those for running and the difference may well relate to the weight-bearing nature of running. Each gram of glycogen stored results in the storage of 2.7 grams of water. This additional stored weight (2.7 g H_2O + 1 g glycogen) creates a 0.5 kg to 2.0 kg increase in total body weight that must be carried at the start of a race, having a larger

Table 11.3 A suggested menu providing 600 grams of carbohydrate as part of a carbohydrate-loading phase.

Food item	Carbohydrate content (g)
Breakfast	
100 g muesli	70
100 g Crunchy Bran®	55
4 × Weetabix/Weet-Bix®	50
Skimmed milk	12
4 × wholewheat toast	60
1 × banana	30
Lunch	
Baked potato	65
Baked Beans (1/2 tin)	30
Glass skimmed milk	12
1 × low-fat yogurt	8
1 × apple	20
Dinner	
100 g wholewheat pasta	70
Pasta sauce (low fat)	5
1 × low-fat yogurt	8
Snacks	
1 × apple	20
1 × banana	30
1 × cup of grapes	30
2 × bagels	60
Total	**635**

impact on weight-bearing sports. It is very important to model any carbohydrate-loading strategy during a practice session or unimportant race rather than employing a new diet before a major event. If a carbohydrate-loading strategy appears to work for you it can then provide a model for subsequent more important events.

Key points

Carbohydrate loading:

➤ increases resting muscle glycogen levels
➤ delays glycogen depletion and fatigue, improving endurance performance

A further aspect to consider for high-intensity aerobic endurance sports is that of in-race carbohydrate feeding. In events lasting more than one hour the consumption of a carbohydrate sports drink or gel has been shown to result in improvements in performance and delaying of fatigue. The use of a carbohydrate-electrolyte sports drink, the most effective for delaying fatigue (Maughan et al. 1989), has not only a glycogen-sparing effect, but also helps to maintain hydration, electrolyte balance and to make fluid intake more palatable. The effects of dehydration can have a major impact on performance in endurance events with a 2% drop in bodyweight (through water loss during exercise) associated with a resultant drop in speed. Consumption of a 6–8% carbohydrate drink during exercise is recommended for improved performance. A higher concentration can affect gastric emptying and lead to discomfort so ideally should be avoided. If employing a carbohydrate-drinking schedule during a race, ingestion should begin within the first 30 minutes of exercise and continue at a rate of $500mL \cdot Hr^{-1}$ hr for the duration of the race. A 6–8% carbohydrate solution would represent an intake of about 30–40 g of carbohydrate per hour (about 6–8 grams per 100 ml).

In addition to carbohydrate, electrolytes are commonly included in drinks consumed during endurance events. As mentioned previously, the primary mechanism of heat loss during exercise is the evaporation of sweat from the surface of the skin. Sweat contains a variety of electrolytes, especially sodium and chloride. The loss of sodium through sweating is of greatest concern to the athlete due to its potential link with muscle cramping. The composition of sweat varies greatly between individuals, hence an athlete must not only work out their sweat rate in different conditions, but also analyse their sweat sodium concentration. This will aid in determining the ideal composition of drink for them.

An additional advantage obtained through the use of a carbohydrate-electrolyte drink relates to the rates of water and sodium absorption which are enhanced when combined with carbohydrate. As with carbohydrate loading, it is important to practise a drink strategy before a major event. An athlete's rate of fluid loss (pre-weight minus post-weight, compensating for fluid intake and urine loss) should be determined. The volume of fluid consumed during prolonged exercise must be sufficient to prevent a loss of body mass of ≥2%. The timing and volume of fluid intake should be individualised to determine what can be tolerated without gastric discomfort.

Key points

A carbohydrate-electrolyte drink consumed during exercise can:

➤ reduce rate of dehydration

➤ have a glycogen sparing effect

➤ maintain electrolyte balance

➤ increase fluid palatability

➤ delay fatigue and improve performance

Caffeine as an ergogenic aid

Caffeine, one of the most widely-consumed drugs, is found naturally in tea, coffee and chocolate. A tea bag contains around 65–100 mg, ground coffee 125 mg per cup and milk chocolate in the region of 50 mg per small bar. Caffeine is a purine, similar in structure to adenine which forms the basis for ATP, and is a central nervous system stimulant. The effects of caffeine are widespread and include increasing mental alertness, concentration, mood state, fatty acid mobilisation, catecholamine release (adrenaline and noradrenaline) and muscle fibre recruitment. Caffeine consumption also results in a decrease in perception of effort, prolongs the time to fatigue and reduces reaction time. As a consequence, caffeine represents the most wide-ranging of the ergogenic aids across the eight chapters in Part II of this textbook. Increases in mental functioning can impact on all sports. Decreases in reaction time, and increases in muscle fibre recruitment and catecholamine release, can result in performance improvements for power and power endurance activities (Chapter 9). The increased catecholamine release and reduced perception of effort represent potential improvements in performance for anaerobic endurance events (Chapter 10). The lowered perception of effort, the glycogen-sparing effect of increased fatty acid mobilisation and usage, along with the delaying of fatigue, can significantly improve performance in intermittent and aerobic activities (Chapters 11, 12 and 13).

The benefits of caffeine ingestion before exercise have been most widely researched and reported for endurance sports. A classic study by Costill and colleagues published in 1978 provides an excellent example of the effects of caffeine on endurance performance. In this study nine cyclists consumed caffeine in one trial, and a placebo in the other trial, during which they cycled to exhaustion at an exercise intensity of 80% of $\dot{V}O_{2max}$. Time to exhaustion was nearly 20% higher during the caffeine trial and the cyclists exhibited a lower respiratory exchange ratio (RER) value indicating a shift towards fat metabolism, thereby sparing glycogen stores. In addition, the athletes reported the caffeine trial as being easier than the placebo trial. Subsequent studies have produced similar findings with caffeine resulting in a 10–20% improvement in time to exhaustion.

At rest, caffeine is a diuretic and this presents a potential problem regarding its use as an ergogenic aid. The diuretic effect, however is negated during exercise due to catecholamine release at the start of exercise that stimulates the release of anti-diuretic hormone; this increases water re-absorption and counteracts the diuretic effects of caffeine. The findings of a variety of studies suggest that an ingestion of 3–5 mg of caffeine per kg bodyweight is sufficient to create an ergogenic effect. For those who consume caffeine regularly, however, any ergogenic effect would not be realised unless the athlete completed a wash-out phase (did not consume caffeine) prior to the event. Research suggests that omission of caffeine from the diet for 5–6 days should be sufficient to establish an ergogenic effect for regular caffeine consumers. For those that do not normally consume caffeine, or when a dose is higher than normally encountered, there are potential side effects which include restlessness, elevated heart rate, insomnia and headaches. Unless consumed in excess doses caffeine ingestion does not generally present a health risk and as such represents an ergogenic aid that can positively affect performance in a wide range of sports.

Caffeine was a restricted substance until 2004 when WADA removed it from the banned list. Although a monitored substance, athletes are now able to use caffeine as a performance supplement. Again, any individual using caffeine as an ergogenic aid has to make a moral decision about its ingestion despite the recent changes in the regulations regarding caffeine and sports performance.

Key points

Ergogenic aids for high-intensity aerobic endurance sports are:

➤ short duration – β-alanine and bicarbonate

➤ longer duration – glycogen loading and in-race feeding

➤ caffeine – can improve time to exhaustion by 10–20%

Check your recall
Fill in the missing words.

➤ Aerobic endurance sports primarily utilise the
_____ energy system; however, a switch to
_____ energy pathways occurs during a finishing
sprint.

➤ The transition from aerobic to anaerobic metabolism is
known as the _____ _____ threshold.

➤ The anaerobic threshold is also referred to as the
_____ threshold.

➤ The point at which _____ begins to accumulate is
commonly used to identify an athlete's AAT.

➤ As a non-invasive measure, _____ _____
corresponding to lactate threshold or maximal lactate steady
state can be used to set training zones.

➤ When performing sub-maximal exercise, steady state
is achieved when energy demand is met by energy
_____.

➤ Beyond a critical level, the _____ threshold, it is no
longer possible to achieve steady state.

➤ The delay in the rise of oxygen consumption at the start of
exercise is termed an oxygen _____.

➤ The elevated oxygen consumption and ventilation upon
completion of exercise is known as the excess post-exercise
oxygen consumption (EPOC), also referred to as the oxygen
_____.

➤ In long-duration endurance sports, fatigue results from
_____ depletion.

➤ A gradual increase in HR during prolonged steady-state
exercise is known as _____ _____.

➤ In short-duration aerobic activities, fatigue results from the
accumulation of _____.

➤ As the exercise intensity falls and duration increases,
_____ depletion becomes the predominant
mechanism behind fatigue.

➤ Aerobic power improvement with training occurs mainly
in the first _____ to _____ months of
training.

➤ Following training, there is a metabolic shift toward
_____ oxidation by muscle fibres.

➤ A regimen commonly used by long-duration aerobic
athletes to enhance performance is that of _____
loading.

Review questions

1. Define the Aerobic-Anaerobic Transition. Why is it important to know the exercise intensity at which this occurs
when training a high-intensity endurance athlete?

2. Why do the increases in exercise intensity need to be
relatively small when conducting an incremental lactate
threshold test? Why will some physiologists have a performer complete a second LT test with smaller intervals?

3. With the use of graphs, discuss the different methods used
to identify the lactate threshold from a lactate curve.

4. How does testing for critical power differ from that carried
out for lactate threshold or maximal lactate steady state?

5. Why are lactate threshold, maximal lactate steady state
and critical power tests more useful to coaches and athletes
than $\dot{V}O_{2max}$ tests?

6. In practice, how are training zones identified during the
development of a training programme for an athlete?

7. What is meant by cardiovascular drift? Explain why it may
occur during high-intensity aerobic endurance activity?

8. Why is it important to consider the sport of an athlete
before conducting aerobic power testing? Why is it difficult to compare meaningfully the $\dot{V}O_{2max}$ scores of sea
kayakers and fell runners?

9. What is an oxygen deficit? Why might the continued elevation of oxygen consumption continue after the oxygen
deficit appears to be repaid?

10. What happens to levels of cortisol and testosterone as a
result of aerobic training? How does this impact on type I
muscle fibres?

Teach it!
In groups of three choose one topic and
teach it to the rest of the study group.

1. Explain the importance of the aerobic-anaerobic transition
to the endurance athlete. What tests can be used to assess
aerobic endurance? In practice, which tests are most commonly adopted with elite athletes?

2. Discuss the structural and functional changes in muscle
tissue with aerobic training, linking the adaptations to
improvements in performance.

3. Taking into account the range of endurance event durations, what are the primary mechanisms of fatigue? Discuss
ways in which the development of fatigue can be delayed
and performance enhanced.

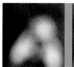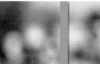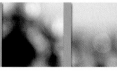

SPORT IN ACTION

Biography: Tim Brabants
Adventure sport: Kayak sprint racing

Tim, a 29-year-old doctor based in Nottingham, is a K1 kayak sprint racing specialist. He started canoeing at the age of 10 when taken by his mother to a come-and-try-it session at Elmbridge Canoe Club. The club has a strong tradition in sprint and marathon racing and it wasn't long before Tim was taking part in domestic competitions. His discipline is K1 1,000 m and he has won titles and medals at national and international levels. In 2008 he won a K1 gold medal in the K1 1,000 m and a bronze in 500 m at the Beijing Olympics to add to his World K1 1,000 gold medal in 2007 and Olympic bronze in 2000. He is the current world record holder for the 1,000 m sprint, a time he set in the heats at the Athens 2004 Olympic Games. He was junior World Champion in 1995, senior European Champion in 2002 and 2006. Away from the 1,000 m distance he joined with Conor Holmes in 1998 to take a K2 silver medal at the Marathon World Championships.

Sydney 2000 Olympic Games

Sprint kayak racing is held on a 2,000 m regatta lake, racing over a distance of 1,000 m or 500 m in single, double or four-man kayaks. Each race has nine lanes with stationary starts and events are organised into heats, semis and finals.

My first shot at qualifying for an Olympic Games was whilst still a junior in 1995, narrowly missing out on competing in the Atlanta Olympics 1996. Three years later I was fitter, stronger and faster and knew that to qualify for Sydney I would need to come in the top eight at the World Championships in 1999. I performed well, finishing sixth. From that moment all my focus was on training and preparing for the Olympic Games in Sydney 2000. I took time out of my medical degree to make more time for training. We work on four-year cycles so this was the big year.

Training two to three times a day, six days a week is tough. The coldest months are the worst when the water freezes on your clothing, kayak and paddles, and your hands hurt for an hour after as they re-warm. Your muscles are aching every day from weight training. Training camps, World Cup and European Championship races are also that year. We race and train in a multitude of climates and altitudes so one has to develop effective ways of acclimatising to each venue quickly and successfully. The physical demands of my sport require a high aerobic capacity combined with good strength endurance as well as an explosive element. Training has to be carefully planned and my coach Eric Farrell was excellent at this. Every day follows the same routine but every day you're closer to your dream of competing in the Olympic Games.

As a nation we had never medalled in sprint kayak racing at the Olympics. The build-up was different from anything I had experienced. All of a sudden there was a large increase in media attention with radio, television and newspaper interviews. Also there was lots of information about the Olympics, travel and boat transport arrangements, measuring for kit etc. It would be easy to become caught up in all of this and get distracted. I knew I wanted to go to Australia and race the best race of my life so far; it wasn't just about competing at the Olympics. To do that would require me to stay focused, train hard and manage my time better with the increased demands. Good quality recovery time enables good quality training.

I'd raced at major events before but I knew this would be different mainly from a psychological

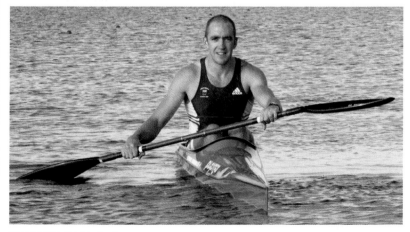

(*Source*: Trevor Chapman)

viewpoint. The other main challenges would be the time difference, climate and length of travel. These we tackled by travelling four weeks before competition to fully acclimatise. This allowed a good block of quality training to sharpen up for the start of racing. We stayed away from Sydney for the first three weeks to avoid too many distractions. The Olympic village is an amazing place. The best athletes in the world all staying in the same place, effectively everyone having their World Championships at the same time. I found it a very positive and motivating experience. Our competition venue was a 2,000 m lake just like everywhere else I race, apart from the 30,000 spectators, high security, TV cameras and media attention.

Come race day I was ready. I was acclimatised and used to the different atmosphere at the Olympics. I'd

watched other people standing on the Olympic podium and that's where I wanted to be too. The elation and look on their faces was very motivating. When I was in my boat on the water, that was my familiar territory. I was there to do what I'd done many times before and had spent many years training for. The first race went well and then I was drawn in probably the hardest of the three semi-finals, up against the European champion and current Olympic and World Champion. Then it was the final, this was it, my first Olympic final. An Olympic rowing friend, Tom Kay, had said to me that if I didn't feel I was going to die when I crossed the finish line then I hadn't done enough. The important thing was to prepare and warm up like I do for any other race. On the start line when the gun went off my gate didn't drop. For a second

I thought that was it, race over. On looking across I was aware that no one else's had gone down either, a system fault. Time to re-focus, paddle round and get back on the start line. I stuck to my race plan not worrying about where anyone else was. With 50 m to go I was in fifth place, really digging deep now, nothing to lose. I gave it everything and in that last 50 m I passed two people to finish third, Britain's first ever Olympic medal in sprint kayak racing. I'd raced the best race of my life and came home with a medal.

Eight years later at the Beijing Olympic Games Tim went on to better this result with a Gold medal in K1 1,000 m and a Bronze in the K1 500 m. He was the first British kayaker in slalom or sprint to win an Olympic gold medal.

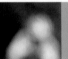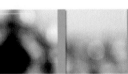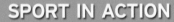

SPORT IN ACTION

Biography: Anna Hemmings
Adventure sport: K1 kayak marathon

Anna Hemmings, for many years Britain's leading female marathon canoeist, six times World and three times European Champion, was told in 2003 by medical experts she might never race again. In 2005, however, she signalled a miraculous return to fitness by regaining her status as the world's leading marathon canoeist at the Marathon Racing World Championships in Perth, Australia. It is her fourth gold medal in the 13-year history of the event, and her ninth World and European Championship

medal, confirming her status as Britain's most successful ever female canoeist. Anna's achievements were recognised at the 2005 Sunday Times Sports Woman of the Year Awards, where she won the Champions Award and in 2010 when she was made a MBE. Anna, 35 years old, from Surrey, was diagnosed with chronic fatigue syndrome which had threatened to end her career. However, reverse therapy enabled her to overcome the illness and return to the highest level of marathon performance. After her success at the 2005 World Marathon Championships Anna she went on to take two further World Marathon gold medals (2006 and 2007) and

compete at the Beijing 2008 Olympic Games prior to retiring in 2009.

Marathon Racing World Championships 2005

The sweetest victory

We were about 150 m away from the final portage when I took the lead; I arrived at the portage (a portage is where you have to get out of your kayak and run with it for 200 m before re-entering the water for the next lap), I leapt out of my boat, and, totally focused, I ran, ready to embrace the hardest part of the race.

Imagine this, you've already been racing for an hour-and-three-quarters, you get out of the boat and

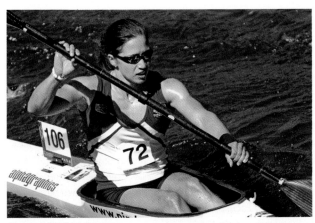

(*Source*: Mark Lloyd)

run with it as rapidly as you can for 200 m, the first 170 m being on grass around a bend and then the last 30 m on sand. Just as your legs are getting tired it gets even tougher – the sand completely zaps the energy from your legs! You get back in, your legs have seized up, your arm is tired from carrying the boat, your lungs are bursting and then you have to pull away and paddle as fast as you can. I managed to establish a 100 m lead but I knew that if I relaxed they would catch me. I paddled hard but this was the bit that hurt – the pain was kicking in big time, then I realised that I'd been there before, in a number of races and in a thousand training sessions. I remembered that this is what I trained for – being able to push through the pain barrier in the last 6 km of the World Championships . . .

How do you prepare yourself for that? When you think about marathon canoeing, most people compare it to running a marathon; however it is more akin to cycling. In the same way that cyclists sit on the slipstream and ride along in the peleton; canoeists 'sit on the wash' (or ride the wave that comes off the side of the boat) and race in a pack. The pack leader changes every so often, thus causing the paddlers to jostle for the best positions in the group. By sitting on the wash you can conserve about 30%

more energy than the person leading the pack. So my plan is usually to sit on the wash as much possible and conserve as much energy as possible!

The idea of riding waves and racing in groups means that the pace fluctuates; there are numerous sprints, particularly as a group approaches a turn or portage or when the pack leader changes. The start of a marathon race is pretty rapid too. Despite the fact that the race is 18 miles (28.8 km) long, if you want to win, it is essential that you make the front group; otherwise you are playing catch up for the rest of the race. With between 20–30 canoeists on the start line the first 1000 m are fairly frantic as everyone sprints to make the front group and fights to gain the best position. Equally a sprint finish is not uncommon. A successful marathon canoeist, therefore, doesn't only require a high level of endurance; a powerful sprint is also of paramount importance.

In order to prepare my body for this, in a typical training week (during the summer) I would clock up around 50–60 km on the water. This would consist of 10–11 individual training sessions; 8–9 of those would be on the water and 1–2 would be running sessions. I would normally do weight training twice a week. However, in the summer of 2005 I was challenged

with a wrist injury which forced me to omit weight training altogether. Although weight training is important for building power and strength, with a number of years of weight training behind me it wasn't going to be detrimental.

I run a couple of times a week for two reasons. The first being that I believe running is a great way to build general fitness and stamina (crucial for marathon racing). The second reason is because we have to do portages which are usually around 200 m long. Although you don't have to be an elite runner, the more comfortable you are running through the portage, the less it will take out of you and affect you when you get back on the water.

If during one week I did eight sessions on the water, they would be broken down in the following way:

5 × endurance sessions, including:

1 × 10 km time trial or 21 km race

1 × long intervals at core aerobic pace (CAP)

2 × intervals at threshold eg 4 × 4 mins on 1 min rest, 3 × 5 mins on 1 min rest, 2 × 6 mins on 1 min rest, with 3-4 mins rest between the sets

1 × 4 km time trial followed by long intervals at threshold

3 × speed session, including:

1 × speed endurance

2 × speed or speed-strength

A speed-strength session is resistance training; in a similar way that a sprinter on the track might run dragging a tyre or some other form of resistance, a canoeist will tie a bungee around the kayak and place 1-3 tennis balls underneath it to create extra drag and resistance.

In my preparation for the world championships, the only time that I paddled the full race distance was at the European Championships. With ➤

➤ so many years of endurance training behind me and the solid base that I built at the beginning of my career, it is not necessary for me to race regularly or train over the race distance.

With all this training in place I was finally ready to head to Australia. I flew out to Perth 14 days prior to the race, this gave me sufficient time to overcome the jet-lag, acclimatise and complete the finishing touches of the training programme. The race was on a Saturday and I completed my final training session on Tuesday evening, this left me with three full days to rest and build up my glycogen stores. I consumed a high-carbohydrate diet and plenty of fluids. Race day arrived; I was rested and ready to endure the toughest part of the race. . .

I raced through the pain barrier and finally I entered the home straight, there was no chance of anyone catching me now, the challenge was maintaining my focus, because all of a sudden I was distracted by the thought of another world title and that made me emotional! This was not the time to be getting emotional, I hadn't won yet! I needed to focus!

I did and finally after 2 hours 16 minutes of racing I crossed the line in first place – world title number four! I threw my arms in the air and gave a yelp of joy and relief. It was the sweetest victory yet. (If you would like to see video footage of me in action please go to my website: www. annahemmings.com.)

CLASSIC RESEARCH SUMMARY

The use of the aerobic-anaerobic transition in determining endurance training intensity by Kindermann et al. (1979)

In the 1970s, many researchers held differing views on the best criteria for the selection of the most appropriate training intensity for endurance athletes. The anaerobic threshold was suggested, in 1978, to be a suitable guideline for the determination of exercise training intensity. Kindermann and colleagues aimed to build on this suggestion by establishing an exercise intensity that could be maintained for prolonged periods of time, yet adequate for endurance training.

Kindermann and colleagues tested seven national-level cross-country skiers. Initially they completed an incremental treadmill test to volitional exhaustion. The treadmill incline was maintained at 5% throughout the test whereas velocity was increased from a starting level of 8 km·h^{-1} by 2 km·h^{-1} every three minutes. Exercise was stopped for 20 s after each three minute period to allow the testers to obtain a blood sample from the ear lobe for the analysis of arterialised blood lactate concentration. In addition, a final blood sample was taken three minutes following volitional exhaustion for the determination of maximal post-exercise lactate concentration. With the use of an Oxycon gas analysis system, $\dot{V}O_2$ and $\dot{V}_E$ were recorded and heart rate was monitored with electrocardiograms. The aerobic-anaerobic threshold was defined in this paper as a blood lactate concentration of 4 mM. Two additional treadmill tests were then completed: (1) 30 min running at the aerobic-anaerobic threshold HR (treadmill speed was continually reduced to maintain HR at this level), and (2) 30 min running at the aerobic-anaerobic threshold velocity. Heart rate was recorded every minute while $\dot{V}O_2$ was continuously monitored, and blood samples were taken from the ear lobe at rest and every 5 min during the 30-min run.

The primary finding of this paper was that running at an intensity sufficient to elevate blood lactate concentration to around 4 mM (as determined with an incremental treadmill test) can be performed by the majority for 45 – 60 min, with a few able to continue for even longer. This exercise elevated HR to an average of 170 beats·min^{-1}, although some individuals experienced HRs in excess of 180 beats·min^{-1}. Kindermann and colleagues suggested that training at an intensity around the 'aerobic-anaerobic' threshold (~4 mM blood lactate) would lead to adaptations in both the cardiovascular system and the muscle cells. It has since been determined that blood lactate measures of the aerobic-anaerobic transition are strong predictors of endurance performance in 30- >60-min races, hence its improvement with endurance training is critical for optimal performance.

Reference: Kindermann, W., Simon, G. and Keul, J. (1979). The significance of the aerobic-anaerobic transition for the determination of work load intensities during endurance training. *European Journal of Applied Physiology*, 42: 25-34.

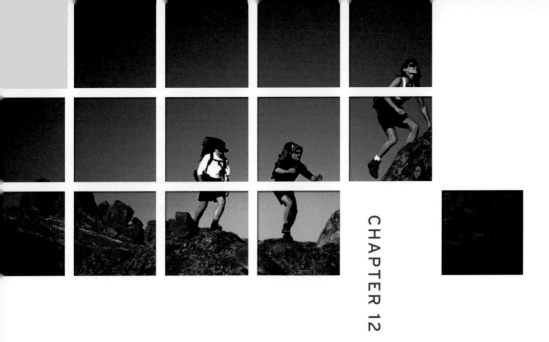

Lower-intensity aerobic endurance sports

Learning objectives

After reading, considering and discussing with a study partner the material in this chapter you should be able to:

➤ explain the structure of mitochondria and the location of aerobic pathways such as β oxidation, Krebs cycle and the electron transport chain

➤ explain the necessity for and the reactions within lipolysis

➤ summarise β oxidation and its role in aerobic metabolism

➤ describe the purpose of deamination as part of aerobic metabolism

➤ teach others about the reactions in Krebs cycle and the by-products of these reactions

➤ explain the processes involved in the electron transport chain

➤ compare the roles of NAD^+ and FAD as electron carriers

➤ discuss oxidative phosphorylation and its connection to the electron transport chain

➤ compare and contrast different protocols for VO_{2max} assessment

➤ describe central and peripheral fatigue

➤ explain the effects of and risks associated with the performance enhancing drug EPO (erythropoietin)

➤ summarise findings regarding altitude training and the particular advantages associated with a live high-train low regimen

Despite being referred to, in the context of this textbook, as lower-intensity aerobic endurance sports, the intensity of the activities in this chapter can vary considerably. In Chapters 9–11, where the intensity was high relative to the duration of the sports, a figure was provided at the start of each chapter to highlight a number of sports within each duration continuum. As the intensity of the sports covered in this chapter can vary, we consider both the intensity and duration of these sports. Figure 12.1 provides a model of the relative intensity and duration of a number of lower-intensity aerobic endurance sports. It is important to recognise, however, that this is an illustrative model, and in reality, the level of the athlete, his or her goals, the intentions of a session, event or journey can greatly alter the intensity and duration of any sport. It is important for any athlete or coach to consider the relative intensity and duration of the activity before making decisions about the physiological demands of the sport.

Aerobic metabolism provides the main source of energy for many sports, especially those that are the focus of Chapters 11, 12 and 13, hence it is important for athletes and coaches to understand the energy pathways underlying aerobic endurance. This chapter begins with a more detailed description of the pathways in aerobic metabolism that were introduced in Chapter 8. Following this, we will consider the physiology of lower-intensity aerobic endurance sports, including tests of aerobic capacity, likely mechanisms behind fatigue, and finally legal and illegal ergogenic aids.

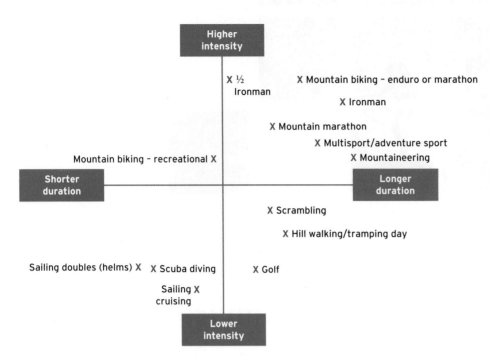

Figure 12.1 Duration and intensity continuum model for lower-intensity aerobic endurance sports. The intensity and duration of each of the sports could vary greatly depending on the ability of the participants and aim of the session/activity.

12.1 Energy supply for aerobic endurance sports

The aerobic system (also known as the oxidative system or referred to as aerobic metabolism or oxidative phosphorylation) represents the predominant energy system for aerobic endurance sports (covered in Chapters 11 and 12). It is also central to recovery and provides energy for lower-intensity exercise bouts within intermittent sports (see Chapter 13). Despite the predominance of other metabolic pathways at the start of high-intensity aerobic exercise, aerobic metabolism underlies the performance of any form of aerobic exercise. Regardless of the name used, the key component for aerobic endurance activities is the presence of oxygen. The phosphagen system (1st gear) and glycolysis (2nd gear) provide the anaerobic mechanisms for ATP production for very short, and short duration, activities. The aerobic system, using oxygen delivered to the cells of the body via the respiratory and cardiovascular systems, provides the 3rd gear, or overdrive, for energy production. The aerobic pathway provides the bulk of the energy necessary to complete a marathon, an ironman triathlon or a day trekking/tramping.

An overview of the processes and pathways that play a role in aerobic metabolism are shown in Figure 12.2. Power and power-endurance (anaerobic) sports fuelled by the phosphagen system rely upon PCr to sustain ATP concentrations, and anaerobic endurance sports predominantly utilise glucose to synthesise ATP during fast-rate glycolysis. It is worth noting that during anaerobic metabolism,

fat and protein must be converted to glucose for use as an indirect (not from dietary intake) energy source. In contrast, the aerobic system can utilise directly all three dietary macronutrients (carbohydrate, fat and protein) to synthesize ATP. As can be seen in Figure 12.2, the use of carbohydrate, fat and protein as sources for ATP production relies on a primary catabolic process within a cell, following digestion and absorption.

After digestion, glucose, glycogen, free fatty acids and amino acids are catabolised through primary and secondary degradation mechanisms to synthesise ATP. Glycolysis, the primary degradation mechanism for glucose and glycogen, was described in Chapter 10. The mechanisms for the primary catabolism of free fatty acids (β (beta) oxidation) and amino acids (deamination) are described in this chapter. After the primary cellular catabolic processes, the products of these reactions are further degraded in the parallel processes of the Krebs cycle and the electron transport chain (ETC) for the synthesis of ATP. The secondary mechanisms for aerobic energy production, along with β oxidation, take place within the mitochondria (the powerhouses for each cell). An individual mitochondrion is illustrated in Figure 12.3. The Krebs cycle and β oxidation take place within the inner matrix of the mitochondria which contains all the enzymes required for these processes. The reactions of the electron transport chain occur across the inner membrane of the mitochondria (see Figure 12.3). Although aerobic metabolism takes longer to provide energy for exercise compared to anaerobic pathways, it provides a relatively inexhaustible supply of ATP to sustain performance.

Cellular energy production begins with the dietary macronutrients

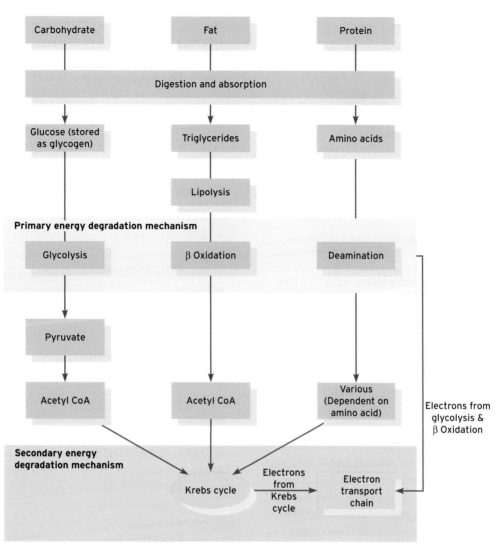

Figure 12.2 Metabolic mechanisms within the aerobic system.

Key points

The products of digestion are catabolised through primary and secondary degradation mechanisms for the production of ATP.

Primary catabolic mechanisms:

➤ Glucose and glycogen – glycolysis (cytosol)

➤ Fatty acids – β oxidation (mitochondrial matrix)

➤ Amino acids – deamination (cytosol)

Secondary catabolic mechanisms:

➤ Krebs cycle (mitochondrial matrix)

➤ ETC (mitochondrial inner membrane)

Pathways for initial substrate catabolism

As a function of digestion, dietary carbohydrate, fat and protein are catabolised to glucose, fatty acids and amino acids (refer to Chapter 2). The primary cellular processes for the further catabolism of these substrates in the process of ATP resynthesis are glycolysis, β oxidation and deamination.

Glucose catabolism

The process of glycolysis, the second of the body's anaerobic energy systems, was described in detail in Chapter 10. During fast-rate glycolysis, required for high-intensity

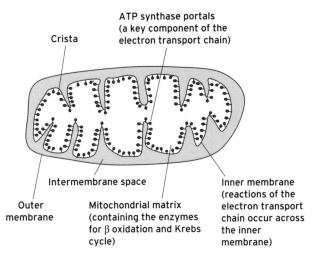

Figure 12.3 Structure of a mitochondrion. The ATP synthase portals provide the channel for H$^+$ ions to return to the matrix. The portals are comprised of two functional F units, F$_0$ stalk which is integrated with the inner membrane and an F$_1$ nodule within the matrix which has ATP synthase attached. ATP synthase is the enzyme that catalyses the reaction to form ATP during oxidative phosphorylation.

short-duration sports, glucose and glycogen are broken down to pyruvate which is then converted to lactate in the sarcoplasm. During lower-intensity aerobic exercise, slower-rate glycolysis also results in the formation of pyruvate which then enters the mitochondria where it is further metabolised within the aerobic pathways. The mitochondrial outer membrane is porous allowing metabolites, such as pyruvate, to pass freely into the mitochondria as far as the inter-membrane space. To enter the inner matrix, however, pyruvate requires a protein carrier to facilitate its transport through the semi-permeable inner membrane. Once within the mitochondrial matrix, pyruvate reacts with coenzyme A (CoA) to form acetyl CoA. This is achieved through a series of reactions catalysed by the *pyruvate dehydrogenase* (PDH) enzyme complex which is illustrated in Figure 12.4. During this process, one carbon

COO$^-$
|
C=O + CoA-SH + NAD$^+$ ⟶
|
CH$_3$

S-CoA
|
C=O + CO$_2$ + NADH
|
CH$_3$

Pyruvate   Acetyl group   Acetyl CoA

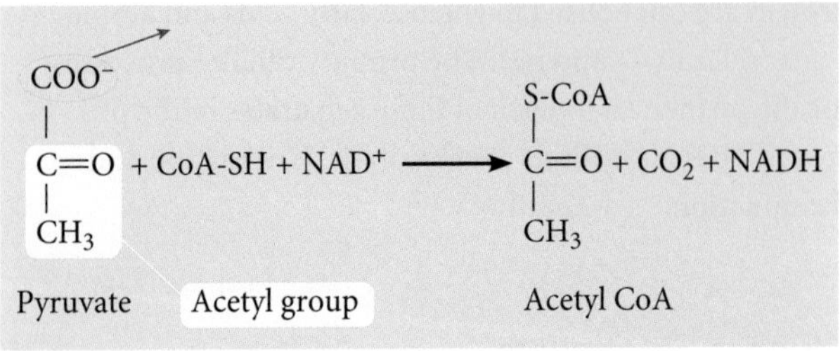

Figure 12.4 The conversion of pyruvate to acetyl CoA catalysed by the pyruvate dehydrogenase enzyme complex. The red arrow indicates the removal of CO$_2$, leaving behind an acetyl group (yellow box).

and two oxygen atoms are removed from pyruvate forming carbon dioxide which is removed from the body through respiration. The removal of CO$_2$ from pyruvate leaves an acetyl group which attaches to the reactive sulfhydryl group (-SH) of CoA to form acetyl CoA with the removal of hydrogen. The hydrogen reduces NAD$^+$, forming NADH which transports it to the ETC resulting in the indirect synthesis of more ATP. Once pyruvate (formed during slower-rate glycolysis) has been converted to acetyl CoA it enters the Krebs cycle within the mitochondrial matrix.

Key points

During lower-intensity exercise:

➤ slower-rate glycolysis produces pyruvate and ATP

➤ pyruvate is transported into the mitochondrial matrix and reacts with CoA to form Acetyl CoA

➤ acetyl CoA enters the Krebs cycle for the production of ATP

Triglyceride catabolism

Stores of glucose and glycogen are limited and provide a relatively short-term energy store that requires frequent replenishment. The storage of fat within specialised adipocytes (fat cells) represents the body's long-term energy store, leading to a plentiful supply of energy rich triglycerides. The properties of fat and its use within the body were discussed in more detail in Chapter 2. Triglycerides, the major storage form of fats, provide over 90% of the lipids used during exercise. Each triglyceride is comprised of a glycerol backbone bonded to three fatty acids. The primary mechanism for the aerobic catabolism of a fatty acid is through β oxidation. However, before this process can take place triglyceride molecules must be broken down into their component parts through a process known as *lipolysis*. Once freed from the glycerol backbone, fatty acids can then be transferred into the matrix of the mitochondria where the enzymes for β oxidation are sequestered. Through the process of β oxidation, the long carbon chain fatty acids are broken down to many two-carbon chain acetyl CoA molecules for entry into the Krebs cycle.

Lipolysis

The process of *lipolysis* takes place within the adipocyte cytosol and involves a series of three reactions. Through the hydrolysis of a triglyceride (i.e. lipolysis), water added to the reactants enables one of the fatty acid (acyl) molecules to be removed from the glycerol backbone in each of the three

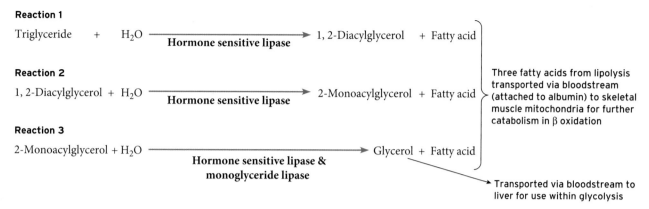

Figure 12.5 The three reactions of lipolysis and the fate of the three fatty acids and glycerol.

reactions. These reactions are illustrated in Figure 12.5. In the first reaction, a fatty acid is removed from the third carbon molecule of glycerol leaving 1,2-diacylglycerol with fatty acids still attached to carbons 1 and 2. The second reaction removes the fatty acid from the first glycerol carbon leaving 2-monoacylglycerol. These first two reactions are catalysed by the enzyme, hormone-sensitive lipase (HSL). In the final reaction, the remaining fatty acid is cleaved from the glycerol molecule, catalysed by monoglyceride lipase along with HSL.

The rate of lipolysis is increased through the action of several hormones on HSL; these are adrenaline, noradrenaline, glucagon, human growth hormone and cortisol. Through their effects on lipolysis, these serve to spare the limited glycogen stores. In contrast, insulin inhibits the action of HSL.

Transport of fatty acids to the mitochondrial matrix

As non-water-soluble structures, fatty acids combine with the blood protein albumin for transport to the skeletal muscles where they become degraded through β oxidation and the Krebs cycle. The remaining glycerol molecule is not reused within the adipocyte but is transported via the blood, primarily to the liver, for use within glycolysis. On reaching the skeletal muscle fibres, the fatty acids must pass through the sarcolemma and the mitochondrial outer and inner membranes before their energy-rich stores can be realised through β oxidation and the Krebs cycle. They pass across the sarcolemma by active transport and easily pass through the porous mitochondrial outer membrane. To enter the mitochondrial matrix, however, each fatty acid must first bond with a CoA molecule (catalysed by the enzyme acyl CoA synthetase). This process requires the energy from the hydrolysis of two ATP molecules to fuel the reaction. The fatty acyl CoA molecule then bonds *reversibly* to carnitine, a small peptide carrier, for transport across the inner mitochondrial membrane. This reaction is catalysed

by carnitine acyl transferase, and results in the formation of acylcarnitine. Once in the mitochondrial matrix, the reverse reaction occurs (also catalysed by carnitine acyl transferase), resulting in the removal of carnitine from acyl CoA which is then available to undergo β oxidation.

β oxidation

All the necessary enzymes for β oxidation are located within the matrix (see Figure 12.3). β *oxidation*, as already mentioned, is a process by which pairs of carbon molecules are detached from the main fatty acid (acyl CoA) until all the energy rich pairs are released (fatty acids always contain even numbers of carbon atoms for example the 16 carbon palmitic acid). This process is called β oxidation because the break in the acyl CoA molecule to form the two-carbon acetyl CoA molecule occurs at the β carbon – the second carbon in the chain. The process of β oxidation involves the four reactions shown in Figure 12.6.

The cycle of reactions in β oxidation continues until the acyl CoA molecule has been fully oxidised to acetyl CoA molecules, each containing two carbons. In the case of palmitic acid, seven cycles of β oxidation would be required for the complete catabolism of the palmitic acyl CoA to create eight acetyl CoA molecules. In the first reaction, catalysed by acyl CoA dehydrogenase, two hydrogen atoms are removed and transferred to the electron transport chain by the co-enzyme carrier flavin adenine dinucleotide (FAD) (see Figure 12.7). In this reaction, therefore, FAD, a derivative of the B vitamin riboflavin and closely related to NAD^+, is reduced to $FADH_2$. The reduction of FAD is shown in Figure 12.7, forming $FADH_2$ by the addition of two hydrogen atoms.

In the second reaction of β oxidation the addition of water hydrates the transenoyl CoA molecule to form 3-hydroxyacyl CoA; this is catalysed by the enzyme enoyl CoA hydratase. The third reaction is similar to the first in that the enzyme, in this case 3-hydroxyacyl CoA dehydrogenase, catalyses

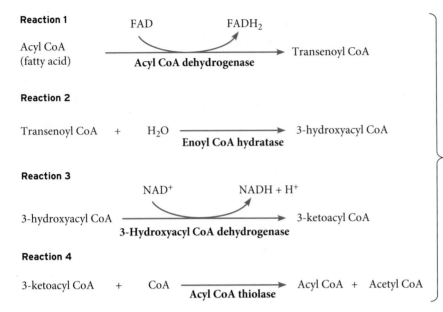

Reaction 1

$$\text{Acyl CoA (fatty acid)} \xrightarrow[\textbf{Acyl CoA dehydrogenase}]{\text{FAD} \quad\quad \text{FADH}_2} \text{Transenoyl CoA}$$

Reaction 2

$$\text{Transenoyl CoA} + \text{H}_2\text{O} \xrightarrow[\textbf{Enoyl CoA hydratase}]{} \text{3-hydroxyacyl CoA}$$

Reaction 3

$$\text{3-hydroxyacyl CoA} \xrightarrow[\textbf{3-Hydroxyacyl CoA dehydrogenase}]{\text{NAD}^+ \quad\quad \text{NADH} + \text{H}^+} \text{3-ketoacyl CoA}$$

Reaction 4

$$\text{3-ketoacyl CoA} + \text{CoA} \xrightarrow[\textbf{Acyl CoA thiolase}]{} \text{Acyl CoA} + \text{Acetyl CoA}$$

The four reactions of β oxidation that lead to the release of a pair of carbons atoms in the formation of acetyl CoA. The reactions take place within the matrix of the mitochondria. The acetyl CoA molecule produced is then available for entry into the Krebs cycle for further degradation within the matrix. The remaining acyl CoA molecule then undergoes the same four reactions to release the next pair of carbon atoms as acetyl CoA. The process of β oxidation continues until all the energy rich carbon pairs are released from a fatty acid. Note that on completion of the final cycle of reactions, two acetyl CoA molecules are the products.

Figure 12.6 The breakdown of fatty acid by β oxidation to form acetyl CoA.

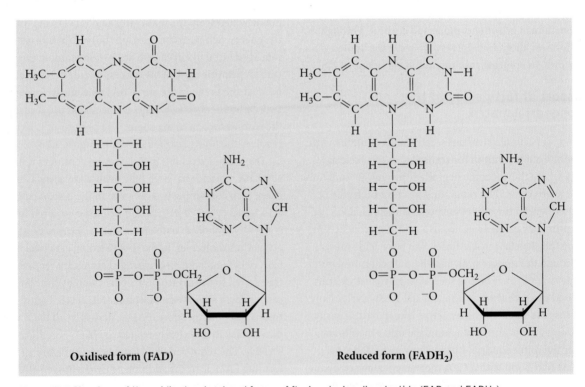

Figure 12.7 Structure of the oxidised and reduced forms of flavin adenine dinucleotide (FAD and FADH$_2$).

the removal of two hydrogen atoms, but the carrier in this instance is NAD^+. In the final reaction, CoA is attached to the final two carbon atoms during their split from the acyl CoA molecule, creating acetyl CoA. This reaction is catalysed by acyl CoA thiolase. The newly formed acetyl CoA molecule is then available to enter Krebs cycle while the new acyl CoA molecule re-enters the β oxidation cycle. For the process of β oxidation to continue, FAD and NAD^+ must be regenerated. This occurs through the transfer of electrons from $FADH_2$ and NADH to the electron transport chain. In common with the Krebs cycle and the ETC, therefore, β oxidation is an oxygen-dependent process.

Key points

Catabolism of triglycerides:

➤ lipolysis – breakdown of triglyceride to fatty acids and glycerol in adipocytes

➤ fatty acids transported in blood (attached to albumin) to skeletal muscle

➤ β oxidation – an aerobic process involving the formation of acetyl CoA in muscle mitochondria

➤ acetyl CoA enters the Krebs cycle and aerobic metabolism

Amino acid catabolism

Deamination refers to the the removal of the nitrogen containing amine group (NH_2) from an amino acid (described in Chapter 2), and this enables the carbon-based skeleton to be utilised as an energy source for aerobic metabolism. The removal of NH_2 can occur through an isolated deamination or through transamination (the removal of an amine group from one amino acid to attach to the carbon-based skeleton of another), as occurs during the glucose-alanine cycle. Twenty amino acids are necessary for human growth and health; these are shown in Table 2.8. The body's amino acid pool (reserve) is contained within the liver, bloodstream and skeletal muscle. The majority of amino acids are deaminated within the liver, although a few can be deaminated within skeletal muscle fibres. Following deamination, the carbon-based skeletons are transported to the mitochondria and enter the matrix via the same carrier protein processes as described for the movement of pyruvate. Once within the matrix, the carbon-based skeletons can contribute to aerobic metabolism by entering the Krebs cycle at one or more points. Each amino acid has a unique chemical composition, hence the removal of the amine group reveals a variety of carbon-based skeletons which can enter the Krebs cycle at varying points; as pyruvate,

Table 12.1 Entry point of amino acids to the Krebs cycle following transamination or deamination.

Aerobic energy system entry point	Amino acids
Pyruvate	Alanine (n) Cysteine (n) Glycine (n) Serine (n) Tryptophan (n)
Acetoacetyl CoA (An intermediary substrate synthesised before the formation of Acetyl CoA)	Leucine (e) Lysine (e) Phenylalanine (e) Tryptophan (e) Tyrosine (n)
Acetyl CoA	Leucine (e) Isoleucine (e) Tryptophan (e)
α ketoglutarate	Arginine (n) Glutamine (n) Glutamic Acid (n) Histidine (e/n) Proline (n)
Succinyl CoA	Isoleucine (e) Methionine (e) Threonine (e) Valine (e)
Fumarate	Phenylalanine (e) Tyrosine (n)
Oxaloacetate	Asparagine (n) Aspartic acid (n)

Note: The larger amino acids – isoleucine, leucine, phenylalanine, tryptophan and tyrosine – can be catabolised to a variety of aerobic metabolism intermediaries and therefore appear more than once in the table. (e) essential amino acid, (n) non-essential amino acid. Histidine is essential for children, but can be synthesised in adults, hence (e/n).

acetoacetyl CoA (an intermediary substrate synthesised before the formation of acetyl CoA), acetyl CoA or as an intermediary substrate in the cycle . Table 12.1 provides the aerobic metabolism entry point into Krebs cycle for the carbon skeletons of the twenty amino acids found in the body, which are illustrated later in Figure 12.9.

Key points

Deamination of amino acids:

➤ removal of amine group forms a carbon-based skeleton

➤ carbon-based skeleton can contribute to aerobic metabolism by forming an acetyl CoA intermediary, acetyl CoA, or a Krebs cycle intermediary

Chapter 12 Lower-intensity aerobic endurance sports

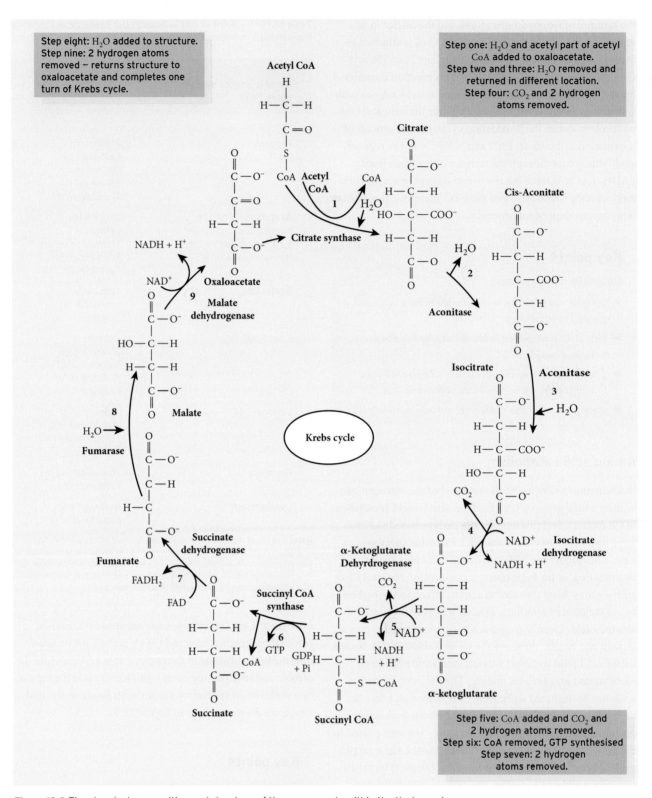

Figure 12.8 The chemical composition and structure of the components within the Krebs cycle.

358

Knowledge integration question

Following the consumption of a high-protein meal, how do the protein molecules enter the blood stream, and from there enter the Krebs cycle for oxidative phosphorylation when required?

Secondary energy degradation mechanisms

Krebs cycle

The Krebs cycle, also known as the tricarboxylic acid cycle or citric acid cycle, involves nine reactions which occur within the matrix of the mitochondria (see Figure 12.3). Through their respective primary metabolic pathways, carbohydrates and fats are converted to acetyl CoA for entry to the Krebs cycle. Protein, if catabolised for energy production, enters the Krebs cycle at a variety of points according to the structure of its carbon-based skeleton. These entry points for protein are shown in Table 12.1. The Krebs cycle, shown in Figure 12.8, was named after Sir Hans Krebs who first identified the nine reactions in the pathway. This process, as with glycolysis and β oxidation, releases hydrogen atoms for use within the electron transport chain. The Krebs cycle employs both FAD and NAD^+ as co-enzyme carriers for the hydrogen atoms removed from substrates. In Figure 12.8 both the reactions and the chemical compositions of the intermediary substrates within the Krebs cycle are illustrated.

One complete turn of the Krebs cycle results in the complete breakdown of a single acetyl CoA molecule. The chemical structure of acetyl coenzyme A is shown in Figure 12.9. The CoA is released in the first reaction, the two carbon atoms are released in reactions four and five as CO_2 and hydrogen atoms plus their associated electrons reduce the co-enzyme carriers FAD and NAD^+ for transfer to the ETC. Upon entry to the Krebs cycle, acetyl CoA bonds with oxaloacetate (a four carbon molecule), to form a six-carbon citrate molecule, consuming one molecule of water during the process. Two further molecules of water are catabolised in reactions three and eight, while one is formed during reaction two. This results in a net water consumption of two molecules to facilitate the complete oxidation of one acetyl CoA molecule.

As a result of reaction one, catalysed by citrate synthase, the released CoA component removed from the acetyl structure combines with α-ketoglutarate to form succinyl CoA in reaction five. Reactions two to eight create a variety of Krebs cycle substrates leading to the formation of a four carbon oxaloacetate molecule in reaction nine. This completes one rotation of the Krebs cycle where oxaloacetate can be combined with a further acetyl CoA for another rotation.

It is interesting to note that the intermediary substrates are effectively not altered by the Krebs cycle, they merely

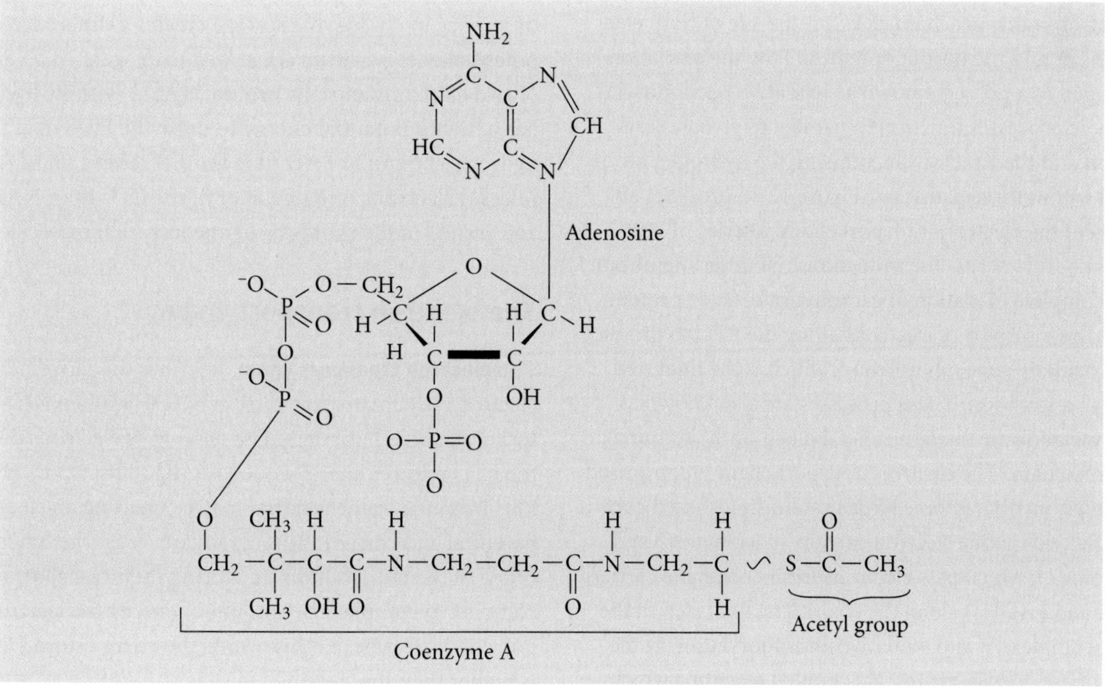

Figure 12.9 Structure of acetyl CoA (co-enzyme A) showing ~ bond between the acetyl group and co-enzyme A.

bond reversibly with the acetyl group through the series of reactions which release electrons and produce one molecule of GTP which is a high-energy nucleotide. The GTP molecule produced by the Krebs cycle can be converted to ATP or, as described in Chapter 9, can be utilised for protein synthesis. Hydrogen atoms, and their associated electrons, are removed from the intermediary substrates in the reactions catalysed by dehydrogenase enzymes; isocitrate dehydrogenase (reaction four), α-ketoglutarate dehydrogenase (reaction five), succinate dehydrogenase (reaction seven) and malate dehydrogenase (reaction nine). In reactions four, five and nine the hydrogen atoms and their electrons reduce NAD^+ to $NADH + H^+$, whereas in reaction seven FAD is reduced to $FADH_2$. These hydrogen atoms are the most important products of the Krebs cycle and are released by the co-enzymes for use within the electron transport chain.

Key points

The Krebs cycle:

➤ involves nine reactions within the mitochondrial matrix

➤ produces one ATP molecule (converted from GTP)

➤ provides an important supply of hydrogen atoms and electrons for use within the ETC

Electron transport chain and oxidative phosphorylation

The electron transport chain (ETC) is the site of both electron transfer and the production of ATP by the oxidation of hydrogen in a process known as oxidative phosphorylation. These processes function in parallel to glycolysis, β oxidation and the Krebs cycle, utilising the hydrogen atoms released within these pathways. Figure 12.10 provides an overview of the electron transport chain, a series of reactions that occurs across the mitochondrial inner membrane.

The complete oxidation of carbohydrate, fat or protein involves the transport of electrons along the ETC to produce ATP by oxidative phosphorylation, which is the final step in cellular respiration. These processes are also known as aerobic metabolism, oxidative metabolism or the terminal respiratory chain. The electron transport chain is comprised of five steps, involving three large protein-lipid-based complexes and two mobile electron carriers (coenzyme Q and cytochrome c), which pass electrons from coenzyme carriers ($NADH$ and $FADH_2$) along the chain. The final step in the chain at complex IV and oxidative phosphorylation at the ATP synthase portals, represents coupled reactions which lead to the formation of ATP and the by-product water. Due

to its importance in the aerobic generation of ATP, we will first reconsider how hydrogen is carried by co-enzymes to the mithochondrial matrix, which is the site of the ETC and oxidative phosphorylation. We will then discuss both the ETC and oxidative phosphorylation.

Hydrogen and the co-enzyme carriers revisited

Hydrogen atoms, as described in Chapter 2, are the smallest atoms and are comprised of a proton and an electron. Hydrogen is represented by the symbol H, protons have a positive charge ($+$) and electrons are negatively charged ($-$). If the electron is removed from a hydrogen atom it becomes a positively charged hydrogen ion (H^+), sometimes referred to as a proton. If a hydrogen atom receives an additional electron it becomes a negatively charged hydride ion (H^-). The pairs of hydrogen atoms released through glycolysis, β oxidation and the Krebs cycle are transported to the ETC by the co-enzyme carriers NAD^+ and FAD. The nature of these two co-enzymes creates a difference in how they bond hydrogen atoms during transport to the ETC. As a positively charged ion, NAD^+ effectively binds with a hydride ion (H^-), forming a neutral NADH molecule. The remaining proton (H^+) remains free in the aqueous environment, such that NADH transfers the proton and two electrons to the electron transport chain. FAD, on the other hand, transfers both hydrogen atoms with their electrons intact and forms $FADH_2$. This difference in co-enzyme storage creates a difference in the potential energy within the stored hydrogen. As a carrier of two electrons and one proton, NAD^+ with its hydrogen has a higher potential energy to drive the ETC than for the hydrogen bound to FAD. It is for this reason that $FADH_2$ releases electrons one step later in the ETC than NADH and results in the synthesis of one less ATP molecule.

The electron transport chain

The **electron transport chain** describes the movement of electrons which are passed from NADH and $FADH_2$ to a series of electron carriers. The passing of electrons down the ETC releases energy which is used to transport H^+ ions from the mitochondrial matrix, creating an electrical potential and concentration gradient across the inner membrane of the mitochondrion. During their transport from complex to complex the amount of energy the electrons possess decreases; in other words the energy stored in step 1 is higher than that retained in step 2 and so on. The energy cascade during the ETC is illustrated in Figure 12.11.

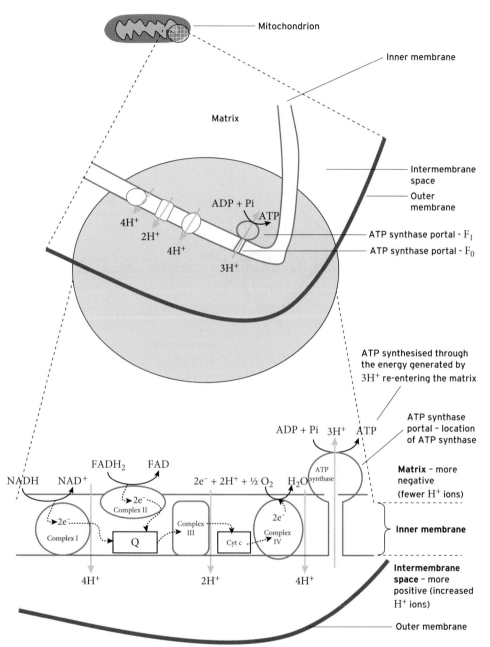

Figure 12.10 Overview of the Electron Transport Chain (ETC) and oxidative phosphorylation.
Q = co-enzyme Q;
Cyt; c = cytochrome c.

The structures within the ETC include three fixed protein-based complexes and two mobile intermediates. The protein-based complexes are aptly named as each comprises a complex arrangement of 4–43 polypeptide subunits. Complex I, also known as NADH-Coenzyme Q oxidoreductase or NADH hydrogenase, contains the cofactor flavin mononucleotide (FMN) to which the electrons are passed prior to eventually being passed to the hydrophobic Coenzyme Q. Coenzyme Q represents the first of the mobile intermediates which, unlike the protein complexes which are fixed within the inner membrane, can move within the membrane. Also known as ubiquinone or simply as Q, coenzyme Q accepts $2H^+$ and two electrons from complex I to form QH_2. Coenzyme Q now passes the two electrons received from complex I to complex III, bypassing complex II. Complex II, which includes the Krebs cycle enzyme succinate dehydrogenase along with three other polypeptide subunits, provides the electron acceptor for $FADH_2$ before passing them to coenzyme Q. Complex III, also known as Q-cytochrome c oxidoreductase, receives electrons from NADH and $FADH_2$ in the form of QH_2 prior to passing them to the second mobile intermediary cytochrome c. Cytochrome c can only be reduced by one electron at a time, so complex III serves as

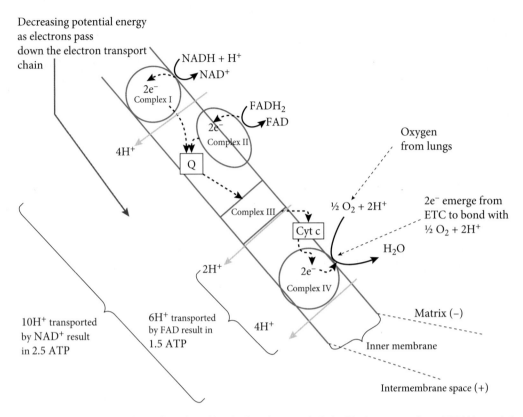

Figure 12.11 The energy cascade as electrons flow down the electron transport chain. Electrons pass from NADH to proteins in complex I while those from $FADH_2$ are passed to Q. The different starting points result in NADH pumping four additional H^+ ions from the matrix. Thus the transfer of electrons from NADH leads to the creation of 2.5 ATP molecules while that from $FADH_2$ create only 1.5 ATP molecules. In the diagram, for ease of understanding, the reactions at the end of the ETC are shown as $2e^- + 1/2O_2 + 3H^+ = H_2O$. In reality, oxygen exists in the matrix as O_2 and therefore the reaction would actually rely on four electrons emerging from the electron transport chain and 6 hydrogen ions from the ATP synthase portals. Thus the reaction is more correctly shown as $4e^- + O_2 + 4H^+ = 2H_2O$. Q = co-enzyme Q; Cyt c = cytochrome c.

a gatekeeper, receiving the electrons from QH2 in a series of reactions in order to pass single electrons to cytochrome c. Cytochrome c passes electrons from complex III, one at a time to the final complex in the electron chain, that of complex IV or cytochrome c oxidase. The reactions within complex IV provide the energy for further H^+ pumping (also achieved by complex I and III) prior to the electrons being transferred to oxygen and forming water.

Until recently, it was believed that each protein complex moved two H^+ ions out of the mitochondrial matrix and that two H^+ were required to phosphorylate each ADP. As such, these figures have been widely used in earlier text-books. Recent research, however, indicates that the protein complexes (I, III and IV) of the ETC move four, two, and four H^+ respectively from the matrix into the intermem-brane space, and three, rather than as previously thought two H^+, are required to synthesise each ATP during oxida-tive phosphorylation. The energy released during the trans-fer of electrons from NADH down the ETC is harnessed, therefore, to transport ten (4 + 2 + 4) hydrogen ions from

the matrix of the mitochondria. As $FADH_2$ transfers its electrons to the chain at co-enzyme Q, six (2 + 4) hydrogen ions are expelled from the matrix for each $FADH_2$ molecule.

Key points

The electron transport chain (ETC):

➤ Involves the movement of electrons, passed from NADH + H^+ and $FADH_2$, along a series of electron carriers (five steps)

➤ Takes place within the inner membrane

➤ Movement of electrons generates an electrical potential which is utilised in the synthesis of ATP (see oxidative phosphorylation)

Oxidative phosphorylation

The theoretical model for **oxidative phosphorylation** was first proposed in 1961 by Peter Mitchell, who won the Nobel Prize in chemistry in 1978 for his description of how the

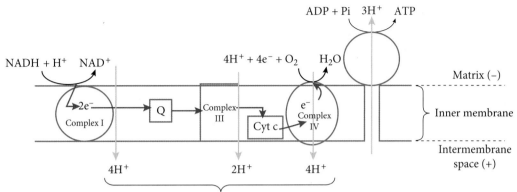

NADH enables the transport of ten hydrogen ions from the matrix to the intermembrane space. This leads to the synthesis of 2.5 ATP.

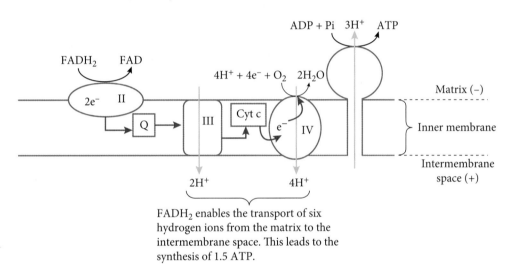

$FADH_2$ enables the transport of six hydrogen ions from the matrix to the intermembrane space. This leads to the synthesis of 1.5 ATP.

Figure 12.12 Oxidative phosphorylation of electrons from NADH and $FADH_2$ resulting in the creation of 2.5 and 1.5 (respectively) molecules of ATP. Q = co-enzyme Q; Cyt = cytochrome c.

ETC leads to the synthesis of ATP. At the end of the ETC the ATP synthase portals (illustrated in Figures 12.3, 12.10 and 12.12) represent the essential structures for oxidative phosphorylation. As is explained in Figure 12.3, the ATP synthase portals are comprised of an F_0 stalk which is integrated with the inner membrane and an F_1 nodule located entirely within the matrix (see Figures 12.10 and 12.12). While the ETC transports protons (H^+) from the matrix to create an electrical potential and concentration gradient across the inner membrane, the ATP synthase portals enable H^+ ions to flow from a high to low concentration and hence back into the matrix. Like water released from a dam, the movement of hydrogen ions into the matrix, due to the charge difference on either side of the inner membrane, provides energy to drive the phosphorylation of ADP to form ATP. In order for this reaction to proceed, oxygen is required as the final electron acceptor at the end of the ETC. Whilst being oxidised, the released electrons are also

reunited with H^+, resulting in the formation of water. In this way, oxygen, gained through respiration, facilitates the phosphorylation of ADP and, consequently, the term oxidative phosphorylation is very appropriate.

As discussed in the previous section, the transfer of electrons along the ETC leads to the oxidation of NADH and $FADH_2$, resulting in 10 H^+ and 6 H^+, respectively, being expelled from the mitochondrial matrix into the intermembrane space. The concentration gradient established provides the potential energy for H^+ to flow through the ATP synthase portals to form ATP. Recent research suggests that three H^+ re-entering the matrix are required to synthesise one molecule of ATP. The Pi required for the phosphorylation of ADP is transferred into the matrix by phosphate transporters (a protein portal), a process which requires a further H^+, so consequently a total of four H^+ are required to synthesise one ATP molecule. With this information regarding the number of H^+ driven out of the matrix and the number of H^+ needed for the generation of one ATP molecule, it is possible to estimate how much ATP can be generated from a single NADH or $FADH_2$ molecule and furthermore from a carbohydrate or fat molecule.

- *Oxidation of one NADH*: It is now thought that when NADH is the electron carrier 10 H^+ are pumped from the mitochondrial matrix. Given that $4H^+$ are required to re-enter the matrix to form one ATP then the oxidation of one NADH results in the formation of 10/4 = **2.5 ATP**.
- *Oxidation of one $FADH_2$*: When $FADH_2$ is the electron carrier, it is now thought that 6 H^+ are pumped from the mitochondrial matrix. Since 4 H^+ are required to form one molecule of ATP, the oxidation of one $FADH_2$ molecule (which leads to the production 6 H^+) produces 6/4 = **1.5 ATP**.

Key points

Oxidative phosphorylation:

➤ Is the production of ATP by the oxidation of nutrients

➤ Occurs during the final two steps of the ETC

➤ Oxygen accepts the transferred electrons and joins with hydrogen to form water as a by-product

➤ This reaction drives the phosphorylation of ADP to form ATP (catalysed by ATP synthase)

➤ Each NADH leads to the synthesis of 2.5 ATP, each $FADH_2$ leads to the synthesis of 1.5 ATP

Oxygen is only required during the ETC

An interesting and important concept to keep in mind is that the reactions involved in glycolysis, β oxidation and the Krebs cycle do not require oxygen. However, for each of these processes to continue over a long duration, such as that during a high- or lower-intensity aerobic endurance sport, oxygen is required to oxidise the electrons emerging from the ETC. The coenzyme carriers NAD^+ and FAD transport hydrogen atoms produced during glycolysis, β oxidation and the Krebs cycle to the ETC where the oxidation process begins. In this way, the ETC is the truly aerobic system or mechanism as it directly consumes molecular oxygen (from respiration) for ATP synthesis. Glycolysis, β oxidation and the Krebs cycle rely on the ETC for removal of hydrogen atoms, and as a consequence, are reliant on the oxygen consumed during the ETC for their continuation. Without the presence of oxygen in sufficient quantities for ETC functioning, the Krebs cycle and β oxidation are inhibited. Glycolysis can continue, as was discussed in Chapter 10, for a relatively short duration without

the presence of oxygen, as the hydrogen atoms produced during the process can be passed to pyruvate resulting in the formation of lactate.

The production of ATP by oxidative phosphorylation

The ETC is the key mechanism for ATP production and is responsible for the generation of over 90% of the body's ATP. The ETC is able to synthesise ATP because the electrons it accepts at the start of the chain from NADH and at step two from $FADH_2$, have a high-energy transfer potential. The ETC utilises this energy to create the electrical difference across the inner membrane, which enables the phosphorylation of ADP to ATP. The oxygen required for the resynthesis of ATP is supplied to the muscles via the blood. Type I fibres are especially adept at aerobic metabolism because they have a dense capillary network, have the highest numbers of mitochondria and contain high levels of myoglobin for oxygen storage within the muscle.

The co-enzyme carriers NAD^+ and FAD are reduced to NADH + H^+ and $FADH_2$ when they accept hydrogen atoms from the reactions in glycolysis, β oxidation and the Krebs cycle. As β oxidation and the Krebs cycle take place within the matrix of the mitochondria, the hydrogen atoms removed from substrates in these processes can be easily transferred to the ETC. The hydrogen atoms removed during glycolysis, however, have to be shuttled from the cytosol to the mitochondrial matrix before they can be transferred to the ETC. The glycerol-phosphate shuttle provides one such mechanism through which NADH enters the mitochondria. In this process the hydrogen atoms are transferred to glycerol-phosphate in the intermembrane space and so can cross the inner membrane. Through the glycerol-phosphate shuttle, however, hydrogen atoms are passed to FAD in the mitochondrial matrix rather than NAD^+ and so result in a lower net ATP production from cytosolic NADH when compared with mitochondrial NADH. Once inside the matrix, hydrogen atoms from glycolysis can enter the ETC.

Steps 1 and 2

The illustration of the ETC in Figure 12.11, reveals the cascade in potential energy as electrons are transferred down the chain. The ETC comprises a series of five steps that are illustrated in Figure 12.12. In step one of the ETC the electrons from NADH are transferred to flavin mononucleotide within complex I. The energy released during this reaction is used to pump $4H^+$ from the matrix. In step two, the electrons are passed from complex I to coenzyme Q (labelled Q in Figure 12.11). $FADH_2$ transfers its electrons to complex II because they have a lower potential energy than those held by NADH; these electrons are then passed co-enzyme Q. As illustrated in Figures 12.11 and 12.12, the later entry by $FADH_2$ to the ETC results in the re-synthesis of one less ATP molecule than is enabled by NADH. It is for this reason that $FADH_2$ results in the production of 1.5 ATP molecules while NADH produces 2.5.

Steps 3-5 and ATP synthase

In the third step, electrons are transferred from co-enzyme Q to a series of protein-based cytochromes comprising heme groups and co-factors known as complex III. In this third step, the transfer of electrons between the cytochrome groups within complex III (cytochrome b to c_1) enables the removal of two further hydrogen ions from the matrix. From complex III, during step 4, the electrons are passed to cytochrome c prior to transfer to complex IV. In complex IV (step 5) the electrons are passed through a final series of cytochromes (cytochrome a – a_3). As a result of the transfers within complex IV, sufficient energy is released to transport four further hydrogen ions from the matrix during step 5.

As a result of the transfer of electrons down the ETC, the transport of hydrogen ions across the inner membrane and into the intermembrane space creates an electrical potential and concentration gradient across the membrane. The intermembrane space becomes more positively charged than the inside of the matrix. The electrical potential creates the mechanism to drive the oxidative phosphorylation of ADP. The events at the end of complex IV and those of ATP synthase portal are coupled. The final reaction of complex IV (step 5) involves the oxidation (joining with molecular oxygen from respiration) of the electrons that emerge from the ETC which then combine with H^+ to form water. This final reaction of the electron transport chain can be represented by the formula $2e^- + 1/2\,O_2 + 2H^+ = H_2O$ or in a more chemically correct formula: $4e^- + O_2 + 4H^+ = 2H_2O$. The action of the hydrogen ions 'rushing' back to the matrix to bond with the oxidised electrons liberates sufficient energy to enable the phosphorylation of ADP to form ATP, a reaction catalysed by ATP synthase (see Figure 12.10). Thus, the end products of the ETC are water and ATP, as illustrated in Figure 12.12.

The fate of ATP

The ATP synthesised through the ETC is transferred from the matrix to the intermembrane space and across the outer membrane to provide energy for muscular contraction during exercise. Although it passes easily through the outer membrane, ATP has to be transported across the inner membrane via an antiport (a protein-based membrane channel). The antiport enables an exchange between ATP and ADP, such that, as an ATP molecule leaves the matrix an ADP molecule enters. A similar type of channel enables phosphate (Pi), along with a H^+, to enter the matrix. Together, these channels present the essential substrates, ADP and Pi, to the ETC for the formation of ATP. As mentioned, the series of reactions in the ETC provide the body's main source of ATP. Table 12.2 provides examples of the potential ATP that can be synthesised from a molecule of glucose glycogen and one of a typical fat, e.g. palmitic acid. The importance of the ETC for ATP production can be seen clearly from the table, where substrate synthesis of ATP (direct from glycolysis and the Krebs cycle) results in only

Table 12.2 ATP production from glucose, glycogen and palmitic acid via direct synthesis and the ETC.

Pathway	Glucose ($C_6H_{12}O_6$)	Glycogen	Palmitic Acid ($C_{16}H_{32}O_2$)
Glycolysis - direct synthesis	2	3^1	-
Fatty acid conversion	-	-	-2^2
β oxidation - direct synthesis	-	-	0
Krebs cycle	2^3	2^3	8^4
ETC	26^5	26^5	99^6
Total	**30**	**31**	**105**

[1]When glycogen is the substrate for glycolysis one fewer ATP molecules is consumed during the degradation process, as a consequence three rather than two molecules of ATP are produced directly.

[2]To convert a fatty acid to acyl CoA - to enter the mitochondria prior to β oxidation - costs two ATP molecules.

[3]Glycolysis results in the formation of two acetyl CoA molecules to drive two rotations of the Krebs cycle, and results in the production of two ATP molecules (or strictly speaking GTP molecules which can be converted to ATP).

[4]Through β oxidation eight acetyl CoA molecules are formed resulting in the production of eight molecules of ATP (from GTP) through the Krebs cycle.

[5]Glycolysis results in the formation of two NADH + H^+ resulting in **3** ATP molecules (hydrogen atoms are transferred to FAD in the mitochondria, 1.5 ATP from each FAD), the conversion from pyruvate to acetyl CoA results in the formation of **5** ATP (resulting from the formation of two NADH + H^+, one for each pyruvate), the Krebs cycle, through two rotations and production of 6 NADH + H^+ and 2 $FADH_2$, results in the formation of **15** ATP and **3** ATP, respectively. Total ATP formation = 26 (3 + 5 + 15 + 3).

[6]As a result of the seven cycles of β oxidation for palmitic acid a total of 27 ATP are produced from $FADH_2$ and NADH + H^+ along with 72 ATP from $FADH_2$ and NADH + H^+ formed during the Krebs cycle making a grand total of 99 ATP through the ETC.

around 10% of the total energy possible through aerobic metabolism. Figure 12.13 provides a visual illustration of the data in Table 12.2 for glucose, glycogen and palmitic acid to show the production of ATP. While looking at Table 12.2 and Figure 12.13 remember that with the ETC, 2.5 molecules of ATP are synthesised from each NADH and 1.5 molecules of ATP are synthesised from each $FADH_2$.

Although ATP production through aerobic metabolism is relatively efficient, only around 25–40% of the total energy released through the complete oxidation of carbohydrate or fat can be harnessed to create ATP. The remaining energy created through the reactions within glycolysis,

β oxidation, the Krebs cycle and the ETC escapes as heat energy (entropy – as described in Chapter 8), which is why body temperature rises during exercise.

Key points

The electron transport chain is the body's main mechanism for ATP production.

Each NADH results in the synthesis of 2.5 ATP, while for $FADH_2$, which enters the ETC further down the chain, results in the synthesis of 1.5 ATP molecules.

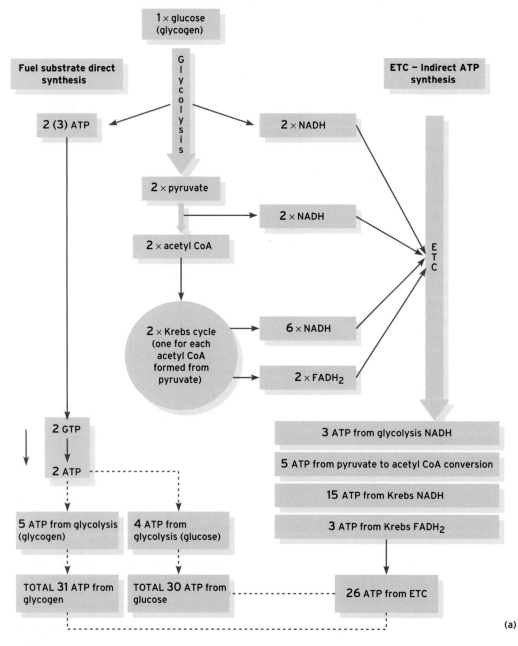

Figure 12.13 ATP synthesis through the oxidation of (a) glucose (glycogen) and (b) palmitic acid.

(a)

Figure 12.13 (continued)

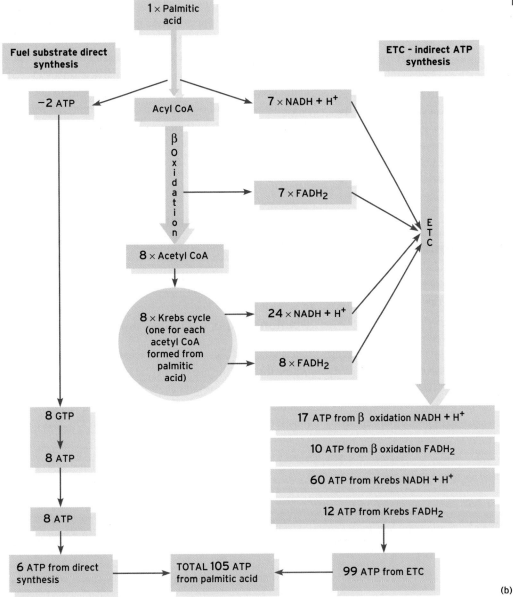

(b)

Knowledge integration question

How are glycolysis and β-oxidation linked with the Krebs cycle, and how are glycolysis and the Krebs cycle linked with the electron transport chain during the generation of ATP from carbohydrate and fat?

12.2 The physiology of lower-intensity aerobic endurance sports

As introduced in Chapter 11, aerobic endurance refers to the body's ability to produce energy in the presence of oxygen. Many sports rely upon a sound level of aerobic fitness for successful performance. One such sport is sailing. A story of the gruelling Sydney to Hobart yacht race is presented in the Sport in Action section on pp. 384–5. In a health context a measurement of cardiovascular fitness is often assessed or estimated to assess an individual's progress on an exercise intervention. This section focuses on appropriate tests of aerobic endurance, prior to examining the effects of exercise on metabolism. Following this, we examine the possible causes of fatigue in lower-intensity aerobic endurance sports and adaptations to training. Several ergogenic aids for low-intensity aerobic endurance sports are then discussed, finishing with a discussion on health and environmental aspects related to these sports.

Aerobic endurance testing

Review of aerobic endurance testing

The use of HR monitors in training to monitor the intensity is widespread among both elite and recreational athletes, and is also becoming popular with those exercising for health benefits. The appropriateness of this method is due to the fact that HR and VO_2 have a strong linear relationship, not surprising as the heart's role is to pump blood containing the required oxygen to the working muscles. The harder you work at increasing exercise intensities, the more oxygen is required by the skeletal muscle and hence the harder the heart has to work.

Due to the expense, and limitations on availability and accessibility of laboratory testing equipment, physiologists have taken advantage of the relationship between HR and $\dot{V}O_2$ and have developed a variety of maximal and sub-maximal tests to predict $\dot{V}O_{2max}$. Table 12.3 provides a variety of tests that can be used based upon their method of assessment. Teachers, coaches, researchers, health professionals and exercise physiologists use different tests according to how appropriate they are for a specific athlete or group.

Where a high degree of accuracy is required a laboratory-based $\dot{V}O_{2max}$ with gas analysis is the most appropriate measure. When a group of performers are to be tested, however, time and financial constraints may mean that the most appropriate test would be one such as the Multi-Stage Shuttle Run Test (MSRT), also known as a Bleep or Beep Test. In the MSRT a number of athletes can be tested at the same time, with each participant's $\dot{V}O_{2max}$ being predicted from the stage at which they drop out or are pulled out from the test. In a clinical setting, or when testing participants to their maximum could be a problem, sub-maximal tests such as the Rockport Walk, the Queen's College step test or the Åstrand-Åstrand aerobic fitness test can be used to predict $\dot{V}O_{2max}$.

Knowledge integration question

What variable is commonly used by coaches and athletes to monitor exercise intensity and what testing is required to elucidate its relationship with exercise intensity?

Pulmonary gas exchange analysis

The analysis of pulmonary gas exchange can be conducted offline through the use of Douglas bags (expired air samples are collected for later analysis) or by online breath-by-breath (b^2) analysis. Figures 12.14 and 12.15 provide illustrations of the equipment necessary for Douglas bag

Table 12.3 Maximal and sub-maximal tests for measuring or predicting $\dot{V}O_{2max}$ that can be employed or modified for aerobic endurance sports.

Maximal assessments of $\dot{V}O_{2max}$	Maximal predictions of $\dot{V}O_{2max}$	Sub-maximal predictions of $\dot{V}O_{2max}$
Laboratory-based tests $\dot{V}O_{2max}$	**Laboratory-based tests – cycle ergometer**	**Laboratory-based tests – cycle ergometer**
1. Douglas bags (off-line)	Åstrand maximal test	Åstrand-Åstrand aerobic fitness test
2. On-line gas analysis	McArdle et al. maximal test	
Common modes of analysis	**Laboratory-based tests – treadmill**	**Laboratory-based tests – treadmill**
Cycle ergometer	Balke protocol	Balke protocol – single stage test
Treadmill	Bruce protocol	Bruce protocol – multi-stage test
Rowing ergometer		
Kayak ergometer		
Useful protocols	**Field-based tests**	**Field-based tests**
Bruce protocol	Multi-stage shuttle run test*	Queen's College step test
Sleivert protocol	Aero test	Rockport walk
Athlete-led protocol		Cooper's 12-minute run
		1.5 mile run test

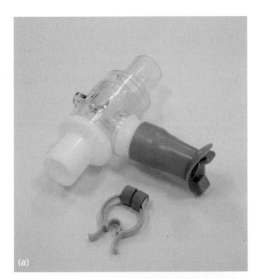
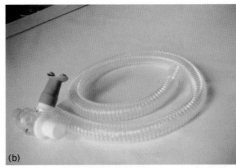
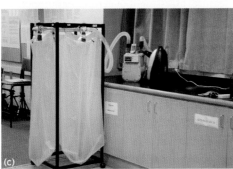
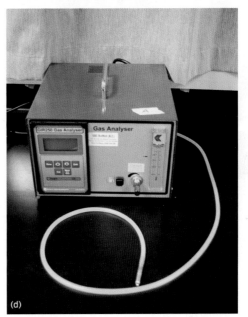
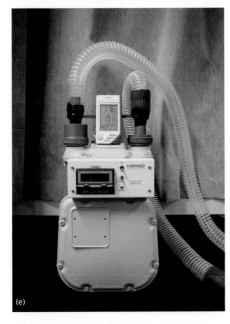

Figure 12.14 Equipment for a Douglas bag collection. During this type of assessment the expired air samples are collected during the test but analysed following completion of the test. (a) nose clip, mouth piece and one-way valve through which the athlete breathes during a test, (b) tubing to connect the mouth piece to the Douglas bag, (c) Douglas bags can be arranged in a rack system depending on the test situation. This photograph shows a Douglas bag rack connected to a gas meter, (d) gas analyser used to assess the oxygen and carbon dioxide percentages in the expired air sample. The gas analysis should always take place before the gas volume measurement and (e) gas meter used to assess the volume of gas expired in a given time period. The tester keeps a record of the timing for each expired air sample. (*Source*: Simon Fryer)

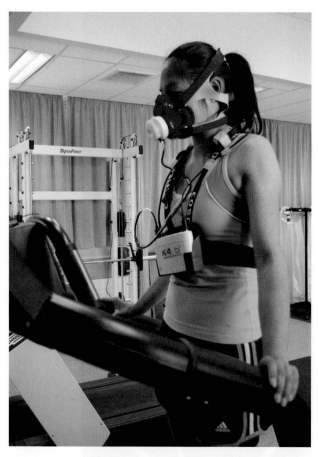

Figure 12.15 Equipment for online gas analysis. During this type of assessment the expired air samples are typically collected breath by breath during the test and analysed throughout the test. Online gas analysis system worn by an athlete during a $\dot{V}O_{2max}$ test. The face mask is designed such that a sample of expired air is sampled with every breath and fed to the gas analyser which in this case is worn on the chest. The athlete has a small battery pack attached to their back and the data can be logged in the system or relayed by telemetry to a receiving laptop computer (allowing the tester to assess oxygen consumption during the test). (*Source*: Simon Fryer)

Key points

A wide variety of maximal and sub-maximal tests has been developed for the measurement, or prediction, of aerobic endurance or power.

The most accurate tests involve the analysis of pulmonary gas exchange by:

➤ Douglas bags
➤ Online systems

Tests of aerobic endurance

The traditional gold standard (seen as the most accurate measure) assessment of aerobic endurance or power is the maximal oxygen uptake ($\dot{V}O_{2max}$) test, as developed by the British physiologist Archibald Hill. In a laboratory setting, the test is carried out using a treadmill, cycle ergometer (an ergometer is a work measuring device), rowing ergometer or kayak ergometer. The selection of ergometer is based upon the mode of exercise that most closely matches the demands of the sport. Maximal aerobic power is most commonly reported in either absolute terms ($L \cdot min^{-1}$) or relative to bodyweight ($mL \cdot kg^{-1} \cdot min^{-1}$). To convert from absolute to relative values simply multiply by 1000 to change from litres to millilitres and then divide by bodyweight. For example, a $\dot{V}O_{2max}$ of 4.2 $L \cdot min^{-1}$ for a 70 kg male would represent a relative $\dot{V}O_{2max}$ of 60 $mL \cdot kg^{-1} \cdot min^{-1}$ ($4.2 \times 1,000/70$). For comparative purposes it is more useful to record data in the relative form rather than absolute figures. By doing this you take into account the body mass of the participants. Female athletes tend to have lower absolute $\dot{V}O_{2max}$, but when converted to relative values differences between $\dot{V}O_{2max}$ scores between male and female athletes of similar abilities tend to be much smaller.

After a warm-up, the athlete being tested completes an 8–12 minute protocol designed to take them to their maximum work rate during this time, with the workload increasing at regular intervals throughout the test. The test format and duration is designed to allow accurate expression of maximal oxygen consumption. The amount of oxygen consumed is monitored and recorded throughout the test by direct pulmonary gas exchange measurement. This involves the analysis of expired air samples from which the percentage of oxygen consumed and carbon dioxide produced can be calculated. The greater an athlete's aerobic power, the longer they will be able to continue in the test and the greater the volume of oxygen they are able to use to produce energy. Figure 12.16 provides an illustration of

and online gas analysis. The advantage of the Douglas bag system is accuracy, although you have to wait until after testing before obtaining results and its use in the field is not practical. Portable online gas analysis systems, such as that shown in Figure 12.15 have an advantage over the Douglas bag system because they can be used relatively easily in the field (a great advantage for some sports) and provide oxygen consumption data during the test. The disadvantage of the online systems is their relative accuracy when compared with Douglas bag gas analysis, although their accuracy is improving with each generation of system that becomes available.

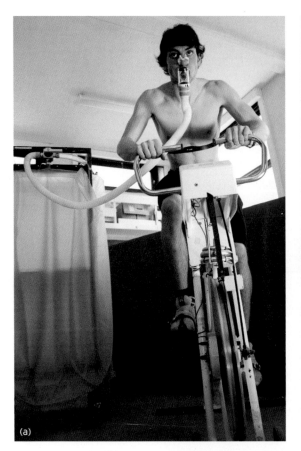

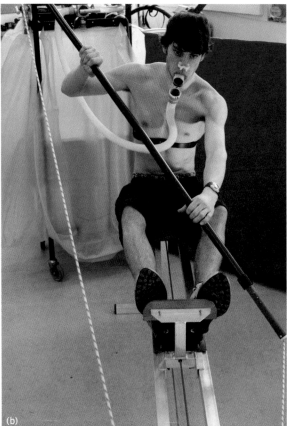

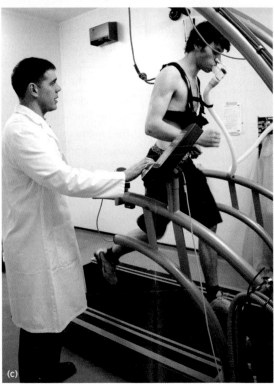

Figure 12.16 $\dot{V}O_{2max}$ tests being conducted on (a) a cycle ergometer, (b) kayak ergometer and (c) on a treadmill. In each case the expired air gas sample is being collected using Douglas bags. (*Source*: Simon Fryer)

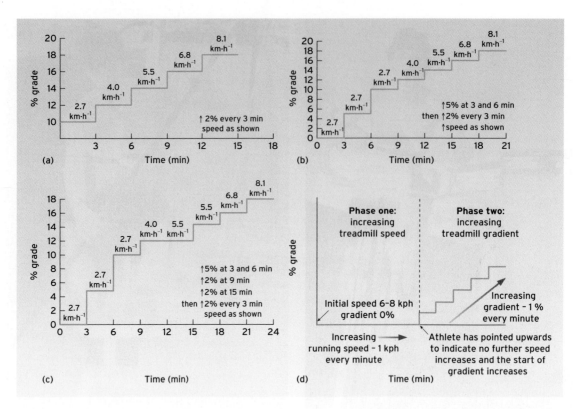

Figure 12.17 Bruce, modified Bruce, adapted Bruce and athlete-led protocols for treadmill assessment of $\dot{V}O_{2max}$. (a) Bruce (Bruce et al. 1973), (b) Modified Bruce (Lerman et al. 1976), (c) Adapted Bruce protocol, (d) Athlete-led protocol.

$\dot{V}O_{2max}$ tests being conducted on a cycle ergometer, kayak ergometer and a treadmill. Tests can either be of a maximal or sub-maximal nature, and can involve the direct measurement of, or the prediction of, $\dot{V}O_{2max}$.

Maximal tests

Figure 12.18 and Table 12.4 provide details of several useful protocols for $\dot{V}O_{2max}$ assessment. Each of these protocols was designed for completion on a treadmill, using either online, or Douglas-bag expired-gas collection. Normal laboratory health and safety regulations should be followed throughout the test, including familiarising participants with regard to the nature of the $\dot{V}O_{2max}$ test and the specific details of the protocol. Following these laboratory protocols, a maximal field test for the estimation of $\dot{V}O_{2max}$ is discussed.

Bruce protocol

The Bruce protocol, illustrated in Figure 12.17, is a standard treadmill protocol that was originally developed in the 1970s. The protocol has a number of versions all of which can be used successfully with normal or high-risk populations. The original Bruce protocol, however, is best used with normal populations, while the modified and adapted versions are best

suited for use with high-risk populations. The tests are walking protocols, until the later stages, and rely on large increases in the gradient as a major component to the increase in load for each new stage. The modified Bruce has two additional stages at the start of the test to provide a staged introduction to the 10% gradient starting after the sixth minute. The adapted version of the Bruce was developed to reduce the load increase in the modified Bruce protocol that occurs at stage 5, where there is a combined treadmill speed and gradient increase. The Bruce protocol is an excellent maximal protocol to use in a health setting with high-risk populations. The following two protocols, the athlete-led and Sleivert, are better for use with athletic populations.

Athlete-led protocol

The athlete-led protocol (ALP) derives its name from the fact that the athlete controls the progression of the test. A summary of the test protocol can be seen in Figure 12.17. The test starts with an initial running speed of 6–8 km·h^{-1} at a 0% treadmill gradient. In this initial phase, the treadmill speed is increased by 1 km·h^{-1} at the end of each minute. This continues until the athlete points up with their index finger (rather than talking due to the presence

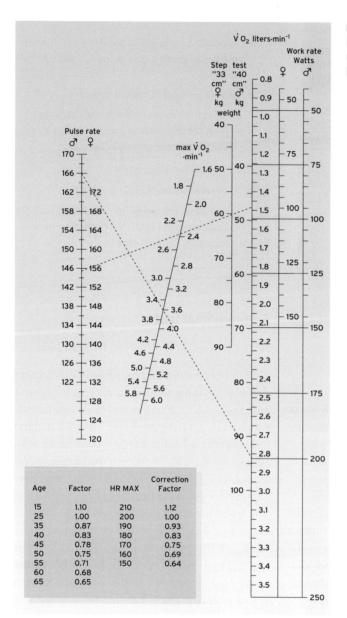

Figure 12.18 Åstrand-Åstrand nomogram. A line is drawn between the workload and heart rate (different for male and female) to reveal a predicted absolute $\dot{V}O_{2max}$ value.

of the mouth piece or face mask), indicating that he or she has reached their maximal cadence (running speed). From this point, the increasing load is applied by elevating the gradient of the treadmill. This commences phase two of the test where at the end of each minute the treadmill gradient is increased by 1%. This phase continues until volitional exhaustion or the tester ceases the test. The ALP is an ideal test protocol to use with runners during their training, including triathletes.

Sleivert protocol

The Sleivert protocol, detailed in Table 12.4, provides a novel method which can be applied to individuals with a wide range of fitness levels. Unlike the standard, one structure for all approach, found in tests such as the Bruce, the Sleivert provides alternative sub-protocols based on performance during the first two stages. The first stage involves walking on the treadmill for two minutes at a speed of 5 km·h^{-1} (0% gradient), which is followed by a four minute running stage at 10 km·h^{-1}. The participant's HR at the end of stage two is then used to decide whether the participant follows sub-protocol A, B, C or D as shown in Table 12.4. For example, if a participant's HR was 145 beats·min^{-1} at the end of stage two, he or she would follow sub-protocol B for the remaining duration of the test. This responsive style of protocol can result in the achievement of a higher $\dot{V}O_{2max}$ for normal or athletic

Table 12.4 Sub-protocols within the Sleivert treadmill protocol.

Sub-protocol A	Sub-protocol B	Sub-protocol C	Sub-protocol D
HR < 140	140 < HR < 150	150 < HR < 160	HR > 160
2 min stages	2 min stages	2 min stages	2 min stages
12 kph	11 kph	10 kph	9 kph
13 kph	12 kph	11 kph	10 kph
14 kph	13 kph	12 kph	11 kph
15 kph	14 kph	13 kph	12 kph
then increase gradient by 2% every 2 minutes until volitional exhaustion.			

➤ Athlete-led protocol (increase in speed followed by increase in gradient, the change occurs when indicated by athlete)
➤ Sleivert protocol (increases in speed)
  • Two initial stages (walking, then running)
  • Then complete one of four sub-protocols depending on HR response during initial stages

Maximal field running test for estimation of $\dot{V}O_{2max}$:

➤ Multistage Shuttle Run Test (MSRT)
  • Run 20-m shuttles in time to an audio cue (bleeps)
  • Time between bleeps decreases every minute, increasing running speed

populations. The test duration in the Sleivert protocol, however, might be too long (more than the ideal of 8–12 min) for experienced runners. In such cases the ALP might provide the most appropriate protocol.

Multi-stage shuttle run test (*MSRT*)

This test was developed as a convenient maximal field test to predict $\dot{V}O_{2max}$ that can be used with one or more subjects being assessed concurrently. A commercial package, which includes a compact disc (CD) to conduct the test, instructions and $\dot{V}O_{2max}$ prediction tables, is readily available and probably is a test familiar to many teachers, coaches and health professionals. It has been used by many sports teams and athletes including the English and New Zealand rugby and British judo teams. The MSRT was introduced in 1988. During a MSRT participants run 20 m shuttles between two marked lines keeping in time with increasingly faster beeps/bleeps on the MSRT CD. The point at which a participant drops out, or is pulled out from the test because of missing the line three times in a row is noted. The shuttle test result can be used in conjunction with a prediction table to identify the participant's estimated $\dot{V}O_{2max}$.

Key points

Maximal laboratory treadmill tests for the assessment of $\dot{V}O_{2max}$:

➤ Bruce protocol (combined increases in speed and gradient)
  • Original protocol – suited best to normal population
  • Modified and adapted protocols – suited best to high-risk populations

Sub-maximal tests

Åstrand-Åstrand aerobic fitness test

This aerobic endurance test, sometimes referred to as the Åstrand-Rhyming aerobic fitness test, is a laboratory-based sub-maximal assessment of aerobic fitness from which $\dot{V}O_{2max}$ can be predicted using a nomogram. The test is conducted using a cycle ergometer for which the applied resistance and cadence (pedal speed) can be altered. Once the seat height and handlebars have been adjusted for the participant they begin to pedal at 50 rpm. The initial workload should be set at 75–100 W for females and 100–150 W for men. The workload is then manipulated such that the participant's HR rises to between 130 and 170 beats·min^{-1}. Once the heart rate reaches the target zone the athlete continues to pedal for six minutes at that intensity. The HR should be recorded at the end of the fifth and sixth minutes. If it differs by less than five beats·min^{-1} the test is complete, whereas, if the difference is greater than this the test is continued until two consecutive heart rates are within five beats·min^{-1}. An Åstrand-Åstrand Nomogram is then consulted to identify the participants estimated $\dot{V}O_{2max}$. Figure 12.18 provides a nomogram where a line is drawn between the pulse rate (mean heart rate for the last two minutes of the test) and the work rate at which the performer was pedalling. The predicted $\dot{V}O_{2max}$ is read from the centre line. As HR has been demonstrated to decrease with age there is a correction factor included in the nomogram to account for differences in age. The score read from the centre line would be multiplied by the age correction factor to arrive at the estimated age adjusted $\dot{V}O_{2max}$.

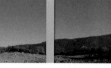

CALCULATION

Rockport walk example

A male aged 40 years with a mass of 85 kg completed the test in 13 mins with a final HR of 88 beats·min^{-1}. Their $\dot{V}O_{2max}$ prediction is calculated below:

$$\dot{V}O_{2max} = 6.9652 + (0.0091 \times 85) - (0.0257 \times 40) + (0.5955 \times 1) - (0.2240 \times 13) - (0.0115 \times 88)$$

$$\dot{V}O_{2max} = 6.9652 + (0.7735) - (1.028) + (0.5955) - (2.912) - (1.012)$$

$$\dot{V}O_{2max} = 3.3822$$

$$\dot{V}O_{2max} = 3.38 \text{ L·min}^{-1} \text{ (to convert to mL·kg}^{-1}\text{·min}^{-1} \times \text{ by 1000 and} \div \text{ by mass)}$$

$$\dot{V}O_{2max} = 39.79 \text{ mL·kg}^{-1}\text{·min}^{-1}$$

Rockport walk

This test is a further sub-maximal field test, the results of which can be used to predict $\dot{V}O_{2max}$. In this simple test participants complete a one-mile walk as quickly as possible. At the end of the test the performer counts their pulse for 15 seconds. This figure is then multiplied by four to give a minute value (beats·min^{-1}). The following equation can then be used to provide a predicted $\dot{V}O_{2max}$:

$$\dot{V}O_{2max} = 6.9652 + (0.0091 \times \text{mass}) - (0.0257 \times \text{age}) + (0.5955 \times \text{sex}) - (0.2240 \times \text{T1}) - (0.0115 \times \text{HR})$$

where mass = weight in kg, age = years, sex 1 = male, 0 = female, T1 = 1 mile walk time (minutes), HR = beats·min^{-1}.

Performance-related tests

In addition to the above measures and estimations of $\dot{V}O_{2max}$ as an assessment of aerobic fitness, a number of performance-related tests involving time to test completion or distance covered have been developed for athletes such as swimmers and rowers. These include race distance, T_5, T_{10} and T_{30} swims (distance swum in 5, 10 or 30 min), and 500 m, 1000 m and 2000 m timed distance tests (rowing). The key concept with these tests is the ability to closely match the requirements of the sport being tested. Research indicates that kayakers score higher, relatively, on a kayak ergometer than they do on a treadmill or a cycle ergometer, and higher still when they are tested in their own boats.

Specificity, which was discussed in more detail in Chapter 8, is as important for testing as it is for training.

Key points

Sub-maximal tests for the prediction of $\dot{V}O_{2max}$:

➤ Åstrand-Åstrand aerobic fitness test
  • Laboratory-based cycle test
  • $\dot{V}O_{2max}$ is predicted using a nomogram (line drawn between HR and work rate)
➤ Rockport walk
  • Field-based walking test
  • Complete a one mile walk as quickly as possible
  • An equation is used to predict $\dot{V}O_{2max}$
➤ Performance-related tests
  • Distance covered in a set time, or time to complete a set distance

Further measures of aerobic endurance

Although the $\dot{V}O_{2max}$ test has traditionally been the gold standard measure of aerobic endurance, it is now more common for exercise physiologists and coaches to use lactate threshold (LT), MLSS and critical power tests to assess aerobic fitness as it relates to race performance. Research indicates that the exercise intensity at which an athlete's LT, MLSS or critical power occurs is a more accurate predictor of race success than his or her $\dot{V}O_{2max}$ for aerobic endurance events such as 10 km running. Lactate threshold, MLSS and critical power testing were described in Chapter 11.

Knowledge integration question

What test would be most suitable to measure, or estimate, aerobic endurance in a group of individuals at risk of cardiovascular disease?

Metabolic rate

Estimation of metabolic rate

Heat from the combustion of the macronutrients can be measured using a bomb calorimeter to determine their calorific content (as described in Chapter 2). Our **metabolism** represents the sum of the reactions that take place within our bodies. The hydrolysis of ATP, which occurs to provide the energy for cellular work, is an exothermic process, resulting in energy being liberated in the form of heat. In theory, a calorimeter could be used to measure directly the heat produced through the reactions taking place in our bodies, i.e. our *metabolic rate*. The process of direct measurement of metabolism through the use of a calorimeter is difficult because humans do not liberate all the heat they produce. As a consequence, researchers have developed methods for the indirect determination of metabolism. One of the most commonly used methods is through gas analysis. The measurement of oxygen consumption ($\dot{V}O_2$) can be used, not only to assess an athlete's fitness ($\dot{V}O_{2max}$) and the predominant macronutrient for performance (RER), but it can also serve to inform exercise physiologists about an individual's metabolic rate.

In the original studies of metabolism, researchers brought participants into a laboratory overnight to examine their basal metabolic rate (BMR). The participants in such studies had to refrain from eating for 12 hours, be in a completely rested state and be assessed in a supine (on their back) position for a ten-minute period during which the gas collection is made. Analysis of the expired air samples was then used to determine the BMR. Subsequent research has shown there is little difference between a resting metabolic rate (RMR – as measured following 10 min of seated rest) and BMR. As a consequence, due to the cost involved in the determination of BMR, most researchers identify an individual's RMR before looking at the effect of exercise on the rate of metabolism. When 1 L of oxygen is used to oxidise a mixture of carbohydrate, fat and protein, about 4.8 kcal of energy is liberated. At rest a litre of oxygen is consumed every three minutes resulting in a consumption of around 20 L of oxygen an hour or around 450–480 L per day. This equates to average daily energy expenditure at RMR of 2,100–2,300 kcal. The recommended daily nutritional intakes (Table 2.11 in Chapter 2) were developed from similar estimates of average RMR. To maintain a stable weight, calorific intake must be balanced with energy expenditure.

Alternative methods of estimating energy expenditure

Metabolic equivalent

A further term often encountered with regard to energy expenditure is that of the metabolic equivalent (MET). The MET represents a further system for classifying the intensity of exercise based on RMR. One MET is equal to a resting oxygen consumption of 3.5 ml·kg^{-1}·min^{-1}. Exercise intensities can then be graded according to the number of MET units required for participation. For example, running at 9.6 km·hr^{-1} (6 miles·h^{-1}), not surprisingly, represents a higher energy expenditure of around 10 METs, than for walking with an energy expenditure of around 3 METs.

Heart rate

The linear relationship between oxygen consumption and heart rate at sub-maximal exercise intensities can be employed as a guide to energy expenditure. In a variety of sports, where it may not be possible to collect oxygen consumption data during participation, this relationship offers a method for the estimation of energy expenditure. If an exercise physiologist knows an individual's oxygen consumption and heart rate across a range of exercise intensities from laboratory testing, it is possible to infer the energy expenditure during exercise in the field from heart rate data. The limitations with this method occur due to the specificity of exercise. The exercise mode used in the laboratory testing must match that of the sport. For instance, research has indicated that for rowing – where there is a relatively high loading on the upper body – the use of treadmill running tests in the laboratory over-predict the oxygen consumption. The HR–$\dot{V}O_2$ relationship may be of limited use for researchers, but it can provide a guide to the energy demands of different sports for athletes and coaches, especially during the development of a body of research knowledge for a particular sport.

Key points

In practice, athletes and coaches commonly use HR as an indication of exercise intensity.

The metabolic equivalent (MET) can also give an indication of exercise intensity for a variety of activities including sports performance (1 MET = resting $\dot{V}O_2$ of 3.5 mL·kg^{-1}·min^{-1}, i.e. RMR).

Factors influencing metabolic rate

A variety of factors can influence resting metabolic rate. Higher levels of fat-free mass, body surface area, body temperature and stress all serve to increase RMR. Increasing age on the other hand has been shown to result in a linear decrease in RMR. It is thought that much of the decrease in RMR with age is related to a decrease in fat-free mass and an increase in fat mass associated with a sedentary lifestyle. Research has indicated that for individuals with an active lifestyle – those who exercise or train regularly – the age-related decrease in RMR is halted or at least slowed. The presence of thyroxine and adrenaline, associated with the onset of exercise, also serve to increase metabolism. In addition to the stimulation of metabolic rate by hormonal increases, exercise stimulates a general rise in metabolism, resulting in an increase in energy expenditure. Table 12.5 provides an overview of energy expenditures for a variety of sports and activities.

Fatigue in lower-intensity aerobic endurance sports

The predominant energy system for lower-intensity endurance activity performance is the aerobic system. The relative intensity of the sports that fall into this category would determine the predominant energy substrate – carbohydrate or fat. As exercise intensity increases above 50–60%

of maximum, fat stores alone can no longer provide the energy for exercise, with an increasing reliance on glycogen stores. The duration–intensity continuum for lower-intensity aerobic endurance sports is illustrated in Figure 12.1. For the sports illustrated within the higher-intensity section of the continuum, a contribution of glycogen supplies in addition to fat metabolism would be expected. This model, however, provides only a guide, and activities below the line could easily, and often by choice are, completed at an intensity level that necessitates a metabolic contribution from glycolysis.

Fatigue in lower-intensity activities occurs primarily due to glycogen depletion, often as a result of the long duration of the activity. The mechanism behind glycogen depletion and its effect on performance was described in Chapter 11. In some sports, such as mountaineering, where night-time starts may be required, the added fatiguing factor of sleep deprivation can impact on performance. This introduces a further aspect to fatigue that has not as yet been covered. In Chapters 9–11 the mechanisms behind fatigue have been described within a physiological context as they pertain to substrate depletion and impaired functioning at a muscular level. These aspects of fatigue constitute **peripheral fatigue**. Since the start of the 20th century researchers have become increasingly interested in the effects of **central fatigue** on performance. Research indicates that sleep deprivation does not have an impact on exercise metabolism (as long as substrate supplies are maintained), cardiovascular performance or muscular strength, but it does significantly increase feelings of fatigue. The feelings of fatigue at the end of a race day's activity, which can include pain, nausea and tiredness, are centrally located expressions of fatigue. Central fatigue involves an increase in the perceived effort required to complete a particular task, and a diminished drive to continue exercise. The complex nature of the physiology and biochemistry of the brain means that the mechanisms behind central fatigue are not fully understood. Any athlete, however, who has felt pain and the desire to stop exercising during a marathon or a day walking/tramping in the hills has felt the symptoms of central fatigue.

The brain monoamines, serotonin, dopamine and noradrenaline (neurotransmitters), play a key role in the transduction of signals between neurons, and exercise-induced changes in these compounds have been related to central fatigue. The exact mechanism of central fatigue remains unknown, although it is likely that interplay between these three neurotransmitter systems is involved. The catecholamines may play the more important role in the development of fatigue as brain dopamine and

Table 12.5 Estimates of energy expenditure for a variety of sports and activities for an individual with a body weight of 70 kg

Sport	Energy Expenditure (METS)	Energy expenditure (kcal·min^{-1})	Energy expenditure (kJ·min^{-1})
Activity promoting video game (e.g. Wii Fit, moderate intensity, aerobic, resistance)	3.8	4.44	18.60
Basketball game	8.0	9.35	39.15
Bicycling (<10 miles·h^{-1}, leisure)	4.0	4.68	19.57
Bicycling (mountain, uphill, vigorous)	14.0	16.37	68.51
Bicycling (RPM / Spin bike class)	8.5	9.94	41.59
Boxing (in ring, general)	12.8	14.96	62.64
Canoeing, rowing (moderate effort, 4.0 - 5.9 miles·h^{-1})	5.8	6.78	28.38
Canoeing, rowing (competition)	12.0	14.03	58.72
Cricket (batting, bowling, fielding)	4.8	5.61	23.49
Dancing (ballet, modern or jazz, general class or rehearsal)	5.0	5.85	24.47
Football (American)	8.0	9.35	39.15
Golf (walking, carrying clubs)	4.3	5.03	21.04
Hill climbing (carrying 15 kg pack)	6.3	7.36	30.83
Hockey (field)	7.8	9.12	38.17
Ice-skating (general)	7.0	8.18	34.25
Kayaking (moderate effort)	5.0	5.85	24.47
Martial arts (moderate pace)	10.3	12.04	50.40
Resistance training (multiple exercises, 8 - 15 reps at varied resistance)	3.5	4.09	17.13
Rock climbing (ascending rock, high difficulty)	7.5	8.77	36.70
Rowing (stationary, general, moderate effort)	4.8	5.61	23.49
Rugby union (competitive)	8.3	9.70	40.62
Running (4 miles·h^{-1})	6.0	7.01	29.36
Running (9 miles·h^{-1})	12.8	14.96	62.64
Running (14 miles·h^{-1})	23.0	26.89	112.55
Running (marathon)	13.3	15.55	65.08
Skiing (cross-country, moderate speed and effort)	9.0	10.52	44.04
Skiing (downhill, moderate effort)	5.3	6.20	25.94
Soccer (competitive)	10.0	11.69	48.93
Squash (competitive)	12.0	14.03	58.72
Swimming (breaststroke, recreational)	4.8	5.61	23.49
Swimming laps (freestyle, fast, vigorous effort)	9.8	11.46	47.96
Tennis (singles)	8.0	9.35	39.15
Track and field (e.g. shot, discus, hammer)	4.0	4.68	19.57
Track and field (e.g. high jump, long jump, triple jump, pole vault, javelin)	6.0	7.01	29.36
Track and field (e.g. steeplechase, hurdles)	10.0	11.69	48.93
Walking for exercise (3.5 miles·h^{-1}, level, brisk, firm surface)	4.3	5.03	21.04
Water aerobics	5.3	6.20	25.94
Water jogging	9.8	11.46	47.96
Water walking (moderate effort and pace)	4.5	5.26	22.02

MET = metabolic equivalent.
1 MET = 0.0167 kcal·kg^{-1}·min^{-1}
1 kcal = 4.186 kJ
Energy expenditure data from the 2011 Compendium of Physical Activities (http://links.lww.com/MSS/A82) as provided in Ainsworth et al. 2011.

noradrenaline levels have recently been reported to influence exercise performance. For more details on the involvement of these brain neurotransmitters on central fatigue and exercise performance at different environmental temperatures, refer to the recent review by Roelands and Meeusen (2010).

Key points

Fatigue in lower-intensity aerobic endurance sports can be due to:

➤ Peripheral fatigue – glycogen depletion

➤ Central fatigue – feelings of tiredness, pain and nausea

  • Linked with brain serotonin, dopamine and noradrenaline levels

---

Knowledge integration question

In what ways do fatigue mechanisms differ between lower-intensity and high-intensity aerobic endurance sports?

Physiological adaptations to aerobic training

The main physiological adaptations to aerobic training were described in Chapter 11. These adaptations would apply equally to the lower-intensity aerobic endurance activities that are the focus of this chapter. However, the extent of any adaptation will be dependent upon the duration, intensity and type of training undertaken. Research indicates that after a relatively short period of time, 6–12 months after training commences, most improvements in $\dot{V}O_{2max}$ will have been realised. After this period an individual can continue to improve their AAT through training at or just above the exercise intensity at which LT or MLSS occurs. After testing to identify an individual's LT or MLSS, the heart rate at which these occur can be used to guide the training intensity for future exercise. To continue improvements with LT/MLSS (and aerobic performance) interval training and continuous training provide the most useful methods to sustain training adaptations.

12.3 Ergogenic aids for lower-intensity aerobic endurance sports

As a result of the prolonged duration of some lower-intensity aerobic endurance sports, and the negative effects of glycogen depletion on performance, this section begins with a brief review of carbohydrate feeding strategies

during exercise. This is followed by a description of methods of improving aerobic performance, legal and illegal, including blood doping, the use of erythropoietin and altitude training.

Carbohydrate and electrolyte replacement during exercise

Employment of the carbohydrate loading strategies described in Chapter 11 provides an optimal glycogen starting point, above and beyond that achieved through a healthy balanced diet. Carbohydrate ingestion during lower-intensity aerobic endurance exercise can further manipulate glycogen stores and blood glucose levels. Thus, in addition to increasing carbohydrate intake prior to exercise, the use of carbohydrate drinks to maintain performance during a race or journey should be considered in a large number of sports. The long duration of many of the lower-intensity sports, such as adventure racing, also necessitates the use of food supplements to maintain performance. In this context the ingestion of a range of carbohydrate sources appears to provide the ideal mechanism for maintaining longer-term aerobic performance. The consumption of food items comprising complex as well as simple carbohydrates appear to help maintain blood glucose supply over time. A combination of breads, sandwiches, biscuits, fruit, snack bars and sweets can help to maintain carbohydrate levels during a longer-duration event or journey.

In addition to the use of carbohydrate drinks to refuel and hydrate the body during longer-duration sports, the replacement of electrolytes lost through sweating should be considered, particularly if exercising in a hot environment where sweating can be substantial. This is commonly achieved by athletes through the consumption of a combined carbohydrate-electrolyte drink. Sodium, potassium and chloride comprise the body's electrolytes. Electrolytes serve to maintain the fluid balance between the body's various intracellular and extracellular compartments. Longer-duration sports, especially those where either the clothing necessary or the environmental temperature encountered can result in prolonged periods of sweating, can lead to a marked sodium and chloride loss. In activities such as a long day walking/tramping or mountaineering, where the duration of exercise can be as long as 10–15 hours, sodium loss through sweating can present a significant problem.

Hyponatraemia, resulting from the ingestion of too much plain water and sodium loss through sweating, represents a potentially life-threatening condition. There have been incidences of hyponatraemia recorded after ironman and ultramarathon races. When extreme levels of sodium are lost through sweating, there is a reduction in the total concentrations available within the body to maintain intracellular and extracellular electrolyte balance. This situation is exacerbated by the ingestion of high volumes of plain water as dilution of the already low extracellular sodium level occurs. The dual effect of decreased sodium levels and intake of water can lead to an upset of sodium regulation in the body leading to a further reduction of extracellular sodium as sodium leaks into the intestine. Hyponatraemia can be prevented through the use of an electrolyte or combined carbohydrate-electrolyte drink during prolonged aerobic exercise. In multi-day events, such as mountaineering, research indicates that sodium levels can be maintained through normal dietary intake. Hyponatraemia is an extreme and relatively uncommon condition, but athletes involved in long-duration (10–15 hours) activities, particularly when they are performed in the heat, should be aware of the condition and its consequences. Maintaining hydration during prolonged endurance activities is crucial to minimise the negative effects of dehydration on performance. As has been illustrated above, the composition of the fluid consumed should be carefully considered to optimise fluid, fuel and/or electrolyte replacement depending on the demands of the sport and the environmental conditions.

Key points

Functions of carbohydrate and electrolyte replacement during low-intensity aerobic endurance exercise:

➤ Replace carbohydrate stores to delay fatigue
  - Food: complex and simple sources
  - Carbohydrate drink

➤ Replace electrolytes lost through sweating (particularly Na^+)

➤ Particularly important when exercising in the heat for a long duration

Knowledge integration question

Taking into consideration fluid, fuel and electrolyte requirements during prolonged exercise in the heat, what ergogenic aids would be most beneficial for performance optimisation?

Blood doping

Blood doping, the use of erythropoietin and altitude training are discussed together in this chapter because they all relate to a potential improvement in oxygen transport capacity. Blood doping, the infusion of red blood cells to improve performance, was first described as a potential ergogenic aid in the 1970s, and became a banned practice in 1984. It was initially developed as a method to improve aerobic endurance performance by increasing the number of red blood cells (increasing the haematocrit) and consequently improving an athlete's oxygen carrying capacity. More recently, research has shown that blood doping may also have a positive effect on thermoregulation.

Blood doping, also known as induced erythrocythaemia, blood boosting or blood packing, can be carried out using a reinfusion of the athlete's own blood or through an infusion of a matched donor's blood. The advantage of using autologous blood doping (an athlete's own blood) is that there is less risk of infection or disease from the re-infused blood. The disadvantages are that the initial donation of blood will have a negative effect on training and performance until the lost erythrocytes are replaced. The removed blood would need to be stored for re-infusion at a later date, a process that leads to damage to some of the blood cells. Conversely, there is an increased risk of disease from infusing a matched sample (heterologous blood doping), but no detraining effect and no loss of erythrocytes through the requirement to store blood.

Initially the results of blood doping studies, which were primarily carried out on autologous blood doping, were equivocal as to the potential benefits of this illegal ergogenic aid. More recent research indicated that a key factor that led to the mixed results was the method of blood storage. If an autologous blood sample (typically 2 units – 900 mL of blood) is stored in a fridge at 4° C around 7% of the red blood cells are lost each week. Given that a minimum period of eight weeks is required to restore the removed cells and to allow for a return to previous fitness levels, this would mean that 40–60% of the red blood cells would be lost (damaged) prior to re-infusion. As a consequence, studies using this method of storage were often unable to show any benefit from autologous blood doping. In contrast, freezing a prepared (centrifuged, removal of RBCs and re-suspension in glycerol) autologous blood sample in liquid nitrogen, enables samples to be stored indefinitely and reduces total erythrocyte loss to around 15%. When the blood is prepared and stored in this way, its re-infusion, whether autologous or fresh heterologous blood, has been seen to result in improved aerobic endurance performance.

The main benefit of blood doping, is an improved oxygen transport capacity. By increasing the number of red blood cells, and as a consequence the volume of haemoglobin, the amount of oxygen able to be transported and made available to the working muscles during exercise is increased. It is important to note, however, that such an improvement would only be achieved if the cardiac output could be maintained. If the increase in red blood cells and consequent increase in blood viscosity (loss of fluidity due to the increased proportion of cellular components) did not reduce cardiac output then the infusion of additional erythrocytes would be performance-enhancing.

A further performance enhancement through blood doping may be achieved due to a potential improvement in thermoregulation. During endurance performance an additional function of blood, besides supplying oxygen to the working muscles, is its thermoregulatory function. When the body temperature rises, particularly during prolonged exercise in the heat, some of the blood volume has to be diverted to the skin to aid heat loss. This blood, diverted to the skin for cooling purposes, would therefore not be available for the transport of oxygen to the working muscles. Through blood doping and the increased oxygen transport capability, a lower volume of blood could supply the oxygen to the muscles, hence the diversion of blood to the periphery for cooling would have a lesser effect on performance. The infusion of two units of blood can provide significant thermoregulatory and performance advantages for an athlete during aerobic endurance sports. Despite any potential performance benefit from blood doping, it is not without risks and is an illegal performance enhancement.

Erythropoietin

As was described in Chapters 2 and 6, erythropoietin (EPO) is a naturally occuring glycoprotein hormone produced primarily by the kidneys. Around 10% is produced elsewhere, mainly in the liver but also minimally by cells within the brain. Erythropoietin is the hormone responsible for the stimulation of red blood cell production and is transported via the plasma to specialist receptors on the surface of cells within the marrow cavity of the long bones. An increase in EPO production is stimulated by cellular hypoxia which can occur through the lysing (breakdown) of red blood cells or through blood loss from the body. On detection of hypoxia, the kidneys and liver are stimulated to increase erythrocyte production. When the normal number of red blood cells is restored the stimulus is removed. In this way a natural steady-state red blood cell level is achieved for each individual.

In the late 1980s a synthetic form of EPO was produced for the first time, originally developed for the treatment of patients with anaemia or renal failure. Recombinant human EPO (rHuEPO), as it is known, was quickly identified by athletes and coaches as a potential blood doping ergogenic aid. In response to this abuse of the drug, the International Olympic Committee (IOC) banned the use of EPO as a performance-enhancing substance. The abuse of EPO has been most closely been linked with the sport of cycling, where there are a number of sudden deaths, mainly through heart attacks, that have been linked with the drug. Tests for rHuEPO have now been developed for urine and blood samples. These tests have resulted in a number of athletes being caught and banned from the sport in which they participate.

The synthetic form of EPO works in the same way as endogenous EPO, stimulating erythrocyte production. This increase in red blood cells leads to a performance-enhancing increase in oxygen transport capacity. The danger associated with the use of this ergogenic aid is that by increasing the red blood cell count, the haematocrit can increase from a normal level of around 45% up to as much as 60% and beyond, and by doing so the viscosity of an athlete's blood also increases. This increase in haematocrit and blood viscosity puts an athlete at risk of stroke or heart attack, a risk that is enhanced as a result of the dehydration associated with aerobic endurance exercise.

Key points

Ergogenic aids to improve oxygen transport capacity:
➤ Blood doping
  • Infusion of blood to increase red blood cell number
➤ Erythropoetin
  • Hormone that stimulates red blood cell production
Although both ergogenic aids can improve performance, they increase the viscosity of the blood (increasing risk of heart attack) and are illegal procedures

Altitude training

Altitude training can bring about similar ergogenic effects as blood doping and EPO, except it is a legal regimen commonly used by elite athletes. Its consideration is therefore included in this section, while the general effects of altitude on physiological functioning are discussed in the following section on health and environmental aspects. As a consequence this section should be read in conjunction with the section on attitude in Chapter 15.

Does altitude training improve performance?

Prolonged exposure to altitude is associated with a rise in the number of red blood cells, and consequential improvement in oxygen transport capacity, which has led athletes to experiment with altitude training as a method for improving endurance performance. The theory behind this is that if an athlete trains at altitude for a period of time before returning to compete at sea level, the improved oxygen transport capacity should improve their endurance performance. In other words, the increase in the number of red blood cells with altitude training leads to an increased oxygen delivery to the working muscles and an improvement in sea-level race performance. As such, altitude training provides a legal method through which to bring about the effects of blood doping or EPO supplementation.

The results of studies, however, have been equivocal as to the success of altitude training. Some studies have reported significant improvements in sea-level endurance performance in response to altitude training. Other researchers have been unable to confirm these results with similar groups of athletes. It has been suggested that the mixed results arise because of the decrease in training intensity achievable during exercise at altitude. Research reveals that the physiological response to exercise is elevated at altitude, hence an athlete has to work harder to maintain any given workload. The average exercise intensity of training is therefore lower at altitude when compared with sea level. As is described in Chapter 15, the lower partial pressure of oxygen (PO_2) is responsible for the decreased ability to train at the same high intensity at altitude as can be performed at sea level. The reduced training load at altitude has been found to offset the benefits of improved oxygen transport capacity. In addition, the recipe for successful altitude training is further complicated by the need to identify (i) how long an athlete should stay at altitude to produce the best results, (ii) the most appropriate altitude at which to stay, (iii) how to offset the upset in an athlete's normal routine enforced by a stay at altitude, and (iv) the intensities of training that bring the best results.

Live-high train-low

The equivocal results achieved with pure altitude training have led researchers to investigate the benefits of live high-train low (hi-lo) strategies. In this type of training athletes spend most of their time living at altitude to stimulate the physiological benefits associated with prolonged altitude exposure, but return to sea level for training, thereby maintaining the intensity of training. Within the literature participants have either lived at altitude for acclimatisation or alternatively resided within a de-pressurised house, while some have slept in a hypobaric chamber or tent. These simulated altitude alternatives provide an opportunity for an athlete to experience the benefits of living at altitude without having to move away from their normal training environment. A research paper by Levine and Stray-Gundersen on the effects of HiLo training has been summarised to provide an insight into the performance benefits of such training (see pp. 385–6).

Knowledge integration question

For sea-level performance, what altitude training regimen is most beneficial, and why?

Key points

Altitude training:

➤ Increasingly used by elite athletes to naturally increase oxygen carrying capacity and improve performance

➤ Reduction in training intensity at altitude may off-set improved oxygen carrying capacity

➤ Live-high train-low strategy
  - Gain physiological benefits from living at altitude
  - Can maintain sea-level training intensity

Check your recall
Fill in the missing words.

➤ The _____ energy system provides a relatively inexhaustible energy supply.

➤ The primary mechanism for aerobic catabolism of fatty acids is _____.

➤ Deamination of _____ _____ leaves a carbon-based skeleton which can be used to generate energy.

➤ The Krebs cycle consists of _____ chemical reactions which take place within the _____ of the mitochondria.

➤ Carbohydrates and fats are broken down to _____ _____ for entry to the Krebs cycle.

➤ The most important product of the Krebs cycle, which is transported to the electron transport chain for the re-synthesis of ATP, is _____.

➤ The electron transport chain consists of _____ chemical reactions that end with the production of ATP and _____.

➤ Approximately _____% of the energy generated during the catabolism of carbohydrate or fat is converted to heat, resulting in increased body temperature during aerobic activities.

➤ The most common method used to determine metabolic rate is that of _____ _____.

➤ At rest, typical oxygen consumption is _____$L \cdot h^{-1}$ which equates to a daily energy expenditure of around _____ kcal. This is the resting metabolic rate (RMR).

➤ Energy expenditure during exercise is sometimes expressed as a metabolic equivalent (MET) value. One MET is equal to _____$mL \cdot kg^{-1} \cdot min^{-1}$, the assumed _____ _____ _____.

➤ Following laboratory testing, metabolic rate can be estimated from _____ _____, so long as the testing mode of exercise was _____ to the sport.

➤ During lower-intensity aerobic endurance exercise, the exercise intensity is generally such that a _____ _____ is reached.

➤ A higher intensity of exercise results in a greater reliance on _____ as the fuel source for ATP production.

➤ Fatigue generally occurs during low-intensity exercise as a result of _____ depletion.

➤ The majority of aerobic power adaptation to lower-intensity aerobic endurance exercise occurs within the first _____ to _____ months of training.

➤ If an athlete is continuously pushed too hard in training then over-reaching and ultimately_____ _____can occur, resulting in a decline in _____.

➤ During exercise, the consumption of a _____ drink and solid food can help to maintain performance.

Review questions

1. What are the primary degradation mechanisms for glycogen, triglycerides and amino acids that allow their use for ATP production in the Krebs cycle?

2. Which hormone catalyses the first two reactions in lipolysis?

3. Which hormones stimulate an increase in the rate of lipolysis?

4. Why is β oxidation aptly named?

5. What are the two products of the Krebs cycle that can be used to support lower-intensity aerobic endurance activity? How do these two products contribute to energy production?

6. How is the electron cascade related to the movement of hydrogen ions during the process of the electron transport chain?

7. Why is the movement of H^+ out of the mitochondrial matrix important for ATP production?

8. Why is oxygen essential to the functioning of the electron transport chain and the process of oxidative phosphorylation?

9. What is meant by Resting Metabolic Rate? What is the daily expected energy expenditure at RMR?

10. What measurement can be used as an indicator of aerobic training intensity other than blood lactate concentration? What physiological relationship justifies its use as a guide of exercise intensity?

Teach it!
In groups of three choose one topic and teach it to the rest of the study group.

1. Explain how the aerobic energy pathway is better suited for lower-intensity aerobic endurance sports than the anaerobic pathways. Describe the systems involved in the aerobic pathway with a focus on the amount of ATP produced.

2. Explain the structure of mitochondria and the location of β oxidation, Krebs cycle and the electron transport chain.

3. Explain the electron transport chain and oxidative phosphorylation.

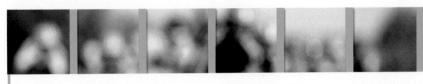

SPORT IN ACTION

Biography: Ben Ainslie OBE

Adventure sport: Sailing

Ben, born in Macclesfield, began sailing at the age of eight at Restronguet, near Falmouth in Cornwall. His father was a successful sailor and Ben quickly found success. At the age of 16 he became Laser Radial World Champion. Supported by his parents Ben was picked for the 1996 Olympic Games at the age of 19 where he won a silver medal. He has continued his career with great success winning many international medals and Gold at the Sydney, Athens and Beijing Olympic Games in Laser (2000) and Finn (2004 and 2008) classes. Ben has won nine European and World titles won the 2008 Finn Gold Cup for a record fifth time, he was also World Match Racing Champion in 2010. Ben has qualified for the 2012 London Olympic Games as well launching his own America's Cup Team BAR Racing, which will compete in the 2013 AC45 Event. He was made a CBE in 2009 and was named ISAF World Sailor of the year in 1998, 2002, 2008 as well as being British Yachtsman of the Year on five occasions.

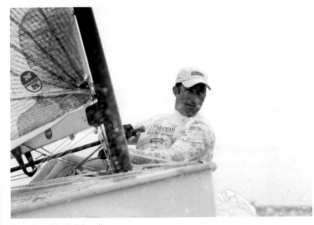

(*Source*: Mark Lloyd)

The 2005 Sydney– Hobart race

The Sydney to Hobart yacht race is often referred to as the world's toughest yacht race and one of the toughest races any in any sport. The history of the race is littered with stories of disasters or amazing feats of seamanship, in extraordinary conditions. This 600-mile race is particularly tough due to the unique and extremely challenging conditions the boats encounter as they cross Bass Straight, the body of ocean between Australia's southernmost tip and Hobart in Tasmania. Bass Straight is notorious to yachtsman around the world as the southerly running currents run against the weather fronts that produce 40-80 mph winds. The waves produced by this phenomenon are quite literally mountainous and the combination of wind and water can be deadly. The most race tragic of races was the 1998 Sydney–Hobart where the fleet of racers were caught in one of the biggest storms to hit Bass Straight in the 20th century. Four yachtsmen were lost, including Glyn Charles, a highly experienced Olympic yachtsman and a close friend.

I was invited to sail in the last Sydney–Hobart race on *Shockwave*, one of the biggest and most technically advanced racing yachts ever built. This boat is a far cry from the single-handed Finn dinghy in which I raced at the 2004 and 2008 Olympic Games. 'Shockwave' is one hundred feet long, ten times the size of my Finn and there were 24 crew in the team. Up until this race my offshore sailing experience was minimal and whilst I had proved myself at inshore racing, this was a big test! My father skippered a boat in the first Whitbread Around the World Race, so in a way I always felt that offshore sailing was in my genes but I wasn't one hundred per cent sure about how the race would play out.

The fleet of over one hundred and fifty boats started in idyllic conditions on Sydney Harbour on Boxing Day 2005. As we reached out of Sydney Heads the spectator fleet and the number of helicopters in the air astounded me. I had been involved in some pretty big races but this was unbelievable!

Normally the prevailing wind is southerly and this gives the boats a beat into the wind all the way to Tasmania. However, the weather gods were on our side and as we headed out to sea we took the lead over our sister ship *Wild Oats* and set a spinnaker, for a downwind sail. I was at the helm steering the boat and a cameraman came up to me to ask what I thought of my first Hobart race? 'Piece of piss, I don't know what all the fuss is about'. As soon as I said it I wished I had been a little more cautious as we still had over five hundred miles to sail to Hobart and I knew the history of the race.

My fears were realised on the second night at sea. The wind had built to 35 knots and the boat was screaming along at 30 knots in pitch-black conditions. I was off watch and below deck asleep as the boat flew into the back of a large wave dropping the speed from 30 knots to 8 knots. The result was that the spinnaker disintegrated into two and the bow frame was ripped away from the boat!! The next thing I knew I was on the bow of the boat in my thermal underwear, a place I really shouldn't have been but I wanted to help. We had no lifelines or any of the equipment we should have had but it was just one of those

situations you just have to deal with. Eventually we recovered the spinnaker and got the boat back on its feet. As we all got back to the safety of the cockpit some one started laughing and eventually the whole crew were laughing at the situation and relief that we had managed to get through it. The wipe out cost us badly and we ended up losing the race record and line honours to the very impressive *Wild Oats*.

Some time later I was watching a movie called the *The Worlds Fastest Indian*. In the movie the character played by Anthony Hopkins talks about risking everything for the buzz of being on his rusty old bike doing crazy speeds and really living, just for one minute! As I sat there I knew exactly what he meant. The experience of being on the edge like that will live with me forever.

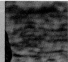

CLASSIC RESEARCH SUMMARY

Live high train low by Levine and Stray-Gundersen (1997)

Results regarding the effects of altitude training on subsequent sea-level performance have been equivocal. It has been suggested that the decreased training intensity associated with exercise at altitude lessens the effect of increased oxygen-carrying capacity. An ideal solution to this problem, to obtain the benefits of altitude living while maintaining the exercise intensity associated with sea-level training, would be to adopt a live-high train-low strategy. Levine and Stray-Gundersen conducted a classic study regarding the effects of a live-high train-low (hi-lo) regime as compared with live-high train-high (hi-hi) and live-low train-low (lo-lo), and their relative effects on performance.

The study, based in Dallas Texas (150m), but also using centres at Deer Valley Utah (high altitude – 2,500m) and Chula Vista, San Diego (sea level), was conducted with 39 male

and female distance runners (27 and 12 respectively). The exact protocol for the study is shown overleaf and included a two-week familiarisation (lead-in) phase where the athletes were brought together and introduced to the types of training to be used and familiarised with all the tests to be conducted during the study. After a four-week baseline training phase in Dallas, the athletes were randomly assigned to one of the three treatments. Twenty-six of the athletes travelled to Utah for hi-hi or hi-lo training while the remaining 13 athletes travelled to Chula Vista, designed to match the climatic conditions in Utah, but without the altitude. Tests conducted throughout the study included 5,000 m (5K) time trials conducted on a 400 m running track, various blood measures (plasma volume, blood volume, red cell mass and haemoglobin content), and assessment of $\dot{V}O_{2max}$.

The results indicated that the hi-hi and hi-lo protocols increased red cell mass (hi-hi: 27.9 to 31.7 ml·kg^{-1};

hi-lo: 26.2 to 29.6 ml·kg^{-1}, compared with a slight decline for the sea level (SL) athletes after the treatment phase) and haemoglobin content (hi-hi: 13.8 to 15.0 mg·dL^{-1}; hi-lo: 13.3-14.8 mg·dL^{-1}; lo-lo 13.6-14.1 mg·dL^{-1}). The alterations in oxygen-carrying capacity led to increases in $\dot{V}O_{2max}$ for the hi-hi (64.2 to 67 ml·kg^{-1}·min^{-1}) and hi-lo (62.4 to 66.3 ml·kg^{-1}·min^{-1}) athletes, whereas the lo-lo athletes decreased slightly (64.4 to 63.7 ml·kg^{-1}·min^{-1}). The physiological alterations, however, led to improved SL performances (5K race time) for only the hi-lo athletes. The performance of the hi-hi and lo-lo athletes decreased with slightly slower mean times recorded than were achieved prior to the treatment phase. The 13.4 second improvement for the hi-lo athletes represented a statistically significant difference than for the hi-hi and lo-lo athletes' times. These results indicate that hi-lo training has a performance advantage for

➤

endurance athletes. Living at altitude (2,500 m), but training at a lower altitude (1,200–1,400 m), results in improved endurance performance when compared with hi-hi and lo-lo training strategies.

This study provides important findings for consideration by coaches and performers taking part in competitive endurance adventure sports.

Reference: Levine, B.D. and Stray-Gundersen, J. (1997). 'Living high-training low': Effect of moderate-altitude acclimatization with low-altitude training on performance. *Journal of Applied Physiology*, 83(1), 102–12.

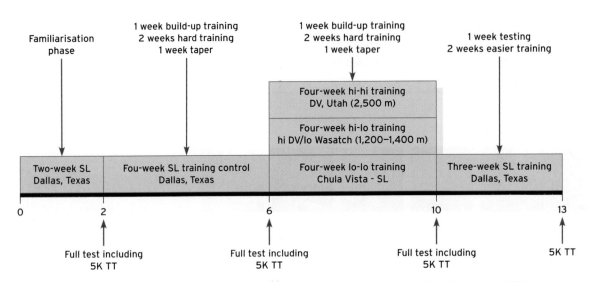

The study phases during the 13-week testing period. (*Source*: Adapted from Levine and Stray-Gundersen (1997))

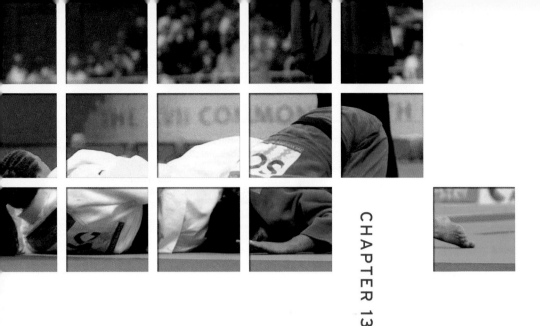

CHAPTER 13

Intermittent sports

Learning objectives

After reading, considering and discussing with a study partner the material in this chapter you should be able to:

➤ discuss the general physiology of intermittent sports in comparison to continuous sports

➤ describe key physiological research findings in the field of intermittent exercise

➤ compare and contrast the physiological demands of a range of intermittent sports

➤ identify a range of sport-specific fitness tests for intermittent sports

➤ apply knowledge of the sport, principles for testing and exercise physiology to adapt existing tests or devise novel tests to assess sport-specific fitness

This chapter covers the physiology of intermittent sports, as the variation in exercise intensities within these sports places demands on both anaerobic and aerobic metabolic pathways. Intermittent sports involve bursts of high-intensity exercise coupled with lower-intensity phases and/or periods of rest. The on-off nature of intermittent sports creates demands on the phosphagen system, glycolysis and the aerobic pathways.

A duration continuum for a number of intermittent sports is shown in Figure 13.1. The duration of intermittent sports can vary greatly for different events, and while the game duration can be as short as 20 minutes, for a canoe polo match, the longest tennis match was over 11 hours 5 minutes' duration (played over four days) between Nicolas Mahout and John Isner at Wimbledon, 2010. In addition to sports, interval and strength training sessions involve intermittent exercise and consequently also place demands on aerobic and anaerobic metabolism.

This chapter begins with a review of the general physiological responses to intermittent exercise and continues with a review of the physiology of a range of intermittent sports. Finally, we examine ergogenic aids for intermittent sports.

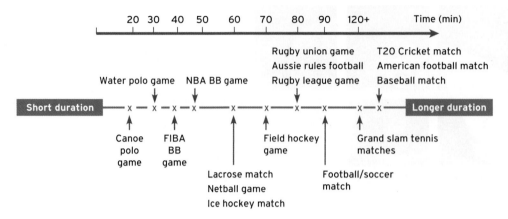

Figure 13.1 The duration continuum for intermittent sports. BB = basketball; NBA = National Basketball Association; FIBA = International Basketball Foundation; T20 = Twenty20.

13.1 General physiology of intermittent exercise

The physiology of intermittent exercise has been increasingly investigated since the 1960s. Intermittent exercise involves periods of exercise interspersed with rest or recovery periods. The past 50 years has seen a growth in the body of knowledge relating to the physiological demands, predominant energy systems and causes of fatigue in intermittent exercise. Researchers have manipulated exercise and recovery periods to examine their effects on oxygen consumption and the various substrates of metabolism, such as ATP, ADP, Pi, and lactate. With regard to exercise protocols, they have varied exercise intensity across three main levels. The exercise intensity has been set sub-maximally (below $\dot{V}O_{2max}$) at the same level as an individual's $\dot{V}O_{2max}$ (maximal), or supra-maximally, at an exercise intensity above the participant's $\dot{V}O_{2max}$. As was discussed in Chapter 9, maximal human power outputs are achieved in the first 2–4 s of activity. The vertical jump or the Wingate anaerobic test (WAnT) (explained in Chapters 9 and 10, respectively) provide laboratory measures of maximal power output. Peak power outputs, which can exceed 1,000 W, are achieved in the first 2–4 s of a WAnT. The $\dot{V}O_{2max}$ test provides a measure of aerobic power, the value of which tends to be around 25–50% of that achieved in a power test such as the WAnT.

The available research data regarding intermittent activities has been largely obtained through laboratory-based studies with careful manipulation of specific variables. The manipulated variables in intermittent exercise studies include the mode of exercise, exercise intensity, exercise duration, recovery duration and the number of work intervals (the duration of the test). Laboratory-based studies have been most commonly conducted on a cycle ergometer or a treadmill. The advantage with these laboratory-based studies relates to control over extraneous variables and

being able to form regularised exercise protocols, e.g. 10 times six-second sprints with a 30-second recovery between each repetition. Through this approach, a great deal has been learned regarding the physiological response to these types of intermittent activity. The disadvantage of this approach, however, relates to the fact that none of the sports covered in this chapter (except in training) have regulated exercise periods. The exercise and recovery periods during rugby or netball, for example, are dictated by the flow of the game. A player may be involved in the game for a period of time before getting a recovery, and each recovery phase will vary in length. This non-regulated pattern is similar to the coffee-grinding required by crew members in match racing (sailing). A crew member may have to make several changes of sail in quick succession, before a longer rest period occurs. This needs to be kept in mind when reading about the general physiological response to intermittent sport.

In the field, researchers studying sports like football/soccer have employed the use of video analysis, heart rate monitors and global positioning system (GPS) tracking devices, along with software such as Silicon Coach, Gamebreaker and Dart Fish to examine the physiological demands of the sport. The data collected provides information regarding the distances covered, speeds of travel during a match and the extent of fatigue within a sport-specific environment. The availability of these forms of technology has enabled a much broader development in field-based research than was possible in the 1960s. The specific physiological responses to a number of sports, often including these forms of technology, are described in the next section.

Physiological demands of intermittent exercise

The duration of a sport will have a direct impact upon the physiological demands and the exercise intensity that can be maintained. Intermittent sports rely on energy production from anaerobic and aerobic metabolism. The predominant energy system for any specific activity is determined by the duration of the sport. For example, a short-duration (20 minutes) canoe polo match will likely involve a higher ratio of high-intensity to low-intensity exercise compared with a longer-duration sport, such as soccer (90 min), hence energy system predominance will differ. Research shows that intermittent sports rely on ATP synthesis via the phosphagen system, fast-rate glycolysis and aerobic metabolism. This section goes on to describe findings regarding the predominant energy system for specific intermittent exercise.

Key research findings

Variations of exercise and recovery characteristics

One of the first studies to examine the physiological responses to intermittent exercise was conducted in 1960 by Christensen and colleagues. The exercise intensity was set at a high intensity level such that exhaustion was reached within 5 min of continuous exercise. During four minutes of continuous running on a treadmill at that exercise intensity the participants were able to complete 1,300 m with a rise in blood lactate concentration to 16.85 mM and a mean oxygen consumption of 5.6 L·min^{-1}. On three subsequent days the participants completed one of the following 30-min intermittent exercise protocols; one with 10 s exercise matched with 5 s recovery (10/5), one with 10 s exercise to 10 s recovery (10/10) and lastly one with 15 s exercise with 30 s recovery (15/30). The exercise intensity was kept the same for the intermittent activity sessions as during the 4-min continuous run. All three exercise protocols resulted in a lower lactate level (4.94 mM, 2.25 mM and 1.80 mM) at the end of exercise than for the continuous exercise (16.85 mM) and the participants were able to complete the 30-min sessions at an intensity that would have caused exhaustion within five minutes of continuous running. The 10/5 intermittent protocol enabled the furthest distance to be covered within the 30 minutes (mean distance run 6,670 m) and included 120 exercise intervals resulting in a total work time of 20 min – this at an intensity that would have caused fatigue within 5 minutes of continuous running.

In 1967 Karlsson and co-workers completed a study examining the effect of varying exercise intensity on the physiological response to intermittent exercise. In this study, with 20 s exercise and 10 s recovery periods, the exercise intensity was manipulated to examine the effect

on rate of fatigue. The influence of exercise intensity on exhaustion was clearly demonstrated through the results of one participant, who ran for one hour at a speed of 22 km·h^{-1}, but could only sustain exercise for 25 min when the intensity was raised to 22.75 km·h^{-1}.

In a study by Margaria et al. (1969), with a supra-maximal exercise intensity that would cause fatigue in 30–40 s of continuous exercise, the recovery interval between the 10 s exercise periods was manipulated. When an exercise-to-recovery ratio of 1:3 (10 s exercise, 30 s recovery) was used, a much lower elevation of blood lactate concentration above resting levels was achieved when compared with a 1:1 (10 seconds exercise, 10 seconds recovery) protocol where lactate concentrations rose progressively throughout the test.

The duration of the exercise, as well as the exercise intensity and recovery duration, were shown to be important in intermittent exercise through research conducted by Saltin and Essén (1971). In their study, exercise intervals of 10 s and 20 seconds with recovery periods of 5 seconds and 10 seconds (2:1 ratio) respectively, initiated only slight rises in blood lactate concentrations above resting levels. When the exercise intervals were for 30 and 60 seconds duration, higher rises in mean lactate concentration were found.

Key points

Sports of an intermittent nature:

➤ Rely on both anaerobic and aerobic metabolism – predominant energy system determined by the duration of the sport

➤ Physiological demands are influenced by

- Exercise intensity – higher intensity, less time to fatigue
- Exercise duration – longer duration, greater rise in blood lactate level
- Recovery duration – shorter recovery, greater rise in blood lactate level

➤ Total work time achievable is greater compared to continuous exercise at the same exercise intensity

---

Knowledge integration question

What effects do exercise intensity and duration, and recovery duration have on the metabolic demands of intermittent exercise?

Energy pathways for intermittent sports

As the intermittent exercise research has developed, researchers have moved on to examine in more detail, and extrapolate from findings, implications about substrate utilisation during exercise. In a study by Essén and co-workers (1977) a comparison was made regarding lactate concentrations, ATP and PCr stores in the muscle, between continuous and intermittent exercise. After identification of $\dot{V}O_{2max}$, the five individuals in the study completed two cycle ergometer protocols, one continuous and one intermittent. The intermittent protocol involved an exercise-to-rest ratio of 1:1 for 1 h. Workload for the intermittent exercise bouts was that which elicited $\dot{V}O_{2max}$ (average of 299 W). During the continuous protocol the participants again cycled for 1 h with the exercise intensity set at 55% of $\dot{V}O_{2max}$ (average of 157 W) to maintain a matched mean intensity for the two tests. In both the continuous and intermittent protocols a small increase in muscle lactate occurred within the first 5 min of exercise with little difference thereafter. Despite little difference in muscle lactate levels, large fluctuations in ATP and PCr stores occurred between exercise and rest throughout the intermittent exercise protocol. After 5 min of exercise the PCr stores, for example, fell to 40% of their resting levels, but during recovery were replenished to 70% of their original level. These changes in PCr stores were similar throughout the hour of exercise for the intermittent exercise protocol. During the continuous exercise, however, the levels of ATP and PCr were maintained at a level that was 50% higher than during intermittent recovery. Indeed, intermittent exercise, conducted at the same mean running speed as continuous exercise, has been shown to be more energy-demanding (Bangsbo, 1994).

Further conclusions drawn by Essén, from this and later research, relate to differences in fat oxidation and muscle fibre type recruitment between intermittent and continuous exercise. Intermittent and continuous exercise tend to result in similar patterns of glycogen usage during exercise; however, fat oxidation appears to be elevated in intermittent exercise.

In 1993 Gaitanos and co-workers published important findings regarding intermittent exercise which feature in the 'Classic research summary' on p. 432. In their study, participants completed ten 6 s sprints on a cycle ergometer at a supra-maximal workload with a 30 s recovery between each sprint. Quantifying the fall in peak power across the sprints they identified a mean drop of 33% between the first and last sprint. Muscle biopsy analysis revealed distinct changes in energy system contribution to total energy production between the 1st and the 10th sprint. Hydrolysis of ATP stores represented a 6.3% (sprint 1) and 3.8% (sprint 10) contribution to total energy utilisation which represented around a 2% change between the 1st and the 10th sprint. The largest metabolic changes, however, from the 1st to the 10th sprint, were the breakdown of PCr (phosphagen system) and glucose/glycogen (glycolysis). The relative energy contribution from glycolysis fell from 44.1% to 16.1% and the magnitude of PCr breakdown rose from 49.6% to 80.1% between the first and last sprint. These findings suggest that, as the duration of exercise increases, the relative contribution of glycolysis to energy production decreases. The relative decrease in glycolysis is reflective of the drop in peak power output during repeat sprints and places a greater relative demand on PCr catabolism and aerobic metabolism.

In 1996 Bogdanis et al. investigated the effects of two repeated cycle sprints on muscle metabolism (30 s duration, with a 4 min recovery between efforts). They found an alteration in the anaerobic and aerobic contributions to total energy production between the two sprints. In the second sprint, where there was an 18% mean decrease in total work, Bogdanis et al. found a 41% mean decrease in anaerobic contribution to total energy production. This decrease was to some extent offset by a 15% mean increase in aerobic contribution. These findings are in agreement with Gaitanos et al. who also found alterations in anaerobic and aerobic contributions to total energy production for repeat sprints. Interestingly, Bogdanis et al. also found a significant correlation ($r = 0.84$) between PCr resynthesis during recovery and subsequent power output. The researchers suggested that the power output that can be achieved in a subsequent sprint is related to the level of PCr resynthesis. This finding links in with recent findings reported by Ostojic et al. (2010) who investigated heart rate recovery (HRR) following maximal exercise for intermittent and aerobic endurance (continuous exercise) athletes. Ostojic et al. found the intermittent athletes had a significantly lower HR during the first 20 s of recovery when compared with the endurance athletes. This data suggests that there is an alteration not only in aerobic and anaerobic contribution between sprints, but this also may result in a trained difference for athletes taking part in intermittent sports.

In the year 2000, the energy expenditure of a continuous run and differing intermittent protocols was investigated by Bisciotti and colleagues. The study participant ran at $5\ m \cdot s^{-1}$ and covered 1 km in the following four protocols: a continuous run, 20 reps of 50 m, 50 reps of 20 m, and 100 reps of 10 m. The continuous run expended 69.3 kcal of energy, which was increased by 32%, 79.9% and 159.8%, respectively, during the intermittent protocols. This study clearly demonstrates that intermittent running increases energy expenditure above that of continuous running, and that an increase in the number of starts and stops increases the amount of muscular work. This is particularly relevant to intermittent sports which include many acceleration and deceleration movements.

Summary of research findings

It is worth summarising the findings of these studies as they reveal much about the physiology of intermittent exercise. It is possible for a performer to maintain a given work intensity for a greater total during intermittent compared with continuous exercise. An individual can perform intermittent exercise for an hour or more at a maximal or supra-maximal exercise intensity, which would cause fatigue within a few minutes if performed continuously. The exercise intensity, length of exercise bout and recovery duration will determine the time to exhaustion and the blood lactate response in intermittent activities. The closer the exercise intensity is to maximal power output and the shorter the recovery periods, the greater will be the drop in peak power output over subsequent sprints. On the other hand, the duration of the intermittent exercise, as well as impacting upon the intensity maintained, will alter the relative contribution of aerobic and anaerobic metabolism to performance.

In the early stages of intermittent exercise, glycolysis plays a greater relative role in energy production when compared with continuous exercise; this is reflected by the higher initial lactate levels. As the duration of intermittent exercise continues, the relative contribution of glycolysis is decreased, while the importance of PCr breakdown and aerobic metabolism (particularly of fat oxidation) is increased. Intermittent exercise has been shown to provide a greater utilisation of fat oxidation than continuous exercise. It is believed that this occurs as a result of the recovery periods in intermittent exercise which enable the replenishment of myoglobin and haemoglobin oxygen stores during each rest period, allowing for greater fat oxidation. In effect this represents an improved 'priming' of the aerobic system. This finding has led researchers to examine the possibilities of intermittent exercise as an improved exercise mechanism for weight loss. The results of such research are presented in the health section in Chapter 4.

It appears that PCr and glycogen provide the main sources of energy during intermittent exercise, while fat oxidation and blood glucose provide the substrates for the recovery periods. With regard to muscle fibre type, research suggests that intermittent exercise results in the recruitment of type I and II fibres as opposed to the mainly type I fibres recruited during continuous exercise. Further research is required, particularly for specific sports, to determine the effects of intermittent exercise in a game or match situation. The key finding to date is perhaps that, whereas for the sports that are the focus of the other chapters in part II of this book (where one energy system tends to be predominant), for intermittent sports aerobic and anaerobic metabolism will predominate at different points in time. The exact contribution of each is determined by the duration and intensity of the exercise periods along with the length of recovery periods. For example, the nature of energy production for a canoe polo game (20 min) might differ from that for a soccer match (90 min). Importantly for training, players, teachers and coaches should be aware of the specific physiological demands of not just the sport itself, but the position a particular athlete plays. The physiological demands for a midfield player may be very different compared to those for a forward within the team. As a consequence, the programme devised for an individual player should reflect the demands of the sport and each unique position.

From research to reality

As is described in more detail below, in the section on tests for intermittent sports players, developments in technology have enabled more in-depth analysis of the time and motion for specific sports, player positions and ability levels. We will examine some of these in more detail in the sport-specific physiology sections which follows later in this chapter. Research findings are now available for a variety of sports and provide useful insights into the dynamics of time and motion. In team sports such as hockey, rugby and football/soccer the duration of maximal sprints is often much less (around 2–3 s) than the 6 s of all-out efforts completed by athletes in the Gaitanos et al. study. This has implications regarding the application of their results to these sports, although research on racquet sports (tennis, badminton and squash) shows that typically, an average of between 5–10 s is spent in high-intensity exercise (rallies), with these findings more closely linked to Gaitanos et al.'s sprint duration.

In reality, the nature of many intermittent sports means that players use a number of different speeds or intensities of effort, rather than all-out effort throughout. Time and motion analyses reveal different patterns of high to lower intensity ratios for invasion (field) and racquet sports. In invasion sports the ratio varies between 1:6 and

1:14, whereas for racquet sports the ratios are more closely grouped between 1:1 and 1:5. The results of time and motion analyses are discussed in more detail below, as they relate to specific intermittent sports. The nature of a sport or position will clearly have implications for the time and motion dynamics which in turn are likely to affect the relative contribution of anaerobic and aerobic metabolism to total energy production.

Key points

Intermittent sports:

➤ Progressive decline in energy production from glycolysis and increased reliance on ATP-PCr system

➤ Recovery periods

- Enable partial restoration of muscle ATP and PCr stores
- Allow for oxygen replenishment – enabling increased fat metabolism compared with continuous exercise

---

Tests for intermittent sports players

There are a number of testing methods which have been developed in recent years to assess intermittent sports players. In this section we describe time and motion analysis (TMA), the intermittent anaerobic running test (IAnRT), the prolonged high-intensity intermittent running sport simulation (PHIIRSS), and the Yo-Yo intermittent recovery test (Yo-Yo).

Time and motion analysis

Developments in technology have enabled researchers to complete detailed analyses of the movement and exercise intensities for a variety of sports. Time and motion analyses are not a new phenomenon in sport, going back to notational analyses conducted in countries such as the former East Germany, where for sports like judo, real-time data was captured by coaches to provide feedback to players based on their performance in a particular fight. The development of video, software programmes, accelerometers and GPS tracking devices have enabled a far more detailed analysis of a player's performance and increasingly, this data is available in real time. These developments enable athletes, coaches and exercise scientists to have a far more complete picture of a player's performance during a game rather than afterwards.

Time and motion analyses have now been conducted for a wide range of sports including football/soccer, Aussie rules football and canoe polo. One of the key aspects that is necessary when comparing data is the methodological differences that exist between studies. For instance, researchers in different studies have set the boundaries for intensities of exercise by different methods (HR relative to HR_{max} versus speed relative to maximal sprint speed) and systems of categorisation.

The developments in tracking systems, such as the VXSport system illustrated in Figure 13.2, provide exciting opportunities for examining more closely the demands of specific sports, players' positions and differences between ability levels. The VXSport units illustrated have been used by the New Zealand All Blacks, Leicester City Football Club, the England cricket team and recently by World Champion surfer Kelly Slater at the Quicksilver Pro Gold Coast. Research findings indicate that the VXSport provides a valid and reliable tracking device for use in continuous sports, as well as for the intermittent sports that are the focus of this chapter. If the exercise intensities can be standardised for each sport (and ideally across sports where possible) this will make comparison between studies an easier process for athletes, coaches and exercise scientists.

Intermittent anaerobic running test

The IAnRT was developed by Psotta et al. (2005), primarily as a test for football/soccer players. It was designed as a sport-specific test of intermittent exercise ability, the protocol for which is shown in Figure 13.3. A test preparation phase is conducted prior to two testing phases. In preparation for the test a 10-min warm-up, including running and stretching exercises, followed by two sub-maximal 20 m sprints, is conducted. Three minutes after completion of the warm-up the participant completes the maximal sprint phase which involves a further two 20 m sprints, this time at maximal speed to assess individual sprint performance. In order to improve the accuracy of timing, gates should ideally be used for each part of the test. The timing gates should be set up 20 m apart with a 10 m run-out at either end for safe deceleration.

The starting line for each of the sprints should be standardised, placed 30 cm behind the line of the timing gates. The recovery between each sprint, as shown in Figure 13.3, should be measured using a handheld stop-watch and the athlete counted down into the next sprint.

The second phase of testing, the IAnRT, starts 2 min after the maximal sprint phase. It involves 10 maximal 20 m sprints with 20 s rest between repetitions. The time for each sprint is recorded. From this data a number of parameters can be calculated to analyse intermittent sports

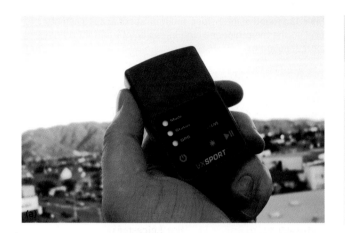
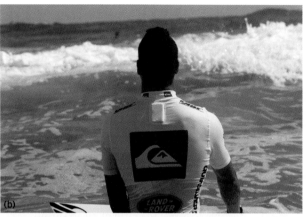
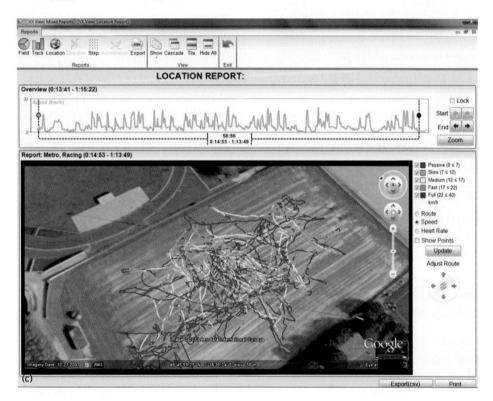

Figure 13.2 (a) Illustration of a performance tracking device, the VX Sport system which can be used as part of time and motion analysis, (b) VX Sport system in use, and (c) sample VX Sport data. (*Source*: Jamie Tout)

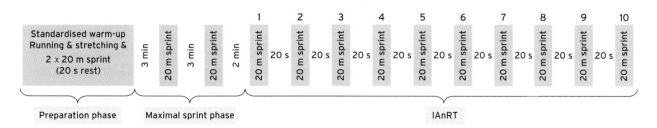

Figure 13.3 Protocol for the Intermittent anaerobic running test. The length of the recovery between each sprint is provided between each sprint box in the figure. (*Source*: Adapted from Psotta et al. (2005))

performance. After conversion of the times to running speeds (velocities), the decline in running velocity (ΔV – change in velocity) during the IAnRT can be calculated by finding the mean velocity of the last two sprints and taking this away from the mean velocity for the first two sprints (mean of sprint 9 and 10 – mean of sprint 1 and 2):

$$\Delta V(m \cdot s^{-1}) = [(V_9 + V_{10})/2] - [(V_1 + V_2)/2]$$

Secondly, the fatigue index, the percentage decline in velocity across the test, can be calculated from the formula:

$$FI\% = (\Delta V/mean\ V_{1+2}) \times 100$$

Lastly, it is possible to assess the ratio of mean sprint velocity (across all 10 sprints) to the mean for the first two sprints, which can be calculated as follows:

$$(mean\ V_{1+2+3+4+5+6+7+8+9+10})/(mean\ V_{1+2})$$

Psotta et al. found the IAnRT to provide a valid and reliable measure of intermittent anaerobic ability for soccer players. However, given the results of time and motion analyses for a number of intermittent sports such as rugby union and rugby league, it may be that the test has application to a number of sports. This premise would require further investigation, and it would also be worthwhile to examine the validity and reliability of the test with adult football/soccer players of varying abilities in a larger-scale study (the study was conducted with 29 adolescent elite level football/soccer players).

Prolonged high-intensity intermittent running sport simulation

The PHIIRSS was developed by Sirotic and Coutts (2007) and is based on time and motion analysis data for the sports of field hockey, football/soccer, rugby union and rugby league. For the sport simulation, five exercise intensities were selected based on maximal sprint running speed to accompany resting/standing periods within a game simulation of 2×15 min. The relative exercise intensities for the simulation are shown in Table 13.1.

Sirotic and Coutts divided the intensities into aerobic (standing, walking, jogging and running) and anaerobic (fast running and sprinting). Results of time and motion analyses were then used to assign a 9.5:1 ratio between aerobic and anaerobic activity, the proportion of time spent in each activity and the duration for each phase, as shown in Table 13.1. A computer software programme is then used to randomise the sequence for each of the 15-min exercise periods such that the pattern of activity

Table 13.1 Relative intensities and time spent at each activity level during the prolonged high-intensity intermittent running sport simulation.

Activity	MSS$_{relative}$ intensity	Proportion of time	Duration of activity
Resting/standing still	0%	17%	8 s
Walking	20%	34%	8 s
Jogging	35%	27%	8 s
Running	50%	13%	6 s
Fast running	70%	4%	4 s
Sprinting	100%	5%	3 s

MSS = maximal sprint speed

matched that for a game situation. The simulation was completed on a non-motorised treadmill, after having previously measured each athlete's maximal sprint speed. Maximal speed was determined by assessing speed for 3×6 s sprints with a 2-min recovery between each sprint. The results of the sprint test were used to determine the required speed for each exercise intensity level. Computer software then provided a beep at the start of each phase and a further beep system indicated the speed for the next phase. Data that can be recorded for each individual during or after the test include mean HR and capillary lactate concentrations. Results from tests can be used to compare between athletes and also between phases of training.

Yo-Yo intermittent recovery test

The Yo-Yo test was developed by Bangsbo (1994) for the sport of football/soccer, but more recently has been validated by Castagna et al. (2008) for use with basketball players. The test involves the use of a pre-recorded audio track which provides beeps to control the pace of the test in a similar way to the multi stage shuttle run test which was described in Chapter 12. The test has been developed with two possible levels, the choice of which is made according to the ability and fitness of the athletes, with level 1 starting at 10 km·h^{-1} and level 2 for fitter participants starting at 13 km·h^{-1}.

The prescribed warm-up for the Yo-Yo should be the first four running bouts of the test carried out 5 min before the start of the test. The participant would then recover ready for the start of the test. The Yo-Yo intermittent

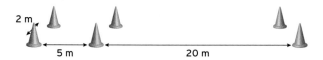

2 m

5 m   20 m

Figure 13.4 The set-up for the Yo-Yo recovery test.

recovery test requires participants to complete 40 m (out and back) shuttles interspersed by a 10 m (out and back) active recovery. The course set-up for the Yo-Yo test is shown in Figure 13.4. A player continues to complete the 2×20 m shuttle followed by 2×5 m recovery sequence until they can no longer keep pace with the audio track.

The stage and speed level at which a player twice fails to reach the finishing line in time should be recorded as his or her result. The booklet accompanying the CD for the test also provides a total distance that would have been covered at each stage and level. These results can be used for comparative analysis with other players or subsequent tests.

Key points

Common tests for the assessment of intermittent sports players:

➤ Time and motion analysis (TMA)

➤ Intermittent anaerobic running test (IAnRT)

➤ Prolonged high-intensity intermittent running sport simulation (PHIIRSS)

➤ Yo-Yo intermittent recovery test (Yo-Yo)

Fatigue in intermittent sports

The mechanisms for fatigue in intermittent sports relate to the duration of exercise. In short-term, higher-intensity intermittent activities a variety of mechanisms for fatigue have been postulated that lead to an interruption in the contractile processes or an inhibition of excitation–contraction coupling. In prolonged intermittent sports of over 90 min duration it is likely that glycogen depletion forms one of the major mechanisms behind fatigue. The specific mechanisms, however, still require further research.

In Chapter 9, Ca^{2+} transport disruption and PCr depletion were described as possible mechanisms for fatigue in power endurance sports. The role of increases in H^+ and Pi concentration, along with citrate leakage

from the mitochondria, were described in Chapter 10 as inhibitors of glycolysis during anaerobic endurance sports. Intermittent exercise research indicates H^+, Pi and citrate concentrations are increased in response to repeated sprints. As a result, each of the above mechanisms, have been cited as possible causes of fatigue in short-term, high-intensity intermittent sports. In addition, recent studies have suggested that the leakage of K^+ from within the sacroplasm into the extracellular fluid (surrounding each muscle fibre) is a possible mechanism for fatigue in high-intensity sports. As was described in Chapter 3, the Na^+-K^+ pump establishes a resting potential for nerve impulse conduction and muscle fibre contraction. The Na^+-K^+ pump, shown in Figure 3.6, transports Na^+ to the outside of the cell membrane into the extracellular fluid and transfers K^+ into the cell. This movement of ions is important for the establishment of a resting membrane potential. Research has identified increased interstitial K^+ concentrations at the point of fatigue and consequently it has been suggested that these rises create a decrease in the resting membrane potential and disruption to excitation–contraction coupling (which was described in Chapter 4).

Glycogen stores in the muscles and liver represent a major substrate for ATP synthesis during exercise. During high-intensity aerobic endurance sports (Chapter 11), lower-intensity but longer-duration aerobic sports (Chapter 12) or prolonged intermittent sports, the body's glycogen stores can become depleted. The depletion of glycogen stores leads to a detrimental decrease in substrate availability and has been linked with fatigue in many high-intensity or long-duration sports. Research indicates that during running, glycogen stores are used 40 times faster than during walking. It is for this reason that an individual's glycogen stores can be sufficient to climb a 1,000 m peak, but can become depleted during a kayak or road marathon. Research shows that performers perceive exercise as more fatiguing when operating in a glycogen depleted state. The feeling of 'hitting the wall' in high-intensity aerobic endurance sports, such as in the later stages of a marathon (at around 17–22 miles) or towards the end of a long day in the mountains, can largely be attributed to glycogen depletion. Glycogen depletion can have a significant negative effect on performance in intermittent sports and lead to increased feelings of fatigue. A number of studies, however, indicate that carbohydrate loading before exercise and glucose intake during exercise can delay the incidence of glycogen depletion. Strategies for delaying or avoiding glycogen depletion were described in Chapter 11 in the section on ergogenic aids.

Key points

Potential mechanisms of fatigue in intermittent sports:

➤ Shorter-duration activities

- Inhibition of excitation–contraction coupling or interruption of the contractile process
- Possible factors involved: increases in H^+, citrate leakage, Ca^{2+} transport disruption, PCr depletion, and K^+ leakage

➤ Longer-duration activities

- Glycogen depletion

Training and recovery in intermittent sports

The adaptations to training for intermittent sport athletes are determined by the nature of the training undertaken. A time and motion analysis such as that carried out by Bussell for canoe polo (described below), is essential to understand the demands of the activity and determine training programme structure. The type of training should match the specific demands of the sport. Training for the adaptation of the anaerobic and aerobic systems is discussed below.

Intermittent training

There are two main forms of intermittent training which vary in the intensity and duration of the load, and hence result in differing physiological adaptations to training. Intermittent aerobic (ITA) training involves working at 100−120% of maximal aerobic velocity (MAV) − as determined with the MSRT or the Yo-Yo test – for 10–30 s (no longer than 1 min). The primary adaptation to ITA training is an enhanced $\dot{V}O_{2max}$ due to factors such as improved myoglobin efficiency, muscle oxygen kinetics (the rate at which $\dot{V}O_2$ is increased to match the increase in energy expenditure) and enzyme levels. The other form of intermittent training, intermittent high intensity training (IHIT), involves higher-intensity loads (120–140% or 150% MAV) of a shorter duration 5–10 s (for sports involving a variety of exercise intensities, durations and frequencies, such as football/soccer, hockey, rugby, basketball etc.). Following ITHI training, the ability to repeat intense accelerations is increased (due to a greater rate of PCr resynthesis), muscle glycogen content is elevated, and the accumulation of lactate during intense effort is reduced. When developing a training programme for an intermittent sport, these variations in adaptations need to be considered alongside the sport-specific demands.

Development of an intermittent training programme

All intermittent sports should incorporate intermittent interval training into their schedule, as indicated by the specificity principle of training. An important point to consider from the start is that the benefits of intermittent exercise depend on the total distance covered during the work bouts (e.g. 120% MAV), as this is related to the number of muscle contractions performed at 'optimal intensities' (sport-specific predominant intensity) (Casas, 2008). The following six steps are involved in the development of an intermittent training programme:

1. Establish MAV
2. Determine which form of intermittent training is appropriate
3. Establish total volume
4. Establish duration of work and rest periods
5. Select the intensity of the work
6. Establish form of recovery periods

Initially, an athlete's MAV must be established with the performance of an incremental test to exhaustion, such as the MSRT or the Yo-Yo test for athletes of intermittent sports. The aim of the training, with reference to the sport-specific demands, is established and the appropriate form of intermittent training selected. Where available, motion analysis or GPS data reported for the sport of interest should be consulted to obtain information on the total distance covered and what movements and intensities are involved. This information, along with the training effects desired, can be used in the establishment of total volume during intermittent training. Following the determination of the type and total volume of training, the duration and intensity of the work and recovery bouts can be established. The duration of work is obviously going to depend on the intensity selected – as the intensity increases the duration will need to be lowered. The duration of the recovery periods is dependent on the work duration and intensity. Common work-to-rest ratios for intermittent training are 1:1 or 1:1.5 (e.g. 10 s × 10 s, 10 s × 15 s, 20 s × 30 s). Additionally, when determining the duration of recovery periods, the physiological aim of the training should be considered. The selection of an active or passive recovery period will likely depend on the fitness of the athlete.

Recovery

Another interesting aspect to consider for those involved in intermittent sports is the form of recovery strategy to employ between exercise bouts. Where possible, an active recovery is recommended (50–60% MAV) over a passive recovery, due to its effects on lactate concentration and perceived exertion (RPE). Research has shown that lactate uptake by skeletal muscle is increased when light exercise is performed in preference to complete rest. There appears to be a dynamic situation with regard to the exchange of lactate as a fuel source across muscle fibres within an exercising muscle and between working and non-working muscle groups. Additionally, a recent study has found intermittent exercise with active recoveries to reduce the blood lactate concentration during exercise compared with passive recoveries (38% higher blood lactate concentration) (Mandroukas et al. 2011). This is supportive of an earlier study which reported a lower blood lactate concentration when 6 s bouts of cycling were interspersed with active recovery compared with passive recovery (Ahmaidi et al. 1996). Whether the reductions in lactate with active recoveries lead to a resultant improvement in performance remains equivocal. In addition to the benefits of active recovery on lowering lactate concentration, performance and rating of perceived exertion (RPE) appear to improve when recovery involves low-intensity activity, compared with a passive recovery.

Intermittent running with active recoveries, however, reduces the time to exhaustion compared with passive recoveries. The additional oxygen required during active recoveries is likely to reduce the oxygen available to reload myoglobin and haemoglobin, to lower lactate levels, and to resynthesise PCr, hence reducing the time to exhaustion (Dupont et al. 2003, 2004).

Knowledge integration question

Should recovery periods during intermittent training be too short relative to the exercise load, what physiological changes will occur that may lead to fatigue?

Further aerobic training protocols for intermittent sports

A high level of aerobic fitness is required by team sport athletes due to the large distances covered during competition and for a fast, efficient recovery between repeated periods of high-intensity exercise. Aerobic training results in both central (cardiovascular) and peripheral (muscular) adaptations which, together, can improve a variety of

aerobic measures, such as $\dot{V}O_{2max}$, LT, exercise economy and oxygen uptake kinetics, all of which are beneficial for performance. As discussed above, planned ITA training can improve aerobic fitness levels. Two further methods of improving aerobic capacity, traditional (planned) and sport-specific (planned or spontaneous) aerobic conditioning, are now considered.

Traditional aerobic training involves continuous or interval exercise with minimal directional changes and involves no skill component, hence it has little specificity for team sports. It does, however, increase aerobic capacity within 4–10 weeks, and can considerably improve team sport performance (increased total distance covered and number of sprints during a match). More recently, aerobic training has developed to include sport-specific activities (movement patterns and skills) such as occurs during small-sided games and dribbling circuits, while still improving aerobic fitness. Whether this sport-specific enhancement of aerobic fitness relates to a greater performance improvement compared to traditional aerobic training remains to be determined.

Traditional training more commonly involves interval running, rather than continuous running, especially in elite team sport athletes who already have a high aerobic fitness level. In general, the intensity of the intervals ranges from 85–95% HR_{max}, while the interval duration is ≤ 4 min, separated by a maximum of 3 min active recovery ($\sim 60\%$ HR_{max}). These conditioning sessions are traditionally performed twice a week for 4–10 weeks. Sport-specific aerobic training is increasingly being implemented within programmes of professional teams. The soccer-specific dribbling test (described in detail in the section on 'physiology of football/soccer') is a good example of sport-specific aerobic training, which includes directional changes, acceleration, deceleration, and ball skills. Due to the skill component involved, sport-specific training may not be suitable for less skilled athletes, as they may be unable to maintain the skill at a fast enough pace to achieve the physiological stress required for fitness benefits. In contrast, highly trained athletes may not achieve a training benefit from small-sided games, unless they are tailored (manipulation of player numbers, field dimensions and game rules) to increase the physical load imposed on the athlete.

The literature suggests that traditional and sport-specific aerobic training both stimulate an improved aerobic fitness and sport performance, although more research is warranted in this area. Sport-specific training, however, has the additional benefit of improving skill level at the same time as aerobic fitness.

Key points

Training for intermittent sports:

➤ As specific to sport as possible

➤ Exercise intensity, duration and recovery intervals should match demands of sport as closely as possible

➤ Intermittent training can be used to improve aerobic fitness (ITA) or repeat acceleration ability (IHIT)

• ITA – less intense (100–120% MVA) and longer (10–30 s) exercise bouts

• IHIT – more intense (120–140% or 150% MVA) and shorter (5–10 s) exercise bouts

➤ Traditional or sport-specific (small-sided games or dribbling circuits) aerobic conditioning enhances aerobic fitness

Recovery during intermittent sports

➤ Active recovery can improve performance by lowering lactate concentration and RPE

➤ May have implications for athletes during game breaks, e.g. half-time

13.2 Physiology of a variety of intermittent sports

In this section an overview of the physiological demands of a range of intermittent sports is provided. Invasion games such as rugby and hockey are described as well as racquet sports, striking and fielding sports, martial arts and adventure sports such as sailing and surfing.

The physiology of football/soccer

As well as being one of the most popular sports worldwide, football/soccer is perhaps the most widely researched intermittent sport. In the rest of this review we will refer to the sport as football, in keeping with the terminology used by the world governing body. Played by two teams of 11 players over a 90 min duration, the game has more than 120 million registered and unregistered players worldwide. There are now over 200 countries represented on the Fédération Internationale de Football Association (FIFA) and as such football can be truly thought of as a worldwide sport.

Distance covered

The development of new technologies has enabled a much closer analysis of the demands of the sport. Depending on the standard of the game, the environmental conditions and the position of the player, footballers typically cover 4–12 km during a match. Playing position accounts for much of the variation in distance covered, with goalkeepers averaging around 4 km, while midfield players typically cover distances of 9–12 km during a game. Research suggests, perhaps not surprisingly, that attackers and defenders (offence and defence players) cover similar distances of around 7–10 km. Typically, wingers and full backs tend to cover a greater distance and with a higher percentage as sprinting than central defenders. The distance covered and indeed the intensity of exercise are normally 7–10% lower in the second half (45 min) than the first. Interestingly, climatic conditions and styles of play also affect the distances covered, with players in South American countries often covering up to 15% less distance during a game than players in some European leagues.

Exercise intensity

Over the duration of a game the overall exercise intensity in football appears to be close to the aerobic-anaerobic transition (see Chapter 11 for more details about this aspect of metabolism), equating to 80–90% of a player's HR_{max}. This, however, is an average value and, as time and motion analysis data reveal, there is a great variation in exercise intensity from one moment to the next. One aspect that affects the intensity of football is the actual playing time. In a typical game the ball is in play for around 60 of the 90 min of a match. When the ball is out of play the intensity of exercise for individual players typically drops. Although there is some variation between studies, researchers investigating the time and motion in football generally categorise movement into time spent or distance travelled standing, walking, jogging, running/cruising/striding, sprinting and sometimes moving backwards. Perhaps not surprisingly, the greatest distance is covered while jogging and walking, with around 20% of the distance covered when running/cruising/striding, while only 5–10% of total distance, depending on the league in which the game is played, is covered when sprinting.

Metabolic demands

The nature of the game means the metabolic demands during a match are both aerobic and anaerobic. While demands of football are predominantly aerobic, some of the most crucial aspects of the game, those that often make the difference between winning and losing a match, require energy synthesised via anaerobic pathways. Tackling, along with sprinting and jumping for a ball, all require anaerobic bursts from a player during a game. Typically, footballers have a high aerobic capacity with a $\dot{V}O_{2max}$, for males of 50–70 mL·kg^{-1}·min^{-1}, females around 40–60 mL·kg^{-1}·min^{-1} and adolescents up to 60 mL·kg^{-1}·min^{-1}. Although oxygen consumption is difficult to measure during a game, a number of studies using portable gas analysers or the HR–$\dot{V}O_2$ relationship suggest that the average oxygen consumption during a game is around 75% of $\dot{V}O_{2max}$. The anaerobic glycolytic component during football matches has been inferred in football studies from the lactate concentrations gathered at the end of the first and second halves of a game, although clearly such results would be heavily affected by the intensity of activity during the last five minutes of play. As a consequence, such findings are not truly representative of the anaerobic contribution to performance across a period of play, but do indicate that anaerobic metabolism clearly plays an important role in the energetics of football. As with the distances covered during a game, lactate concentrations for footballers are typically lower in the second half of a match than in the first and lend support to the notion of a generally lower intensity during the second half of a match. The literature suggests that lactate concentrations at the end of the first half of a game are between 5–8 mM, while those at the end of the second half are typically between 2–4 mM, depending on the player's competitive level.

Football-specific tests

Comparative analysis between studies indicates that the fitness level of professional footballers and indeed the demands of the sport have increased over time. The alterations are perhaps most reflective of the changes in the coaching and training methods used, particularly for clubs at the elite level. In parallel with these changes in training methods, such as the increased concentration on speed agility and quickness, there has been a rapid rise in number of football-specific fitness assessments that have been developed. Examples include the Yo-Yo intermittent recovery test which was described above, football-specific $\dot{V}O_{2max}$ tests, the soccer-specific dribbling (or Hoff test) and the soccer-specific intermittent-exercise test (SSIET). As a football apprentice at Huddersfield Town, England, Matt Crooks has recently been involved in fitness testing, including the yo-yo test, as mentioned in the Sport in Action piece on pp. 429–30.

The soccer-specific dribbling test (also known as the Hoff test) was developed by Hoff et al. (2002) and is conducted on a football field, using a section measuring 55 m by 30 m. The test is conducted over 10 min, during which time a player has to complete as many circuits of the course as possible (course set-up is illustrated in Figure 13.5). The player must keep a ball at their feet (dribbling) for the entirety of the test, which includes sections involving dribbling round cones, over hurdles (the ball and the player must pass over the hurdles), between cones and at one point travelling backwards

with the ball at the feet. Each lap of the course represents a total distance covered of 290 m with elite footballers able to complete over 7 laps (2030 m) during the 10 min of the test.

The soccer-specific intermittent-exercise test was developed by Oliver et al. (2007) and, like the PHIIRSS (which was described above), is conducted on a non-motorised treadmill (NMT). The use of a NMT enables the researcher to collect data on both the velocity of the treadmill belt and the horizontal force produced. In this test, players complete 3×14 min exercise bouts with a 3 min recovery between each exercise period. The test was designed in this way to match, approximately, the time duration of one half of a football match (45 min). The rest periods are provided to enable the researchers to collect capillary blood samples for lactate concentration analysis, and to allow the player to have a drink of water.

Prior to starting the test, the player warms up using the NMT for 5 min at a speed of 8 km·h^{-1} with the inclusion of two < 4 s sprints. This aspect of the warm-up is followed by a 5 min stretching period prior to commencement of the test. The pattern of exercise is the same for each 14 min exercise phase, with each of these broken down into repeated 2-min exercise cycles. Within each 2-min cycle (repeated 7 times in each 14-min exercise bout) a player completes one 5 s maximal sprint accompanied by periods of being stationary, walking, jogging and cruising. The intensity and duration of each of the sub-maximal aspects of the protocol was determined from previous time and motion analysis studies.

Key points

Football (soccer) physiology:

➤ Typical distance covered during a 90-min match is 4–12 km
  • Depends on playing position, environmental conditions, playing level and playing style
➤ Average exercise intensity close to aerobic-anaerobic transition (80–90% of HR$_{max}$), but great variation from one moment to the next
➤ Primarily reliant on aerobic metabolism, but also involves spells of anaerobic metabolism
➤ Average $\dot{V}O_2$ during a game is ~75% $\dot{V}O_{2max}$
➤ Distances covered, exercise intensity and blood lactate concentration are typically lower in the 2nd half of a football match
➤ Fitness can be assessed by several football-specific tests
  • Yo-Yo intermittent recovery test
  • Football specific $\dot{V}O_{2max}$ tests
  • Soccer-specific dribbling or Hoff test
  • Soccer-specific intermittent-exercise test (SSIET)

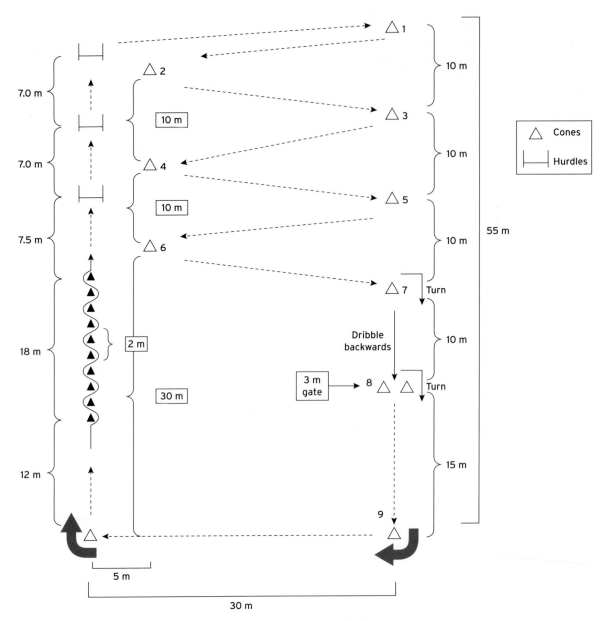

Figure 13.5 The Hoff test: a soccer-specific dribbling test.

The physiology of rugby league

Rugby league was established as a separate rugby code in 1895 when 21 clubs in the north of England formed their own league in a split from the (English) Rugby Football Union (RFU). The clubs broke away from the RFU in a dispute over compensation for wages lost when playing in matches. As part of the split, the new league developed their own rules which included changing the number of players on each team, the requirement to play the ball immediately a tackle is made and the removal of line-outs from the procedures of play. The game is now played in many countries worldwide, but is played most widely in Australia and England. As well as these two countries, others playing rugby league internationally now include New Zealand, France, Russia, Wales, Ireland, Scotland, South Africa, Samoa and Fiji.

The full game of rugby league is played by two teams of 13 players over 80 min with typically twelve interchanges (rotation of players and substitutes) allowed during the professional game (interchanges are often unlimited at junior level and in amateur leagues). Rugby league is a physical contact, collision sport that requires varying intensities of exercise. The playing time is divided into two 40-min halves normally separated by a 10-min half-time break. There are two groups of players in each team, the six forwards who are primarily involved in collisions and tackles, and the seven backs who are normally given the ball in more open play where they can use their speed to exploit gaps in the oppositions defence.

Distance covered

Interestingly the change in the defensive retreat ruling, requiring the defensive team to retreat 10 m rather than 5 m, has led to a change in the work to recovery ratio. Prior to the ruling change, research suggested the work to recovery ratio varied between 1:6 and 1:8. Since the change, more recent findings indicate the work to recovery ratio has risen to between 1:10–1:28 depending on the player position. This ruling change, and the consequential increase in the time spent in recovery, has directly affected the physiological demands of the sport. Time and motion analysis data suggest that the distance players travel during a game has substantially increased as a result of this ruling change. Prior to the introduction of the 10 m defensive ruling players ran ~7 km during a game. Following the rule change, the average distance covered has typically increased to 9–10 km per game. While the decrease in the work-to-recovery ratio suggests that players typically have longer to recover between work efforts, the introduction of limited interchanges at the professional level has resulted in an increase in the physiological demands on players. These changes to the game need to be kept in mind when considering the physiology of rugby league.

Body mass and composition

As a physical contact or collision sport the size of players is important. Rugby league players at the senior level typically have a body mass between 85–90 kg, with forwards (17.5%) having a higher mean body fat percentage (%BF) than backs (15%). As would perhaps be expected, amateur players tend to have a higher %BF (forwards and backs), than semi-professional players who in turn have higher reported mean %BF than professional players.

Aerobic fitness

The intermittent high-intensity nature of rugby league and the length of matches require players to have good levels of aerobic and anaerobic fitness. Professional rugby league players who train 5–6 days per week have been reported to have a $\dot{V}O_{2max}$ of between 55–60 mL·kg^{-1}·min^{-1}.

Interestingly, later research, despite the previously described differences in the roles of forwards and backs, indicates that the aerobic power of the two groups of players is very similar. It has been suggested that the lack of difference between positional groups may relate to non-differentiation in training for forwards and backs, even at a professional level. Alternatively, it may simply be that the nature of the game requires a high level of aerobic fitness for both forwards and backs.

Injury risk

As might be expected, collision sport players tend to have an increased injury risk when compared to non-collision and non-contact sports. Additionally, however, research suggests that rugby league players have a greater risk of injury than players of other collision sports. In some studies the injury incidence rate has been reported as more than double that found in other sports. It has been suggested that at the elite level the increased injury risk is related to the intensity at which the game is played, with the collision-based nature of the sport resulting in head and neck injuries being those most commonly sustained.

Rugby league-specific tests

A number of different tests can be used to analyse the fitness of rugby league players (Gabbett et al., 2008, 2010). Gabbett (2005) suggested that rugby league players require highly developed speed, agility, strength, muscular power and aerobic power, and a number of tests have been employed to assess these aspects of fitness for rugby league. Tests used include the 5 m, 10 m and 20 m sprints, vertical jump test, reactive agility test, L test, 505 test and the modified 505 test. The set-ups for the agility tests (reactive agility test, L test, 505 and modified 505 tests) are shown in Figure 13.6.

Agility tests

The reactive agility test (RAT), developed by Sheppard et al. (2006), involves anticipation and decision-making components. The test, also used with Australian Rules Football players, requires participants to complete 12 trials, of four possible scenarios, involving a forward movement followed by a change of direction in response to movement of the tester (who stands opposite the participant, refer to Figure 13.6a). Upon forward movement of the tester (starts the timer) the participant has to move forward and then either left or right, following the movement of the tester, through a set of timing

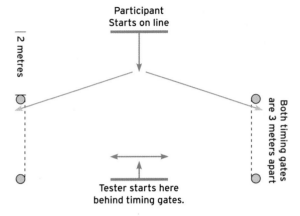

(a) Set-up for the reactive test

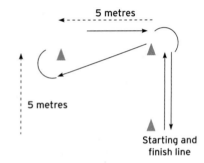

(b) Set-up for the L test

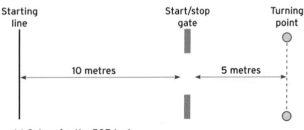

(c) Set-up for the 505 test

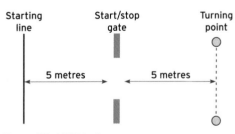

(d) Set-up for the modified 505 test

Figure 13.6 Set-up for a variety of tests suggested for rugby league players: (a) reactive agility test and (b) L-test (c) 505 test (d) modified 505 test.

gates (stops the timer). The recorded score is the mean time of all 12 trials.

A further test of agility is the L run, in which an athlete has to complete an out and back run around cones set in

an L shape (illustrated in Figure 13.6b). The time to completion of the course is recorded for comparison between individuals or for an individual at different stages within the season. The 505 test and modified 505 are, not surprisingly, very similar tests of agility. From the starting line (set either 5 m (modified test) or 10 m (original test) from the timing gates) a participant runs through the timing lights (triggering the start of the test) to the turning point and back though the timing lights, thereby finishing the test. The time for the out and back 5 m course (10 m total distance) is recorded for each participant. For the L test and the 505 tests each participant is allowed three trials, with his or her best score being recorded for that battery of testing.

> ## Key points
>
> Rugby league physiology:
>
> ➤ Typical body mass of 85–90 kg, %BF higher in forwards (17.5%) than backs (15%)
>
> ➤ Work to recovery ratio ranges from 1:10 to 1:28 depending on position
>
> ➤ Cover 9–10 km per game
>
> ➤ High aerobic fitness: $\dot{V}O_{2max}$ 55–60 mL·kg^{-1}·min^{-1}
>
> ➤ Greater risk of injury compared to other collision sports
>
> ➤ Tests to assess rugby league players
>
>   • Short sprint tests (5, 10 and 20 m)
>   • Vertical jump test – leg power
>   • Agility tests
>   • Reactive agility test
>   • L test
>   • 505 and modified 505 tests

The physiology of rugby union

The origins of rugby union football date back to the middle ages and are closely linked to a number of games played in Europe. The formal history of the game, while being closely linked with the possible first carrying of the ball by William Webb Ellis at Rugby School, certainly dates back to the formation of the Rugby Football Union in 1871 and the subsequent split in 1895 when the two codes, union and league, were formalised for the first time over a payments dispute. Indeed, rugby union remained the amateur code until 1995 when, for the first time, sport allowed professional players.

The full game of rugby union is played by two teams of 15 players, while a smaller version (rugby 7s) is played by 7 players. At the turn of the 20th century rugby was played in the Olympic Games until it was dropped after the 1924 Olympics. In 2016, rugby 7s will return to the Olympics at the Rio de Janeiro Games. Both forms of the sport are played in an increasing number of countries worldwide, including Ireland, Scotland, Wales, England, France, Italy, Argentina, New Zealand, South Africa, Australia, Samoa, Fiji and Tonga. The International Rugby Board now has over 95 member nations worldwide. Due to the amount of research available the concentration in this section will be upon the full, 15-a-side version of rugby.

The full game is played over 80 min, in two 40-min halves separated by a 10-min interval. The ball is typically in play for around 60 of the 80 min of a game. As for rugby league, teams can be split into forwards and backs, with the forwards being responsible for winning and running with the ball and backs for running longer distances with the ball, often at higher speeds. The forwards are numbered from 1 to 8, while the backs are numbered from 9 to 15.

Body mass and composition

In terms of body mass, forwards are usually heavier than backs. Recent research indicates that both groups have become heavier since the advent of professionalism within the sport. In addition, professional players are normally heavier than amateur players and university sides. Interestingly, when compared with rugby league, in rugby union there are more distinct differences in the body mass of forwards and backs. While rugby union backs are often reported to have similar body masses to those playing rugby league (85–90 kg), the forward players in rugby union are all normally over 100 kg in mass (range between 108 and 112 kg). This tendency for increased body mass in the forwards is also reflected with female rugby union players, where forwards have been reported with mean body masses of 70 kg while backs are around 10 kg lighter. Andy Ellis, a current New Zealand All Black, believes that to be successful at the international level a scrum half (half-back) must weight at least 90 kg. To achieve this, Andy performs resistance and power training which he discusses in the Sport in Action section on pp. 430–1.

A significant change in the body mass of elite players reflects the body composition of forwards. Research indicates that while heavier, modern-day forwards are leaner than previous generations in the sport. The decrease in relative body fat measured in forwards in the modern game has been linked to their improved speed, mobility and scrummaging success. Changes in forward players' body compositions mean that differences in %BF between forwards and backs have narrowed in recent years. At the professional level forwards have a mean %BF around 11–13%, while backs have a mean of 10%.

Exercise intensity and distance covered

Recent changes in the rules, which have attempted to increase the pace and flow of the game, have changed the time and motion analysis of the game. Results of recent studies suggest that rugby union players have a work-to-rest ratio of 1:2 or 1:3, with around 85% of the work time being involved in lower-intensity activity and 15% as high intensity (running, sprinting, tackling, pushing and competing for the ball). In response to the demands of a game, mean HR responses for players have been found to be higher for forwards than backs, indicating that the work intensity is higher for forwards. In one study researchers found forwards to spend over 70% of time at a HR above 85% of maximum, while backs spent 45% of time in this zone.

A time–motion analysis study on elite English rugby union players during match play reported the total distance covered by the backs (6127 m) to be greater than that covered by the forwards (5581 m) (Roberts et al., 2008). Researchers from the University of Chester, commissioned by the RFU, have recently reported data from Premiership rugby matches which similarly indicate a greater total distance covered by backs (6.84 km scrum half) compared to forwards (4.45 km front row). These distances reported for rugby union players are less than those covered by players in games such as soccer.

Metabolic demands

The intermittent nature of the game, with individual activity efforts typically being 4–10 s, requires rugby players to have high levels of aerobic and anaerobic fitness. Indeed, results of $\dot{V}O_{2max}$ assessments indicate a high aerobic endurance fitness of rugby union players, with backs (55–60 mL·kg^{-1}·min^{-1}) having slightly higher levels than forwards (50–55 mL·kg^{-1}·min^{-1}). The duration and intensity of efforts determine which energy system is predominant in the generation of energy during the game. The short-duration, high-intensity movements (jumping, tackling, kicking etc.) place demands on the phosphagen system, whilst incomplete recoveries (i.e. ATP and PCr stores not fully restored) would necessitate a significant energy production via glycolysis, with aerobic metabolism playing an important role in recovery and lower-intensity activity (walking etc.). It appears that forwards may have a greater reliance on anaerobic metabolism than backs, as they have been found to have higher post-match blood lactate concentrations, ranging between 3–6.5 mM. However, again, this is dependent upon the activity of players immediately before the end of the match.

Rugby union-specific tests

Physiological tests advocated for use with rugby union players are similar to those for rugby league players and include anthropometric measurements such as mass, height and body composition along with measurements of strength, power, speed and aerobic endurance. To assess power, the vertical jump test has been advocated as a simple measurement, whilst bench press and squat (1 RM) could be used to assess strength. A variety of distances could be used to assess speed (10 m, 20 m, or 40 m), while the MSRT or Yo-Yo test are used widely to assess aerobic endurance performance.

Key points

Rugby union physiology:

➤ Work-to-rest ratio 1:2 or 1:3

➤ Exercise intensity

  • Work intensity is higher for forwards than backs

  • 85% of work time – lower-intensity activity

  • 15% of work time – high-intensity activity (running, sprinting, tackling, pushing and competing for the ball)

➤ Distance covered during a game is higher for the backs (6 km) than the forwards (4–5 km)

➤ All three energy systems required – phosphagen, glycolysis, aerobic

➤ Require high aerobic and anaerobic fitness

  • Backs have slightly higher aerobic fitness than forwards ($\dot{V}O_{2max}$ of 55–60 and 50–55 mL·kg^{-1}·min^{-1}, respectively)

  • Forwards may have greater reliance on anaerobic metabolism

➤ Tests of fitness

  • Power – vertical jump

  • Strength – bench press and squat 1 RM

  • Anaerobic sprint ability – 10, 20 or 40 m sprints

  • Aerobic endurance – MSRT or Yo-Yo test

The physiology of Australian rules football

Australian rules football, also known as Aussie rules football, dates back to at least 1858 when the first rules were established; however, the exact origins are not clear. Although primarily played in Australia, Aussie rules football is also played in over 30 additional countries worldwide including New Zealand, the USA, Canada, Samoa,

Tonga, the UK and South Africa. The governing body for the sport in Australia is the Australian Football League (AFL) who organise the main competition which culminates each year in the AFL Grand Final, one of the most highly attended championship finals for any sport.

Aussie rules is an intermittent contact sport played over four 20 min quarters by two teams of 18 players (with four interchange reserves allowed). The field of play is typically oval with a length of 135–185 m and a width at midpoint of 110–155 m. The aim of the game is to kick goals which are worth 6 pts or behinds which are worth 1 pt. The scoring area consists of four posts situated at each end of the oval. To score a goal the ball must be kicked between the central posts, while a behind is scored when the ball crosses the goal line between the outer and inner posts on either side of the goal. The distribution of players is such that there are six forwards, six midfielders and six backs. The forwards catch the ball on the full and then attempt to kick a goal; the backs try to disrupt the opposing forwards, while the midfielders' role is to move the ball down the pitch from the backs to the forwards.

There is an increasing research base for Aussie rules football, with papers published relating to aspects such as injuries in the sport, training methods, physiological characteristics of players and sport-specific tests. Research indicates that the ball is typically in play for around 60% of the time and while players spend over 50% of the time engaged in low-intensity exercise they still cover over 10 km during a game. More recent studies have found players covering distances of over 15 km during a game. Midfielders normally spend the most time engaged in high-intensity exercise with about 5–10% of their time spent running or sprinting. Individual high-intensity bursts are typically of 4–6 s duration. These research findings suggest that the key mechanisms of energy production for Aussie rules players are the phosphagen system for the short high-intensity efforts and the aerobic system for recoveries. High aerobic endurance fitness is demonstrated by AFL players, with a $\dot{V}O_{2max}$ in the region of 55–65 mL·kg^{-1}·min^{-1}. Similar to rugby league players and rugby union backs, Aussie rules players have been found to have body masses of 85–90 kg. In contrast to these sports, however, research to date suggests that there is no consistent pattern of differences in %BF between playing positions for AFL players.

With regard to physiological assessments, researchers, trainers and coaches have used a variety of fitness tests. The MSRT and the Yo-Yo test have been widely used to monitor aerobic endurance ability, while sprints of varying distances, including 5 m, 10 m and 20 m, have been used to assess anaerobic sprint ability. In addition, tests such as vertical jump, a number of agility tests and 1 RM and 3 RM for bench press, leg press and chin ups (with a weight attached) have been used to assess a player's power, agility and strength.

Key points

Australian rules football physiology:

➤ Exercise intensity
  • Over 50% of time in low-intensity exercise
  • Midfielders spend most time in high-intensity exercise (5–10% of time)
  • High-intensity bursts are 4–6 s duration
➤ Cover up to 15 km a during game
➤ Key mechanisms of energy production are phosphagen system (short high-intensity bouts) and aerobic system (recovery)
➤ High aerobic endurance fitness: $\dot{V}O_{2max}$ 55–65 mL·kg^{-1}·min^{-1}
➤ Fitness tests
  • Aerobic endurance – MSRT and Yo-Yo test
  • Anaerobic sprint ability – 10, 20 or 40 m sprints
➤ Power – vertical jump
➤ Strength – bench press, leg press and chin ups 1 RM and 3 RM
➤ Agility tests – variety

Physiology of field hockey

Historical background

The roots of field hockey have been traced back to 4000 years ago when a crude form of the game was played in Egypt. Evidence suggests a form of the game was later played in Ancient Greece, from which the Romans developed the game and passed it on to the European nations. Some sports historians believe Irish hurling (thought to be the oldest of the stick-and-ball games) to be the true ancestor of hockey.

The modern form of field hockey was developed in England in the mid 18th century, with the Hockey Association formed in 1886. National Associations were subsequently founded in France (1887), Ireland (1893), Wales (1897), The Netherlands (1898), Scotland (1901), New Zealand (1902), Belgium (1907), Denmark (1908) and Austria (1910). Although hockey was first included in the Olympic Games in London in 1908, it was subsequently dropped from the next Games in Stockholm (1912),

reinstated in Antwerp in 1920 just to be banned again from the Paris Olympics in 1924. Hockey was refused by the organisers of the Paris Games on the grounds that it had no international federation. As a result, the most important step in the history of hockey was taken in 1924 when the sport's international governing body, the International Hockey Federation (FIH), was founded. Hockey was also becoming very popular with women, hence, not long after, the International Federation of Women's Hockey Association (IFWHA) was formed in 1927. It wasn't until 1982 that the two organisations joined to form what we currently know as the FIH. The FIH of today consists of five Continental Associations and has 127 member associations. The sport of hockey has grown considerably since its development in the late 1800s, and has become the main field game for secondary school girls in many European countries. Originally, hockey was primarily played on a grass pitch; however, synthetic pitches were introduced in the 1970s. Despite this early introduction, synthetic pitches were not universally accepted by the world of hockey until the early 1990s, and today all international competitions must be played on a synthetic surface.

An introduction to the sport of hockey

Field hockey is commonly known simply as 'hockey', apart from in countries where hockey refers to an alternative form of hockey, such as ice hockey. For simplicity, the term hockey will be used within this chapter. Hockey can be played as an outdoor or an indoor sport; however, not all member associations of the FIH play both variations. For this reason, the focus in this section is on outdoor field hockey. Hockey is played between two teams of 11 players, with both teams attempting to score goals by moving a ball into the opposing team's goal with a stick. The ball is hard, spherical and made of plastic, and more often than not it is covered with indentations. Teams are allowed five substitutions (i.e. a total of 16 players) who can enter the game at any time (apart from during a penalty corner). Substitutions are unlimited, hence a player can be substituted off for a recovery period, then rejoin the game later. A hockey match consists of two 35-min halves (total duration of 70 min) separated by a 10-min halftime. Only the front flat side and the edges of the stick can be used to play the ball. The ball can be moved, depending on the situation, by pushing, hitting, slapping, flicking or drag-flicking the ball. The hockey pitch is 91.40 m × 50 m, with a goal at each end of the pitch, measuring 2.14 m high, and 3.66 m wide with a 45.7 cm high backboard. The shooting semi-circle is 14.63 m from the goal within which is the penalty spot (0.15 m diameter) 6.49 m from the centre of the

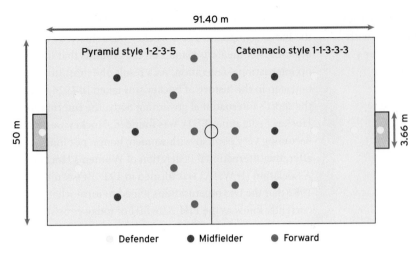

Figure 13.7 Basic dimensions of a hockey pitch and examples of two playing formations.

goal. The general dimensions of the hockey pitch are illustrated in Figure 13.7.

The team of 11 hockey players is generally divided into defenders (fullbacks), midfielders (halfbacks) and forwards. There are numerous formations which are currently used by international hockey teams. Two of these, the traditional pyramid style (1-2-3-5 the number of players starting from the back) and the catenaccio style (1-1-3-3-3), are illustrated in Figure 13.7. The pyramid formation allows for a fast, open, attacking style of play and has been successfully used by the Pakistan and Indian National Teams. In contrast, the catenaccio formation, typical of many European countries, is a more defensive approach relying on fast counter-attacks. The modern game of hockey involves much inter-switching of positions at the elite level with players capable of playing within many different areas of the field.

The physical demands of field hockey

Hockey is a high-intensity intermittent team sport, placing large physical demands on the players. The intermittent nature of hockey is demonstrated by the finding that an average of 1148 motion changes are made per match during elite male competition (Lythe & Kilding, 2011). Several major developments have been made in the sport within the last couple of decades, all of which are likely to have impacted on the demands of the sport. These include advances in stick construction, the advent of the synthetic pitch (and associated technical and tactical changes), and rule changes. The synthetic pitch places more strain on the joints during sudden changes in direction and speed compared with the earlier grass pitches, and additionally, due to its flatness, allows for much better ball control thus increasing the pace of the game. Indeed, Malhotra et al. (1983) demonstrated that the

physical demand of playing hockey on a synthetic pitch was considerably greater (18%) than playing on a grass surface. Several rule changes have occurred in recent years, impacting on the physical requirements of individual players: unlimited (rolling) substitutions in 1992, the offside rule was abolished in 1996, and the recent 'self-pass' at a free hit to improve the flow of the game (2009).

Distances covered and exercise intensity

As discussed previously in this chapter, the use of time-motion analysis in intermittent sports is becoming more popular, with several TMA studies existing for hockey. Due to the recent developments in hockey, some of the data presented in these studies may no longer be accurate for the sport of today. In addition to TMA, GPS technology has recently been used to quantify objectively the movement of elite male and female hockey players during competition and training. Such studies have reported distances covered by individual players and speed of movements, alongside the total duration of varying intensity activities (Gabbett, 2010; Lythe & Kilding, 2011). On average, the mean match time for elite male hockey players is 51.9 min, that is, 74% of total match duration. Only about 3.6% of time during a hockey match is involved with the ball, the majority of which lasts less than one second (Lothian and Farrally, 1992). This finding is similar to that reported by Wein (1981) who found 61% of time on the ball to last from 0.5–2.0 s with only 5% lasting longer than 7 s. In 1988, Hughes compared the performance of elite female players on a grass surface to that on a synthetic surface. The study revealed that, when in possession, the player ran with the ball more on the synthetic pitch. The consistent surface characteristics of the synthetic pitch make the execution of individual skills easier, hence players are able to retain possession for longer, even when under pressure by the opposition. Due to the change in playing surface and the technical and tactical developments in hockey, it may be suggested that time spent on the ball is likely to have increased since the earlier studies. Recent studies, however, did not include an analysis of this aspect of the game, hence the amount of time spent in possession of the ball in the modern game remains to be determined.

The average total distance covered by individual players during a hockey match is 6.8 km for males and 6.6 km for females. A wide range, however, exists for both genders (3.4 km–9.5 km reported for females), with distance covered by defenders (full-backs) significantly less than all other positions in males. Time–motion analysis and GPS have been used to determine the proportion of time players spend within different intensity zones, providing important information to coaches in terms of what energy systems are utilised and what activities should be focused on within training. Similar to before the pitch and rule changes, low-intensity activity predominates the modern game of hockey. Comparison between studies can be difficult, however, due to the employment of different categorisations of exercise intensity. Low- to moderate-intensity activities have recently been reported to account for the majority of the total distance covered in a hockey match (males 93.9%, females 97.3%) (Gabbett 2010; Lythe & Kilding, 2011), supportive of earlier findings that low-intensity movements accounted for 85–95% of match duration (Johnston et al., 2004; Spencer et al., 2004, 2005).

As in many other intermittent sports, however, the low-intensity periods of the game are interspersed with frequent short bursts of high-acceleration, high-velocity activity. The proportion of the elite female game spent in high-intensity (> 5 m·s^{-1}) activity is low (1.7%). Elite female midfielders have been found to conduct a greater number of high-velocity and high-acceleration efforts over the course of the match, involving more time in high-intensity running and covering a greater total distance, compared with strikers and defenders. Across all playing positions, the number of high-velocity (> 5 m·s^{-1}) activities range from 43 to 53, and high-acceleration (> 0.5 m·s^{-2} lasting for ≥ 2 s) activities range from 36 to 44, during elite female competition. The typical distance covered (up to 20 m) during each high-intensity effort, however, is similar between player positions. Elite male hockey players complete, on average, 34 sprints per game, with a mean duration of 3.3 s. Recovery between sprints was shown to be 113 s on average. Due to their roles within the game, it is not surprising that strikers perform the most sprints (46.9), and fullbacks the fewest sprints (19.8). On average, 84.9% of a players' maximum speed is reached during matches, with strikers being the fastest (mean 28.2 km·h^{-1}) and reaching speeds closest to their maximum (89.2%). An important fitness component of team sports, including hockey, is that of repeated sprint ability. As many as seven sprints may be involved in a repeated sprint bout in an elite male hockey competition, with a 10–20 s recovery between sprints (Spencer et al., 2004). It is clear from this data that hockey requires a high aerobic capacity to allow the players to cover the high distances required at the elite level, and to aid in the recovery between high-intensity bouts. Training of the anaerobic pathways is also required for the generation of energy during the multiple fast accelerations and sprints involved in the game.

Early studies in hockey suggest there is a reduced energy cost during the second half of a hockey match due to a reduced time spent in high-intensity activity (Lothian and Farrally, 1992, 1994). Recently, however, despite a small reduction in the total distance covered between the first and second halves, the distance covered during high-intensity activity remained unaltered in elite male hockey players (Lythe & Kilding, 2011). This is supportive of the findings of Spencer et al., (2004), who similarly reported no change in the amount of striding and sprinting that occurred in the first and second halves of a hockey game. This is an important finding, as it is during periods of high-intensity activity that match-deciding events occur.

A further factor relating to the demands of hockey that requires consideration is the fact that international hockey tournaments often require teams to play three games within a period of four days. To determine the effects of this type of competition schedule on the amount and type of activity within a match, Spencer et al., (2005) documented changes in time–motion analysis of 14 elite male Australian hockey players. The proportion of time spent standing was found to increase across the three games, accompanied by a fall in the time spent jogging. The percent time in striding increased in the final game while the frequency of repeated-sprint bouts decreased across the three games. These findings suggest that a residual fatigue may remain when hockey games are played with only 24–48 h recovery.

The physiological demands of field hockey

As mentioned above, hockey places demands on both the aerobic and anaerobic pathways of energy generation.

Due to the demands of the sport, both male and female hockey players have a high aerobic power ($\dot{V}O_{2max}$: males, 55.8–64.9 mL·kg^{-1}·min^{-1}; females, 46.6–59.3 mL·kg^{-1}.min^{-1}) (Gabbett, 2010; Hinrichs et al. 2010; Lythe & Kilding, 2011; Ready & van der Merwe, 1986). Additionally, due to sudden changes in direction and speed, leg power is an important fitness component for hockey. In addition to the benefits of leg strength to hockey, a high level of upper-body strength allows players to pass the ball over long distances at speed and to shoot at goal more powerfully.

Hockey is a game with inbuilt asymmetry as only the flat surface of the stick can be used to play the ball. This acts to raise the physiological demands of the game since players are forced to pay greater attention to body position in relation to both the ball and the opponent. The maintenance of correct positioning will serve to increase the work-rate when playing and, in particular, defending. The mean HR of female hockey players during a match was found to be 171 beats·min^{-1}, a work intensity similar to cruising (Lothian and Farrally, 1992). Elite males have been found to have an average HR of 161 beats·min^{-1} (85.3% HR$_{max}$) during competition, with a mean peak level of 196 beats·min^{-1} (96.3% HR$_{max}$). During the game, 90% of time was spent above 75% HR$_{max}$, 60% of time above 85% HR$_{max}$, and 4% of time above 95% HR$_{max}$ (Lythe & Kilding, 2011).

A unique physiological requirement of field hockey is the semi-crouched position adopted whilst dribbling the ball. Fox (1981) described running in this semi-crouched position as 'an ergonomically unsound posture for fast locomotion'. A study by Reilly and Seaton (1990) found that dribbling a hockey ball increases the energy expenditure by 15–16 kJ·min^{-1} (approximately 15% $\dot{V}O_{2max}$) above that observed in normal running, and increases heart rate by 15% of the maximal heart rate. The HR increases for dribbling a hockey ball are greater than those observed by Reilly and Ball (1984) for dribbling a soccer ball. The additional energy cost in field hockey is partly due to postural factors, and partly to the weight of the hockey stick (600–750 g) and the arm and shoulder exercise in its use. The stooped position adopted places a great load on the spine with spinal shrinkage found to occur at a rate of 0.4 mm·min^{-1} while dribbling a hockey ball (Reilly and Seaton, 1990), approximately four times the rate observed in running (Leatt et al. 1986). In summary, the posture adopted whilst dribbling a hockey ball imposes a physiological strain over and above that of normal running.

Field hockey-specific tests

Three hockey-specific tests will be described in this section, one is a skill test and two are tests involving a combination of skill and physiological characteristics: the shuttle sprint and dribble test (ShuttleSDT) and the slalom sprint and dribble test (SlalomSDT).

The skill test was developed, and tested for reliability and validity, by a group of researchers at Loughborough University (Sunderland et al. 2006). It was designed to include many of the technical elements of hockey, incorporating dribbling, passing, receiving, decision making and shooting. The set up of the test attempted to simulate the sport as closely as possible, with a section of water-based sportsturf used as the surface, and the shooting target the width of a hockey goal and the height of the goal backboard. The player starts 14.63 m from the goal and, as illustrated in Figure 13.8, dribbles the ball round the cones. As the player passes the final line of cones, they break an infra-red beam (positioned on the left indoor board) which triggers one of the lights on the goal to come on and a computer timing system is started. The player then passes

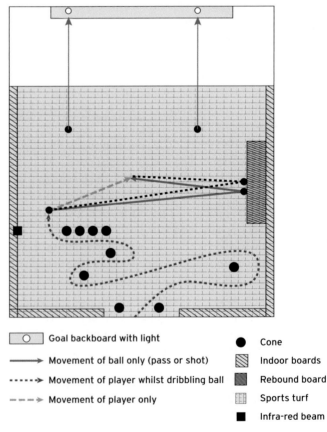

Figure 13.8 Schematic representation of the field hockey skill test.

the ball onto, and receives back from, the rebound board, before shooting at the goal target on the opposite side to the light. The sound of the ball hitting the goal stops the timing system. The time recorded by the computer is the 'decision making' time. The player completes the skill set six times, with one foot touching the start line between each set and to complete the test. A two second penalty is enforced for each of the following errors; the ball touches a cone, the ball touches the player's foot, the player misses the target on the goal. The measure of performance is the overall time, i.e. the total time for the six sets plus any error time. The decision-making time is the average of the six sets. The hockey skill test was shown to be a reliable measure of performance, across a wide range of abilities, and for both males and females. It is also valid as a predictor of coach-assessed hockey performance. Despite this, the test is complex in terms of its set-up and cannot be easily run outdoors with a large number of athletes.

The shuttle sprint and dribble test (ShuttleSDT) is a measure of hockey-specific shuttle sprint ability and ball dribbling performance. It involves the completion of three maximal sprint shuttles (total distance of 32 m), commencing every 20 s, while carrying a hockey stick. The total distance of 32 m is divided into a 6 m and a 10 m shuttle (6 m out and back = 12 m; 10 m out and back = 20 m). After the third sprint, the player is given a 5-min walking recovery, before repeating the three sets of shuttles, only this time the player dribbles a hockey ball. The times of each sprint are ideally measured by electronic timing gates. Individual sprint and dribble times, peak sprint and dribble times, and total sprint and dribble times are recorded. Delta shuttle time (difference between the total dribble and sprint times) is then calculated.

The slalom sprint and dribble test (SlalomSDT) is based on tests of agility and dribbling skills. It involves a 30 m maximal slalom sprint while carrying a hockey stick, a 5-min walking recovery, and a maximal slalom dribble of 30 m. Twelve cones are placed in a zigzag pattern between the start and finish line. Slalom sprint time and slalom dribble time are recorded, following which the difference between these times (delta slalom time) is calculated.

The ShuttleSDT and the SlalomSDT are both useful tests of hockey performance due to the alteration of high and low exercise intensity, and the inclusion of agility, speed and technical skills. They are practical tests in that they are simple to set up, easy to administer, and can be conducted outdoors as part of a training session. The weather conditions, however, should be recorded if test results are to be compared to those at a different stage in an athlete's season.

Key points

Hockey physiology:

➤ Total distance covered – males 6.8 km, females 6.6 km (range 3.4–9.5 km)

➤ Low-intensity activity is predominant (males 93.9%, females 97.3%)

➤ High-intensity activity low (females 1.7%)
  - High-intensity efforts primarily cover up to 20 m
  - Mean sprint duration of elite males 3.3 s
  - Sprint recovery – average of 113 s

➤ Aerobic and anaerobic metabolism required for energy regeneration

➤ Aerobic power ($\dot{V}O_{2max}$) – males, 55.8–64.9 mL·kg^{-1}· min^{-1}; females, 46.6–59.3 mL·kg^{-1}·min^{-1}

➤ During a game, average HR of 161 beats·min^{-1} in males and 171 beats·min^{-1} in females

➤ Fitness tests
  - Shuttle sprint and dribble test
  - Slalom sprint and dribble test

The physiology of basketball

Whereas there is some mystery around origins of rugby union, the history of the sport of basketball dates back to its invention in 1891 by Dr. James Naismith who was a physical education professor from Canada. Naismith taught physical education at Springfield College in north eastern USA and invented Basket Ball as a game for his students to play during the long cold winter months. While similar to modern day basketball, the original game did not include dribbling, which was added to the game in the 1950s. The international governing body for the game is the Fédération Internationale de Basket-ball (FIBA), the A in FIBA standing for amateur, although since 1989 FIBA has governed the sport internationally for amateur and professional players. Basketball is now played all over the world and FIBA has over 210 member nations.

As can be seen in Figure 13.1, the duration of a basketball game varies depending upon the rules under which it is played. Under FIBA regulations a basketball game consists of four 10-min quarters, with a 15-min break between the second and third quarters (half-time) and 2 min between the first and second and the third and fourth quarters. Under the National Basketball Association (NBA) regulations, the quarters last for 12 min. Basketball teams consist of five players, with the taller and heavier players being selected to play closest to the basket. Typically, the *point guard* is responsible for shooting, the *off-guard* (or shooting guard) for distance shooting, the *small forward* shooting at distance and close to the basket, the *power forward* close to the basket shooting and re-bounding, while the *centre* coordinates defence and is a close range shooter. In a game situation, however, players must be able to switch positions and responsibilities such that a power forward should be able to play as a centre or an off-guard play as a small forward.

Exercise intensity

During a game of basketball the game is usually live for about 50% of the time. The nature of the game of basketball, involving quick changes in direction and small movements, make it difficult to measure accurately the distance covered during a game. Research, however, indicates that basketball players spend about 15% of game time in high-intensity movements, during which players can reach HRs of 90–95% HR_{max}. Basketball matches can be played at an intensity such that players spend over 75% of the game with their HR at, or above, 85% of maximum. The intensity of the game is such that playing basketball places significant demands on the glycolytic pathway and research has found that players' lactate concentrations can remain elevated throughout the duration of a game. Findings suggest that, while some positions result in higher concentrations than others, mean lactate concentrations of over 8 mM occur in male basketball players.

During a game, guards typically spend a marginally higher percentage of the game in high-intensity activities than forwards, and forwards are more active than centres. For all players sprints are of such short duration that it is not possible to reach maximum speed. The game in reality consists of intermittent accelerations and decelerations of less than 4 s duration where significant amounts of energy are expended to overcome inertia.

Physiological characteristics

Both male and female basketball physiological characteristics vary by position. Average body masses for male guards, forwards and centres are 90, 100 and 110 kg, while for females the values are 65, 70–75 and 80 kg, respectively. Body fat percentages follow the same trends in the region of 9–11, 10–11 and 11–14% for male guards, forwards and centres and 14, 17 and 20% for female counterparts. In both

cases, while centres have the highest %BF, they also tend to have the highest lean body masses relative to other players on the team. In research published to date, mean $\dot{V}O_{2max}$ for females have typically been in the region of 45–50 mL·kg^{-1}·min^{-1} and males 50–60 mL·kg^{-1}·min^{-1}. These values are lower than compared to other invasion games such as rugby or football and perhaps reflect differences in the nature of the game. The results of lactate concentration analyses are also supportive of such a difference existing between these sports, with the higher values obtained in basketball studies perhaps suggesting an increased reliance on the glycolytic pathway when compared with rugby and football.

Basketball-specific tests

Physiological tests used in basketball include a range of aerobic endurance tests, such as the modified Yo-Yo test, along with tests of the glycolytic system such as the basketball sprint test which was illustrated in Figure 10.12 in Chapter 10. Vertical jump tests have been commonly used to assess power, bench press and squat to assess strength, along with sprints of 10–20 m to assess speed.

Key points

Basketball physiology:

➤ Exercise intensity
  - High-intensity movements – about 15% of the game
  - During high intensity, HR can reach 90–95% HRmax
  - Over 75% of game can be played at heart rates $\geq$ 85% of HRmax

➤ Significant demands on glycolytic pathway
  - Lactate can be elevated for duration of game
  - Male players – lactate concentration over 8 mM

➤ Aerobic fitness ($\dot{V}O_{2max}$) lower than other invasion games (males, 50–60 mL·kg^{-1}·min^{-1}; females, 45–50 mL·kg^{-1}·min^{-1})

➤ Fitness tests
  - Aerobic endurance – modified Yo-Yo test
  - Glycolytic system test – basketball sprint test
  - Anaerobic sprint ability – 10–20 m sprints
  - Power – vertical jump test
  - Strength – bench press and squat

The physiology of netball

As discussed in the previous section, James Naismith invented basketball in 1891. In 1895, Clara Baer, a sports teacher in New Orleans, wrote to Naismith asking him for a copy of the rules of basketball. Naismith subsequently provided Baer with information which included a drawing of the court with pencil lines drawn across it, suggesting the areas of the court which players could best guard. These lines, however, were misinterpreted by Baer who thought they indicated that players could not leave those areas. In 1899, this mistake was included into the rules of women's basketball. In its origins, ball dribbling was not allowed in basketball and this remained the case in the women's game. Netball originates from basketball and was formed and was first played in England in 1895. Despite this, the governing body for netball, the International Federation of Netball Associations (IFNA), originally named the International Federation of Women's Basketball and Netball, was not formed until 1960. Netball became a recognised Olympic sport in 1995 and was included in the Commonwealth Games programme in 1998. The IFNA now has 67 national members which are divided into five Regional Federations including the Americas, Africa, Asia, Oceania and Europe.

An introduction to the sport of netball

Netball is played between two teams, with the aim of the game being to score as many goals as possible by throwing a ball through an elevated goal ring. A netball team consists of 12 players, although only seven are allowed on the court at one time. The positions of netball are goal shooter (GS), goal attack (GA), wing attack (WA), centre (C), wing defence (WD), goal defence (GD) and goal keeper (GK). Depending on position, each player is only allowed within certain areas of the court. Only two players, GS and GA, are allowed within the goal circle (semi-circle centred on goal line) and are therefore responsible for scoring all the team's goals. A netball court is 30.5 m $\times$ 15.25 m and is divided into thirds along its length. There are two goal thirds and between them is the centre third. The centre circle, from which play is started at the start of a game or after a goal is scored, is in the middle of the centre third and has a diameter of 0.9 m. There is a goal circle (semi-circle) at each end of the court with a radius of 4.9 m. Goal posts are placed at the mid-point of each goal line. They are 3.05 m high, from the top of which a goal ring, with an internal diameter of 38 cm, projects (15 cm) horizontally. The netball itself is made of leather, rubber or a similar material, with a 69–71 cm circumference and a weight of 400–450 g.

Netball is a fast, skilful team game which involves running, jumping, throwing and catching, with multiple changes of direction and very short, sharp accelerations required to lose the opposing marking player and become available to receive a pass. A netball game consists of four 15-min quarters. There is a 3-min interval between the 1st and 2nd quarters, and between the 3rd and 4th quarters, with a 5–10 min half-time interval. Netball is predominantly played by females, while male and mixed competitions are increasing in popularity. It is the most popular female team sport in Australia and New Zealand.

Physical demands of netball

Despite its popularity and high incidence of injuries, the sport of netball has received little attention in the literature with regard to fitness testing, training variables and body composition. Netball is a physically demanding intermittent sport which requires strength, power, speed, agility, muscular endurance, aerobic endurance, and flexibility. It requires rapid changes in speed and direction to break free from an opponent, and in combination with high jumps, to receive a pass, intercept an opponent's pass or retrieve the rebound after a shot at goal. Most netball players have a tall, powerful physique, with a high lean body mass and a low percentage of body fat. Physical properties, however, appear to be position-specific in netball. The attackers (GS, GA) and defenders (GD, GK) are taller and heavier than the centre court players (WA, C, WD). Centre court players cover the greatest distance, hence they tend to have a slimmer physique, advantageous for stamina and agility.

The height of elite netballers ranges from 161.8 to 182.4 cm, with body mass ranging from 61.0 to 71.7 kg. An average %BF for all netballers is 24.5%; however, centre court players have a lower level of adiposity. The short work intervals in netball have been suggested to be less than 10–15 s, and are interspersed with recovery periods of at least three times the duration of the work period (work-to-rest ratio of 1:3) (Allison, 1978; Otago, 1983). Due to the nature of netball, with each position only allowed within specific areas of the court, the average sprint times of 1.43–1.84 s are shorter than those reported for other intermittent sports. The proportion of time spent sprinting is position-dependent with WA and WD spending the most time sprinting (16.3%) and completing the most number of sprints (336), in comparison with GS and GK who spend 4.1% of time spent sprinting with 82 sprint efforts (Allison, 1978).

Woolford and Angrove (1992) conducted research investigating position-specific energy demands during netball games. They tested four of the seven positions: GA, WA, C, WD. GA, C, and WD spent the majority of time with a HR above 85% of maximum, while WA spent the majority of time above 75% HR_{max}. The movement patterns demonstrated during netball match play were also identified in 1991 by Steele and Chad. The shooters (GA and GS) were found to spend a high percentage of time catching and rebounding the ball. In contrast, the centre court players (WA, C and WD) spent a high percentage of time jogging, running and shuffling, with less time available for recovery. In addition, WD was also highly involved in jumping. As would be expected, the defenders (GD and GK) were mostly involved in jumping, rebounding and guarding. These findings indicate the requirement of high aerobic and anaerobic fitness during elite netball games. Due to the position-specific movement patterns, training should be tailored to meet the specific requirements of each position. Muscular strength and power are also important attributes of netball players, allowing them to catch and throw the ball, contest a rebound, accelerate at speed and jump high. Indeed, a netballer's power, as measured during a bench press, has been found to be a strong predictor of chest pass performance (Cronin & Owen, 2004). The start/stop nature of netball combined with regular pivoting is illustrative of the high agility requirement of the sport.

An important rule of netball refers to stepping following catching the ball. The landing foot must either stay on the ground or in the air until the ball is passed to another player. If the landing foot is re-grounded a second time before the pass is made it is a step, and the player will be penalised. The elite netball players of today make the landing and passing sequence appear very fluid with the use of a 'run-on' landing technique. This technique appears to be the most beneficial, compared with pivot and two foot landings, for reducing the loads experienced by the lower limbs (Otago, 2004). This is an important factor in the game of netball as landing has been associated with the majority (72.4%) of anterior cruciate ligament (ACL) injuries (Steele, 1987).

Netball-specific testing

The 505 test is a commonly used measure of agility in netball. However, this test involves a set protocol where the athletes know they have to sprint as fast as they can for 5 m, turn 180°, and sprint back 5 m. Unlike the agility measured in this test, movements during a game are not predictable but are triggered by the actions of teammates and the opposition. This reactive aspect of performance has recently been included in a netball-specific test of agility through the addition of a visual-perceptual test component (Farrow et al., 2005). This test of reactive agility can be completed on an indoor netball surface. It involves the completion of a netball-specific agility pattern, including a shuttle time and a sprint time, and a decision-making time in response to a pass from a netball player shown in video footage. The movement pattern involved is shown in Figure 13.9. The player starts by sidestepping to the left then the right, sprints forward 1 m, makes a change of direction (~ 45 ° angle) and sprints 4.1 m through a finishing gate. The change of direction is determined in response to a pass produced by a player on a video display. The cue from the video indicating the direction of the pass occurred when the player began the forward sprint. Results of the test include shuffle time (start to gate 2), sprint time (gate 2 to gate 3 or 4), total time (shuffle + sprint time; measure of agility performance), decision time (number of video frames between moment of pass and player's movement initiation) and movement direction accuracy (did the player move to the correct finish gate?). With this test, highly-skilled netball players have been shown to make faster decisions than lesser-skilled players (Farrow et al., 2005).

Lower-body power is commonly tested with vertical jump and horizontal jump tests. Speed is assessed with a 5, 10 or 20 m sprint, while anaerobic capacity is tested with some form of repeated sprint test. Aerobic power is estimated with the MSRT or Yo-Yo test. A skill test performed by netball players in New Zealand is the wall pass test. This assesses the player's ability to perform passes against a wall (3 m away) with good technique for one minute duration. The number of passes completed is the player's score; however, the quality of the passes is also taken into consideration.

Key points

Netball physiology:

➤ Movements include: running, jumping, throwing, catching, directional changes, rapid acceleration

➤ Aerobic and anaerobic metabolic pathways required for energy generation

➤ Early studies suggested a work-to-rest ration of 1:3

➤ Average sprint time: 1.43–1.84 s

➤ Proportion of time spent sprinting is position specific (4.1% for GS and GK; 16.3% for WA and WD)

➤ Most players spend the majority of time with a HR > 85% HR_{max}

➤ Fitness tests

  • Aerobic endurance – MSRT or Yo-Yo test
  • Anaerobic sprint ability – 5, 10 and 20 m sprints
  • Power – vertical and horizontal jumps
  • Agility – 505 test, reactive agility test

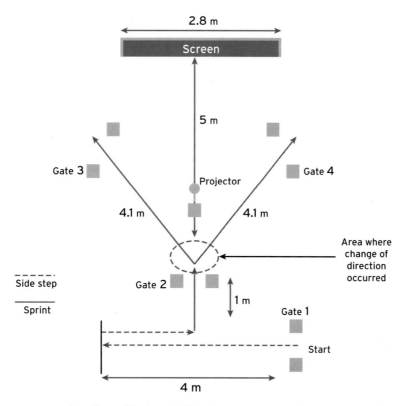

Figure 13.9 Reactive agility for netball test set-up.

The physiology of volleyball

Volleyball was invented by William Morgan, a physical education teacher in Holyoke Massachusetts, USA in 1895. Invented four years after and in the same state as basketball, volleyball was intended to provide a less strenuous alternative form of exercise. The game has grown substantially from these origins and is now played in over 220 countries worldwide, is overseen by the Fédération Internationale de Volleyball (FIVB) and two forms of the game now feature in the Olympic schedule. Volleyball is played by two teams of six players on an indoor court measuring 18 m × 9 m, with each team playing on either side of a net that is 2.43 m above the ground (from the ground to the top of the net in the centre of the court) and 1 metre in depth. While six players are allowed on the court at any one time, a volleyball squad can consist of up to 12 players. Beach volleyball, the most recent form of the game, is played between two pairs of players, most often on an outside sand-covered court measuring 16 m × 8 m. The beach form of the game was first played in the 1920s in California, USA and became an Olympic sport in 1996. The objective of both forms of the game is to ground the ball within the opposing team's court area or to force a mistake from the opposition, such as hitting the ball into the net

or outside the court area. After the serve, each team has three hits to set up their attack, in which the third hit must return the ball across the net. Vertical jump, the ability to rapidly change direction and to dive for the ball are important attributes to support the serving, blocking, passing and spiking required in the sport.

Physiological characteristics

The physiological demands of volleyball require players to have high levels of muscular power (upper and lower body), speed, agility and aerobic endurance. Research indicates that players vary in size and physiological characteristics according to their playing positions. Volleyball playing positions can be grouped to distinguish setters, hitters (right and left side), middles and more recently liberos. For male players at the elite level, middles tend to be the tallest players on the team (often over 2 m), followed by hitters at between 1.9–2.0 m, setters at around 1.9 m, with liberos often being the shortest players (around 1.8 m). With regard to body mass, hitters and middles can be up to 100 kg (usually 90–100 kg), while setters and liberos are typically between 80–85 kg. For female players the studies follow a similar pattern, with liberos representing the shortest and lightest members of teams (1.7 m, 60–65 kg), followed by setters (1.7–1.75 m, 65–70 kg), with hitters and middles representing the tallest and heaviest players (1.8 m, 70–75 kg). From the more limited results available, data suggest that beach volleyball players are lighter and shorter than the middles and hitters. A mean height of 1.87 and body weight of 77 kg were reported for the elite male beach volleyball players involved in a study conducted by Magalhães et al. (2011).

With regard to aerobic endurance capability, research indicates that court volleyball players have high levels of fitness with mean $\dot{V}O_{2max}$ values of 55–65 mL·kg^{-1}·min^{-1} for male players, 45–50 mL·kg^{-1}·min^{-1} for female players and male beach volleyball players average 55 mL·kg^{-1}·min^{-1}. The mechanical power of the leg extensors, which relates to vertical jump height, is greater in volleyball players compared to athletes in other sports (e.g. marathon runners, soccer players, swimmers).

Metabolic demands

Research to date for both forms of the game and for males and females suggest that, as an intermittent sport, volleyball places the predominant energy demands on the phosphagen system and aerobic system. The length of individual plays, the vertical jumping required for serving, blocking and hitting, place demands on ATP and PCr stores. The relatively long breaks between activity, typically on a 1:1 work-to-rest ratio (or better), enable replenishment of these stores through aerobic pathways. Results of data collected during matches suggest that lactate concentrations rarely rise above 2 mM, which lends support to the notion of less demand being placed on the glycolytic pathway during a volleyball game.

Key points

Volleyball physiology:

➤ Players require a high level of muscular power (upper and lower body), speed, agility and aerobic endurance

  • High aerobic fitness ($\dot{V}O_{2max}$) – males, 55–65 mL·kg^{-1}·min^{-1}; females, 45–50 mL·kg^{-1}·min^{-1}; male beach volleyball players, 55 mL·kg^{-1}·min^{-1}
  • High leg power (vertical jump) – males, 55–65 cm; females, 50–55 cm; beach volleyball players, 56 cm

➤ Predominant energy demands of the phosphagen system (vertical jumping, spiking) and aerobic system (recovery breaks)

The physiology of water polo

Water polo, developed by Scotsman William Wilson, was first played in the UK during the mid-to-late 19th Century and was initially played as a water-based form of rugby. Water polo became an Olympic sport for the first time in 1900, although it was not until 100 years later at the Sydney Games that female teams were included in the Olympic programme. The governing body for water polo, as for swimming, is the Fédération Internationale de Natation (FINA), which has over 200 member countries worldwide. Although the duration of game can vary, at international level games consist of four 8-min quarters (7 min for some leagues) separated by 2 min intervals. When stoppages in play are taken into account the duration of matches is around 55 mins, with each quarter typically being completed in around 12 mins.

Water polo teams consist of seven players on the field of play at any one time, with teams typically having six reserves who can be rotated on after a goal, penalty, exclusion or time-out, and in between quarters. The pitch size for a water polo game is slightly larger for males than for females, at 30 × 20 m and 25 × 17 m, respectively. The goals measure 0.9 × 3 m, with the ball being slightly larger (circumference) and heavier (mass) for males than females (typically 68–71 cm, 450 g versus 65–67 cm, 400 g).

Exercise intensity

Water polo games are played at a high intensity, with work-to-rest ratios for outfield players being around 5:3 and 2:5 for goaltenders. Results of time and motion analyses indicate that games are broken down into distinct bouts of activity typically lasting less than 20 s duration and requiring 7–14 s of intense activity such as sprinting. The nature of these efforts and the patterns of play mean that outfield players spend almost all the playing time with their HR above 80% of HR$_{max}$, including periods where HR is between 90–95% of maximum. In terms of oxidative demand, results of previous studies suggest that players operate at around 80% of $\dot{V}O_{2max}$ during peak activity. Lactate concentration data analysed from samples taken during games suggest that players can achieve concentrations as high a 9–12 mM. These results indicate that in addition to energy supplied via the phosphagen system and aerobic pathways, the intensity of the game is such that water polo also places moderate demands upon the glycolytic pathway.

Physiological characteristics

Although there are a limited number of studies published in the field, male water polo players have been suggested to have a body mass of between 75–90 kg, mean %BF around 12–15% and $\dot{V}O_{2max}$ of between 55–60 mL·kg^{-1}·min^{-1}. Female players have been found to have a body mass of around 65–69 kg. Players have been found to cover between 1,000–2,000 m during a game, dependent on their position and the nature of a specific game. These distances are largely covered during swimming phases, where the body is horizontal, which typically comprise about 50% of game time. During these swimming bouts, approximately half of that time involves sprint activity, close to maximal speeds.

Water polo-specific tests

A number of sport-specific performance measures have been developed for water polo and these include the swimming anaerobic power test (SAPT), the 30 s crossbar jump test (CJ$_{30}$) and the water polo intermittent shuttle test (WIST). The SAPT, also known as the SWIM test, involves completing 14×25 m swims, one every 30 s. The time for each 25 m is recorded to the nearest 0.1 s for each participant, from which the velocity for each sprint, mean velocity and fatigue rate can be calculated in a similar way to the IAnRT test (which was described in the section on tests for intermittent sports players). The CJ$_{30}$ requires participants, from a treading water starting position, to jump and touch two-handed the crossbar of a water polo goal (0.9 m) as many times as possible in 30 s.

The WIST is an intermittent shuttle test, conducted in the water, but similar in nature to the Yo-Yo test which was described earlier in this chapter. Water polo players are required to complete out-and-back 7.5 m swims at a progressively increasing speed. The speed for each swim is controlled by a series of audio beeps which indicate the start of each subsequent shuttle. Players are required to complete the test between two lane ropes set 7.5 m apart and a minimum of 2 m away from the side of a pool. In between shuttles players must remain active but stationary during the 10 s recovery prior to starting the next shuttle. The participant must keep pace with the audio signals such that they start to swim when they hear the first beep, touch the lane rope in time with the second beep and return to the end of the course in time for a third beep. Players can swim with their heads in or out of the water, but must lift their heads at the end of each 7.5 m effort to hear the beep. The test starts at a pace of 1.03 m·s^{-1} and a participant continues in the test until he or she fails to be within one arm stroke of the lane rope at the start/finish line, at which point they are given a warning. If the participant fails to finish the next shuttle within one arm stroke the test is terminated and his or her level and stage recorded. From this data it is possible to calculate his or her total distance swum.

Key points

Water polo physiology:

➤ High-intensity sport – work-to-rest ratios of 5:3 (outfield players) and 2:5 (goaltenders)

- Outfield players – majority of playing time HR > 80% of HR$_{max}$, includes periods where HR is 90–95% of HR$_{max}$
- During peak activity, intensity is around 80% of $\dot{V}O_{2max}$
- 50% of game time spent swimming – around half that time involves sprint (near maximal) activity

➤ Cover 1,000 to 2,000 m during a game – position-specific

➤ Metabolic demands

- Energy supplied by all three pathways – phosphagen, glycolysis, aerobic
- During games – Lactate concentration of 9–12 mM

➤ Fitness tests

- Swimming anaerobic power test (SAPT)
- 30 s crossbar jump test (CJ$_{30}$)
- Water polo intermittent shuttle test (WIST)

The physiology of canoe polo

Canoe polo, rapidly increasing in popularity, is a fast and dynamic game played by two teams of five players. The origins of canoe polo, like water polo, date back to the late 19th Century in the UK. In the early forms of the sport, players sat astride barrels or stood upon their canoe poling to get to the ball. In the 1920s the German Canoe federation introduced 'kanupolo' as a way to introduce new members to the sport and the modern sport has developed from these origins. The international governing body for the sport is the International Canoe Federation which has around 150 member nations worldwide. Each team is comprised of eight players in total, with five allowed on the field of play at any one time. Substitutions are made on a rolling on-off basis. Canoe polo is a classic intermittent activity with sprints of varying distance and intensity interspersed with variable duration recoveries. Many of the aspects important to performance in canoe polo can be derived from the preceding sections that have described the physiology, most likely causes of fatigue, nutritional strategies and training methods for intermittent activities. To date, however, there has been less research focus upon the physiology of canoe polo.

Exercise intensity

One of the few studies in this area was a motion analysis completed by Chris Bussell. In this study covert filming of Great Britain players taking part in National League Division One canoe polo matches was completed. Five matches for the goalkeeper and ten matches for the three defenders and four attackers were recorded during data collection for the study. The filming was completed covertly so as to minimise any influence on the playing patterns for any of the participants taking part in the study; however, once filming was completed all participants consented to their involvement. A time and motion analysis was conducted from the video footage, beginning with velocity calculations for each of the participants. Movement was categorised according to whether it was of high intensity (sprinting forwards or backwards), intermediate intensity (tackling, turning the boat or restraining a player), low intensity (slow paddling) or stationary/drifting (little or no exercise being completed by the performer). The results of the study indicated that across the game the attackers travelled at a higher velocity than the defenders; however, for players in both positions there was a general decline in intensity from the first to second half of the match. The defenders in the study appeared to have more balanced performance across the whole game, with just over 10% of their time in both halves spent engaged in high-intensity exercise. The attackers, on the other hand, completed the first half of the game with close to 20% of their time spent at high intensity, but in the second half this percentage fell to just over 6%. The goalkeeper spent 15% of the time in the first half and 12.5% of the second half engaged in high-intensity exercise. For players in all positions, around 70% of time was spent within the low and stationary/drifting categories. In the second half all players spent a slightly increased amount of time in intermediate and low-intensity exercise or stationary/drifting. These results suggest that attention in training may require a focus on the maintenance of physiological performance during the second half of a match, particularly for the attackers.

Special considerations for canoe polo players

Further research, perhaps additionally utilising heart rate monitors and studying players from other countries, would be beneficial prior to decision making regarding fitness programme development for canoe polo players. Nevertheless, in the time before such findings are available research from other similar intermittent activities could be employed to formulate training strategies for attackers and defenders in canoe polo. There are a number of canoe-polo-specific factors that would need to be addressed in making decisions regarding the physiology of canoe polo. Typically, National league and international competitions are organised such that several games are played on the same day. For instance, international competitions may consist of players taking part in 4–5 games in a day for up to 3–4 days and as such, a canoe polo training programme should reflect the demands not just of one match but of a whole day's matches. Some competitions and many internationals take place on open water, rather than in a swimming pool, which can place additional environmental stresses (wind and ambient temperature primarily) on canoe polo players. Further research regarding the physiology of canoe polo would be beneficial to improve understanding of the physical demands of the sport.

Key points

Canoe polo physiology:

➤ Exercise intensity
  - Attackers travel at a higher velocity than defenders – this drops for both groups of players in second half
  - Defenders – just over 10% of time engaged in high-intensity exercise (both halves)
  - Attackers – around 20% of time in 1st half, and just over 6% in 2nd half in high-intensity exercise
  - Goalkeeper – 15% of time in 1st half, and 12.5% in 2nd half, in high-intensity exercise
  - All players – ~70% of time spent in low-intensity and stationary/drifting (little or no exercise)
  - Intensity lower in 2nd half for all players

The physiology of racquet sports

The origins of racquet sports date back to the Middle Ages, most likely 12th-century France, and as a consequence they represent some of the oldest sports played in a modern context. In contrast, the development of games such as speedminton, mean that racquet sports also represent some of the newest intermittent sports developed. Racquet sports include Olympic disciplines such as badminton, table tennis and tennis, as well as squash, racquetball and real tennis. Each of these racket sports, along with speedminton, is typically played as singles or doubles matches, between two or four players. The object of each of the games is to propel a missile (ball or shuttlecock) in such a way that the opponent(s) is unable to make a return. The scoring system is specific to each sport and more recent rule changes in sports such as squash, table tennis and badminton have been developed to improve the speed of play and the spectacle for audiences. Such changes have impacted on the physiological demands of each sport and should be taken into account when reading the information provided in this section and for planning an athlete's training programme. Due to the research data available we will concentrate this section on the sports of tennis, badminton and squash as indicative of the physiology of racquet sports.

Tennis

Tennis is played on a 23.78×8.23 m court for singles, and a 23.78×10.97 m court for doubles, with a net 0.914 m high (at centre court) and spanning the midpoint of the court (i.e. 11.89 m from either end). The mean time for each point is around 7–10 s, with a work-to-rest ratio around 1:3 or 1:5. The length of a tennis match can vary considerably, depending on the ability of the players, the type of surface and the number of sets over which a match is played. A match can be over in as little as 40 min or last over 11 h, as was the case in the record-breaking match between Nicolas Mahout and John Isner, highlighted at the start of this chapter. High-level tennis players have been found to have a $\dot{V}O_{2max}$ of between 55–65 mL·kg^{-1}·min^{-1} for males and 50–55 mL·kg^{-1}·min^{-1} for females. Research regarding match performance suggests that overall intensity of a game is around 60–70% of $\dot{V}O_{2max}$, with HR between 140 and 160 beats·min^{-1}. Mean lactate concentrations have been reported to be around 3 mM during a game; however, after a long rally, values have been shown to rise to 7–8 mM. Research findings to date suggest that, depending on the nature of the game and the particular point being played, tennis will place demands for energy on anaerobic (phosphagen system and glycolysis) and aerobic metabolism.

Badminton

Badminton is played on a 13.4×5.18 m court for singles, and a 13.4×6.1 m court for doubles, with a net 1.524 m high (measured at its centre) and spanning the midpoint of the court (i.e. 6.7 m from either end). The mean time for each point is around 6 s with recoveries of around 12 s between each point, making a 1:2 work to rest ratio. The mean height of elite badminton players in the studies published to date is 1.75 m (males) and 1.65 m (females), with body masses of 67–73 kg and 60 kg for males and females, respectively. Elite level badminton players have a $\dot{V}O_{2max}$ of around 60 mL·kg^{-1}·min^{-1} for males and 50 mL·kg^{-1}·min^{-1} for females, with games played at 73% of $\dot{V}O_{2max}$ and 89% of HR$_{max}$. Post-match lactate concentrations of between 3.0–5.0 mM have been recorded for badminton players, although, typically, concentrations are lower and sometimes closer to 2 mM. Since the introduction of the rally point scoring system the mean duration of matches is normally between 30–35 min in elite level competitions. Researchers to date suggest that the phosphagen system and aerobic system provide the most important metabolic pathways during a badminton match.

Squash

Unlike tennis and badminton, squash is not played by hitting the missile over a net, but by hitting it against a wall in a 4-sided court with the dimensions 6.4×9.75 m. This difference has significant implications for the tactics within the sport and the physiological demands. Squash matches have been found to result in the highest lactate concentrations of the racquet sports, rising to 10 mM at the end of a game or match. The rises in lactate concentrations and increased relative reliance on glycolysis, is closely linked with the duration of points, which is typically between 5–20 s, with short rests periods between points. Games last around 8 min with matches lasting between 30–40 min.

Research indicates that squash is played at a high intensity, around 90% of HR$_{max}$ and around 80% of $\dot{V}O_{2max}$. The mean height of the elite squash players studied to date (1.72–1.77 m for males) is shorter than that of other racquet sports and may reflect the tactical differences between the sports. While being taller can be a distinct advantage for tennis, when moving in the confines of a squash court, relatively shorter players may have an advantage. Results of studies to date suggest that elite squash players have a $\dot{V}O_{2max}$ of 50–60 mL·kg^{-1}·min^{-1}.

Sport-specific tests for racquet sports

There are a number of sport-specific tests which have been developed to assess fitness for badminton, squash and tennis players. For the sport of badminton, two agility tests

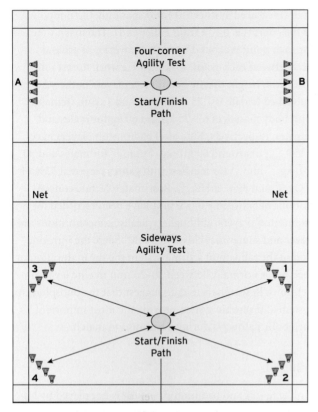

Figure 13.10 The set-up for the FCAT and SAT badminton tests. (*Source*: Adapted from Ooi et al. (2009))

were reported by Ooi et al. (2009), which are the four corners agility test (FCAT) and the sideways agility test (SAT); these are illustrated in Figure 13.10. In both tests shuttlecocks are required to be placed as shown. A squash-specific

graded test, developed by Girard et al. in 2005, is illustrated in Figure 13.11 and discussed.

Both tests involve the player starting from a badminton-ready position, crouched with feet either side of the centre line and facing the net. Neither of these tests requires a racquet. However, players should move using badminton-specific movements and strike each shuttlecock, as shown in Figure 13.10, with their dominant hand. For the FCAT players are required to move from the start/finish position in the sequence as shown 1–4, such that the player moves from start/finish position to point 1 and strikes at a shuttlecock before returning to the start/finish position. In total, players are required to strike 16 shuttles, four at each point, with the time being measured for the total duration of the test. The test is finished when the athlete places one foot on the centre line at the start/finish position. The best of two trials is recorded for each player. The SAT involves players moving from side to side on the court, passing through the start/finish position on each occasion making a total of 10 repetitions (5 to each side of the court). Each time they reach the right or left sideline, the player must strike a shuttlecock with their hand. Again, players would be timed for two trials with the best time recorded.

The squash-specific graded test (SSGT) was developed by Girard et al. (2005) as a game-specific incremental test. The set-up for the test is shown in Figure 13.11 and requires players to move from the T position to one of the points shown in the figure – requiring forward diagonal, lateral or backward diagonal movement and back to the T position. The player must move at all times using squash movement and, with his/her racquet, play a stroke at an imagined ball

Figure 13.11 The set-up for the SSGT. (*Source*: Adapted from Girard et al. (2005))

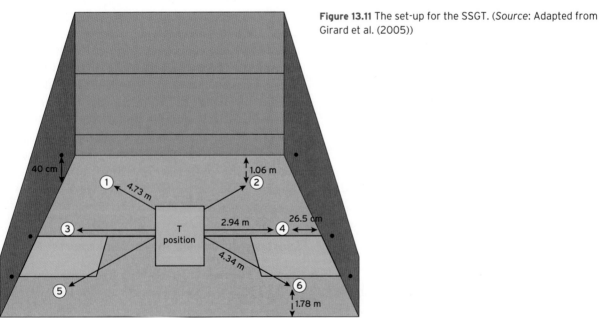

prior to returning to the T position (shot played between 0 and 40 cm above the floor). The sequence of the movements was determined randomly by a computer software programme, with nine movements (two front court, three lateral and four backcourt) in each stage or level. The first three stages provide a warm-up for the player to be tested. Each of the stages has a 10 s recovery prior to the start of the next, with the exception of stage three where, following the warm-up, a 30 s recovery is included. From a starting duration of 38 s for the first stage the time is decreased by 1.8 s for each stage in the warm-up and then by 0.9 s for each subsequent stage. The software programme on each occasion provides the direction required for each shuttle and players continue in the test until they miss the target by 1 m. The competition ranking of squash players is correlated with the time to exhaustion in the SSGT.

Key points

Racquet sport physiology:

➤ Aerobic fitness ($\dot{V}O_{2max}$) – around 50 mL·kg^{-1}·min^{-1} for females and 60 mL·kg^{-1}·min^{-1} for males

➤ Exercise intensity

  • Increases from tennis (60–70% $\dot{V}O_{2max}$), to badminton (73% $\dot{V}O_{2max}$), to squash (80% $\dot{V}O_{2max}$)
  • Highest lactate concentrations found at the end of squash game (10 mM)
  • Tennis and badminton typically produce lower lactate levels (2–5 mM), although this is increased after a long rally (7–8 mM)

➤ Demands placed on both aerobic and anaerobic metabolism

➤ Sport-specific tests

  • Badminton – four corners agility test, sideways agility test
  • Squash – squash-specific graded test

Knowledge integration question

In relation to the demands of the sport, why, in general, is blood lactate concentration greater following a squash match than following a tennis match?

The physiology of cricket

Cricket is another of the older intermittent sports and is also one of the earliest to receive research attention. As early as 1955 a study examined the exercise intensity of the 1953 Ashes Test series between Australia and England during the five tests in the series which was played in England. The origins of cricket can perhaps be traced back to medieval Britain as a game developed and played by children. From these beginnings cricket began to be played by adults around the 16th century but was first played as an international game in 1844, with Test cricket commencing from 1877.

Cricket is a striking and fielding game played between two sides of 11 players who take it in turn to bat and field during the game. The central components of the game include bowling, batting and fielding, with the aim of the game for the fielding side to dismiss (get out) 10 of the 11 players on the batting side, while the batting side attempt to score as many runs as possible from the fielding team's bowling. In the modern day there are several versions of cricket matches played including 5-day test matches, 3-day matches, as well as one-day and Twenty20 matches.

Fletcher's 1955 study examined the average energy expenditure for the players involved in the 1953 Test series. Through his analysis he found that from the potential 150 h of cricket, 46 were lost to the weather and four to breaks in play which meant that just over 100 h involved play. Over the 100 h, 4,363 runs were scored at an average of 43.6 runs per hour, requiring players to run 500 metres each hour between the wickets while batting. He went on to analyse his data further and found that, when averaged, a player expended around 86 kcal·m^{-2}·hr^{-1} scoring 14 runs in 38.5 min, bowling 4.2 overs during 14 min of bowling and fielding 16 balls during 116 min in the field. Fletcher's data indicated that Test match cricket required just a little more energy than required for standing for the same time period. Fletcher's analysis of the game matched many people's impressions of the game; however, recent research suggests that the modern game places greater physiological demands on players.

During a one-day match mean HR for fielding and batting has been found to average 120 beats·min^{-1} while, perhaps not surprisingly, data for fast bowling revealed higher exercise demands. HR data for 12 overs of fast bowling have been found to result in a mean HR (around 172 beats·min^{-1}) that is similar to exercise intensities found in marathon running. Researchers suggest that physiologically cricket places demands primarily on the phosphagen system and aerobic metabolism as the predominant metabolic pathways and also to restore PCr stores prior to the next higher intensity effort.

Although cricket is primarily a lower-intensity intermittent sport, one where skill-related perceptual motor rather than physiological aspects predominate, cricketers usually maintain relatively high levels of fitness to maintain their performance in the sport. Research has shown that the mean aerobic endurance ability of international cricketers is similar to those in higher-intensity sports such as rugby, with a $\dot{V}O_{2max}$ around 60 mL·kg^{-1}·min^{-1}. Typically, bowlers have a slightly lower $\dot{V}O_{2max}$, and are slightly taller and heavier than batsmen.

Key points

Cricket physiology:

➤ Exercise intensity
  • Fielding and batting – average HR 120 beats·min^{-1}
  • Fast bowling – average HR 172 beats·min^{-1}

➤ Despite relatively low intensity of the sport, cricketers maintain high aerobic fitness ($\dot{V}O_{2max}$ ~60 mL·kg^{-1}·min^{-1})

➤ Metabolic demands primarily on phosphagen system and aerobic pathways

---

The physiology of combat sports

Combat sports form some of the oldest sports that are still practised today and include Olympic disciplines such as boxing, fencing, judo, taekwondo and wrestling. These intermittent sports involve athletes in one-to-one, usually unarmed, combat, the roots of which can be traced back to ancient civilisations pre-Christianity. Since these early times humans have enjoyed taking part in and watching these head-to-head clashes where opponents match technique, tactics, and fitness to gain victory over an opponent. While different codes, forms and styles have developed, the aim has remained the same, to develop the skills and fitness to defeat your opponent.

Boxing

The history of boxing or fist fighting can certainly be traced back to Sumerian civilisation around 3000 (BCE), but can perhaps be dated back further to ancient Mesopotamia (~5300–7000 BCE). Ancient carvings and paintings have been found of fist fighting from these times. In addition, there are frescos still existing from ancient Greece (~1000 BCE) depicting gloved fist fighters. After its origins as an Olympic sport in ancient Greece, modern boxing is most closely linked with prize fighting in the UK. In 1743 heavyweight champion Jack Broughton made rule changes for prize fighting which introduced the wearing of padded gloves (mufflers as they were known), banned hitting when someone was on the ground and also the landing of low blows. The rules of boxing were developed further during the next century, and were laid down formally in the Marquess of Queensberry rules published in 1867. The rules of modern day boxing grew from these roots, although there a number of differences between the amateur and professional rules of boxing, such as the use of protective headgear and the length of matches. Within the Olympic Games boxing remains an amateur sport, with athletes often turning professional after Olympic or World success at amateur level. Examples include Cassius Clay (later known as Muhammad Ali) in 1960 and George Foreman in 1968. At the London 2012 Olympics there will be 10 weight categories for men and for the first time as a full event, three weight categories for women. At the London Games the matches for men will take place over 3 × 3 min rounds, while women will compete over 4 × 2 min rounds.

Combat sports often divide competitors into different categories based on their weight, because generally, the larger the body mass of an individual, the greater their strength and power. Although reporting body mass, and to some extent height, lend little to understanding the requirements of these sports, body composition, and strategies to stay within a weight category, can provide valuable information for exercise physiologists that may relate to competition performance. Elite level boxers have been found to have %BF similar to other combat sports such as judo and wrestling, with males (with the exception of heavyweights) having a mean between 5% and 10%. To date there is less data available for female boxers, perhaps because of the relatively short duration for which the sport has been included in the Olympic programme.

$\dot{V}O_{2max}$ tests reveal that elite male boxers typically have an aerobic power between 55 and 65 mL·kg^{-1}·min^{-1}. The relative intensity of boxing, similar to that of judo and wrestling, has been suggested to be higher than for a combat sport such as fencing. Results for female boxers indicate that average HR rises linearly across the three rounds of a contest with a range of 171–184 beats·min^{-1}, similar to that reported for male boxers (175–180 beats·min^{-1}). During a bout, blood lactate concentrations increase by 4–6 mM between rounds and by 8–9 mM by the end of the contest, compared to baseline levels. This data supports the notion that boxing is a high-intensity intermittent sport and indicates that fast-rate glycolysis is an important source of energy during a contest.

Key points

Boxing physiology:

➤ Aerobic power ($\dot{V}O_{2max}$) 55–65 mL·kg^{-1}·min^{-1}

➤ HR rises across three rounds of contest: females, 171–84 beats·min^{-1}; males 175–80 beats·min^{-1}

➤ Fast-rate glycolysis

- Predominant energy generating pathway
- Elevates blood lactate concentration (8–9 mM at end of contest)

Fencing

In a historical sense fencing can be traced back to ancient civilisations where swords were used as weapons of war and training was for battle as well as for sport. In a modern context fencing can be traced back to the schools of fencing that grew up across Europe from the 12th century onwards, including influential schools such as the French School of Fencing in the 18th century. Fencing is one of the rare sports which has featured at every Olympic Games in the modern era. There are three disciplines within the sport which relate to the choice of weapon; foil, epée and sabre. With the foil and epée weapons, points are scored by hitting the opponent within the tip of the weapon only, while in sabre the edge of the blade can be used as well. In epée, fencers can score simultaneously; however, for foil and sabre only one fencer can score at a time. For each of the disciplines at the Olympic Games, fencing bouts are held over three rounds of 3 min or until one fencer reaches 15 pts. While a team event features in the Olympic fencing schedule, all contests take place between two individuals at a time.

Fencing tournaments can last up to 11 hours, of which the bout time for a fencer could be between 47–122 min. During a bout each point typically lasts 5–15 s with a work to break recovery of around 1:1 to 1:3. The movements required in fencing mean a fencer typically covers a distance of 250–1,000 m. Lactate concentration appears to rise significantly during a fencing bout, with post-bout levels generally reaching at least 4 mM. The winner of one competition, however, reached a lactate concentration as high as 15.3 mM at the end of the final. Interestingly, during training lactate concentrations do not appear to rise to the same extent, which has led researchers to suggest that there may be a sympathetic driven elevation in anaerobic glycolysis during competition. The aerobic endurance ability of fencers appears to be consistently lower than endurance-trained athletes, but comparable with other intermittent sport players with a mean $\dot{V}O_{2max}$ of between 55–60 mL·kg^{-1}·min^{-1} for males and 45–50 mL·kg^{-1}·min^{-1} for females.

Key points

Fencing physiology:

➤ During a bout – work-to-rest ratio of 1:1 to 1:3

➤ Lactate concentration post-bout $\geq$ 4 mM, as high as 15.3 mM has been reported

➤ Aerobic power ($\dot{V}O_{2max}$) – males, 55–60 mL·kg^{-1}·min^{-1}; females 45–50 mL·kg^{-1}·min^{-1}

Judo

The origins of judo can be traced to Japan, the martial art of jujutsu and the ideas of Kano Jigoro/Jigoro Kano. Kano studied jujutsu under a number of teachers before beginning to develop his own style where the focus was upon maximal efficiency, minimal effort. In 1882 Kano founded his own school which later became the Kodokan at which he taught his form of jujutsu, which he called judo. The sport consists of throws, hold-downs, chokes and strangles which can be used individually or in combination to score against an opponent or to force a submission. Contests are of 5 min duration with extra time added should a contest finish in a draw.

As a sport where contestants are divided into weight categories, body size and composition are important aspects of the sport. The importance and difficulty in reaching the optimal weight for compitition is clearly illustrated in Karen Roberts' 'Sport in Action' section on pp. 428–9. Somatotype data indicate that judo players are heavily mesomorphic athletes, with a slightly higher tendency to endomorphy than ectomorphy. The body composition of judo players is related to weight category, with the lighter-weight-group athletes typically having the lowest %BF. Male players below 71 kg typically have a %BF below 10%, while those above this weight have a slightly higher %BF (10–15%). Female judo players, with the exception of heavyweight players, generally have a %BF between 15–20%. Similar trends are found for aerobic endurance capacity, with lower-weight players tending to have the highest $\dot{V}O_{2max}$, although this is not always the case. The $\dot{V}O_{2max}$ for judo players tends to be in the range 55–65 mL·kg^{-1}·min^{-1} for males and 45–50 mL·kg^{-1}·min^{-1} for females.

Taekwondo

Taekwondo is the national sport of South Korea and means the 'way (do) of striking with foot (tae) or fist (kwon)'. The history of the sport is shrouded in some mystery with some researchers claiming the sport dates back to the hwarang military group in medieval times. Others suggest the roots come from karate which was introduced to Korea after World War II, with difference in rules and movements being developed to make the sport uniquely Korean. The objective of taekwondo is to throw scoring kicks and punches on your opponent's scoring zone. One point is scored for a kick or punch to the torso, two points for a spinning kick to the head and four points for a turning kick to the head. Contests in the Olympic Games are held over 3×2 min rounds.

Taekwondo, like boxing, judo and wrestling, is a sport where competitors fight in different weight categories and consequently relative body composition is an important aspect of the sport. Elite female taekwondo players have been shown to have a %BF of 15–18%, while values for males are typically 7–12%. With regard to the aerobic capacity of taekwondo athletes, the reported $\dot{V}O_{2max}$ of 54–61 mL·kg^{-1}·min^{-1} for males and 42–50 mL·kg^{-1}·min^{-1} for females are similar to those of other combat sports, and indeed other high-intensity intermittent sports.

Key points

Judo and Taekwondo physiology:

➤ Aerobic power
- Judo – males, 55–65 mL·kg^{-1}·min^{-1}; females, 45–50 mL·kg^{-1}·min^{-1}
- Taekwondo – males, 54–61 mL·kg^{-1}·min^{-1}; females, 42–50 mL·kg^{-1}·min^{-1}

Wrestling

Wrestling, like boxing, can be traced to ancient civilisations pre Christianity, with evidence of wrestling in artwork being found in ancient Egypt around 2000 BCE. Wrestling was popular in Greek civilisation and was one of the sports of the ancient Olympic Games. The sport also has links with, and similarities to, sports like jujutsu in Japan and jiao li in China. Since the advent of the modern Olympic Games, Greco-Roman and freestyle (from 1904) wrestling have featured in every Olympiad except the 1900 Games. In 2004 women's freestyle wrestling was added to the Olympic schedule as a full sport. In the Greco-Roman form of the sport wrestlers can use only their arms and upper bodies to defeat their opponent, whereas in freestyle wrestling the legs can be used as well. In the Olympic Games, wrestling matches take place over 3×2 min rounds with a 30 s break between rounds.

As a weight category sport, similar in that sense to judo and taekwondo, wrestling requires athletes to maintain their body mass below a specified value. Typically, male wrestlers have a %BF of 5–10%, with the exception of heavyweight competitors who have a higher percentage body fat. The intensity and nature of wrestling is such that significant demands are placed on fast-rate glycolysis, as indicated by post-wrestling bout lactate concentrations of 10–15 mM regularly found for wrestlers. With regard to aerobic endurance capacity results for male wrestlers have identified elite athletes to have a $\dot{V}O_{2max}$ of 53–56 mL·kg^{-1}·min^{-1}.

Key points

Wrestling physiology

Aerobic power ($\dot{V}O_{2max}$) – 53–6 mL·kg^{-1}·min^{-1}

High demands on fast-rate glycolysis – post-wrestling bout lactate concentration of 10–15 mM

The physiology of sailing

Sailing is a very popular recreational activity but additionally is a highly competitive adventure sport with events held at European and World level and is included in the Olympic schedule. Furthermore, some classes in sailing are amongst the most expensive and technically sophisticated of any sport. Until recently, however, the physiological demands in sailing – hiking, trapezing, sail pumping and coffee grinding – were largely overlooked. Single-handed dinghy sailing for instance was considered a relatively static sport with the main physiological challenge being the isometric contractions of the legs and abdominal muscles required during hiking. More recent research has challenged the traditional view and provided information about the physiological demands in sailing.

Research suggests that sailing provides greater physiological demands than was previously thought, with the requirements for the helm (skipper) and crew being dependent upon the class of boat sailed. The different roles played by the helm and crews in each sailing class, along with the dramatic changes in physical stresses brought about by an accidental capsize, make it essential that training is based around the physiological demands for the individual crew member. In most classes, the training programmes for the helm should be different from those for the crew to reflect the differing physiological demands of each role.

The diversity of physiological demands in sailing is reflected by the fact that the roles for dinghy double-handers, single-handers and match-racing crews can be considered as intermittent activity. In contrast, typically for dinghy double-hander and match-racing helms, where technical and tactical consideration are paramount, the physiological demands are perhaps best categorised as lower-intensity aerobic endurance (except in the event of a mid-race capsize!). Despite these groupings, the physiological demands and the development of a training programme for any sailor should be individually developed and based upon the current fitness level of the athlete along with the boat demands of their role.

Hiking and trapezing

The main physiological challenges in sailing include hiking, trapezing, sail pumping and coffee-grinding. Table 13.2 provides a summary of the predominant demands for both helm and crew for each class. During upwind sailing, **hiking** is required to counteract the heeling effect or capsizing moment created by the wind's effect on the sail. This involves the helm, crew or both, moving to and then sitting out on the windward side of the boat to provide a

counteraction to the force of the wind, thereby righting the boat. During hiking the muscles of the legs and abdomen are primarily stressed. In double-hander boats, such as 470s and 49ers, the heeling effect is countered by the crew (and helm in 49ers) trapezing. **Trapezing** involves the crew, and additionally the helm in 49ers, suspending their body over the side of the boat. In order to achieve this position a harness is worn which is attached to a wire from high on the mast. The roles of the helm and crew change during upwind and downwind sailing. For example, in the 470 class, during an upwind leg the helm will hike while the crew is relatively less physiologically stressed trapezing, while on a downwind leg the helm may be involved in pumping the mainsail (within legal limits), which is normally quite lightly loaded, while the crew is working relatively harder pumping the spinnaker which has a heavier loading.

Windsurfing and sail pumping

The new Neil Pryde RS:X class represents the only windsurfing class in the Olympic Programme, having recently replaced the Mistral windsurfing board as the Olympic board. The Mistral class was adopted as the windsurfer for the 1996 Olympic Games and was used in all subsequent Games up to Athens. After the Athens 2004 Olympic Games the Neil Pryde RS:X board was adopted as the Olympic board, which remains the board of choice for the London 2012 Olympic Games. The RS:X class is unique to

Table 13.2 Predominant physiological demands by sailing class.

Class	Sailors	Predominant physiological demand
Laser (dinghy)	Single-handed	Hiking
Finn (dinghy)	Single-handed	Hiking
Europe (dinghy)	Single-handed	Hiking
470 (dinghy)	Double-handed	Helm - hiking, crew - trapezing
49er (dinghy)	Double-handed	Helm and crew - trapezing
Tornado (catamaran)	Double-handed	Helm and crew - trapezing
Neil Pryde RS:X (windsurfer)	Single-handed	Sail pumping
Star (keelboat)	Double-handed	Helm - hiking, crew - hiking (harness-assisted)
Yngling (keelboat)	Triple-handed	Helm - hiking, crew - hiking (hobble-assisted)
Yachting (match racing)	Single - multi-handed	Helm - dependent on no. of crew, crew - coffee-grinding

(*Source*: Adapted from Cunningham, P. (2004)).

Olympic sailing, with all the boards and sails made in the same factory meaning all windsurfers are using the same basic craft to sail. Prior to the Atlanta Olympics (1996) a decision was taken to allow unrestricted sail pumping for windsurfing competition. **Sail pumping** involves drawing the sail to and from the windsurfer to use the sail as a 'wing' resulting in an increase in speed. Research indicates that sail pumping can result in substantial increases in speed, perhaps up to three-fold in some wind speeds. The use of sail pumping creates a significant rise in the physiological demands placed upon the windsurfer.

Coffee-grinding

Winches are used on the larger keel boats for hauling and adding tension to sails. In match racing yachts, pairs of cranks are attached to a pedestal and are used to power the winches. The cranks are moved in a bicycle action referred to as **coffee-grinding**. The winching systems on larger sailboats have a gearbox to provide multiple speeds for use with the large sails required to maximise speed in match racing and to allow the power to be transferred to alternative winch systems. A key role for match racing crews is to provide the propulsive force required in coffee-grinding. Coffee-grinding on yachts during a race represents a high-intensity intermittent activity where upper-body strength and a good aerobic base and anaerobic fitness are essential.

Physiological characteristics

In the Olympic classes, sailing competitions tend to have two races per day, although the target time for race duration is different for each class. Typically, windsurfing races at the Olympics will take place over 35–45 min, Laser races over 60 min, Finns over 75 min, and Star races over 90 min. The required wind speed is normally 5–30 knots for racing to be allowed. With two races per day it means that sailors can be on the water for up to 4–6 hours per day which increases the physical demands and has implications for nutritional strategies. In addition to the physical demands associated with each sailing class, environmental stresses of cold and hot ambient temperatures, the effects of wind exposure and possible water immersion can impact upon physiological functioning. All these issues must be addressed when planning a training programme for a sailor. Many researchers believed that dinghy sailing placed relatively low physiological demands upon the sailor. Spurway and Burns (1993) suggested that the major demand arose through hiking and that isometric contraction of the muscles involved in hiking should predominate in training.

Vogiatzis and colleagues (1994), in agreement, suggested that aerobic training should not be emphasised for dinghy sailors (Laser class). More recently, however, research has suggested that the movement required in hiking and trapezing places demands upon the aerobic capacity of the sailor. This concept is not new, as Harrison and co-workers in 1988 suggested that hiking in a static position was a rarity due to changes in wind speed and direction that would necessitate continual movement on the part of the sailor to counteract changes in the heeling effect. As a result of their research Devienne and Guezennec (2000) concluded that, in contrast with the majority of previous research, aerobic capacity should be considered as an important performance factor for sailors. Indeed research by Cunningham(2004) with British Olympic sailors suggests that hiking on a specifically designed hiking ergometer can result in an oxygen consumption rate equivalent to 65–70% of $\dot{V}O_{2max}$ during single-handed race simulations (Laser class). In agreement with this, Castagna and Brisswalter (2007) found very similar results in an on-water study, with hiking during a simulated race requiring up to 69% of $\dot{V}O_{2max}$.

Sail pumping in the RS:X windsurfing class of sailing has been suggested to be a physically demanding activity that places significant demands upon the aerobic system (Vogiatzis et al., 2002). In their study, Vogiatzis and colleagues compared the physiological cost of windsurfing with and without sail pumping (SP) and found that the mean oxygen cost more than doubled for both males and females (males: 19.2 mL·kg^{-1}·min^{-1} compared with 48.4 mL·kg^{-1}·min^{-1}; females: 15.7 mL·kg^{-1}·min^{-1} compared with 40.2 mL·kg^{-1}·min^{-1}, without and with SP, respectively). These oxygen costs of sail pumping represented between 77–87% of each sailor's $\dot{V}O_{2max}$. This result is in agreement with research by De Vito and colleagues who found windsurfing with sail pumping required 75% of the sailors' $\dot{V}O_{2max}$. It is thought that the new Olympic windsurfing class of the Neil Pryde RS:X will show very similar physiological demands to the Mistral class. The results of recent research for both windsurfing and dinghy sailing have indicated the importance of aerobic capacity for sailors and led to changes in emphasis for training programmes.

Exercise that assists in maintaining a steady or decreased body mass, along with hand-eye coordination and agility activities, could be considered for helms in addition to tactical and technical development. For dinghy and yacht racing crews the intermittent activities chosen for training should match both the nature of the rest-exercise intervals during sailing and be as specific as possible to the exercise during sailing. For windsurfers, where the activity during racing can be classified as high-intensity aerobic endurance (the focus of Chapter 11), the major emphasis should be lactate threshold training. In addition, work to develop strength (resistance training based around the Olympic lifts) and maintaining an aerobic base appear to be beneficial to performance.

Key points

Sailing physiology:

➤ Hiking – sitting on windward side of boat to counteract force of wind

- Can involve isometric muscle contractions
- Oxygen consumption rate can reach 65–70% $\dot{V}O_{2max}$

➤ Trapezing – suspending body over side of boat by means of a harness

➤ Sail pumping – drawing sail to and from windsurfer

- More than doubles the oxygen cost of windsurfing
- Results in oxygen consumption of 75–87% $\dot{V}O_{2max}$

➤ Coffee-grinding – movement of cranks to power sail winches

- Aerobic and anaerobic fitness, and upper-body strength essential

➤ In addition to physical demands, sailors are exposed to environmental stresses

---

The physiology of surfing

Developed many centuries ago, surfing has seen a dramatic rise in its popularity in more recent years, although there is a limited availability of research regarding the physiology of surfing. Since the 1980s studies have been conducted regarding the physiological characteristics of surfers, time and motion analysis and common injuries during surfing. Research indicates that male and female surfers are generally shorter and lighter than athletes involved in other water-based activities such as swimming and water polo. Elite level male surfers have been found to have a mean height of 173–5 cm and females between 162–6 cm as compared with means of 183–6 cm and 171–2 cm for male and female swimmers and polo players. With regard to mass, elite male and female surfers have been found to have means of 68 kg and 57–9 kg, while those for swimmers and water polo players have been recorded as between 78–86 kg for males and 63–4 kg for females. Body

fat percentages of 10.5% for males and around 21% for females have been reported.

Research data suggests that, not surprisingly, surfers have higher recorded oxygen uptakes when compared with untrained individuals. These data have been collected using arm-crank ergometers (similar to a cycle ergometer, as was shown in Chapter 12, but moved with the arms rather than the legs), tethered board paddling and using a prone swim bench (a form of dry-land swimming ergometer where front crawl is the assessed stroke). Values of 40–54 mL·kg^{-1}·min^{-1} have been recorded for surfers with maximal heart rates during testing of around 180 beats·min^{-1}. Maximal on-water heart rate values of around 171 beats·min^{-1} have been reported, with an average during surfing of about 135 beats·min^{-1}. This provides evidence for the inclusion of surfing as an alternative method for improving cardiovascular endurance and indeed some schools, in Australia, New Zealand, the UK and the USA, include surfing within the physical education curriculum. A suggested model for the demands of surfing, that includes physiological, psychological and skill-related factors, along with the environmental issues that may be present is shown in Figure 13.12.

A number of studies have used time and motion analysis to report the relative times spent paddling out (sometimes referred to as arm paddling), stationary and wave riding. Similar values for elite and recreational surfers have been identified. A study of recreational surfers reported that, of the time spent surfing, 44% was spent paddling out, 35% stationary and 5% wave riding. A study of 42 male surfers in a professional surf competition recorded values of 51%, 42% and 3.8%, respectively. Taken together, these findings suggest that during a typical surf session perhaps as much as 50% of the time is spent paddling out, 40% stationary and 5% actually surfing (none of these values add up to 100% as each includes a miscellaneous category where activity was not clearly related to paddling out, being stationary or wave riding. An example of a miscellaneous activity would be turning the board to check incoming wave sets and setting position ready to take-off for a wave). Of a typical 3–5 h session, these values indicate that surfers spend somewhere around 9–15 minutes actually riding a wave. The most common injuries reported in surfing are cuts and grazes occurring through contact with other surfers and their boards, the beach or groynes. With regard to overuse injuries, shoulder, lower back and neck injuries represent those most commonly reported and appear to be closely linked with paddling out and departure from the board.

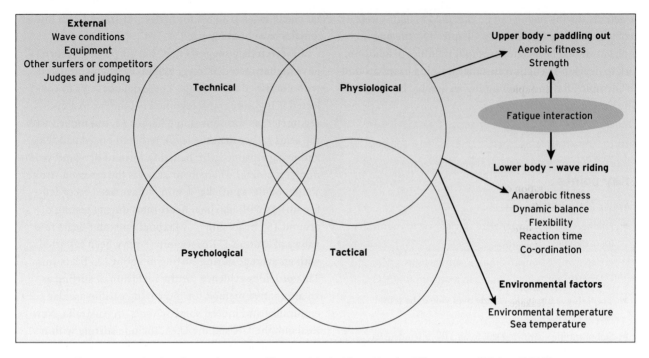

Figure 13.12 The components of surfing performance. (*Source*: Adapted from Mendez-Villanueva and Bishop (2005))

Key points

Surfing physiology:

➤ Aerobic power ($\dot{V}O_{2max}$) – 40–54 mL·kg^{-1}·min^{-1}

➤ Average HR during surfing 135 beats·min^{-1}, maximal values of 171 beats·min^{-1} have been reported

---

13.3 Ergogenic aids for intermittent sports

Beyond the adoption of a normal healthy balanced diet for those involved in intermittent sports, possible dietary manipulations should be determined by the duration and metabolic demands of the intermittent sport. Some intermittent sports, such as soccer or rugby, involve short-duration high-intensity bursts, where the phosphagen system is important for ATP synthesis. These are followed by longer recoveries which enable aerobic metabolism to restore ATP and PCr concentrations ready for a subsequent high-energy burst. For such sports ergogenic aids that improve resting PCr stores, such a creatine monohydrate supplementation, along with carbohydrate feeding to maintain blood glucose levels for aerobic metabolism, may

be beneficial for performance. Creatine monohydrate supplementation was described in Chapter 9.

Athletes involved in intermittent sports that require extended high energy bursts, such as those required for sports like judo or wrestling, might additionally consider the use of a buffer such as bicarbonate or β-alanine to help delay fatigue (as described in Chapter 10). For longer duration intermittent sports, and for those taking part in tournaments, dietary manipulation of carbohydrate intake has been shown to result in improved endurance performance. These manipulations can include pre-exercise carbohydrate loading and during-activity carbohydrate feeding through the use of sports drinks. Each of these manipulations could be beneficial to an intermittent sport athlete. As with any alteration in training, any new supplement should be trialled prior to use before an important event. Practising a supplementation strategy can help to avoid any possible side effects that might be deleterious to performance.

Knowledge integration question

What is the predominant energy system required during high-intensity short bursts of activity in sports such as football and hockey? In what way can an ergogenic aid help with the functioning of this system and hence improve performance?

Check your recall
Fill in the missing words.

➤ Intermittent sports include brief periods of _____ intensity exercise coupled with periods of partial or complete rest.

➤ During intermittent exercise, a much greater volume of work can be completed before exhaustion than during continuous exercise of the same _____.

➤ Increasing the duration of rest periods in intermittent exercise will function to _____ lactate accumulation.

➤ In prolonged intermittent sports (> 90 min), _____ depletion plays an important role in fatigue.

➤ In high-intensity, short-duration intermittent sports, H^+ increases, citrate leakage, _____ transport disruption and _____ depletion all play a potential role in fatigue.

➤ The two main forms of intermittent training are intermittent aerobic (ITA) and _____ _____ _____ (IHIT).

➤ Time–motion analysis and _____ data provide vital information for the development of an intermittent training programme.

➤ During intermittent sports such as soccer, rugby or hockey, the _____ system is important for ATP synthesis during high-intensity bursts of activity.

➤ Two sport-specific tests for badminton are the four corners agility test (FCAT) and the _____ _____ _____ (SAT).

➤ The main physiological challenges in sailing include hiking, sail pumping, _____ and _____ _____.

➤ An ergogenic aid, such as _____ _____, may improve resting PCr stores and hence benefit intermittent sports performance.

Review questions

1. Which factors in relation to intermittent activities will have an impact on the physiological processes that underlie performance?

2. Why is fat oxidation likely to be greater during intermittent exercise than during continuous exercise? What role does fat oxidation play in sustaining performance?

3. Why might increased interstitial K^+ concentrations contribute to fatigue in intermittent activities?

4. Why is it important to match the demands of training to the specific demands of a performer's sport? What might the first stage of this process be?

5. What are the physiological adaptations following intermittent aerobic and intermittent high-intensity training?

6. Why might light exercise be more beneficial than complete rest in some intermittent activities? How have physiologists defined 'light exercise' during studies?

7. What are some general examples of sport-specific aerobic conditioning activities? Name an example for a specific sport.

8. Why are time and motion analyses useful for intermittent sports?

9. Explain how the rule changes in rugby league have affected the physiological demands on professional players.

10. Explain the physiological differences between basketball and football (soccer).

Teach it!
In groups of three, choose one topic and teach it to the rest of the study group.

1. Intermittent sports rely on ATP synthesis via the phosphagen system, fast-rate glycolysis and aerobic metabolism. What variables can be manipulated within an intermittent training programme to change the predominance of the energy systems and obtain physiological adaptations specific to the sport?

2. In a typical intermittent sport, such as football, what demands are made on the metabolic pathways? What is a common test used to assess the aerobic fitness of football players and how could this component of fitness be developed through sport-specific training?

3. Explain the key research findings that indicate that performance during intermittent exercise differs from continuous exercise.

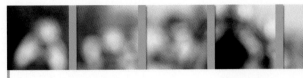

SPORT IN ACTION

Biography: Karen Roberts
Sport: Judo

Intro to me

I first stepped on to the judo mat aged 7 at a local sports centre. It was not long before the coach made the recommendation for me to join the renowned Pinewood Judo Club under the direction of sensei Don Werner. At the age of 14 I made my GB debut at the European Youth Olympics, securing the bronze medal. The following year my family and I attended the Barcelona Olympics to support club mate Nik Fairbrother, my exposure to the Olympic experience was inspirational. A few months later I became the Junior World Champion in Argentina at the age 15, remaining the youngest Junior World Champion to date. I went on to become an Olympian myself in Sydney 2000 and a Senior European and World medallist, before becoming Commonwealth Games Champion in 2002.

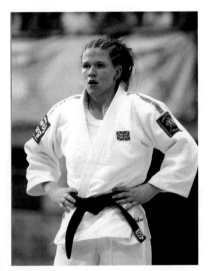

(*Source*: Bob Willingham)

Judo story

Every sports person says it about their sport and I will say it about mine – judo – it is different from anything else out there! To explain why I believe I can say this I will explain a typical competition day. Firstly, the day begins with competitors being weighed to ensure they are within the tolerances for their discipline-mine was under 63 kg; I could weigh anything from 57.1 kg to 63 kg – not a gram more. Generally, and unsurprisingly, the advantage comes from being right at top of the weight limit, so before your competition even starts you are modifying your body composition. The reason I feel it is important to explain this is because often this can be the key to why a day may go well or not.

Following 'weighing-in' you have a minimum of 2 hours to replenish fluids and fuel for the day. To win a gold medal you typically will have five contests in one day with varying rest in between but a minimum of 10 mins. Contest times have changed over the years for women from 4 to 5 minutes, and also a 'golden score' came into play in 2001, if there is no score in the first 5 mins then you fight for another 5 and the first to score wins (another record I believe I hold is the longest fight, I managed to pin my opponent in the final seconds of the golden score and kept her there for the extra 25 secs!). Golden score has now reduced to 3 mins.

Within an individual contest you clearly require an aerobic base, but within the contest a throw requires explosive strength, and the gripping patterns static strength. Perhaps your aerobic base can be less of an issue if you have the ability to throw quickly and accurately. To win a contest you may throw, hold, armlock or strangle your opponent for ippon, which immediately ends the fight. If you throw or hold for a lower score then you continue until the time runs out. These are active ways to score, you can also apply tactics to impose pressure on an opponent so that they receive penalties or your opponent makes mistakes and receives penalties. All of these various connotations occur while your opponent is trying to do exactly the same thing to you!

Due to the various ways to win, you can encounter a wide range of styles of fighters – this is then supported by the necessary physical qualities.

I am sorry for the detailed explanation of the workings of the sport, I am an engineer by trade and this helps me rationalise my personal performance.

I was capable of using various techniques but not known for throwing for maximum points. I was particularly strong in the newaza aspect – hold, armlocks and strangles. As I had no guarantee of a quick finish I had to build a strong aerobic base so that when the opportunity arose in newaza I was still in condition to take it. When I say condition, I suppose this means that despite being fatigued my mind still had to be sharp enough to see a chance and take it – accurately.

On reflection this worked well in my career . . . as long as the other aspect of the competition preparation was done well, weight management. I remember one occasion in Moscow, where my weight had been high coming into the final week of tapering, so I had to maintain 'weight-making' sessions, i.e. long slow runs every day. I made my weight, I had a good draw, but when I went in for my first contest I knew I was feeling the effects. My aerobic base was clearly there, but my decision-making was lousy. Clearly missing the correct taper into the event I had lost my sharpness, but it was more than that – it didn't matter how good my aerobic base was, it felt like it had been stretched too far. I won the first

contest but the second was where it was seen – a clear opportunity to hold my opponent and I couldn't take it. It was a lesson.

I suppose the best example I could find to show the lesson was learnt would be in the final of the 2002 Commonwealth Games. Weight managed well, final taper completed and most importantly I had the condition to finish the day the way I started. I

had a particularly strong opponent in the final – she had beaten me before, and I had beaten her. The opportunity came in the latter stage of the fight – I didn't miss it, she had attacked me with a throw, I avoided it and counter-attacked to take her to the ground and straight on to the arm to force a submission and gain the Commonwealth Games title.

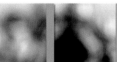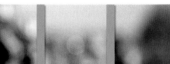

SPORT IN ACTION

Biography: Matt Crooks
Sport: Football/soccer

Matt started playing football at the age of six years with Lepton Badgers. Whilst playing there he was spotted by a Manchester United trainer and asked to train with them. At the age of eight years, Matt,

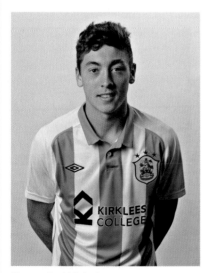

(*Source*: David Sykes)

along with 63 other boys, was chosen for assessment and he trained with Manchester United until he was 15 years old. Out of the 64 boys the club only kept two players: although Matt reached the final four it was now time to move on. Matt chose to play for his home club, Huddersfield Town AFC, where he has just completed his first year as an apprentice, for which he was awarded 'young player of the year'.

My time at Manchester United

What can you say about being with one of the biggest clubs in the world? The training is great – I was training with other good, skilled young friends, boys who have just won the FA Youth Cup. The Carrington training facility for the academy included one outdoor and one indoor full size 3G pitches, plus 10 outdoor pitches like green carpets! We had the use of the senior gym with an indoor swimming

pool which we used if injured or for recovery sessions. Manchester United's style was never to put pressure on us . . . the only pressure I felt was that which I put on myself.

My years at Manchester United involved a lot of travelling and staying on top of my schoolwork was a challenge. I would sometimes be doing my homework very late at night or first thing in the morning. My typical day involved leaving home at 7:30, attending school from 9:00–16:00, straight onto the coach to arrive home at 17:00, and then travelling by car to (while changing into training gear and eating sandwiches) to Carrington for a 2-hour training session, then travelling back to Huddersfield arriving home at 22:00. There were three training sessions mid-week plus sessions on Saturday and Sunday. Although it was hard, the experience will last me a lifetime. I didn't realise how lucky I was to have had the chance to train with Manchester United until I left.

➤

My time at Huddersfield Town

My most memorable game, funnily enough, was not with Manchester United, but against them! I was playing my preferred midfield position for Huddersfield Town in an under-16 game. I wanted to prove myself to Manchester United in this position (they had moved me to centre half in my last year with them, but I don't like defence) and I wanted to impress. That is what I did when I scored the best goal of my career to date . . . it was 'a screamer' from 25 yards out, dropping the shoulder and cutting inside on to my right foot with rising effort. Bang! Into the top right hand corner. We won the game 2–0.

Training as an apprentice is more tactical-based than skill-based. Now that I have moved up to training with the first team standards are higher. The other players have better ball skills and are faster on the ball. The start of training on the 1st July has been the hardest training I have ever done . . . I was exhausted. Our new fitness coach recently tested our speed over 40 yards (using timing gates). My performance (5.07 s) was close to the best (4.9 s). Some other testing involved the Yo-Yo test to assess our cardiovascular fitness and capturing video and photo data to monitor our mobility overtime as an injury prevention measure. In training, not surprisingly we do lots of running, VO_2 runs and match specific sessions, along with flexibility sessions and plyometric work with exercises such as lunges, jumps off one foot and one-foot hops.

My weekly schedule includes 2-hour intensive fast training on Monday and Tuesday, a rest day on Wednesday, a 2-hour morning session and a 1.5-hour afternoon session on Thursday, a 2-hour session on Friday, a match on Saturday and a 1-hour recovery session on Sunday. In addition to these soccer-specific sessions I do a weights session at the gym three times a week. We also have a food guideline to follow to ensure we have sufficient and appropriate nutritional intake. Since the start of the new training programme I feel fitter and faster.

The first team manager and coaching staff are developing a team that will hopefully become champions of league one this year and move into the championship next season. The future is bright!

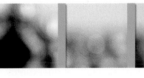

SPORT IN ACTION

Biography: Andy Ellis
Sport: Rugby union

Born in Christchurch, New Zealand, Andy Ellis currently plays half back (scrum half) for Canterbury in provincial rugby and for the Crusaders in the Super 14 league. He was selected for the NZ under-21s side in 2005. However, due to injury in the Super 14 semi-final, was unavailable for international selection until the 2006 end of year tour when Andy made his All Blacks debut playing against England at Twickenham. Since then, Andy has been a regular selection for the All Blacks team, including selection to play in the Rugby World Cup, 2007 and 2011.

Training for rugby union at the elite level

(written with Ashley Jones, strength and conditioning coach for the Crusaders)

Strength and power conditioning

To be a successful international half back, able to withstand the physical demands of the position, and to additionally act as an extra loose forward at times (both in ball-carrying and defending around the edges of the ruck/maul and scrum), I believe my body mass must be at least 90 kg. To this end I perform a weight-training program specific to my position, to maintain upper-body size and strength. This is either added to full body strength training or a power program, or is an

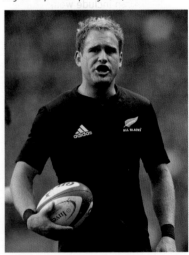

(*Source*: Georgie/RugbyImages)

additional workout at least once a week, involving alternation of two exercises with repetitions declining across sets and weeks (see examples below).

Bench Press super setted with Weighted Chins

- Week 1-6, 5, 4, 4
- Week 2-5, 4, 3, 3
- Week 3-4, 3, 2, 2

Incline Hammer Press super setted with Hammer Strength Low Row

- Week 1-12, 10, 8, 8
- Week 2-10, 8, 6, 6
- Week 3-8, 6, 4, 4

Lower-body strength and power are also extremely important in order to produce explosive running efforts of a short acceleration nature. This is a large part of my game as gaps open up and shut quickly in my position. GPS research studies suggest that I perform in excess of 30 sprints in a game, at a pace above 6 m.s^{-1} and an average distance of 15 m. Some methods I use to develop lower-body strength and power include weights and short acceleration speed sessions. Heavy power training involves rapid movements to switch on a large number of the fast-twitch muscle fibres and can include weight sessions such as:

- power cleans from blocks (5 × 3 reps at 70–80% of max) alternated with knees-to-feet jumps (6 reps per set)
- band box squats (5 × 3 reps at 60% of max) alternated with box jump ups (6 reps per set)
- push press (5 × 3 reps at 70–80% of max) alternated with medicine ball throws against a wall

I also do a short acceleration speed session each week. The session begins with a 15-min warm-up including a range of movement drills (e.g. high knees, carioca, marching) with a gradual increase in speed till you are at around 85% of top speed and are ready for maximal sprinting. The warm up is followed by two of the following sessions:

- Resistance sprint – sprint with resistance (parachute or sled) for 30 m, release resistance, sprint resistance-free for 30 m.
- Flying 30's – build up pace over 22 m to hit top pace, hold pace through to the half way line, walk to the other end of the pitch, repeat to complete four reps.
- One v One – facing the same way, one player (with the ball) starts about 5 m behind the other player; within a 15 m × 50 m area of the field, the player behind attempts to turn the defender (front man) both ways and then, when he sees a gap, sprints past him and races to the 50 m line.

Aerobic conditioning and recovery

The other most important aspect of my physical development is aerobic fitness, as GPS data show that, as a half back, I cover on average > 7,500 m in a game at a variety of intensities. Most of this training is in the off-season to develop a fitness base for higher-intensity training during the season, but each week of the playing season is topped off with a short repeated speed session (e.g. 10 × 50 m every 30 s followed by 20 × 25 m (lying start) every 15 s). Small-sided modified-rules-conditioning games are also used to stimulate

further improvements in fitness, but have the added bonus of developing ball skills and vision concurrently. Some methods employed in the off season are fartlek running (interspersing higher intensities of running with jogging) over a varied terrain for 40-60 min, and cross training on bikes and rowing machines – useful to avoid overloading the legs but still work the heart and lungs appropriately.

I have learnt that as the year/ season lengthens, recovery is very important to maintain both mental and physical components for successful rugby. This means that in some weeks I may not do extra fitness, speed sessions or heavy weights, but instead have a massage, do extra stretching, have extra ice baths, do a light bike spin or pool swim.

Additional stresses during games in South Africa

Games that always stand out for me personally, are when we travel to Pretoria and Johannesburg in South Africa, where it is hot, dry and at altitude. Gasping for oxygen and water are a normal part of a day out on the playing field. Not only are the conditions so different but the people are very passionate and the stadiums are like fortresses. When our bus arrives the crowd hurtles cans of beer and shake our bus. We have full police escorts and the run from the bus to the changing shed is always daunting. Then there are the opponents, again big strong men that carry the ball as hard as any other men in world rugby. Although a tough place to play, it is up there with the most enjoyable games, and is always a test of both character and our physical preparation.

Intermittent maximal exercise by Gaitanos and colleagues (1993)

Many people take part in intermittent exercise sports. Intermittent sports are characterised by short bursts of maximal effort punctuated by rest or sub-maximal exercise. Gaitanos and colleagues made the point that more people engage in intermittent sports (football, tennis, basketball, hockey etc.) than are involved in prolonged continuous exercises (e.g. running, cross-country skiing or distance swimming). In adventure sports there are many examples of intermittent activities or forms of training that include intermittent exercise. Sport rock climbing and bouldering sessions, canoe polo matches, surf kayak, free-style kayak and river running (canoe or kayak) are examples of adventure sports that either inherently involve or can be carried out to involve inter-mittent exercise. Despite such partici-pation numbers less is known about the physiology of intermittent sports when compared with prolonged exer-cise. The aim of the study by Gaitanos and co-workers was to describe the metabolic changes that arise in response to repeat sprint exercise.

The eight male participants took part in 10 repeat sprints of six seconds duration with a 30-second recovery between each one. The mean age, height and mass of the participants was 26.7 years, 175.6 cm and 71.8 kg. Prior to the test, partici-pants were familiarised with the testing procedure and instructed to refrain from exercise the day before testing. The protocol for testing included a rest period for pre-test blood and muscle biopsy sampling, standardised warm-up, the repeat sprints and a 10-min post exercise recovery period. The peak power output (PPO) and mean power output (MPO) for each sprint were recorded. Venous blood samples were taken pre activity, post sprint 1, post sprint 5, post sprint 9, post sprint 10 and at 3, 5 and 10 min during the recovery. Blood samples were analysed for blood lactate concentration, glucose, adrenalin and noradrenalin. Muscle biopsies were taken from the vastus lateralis of the quadriceps muscle pre activity, post sprint 1, post sprint 5 along with pre and post sprint 10. The muscle samples were analysed for a wide variety of metabolites which included ATP, ADP, AMP, PCr, crea-tine, pyruvate and lactate.

The key results for the study are shown in Table 1. The PPO and MPO for the first sprint were 1,253 W and 870 W. The PPO fell by 16% by the 5th sprint and 33% by the 10th sprint. The MPO fell by 13% and 27% at the same points. The PCr concentration fell by 57% after the first sprint, while glycogen and ATP fell by 13 and 14% respectively. By the end of sprint 9 the PCr concentration was 51% of the resting value and decreased a further 16% post sprint 10. At the same stages ATP and glycogen concentrations were 32% and 30% of resting values, respectively, but while glycogen concentration fell by almost a further 9% there was no change in the ATP concentration at the end of sprint 10. From these results Gaitanos and colleagues calculated that the percentage contri-bution from PCr degradation rose from 49.6% in sprint 1 to 80.1% in sprint 10, while the percentage contri-butions from glycolysis and ATP catabolism fell from 44.1-16.1% and 6.3-3.8% respectively.

The results of this study show a progressive decline in power output (peak and mean) across the 10 sprints decreasing by 33 and 27% respectively. As Gaitanos and co-workers point out, however, the MPO for sprint 10 still represented 73% of the value for sprint 1. The slight decrease in lactate production between sprints 9 and 10 is sugges-tive of an inhibition of fast-rate glycolysis. The identified decline in fast-rate glycolysis in sprint 10 placed an increased relative reliance on PCr degradation and increased role for aerobic metabolism. The findings of Gaitanos and colleagues provide evidence to suggest that for intermit-tent exercise there is an increased reliance upon PCr catabolism and aerobic metabolism with increasing duration.

Reference: Gaitanos, G.C., Williams, C., Boobis, L.H. and Brooks, S. (1993). Human muscle metabolism during intermittent maximal exercise. *Journal of Applied Physiology*, 75(2), 712-19.

Table 1 Mean values for power output, blood lactate, plasma catecholamine and key muscle metabolites.

	Pre	Sprint 1	Sprint 5	Sprint 10
PPO (W)	N/A	1253.3	1054.03	834.7
MPO (W)	N/A	870.1	760.47	638.65
BLa (mmol·1⁻¹)	0.6	1.9	9.2	pre 12.6/post 12
Adrenalin (nmol·1⁻¹)	0.4	1.9	4.2	5.1
Noradrenalin (nmol·1⁻¹)	1.7	3.3	15.7	22.3
ATP (mmol/kg dry wt)	24	20.9	N/A	pre 16.4/post 16.4
PCr (mmol/kg dry wt)	76.5	32.9	N/A	pre 37.5/post 12.2
Glycogen (mmol glucosyl units/kg dry wt muscle)	316.8	273.3	N/A	pre 221/post 201

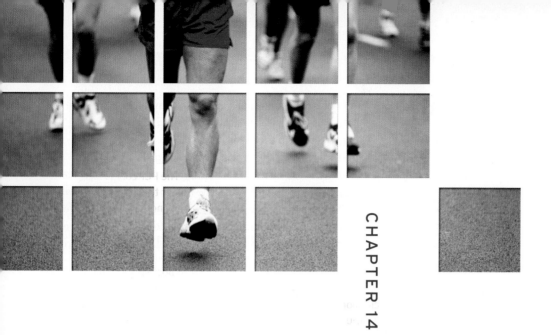

CHAPTER 14

Applied exercise physiology and health

Learning objectives

After reading, considering and discussing with a study partner the material in this chapter you should be able to:

➤ explain a range of short-term and medium-term health factors associated with taking part in sport or exercise, such as delayed-onset muscle soreness (DOMS), a stitch, muscular cramp and over-training

➤ discuss the effects of health issues such as asthma and McArdle's disease for people who take part in sport and exercise, and treatments to help

➤ describe the health benefits associated with taking regular exercise

➤ explain how physical inactivity is associated increased risk of cardiovascular disease, diabetes, obesity and metabolic syndrome

➤ teach to others the health phenomenon known as the female triad

➤ identify how different countries quantify regular physical activity

➤ compare and contrast the merits of high intensity interval training as a time efficient form of physical activity

This chapter considers a wide variety of health issues that relate specifically to, or are associated with, exercise and exercise physiology. The health of students or athletes involved in sports programmes is an important consideration for any physical education teacher or coach. Sometimes those we teach or coach will ask questions about why we get stitches or muscle cramps and we should be able to answer these questions. Alternatively, at any time we might teach or coach someone with asthma or have to teach about curricular aspects such as the effects of exercise as a preventative measure against the development of cardiovascular disease. This chapter covers a range of health issues from short-term sports-related aspects, such as delayed onset muscle soreness to longer-term illnesses such as diabetes or depression and the role that exercise can play as a prevention or treatment. We begin this chapter by focusing on short-term health aspects and then move on to cover longer-term health issues from an applied exercise physiology perspective.

14.1 Sport and exercise-related aspects of health

Delayed onset of muscle soreness

The exercise adage of 'no pain, no gain' can be evidenced immediately after activity and as a delayed response. The immediate feeling of fatigue and 'pain' after exercise (sometimes referred to as the 'pump') results from the accumulation of exercise metabolites such as hydrogen ions in the muscles and, in the case of rock climbing, sailing, pumping and intense weight-training, the pump is caused by blood pooling in the working muscles. These feelings normally subside within minutes or an hour or two after exercise. Intense exercise, however, can result in a delayed onset of muscle soreness known as DOMS which normally occurs within 1–2 days of the exercise and lasts for up to a week post exercise. The symptoms of DOMS include muscle stiffness and soreness, and often leave the areas affected feeling tender to touch. These symptoms tend to peak at onset, dissipating over the following days.

Exercise associated with DOMS

Eccentric muscular contractions, as occur with downhill running (e.g. fell running), or resulting from weight training where a relatively heavy load is taken through a full range of motion (as with lifts such as bench press or squats), are particularly associated with the occurrence of DOMS. In addition to eccentric muscular contractions, DOMS is also associated with an increase in training volume and intensity. This could include situations such as returning to training after a break or the commencement of a new training programme, such as resistance or sprint training. As an example, an athlete who has just completed the first session of a new sprint training programme will experience acute muscle soreness (normally associated with exercise) which will dissipate within 1–2 hours after training. After an asymptomatic period, however, the effects of DOMS will appear 24–48 hours after the sprint session.

Mechanisms of DOMS

The exact cause of DOMS is undergoing further investigation. However, the two prime mechanisms appear to be muscle tissue damage and inflammation around the affected areas. Evidence of DOMS can be assessed through microscopic examination of tissue samples or through the assessment of creatine kinase and the presence of myoglobin in the blood. In instances of DOMS, microscopic muscle tissue examination reveals sarcolemma (muscle cell membrane) rupture along with possible tearing of sarcomere Z-discs (the links between neighbouring sarcomeres) and damage to the myofibrils. The rupture of the sarcolemma allows cell contents to leak out which is why myoglobin and creatine kinase can be detected in the blood during an episode of DOMS.

The muscle fibre micro-trauma occurring in DOMS induces an inflammatory response in the area of tissue damage. Blood analysis during DOMS reveals elevated leukocyte (white blood cell) levels, an immune system response to the trauma and subsequent inflammation. Granular neutrophils and macrophages (which form from monocytes – agranular leukocytes) move into the area of tissue trauma. Neutrophils release oxidants (free radicals) that attack invading micro-organisms and release proteins that have an antibiotic effect in the damaged cells, while macrophages consume the cellular debris that results from the trauma. It is important to note that the free radicals released during DOMS serve a beneficial function. In other instances, however, free radicals can be detrimental to our health, especially those introduced through smoking and air pollution.

DOMS and performance

Research indicates that the muscle micro-trauma and inflammatory response associated with DOMS has a negative effect on maximal strength while its effects remain within the body. These effects are thought to occur as a direct consequence of the tissue trauma and interference with the excitation–contraction coupling of motor units within the traumatised area. Research also indicates that fast-twitch muscle fibres, which are closely associated with maximal contractions and expressions of power and strength, are more susceptible to the effects of DOMS. For sub-maximal exercise, however, there appears to be no negative physiological effect on performance, although, due to the soreness and stiffness, the work is perceived as harder by athletes. Antioxidant supplementation, particularly vitamin E, has been suggested as beneficial in recovery to avoid tissue structure damage associated with excess free radicals released by the neutrophils at the trauma site. The main recommendation for recovery from DOMS is through the light exercise and stretching of the affected area. Once the muscle cells have repaired themselves there appear to be some benefits from an episode of

DOMS. Research indicates that an occurrence of DOMS is a precursor to subsequent gains in strength associated with muscular hypertrophy (increase in muscle size). In addition, a single incidence of DOMS appears to protect the body from subsequent occurrences during a particular phase of training. Although the effects of DOMS can be reduced through training programme management, the commencement of a new programme, new phase of training or new form of exercise often appears to result in an episode of DOMS.

Key points

Delayed onset muscle soreness (DOMS):

➤ Stiffness, soreness and tenderness of muscles

➤ Occurs 1–2 days after training

➤ Symptoms remain for up to one week post-exercise

➤ Results from muscle tissue damage and inflammation

➤ Light exercise and vitamin E supplementation may aid recovery

Muscular cramps

Muscular cramps, painful abnormal muscular contractions of a single muscle group, are not fully understood by researchers. The original theory as to the cause of muscular cramps was based around fluid and electrolyte imbalances within the body associated with exercise in the heat for a long duration. The incidence of muscular cramps during periods of rest and when fluid and electrolyte levels were balanced, has led to further research in the area. For adventure sports performers where the legs are either highly active during the activity (walking, climbing, etc.) or held stationary for long periods (kayaking and canoeing) the muscle groups in the upper and lower leg are particularly prone to muscular cramps. Muscular cramps are thought to be triggered by an irritation to a muscle group. The irritation results in the hyperexcitability of the motor neuron(s) innervating that motor unit bringing about an uncontrolled muscular contraction (cramp). Several factors may be involved in the initiation of cramp including muscle over-use associated with fatigue, fluid imbalances, electrolyte imbalances (particularly potassium), holding a position for too long (such as sitting in a kayak or kneeling in a canoe) and, associated with that, a lack of blood flow to the muscle group. The immediate treatment for muscular cramp is to stretch the muscle and, if appropriate, the replacement of fluids and electrolytes. The most successful preventative measures in the incidence of cramp appear to be regular stretching of the commonly affected muscle groups, which could be implemented within cool-downs, and the maintenance of electrolyte levels, particularly potassium.

Key points

Muscular cramp:

➤ sudden, painful muscular contractions

➤ due to irritation of muscle fibres: dehydration, electrolyte imbalances, remaining static for too long, reduced blood flow

Methods for decreasing the incidence of cramp include:

➤ regular stretching of commonly affected muscle groups

➤ maintain electrolyte balance (particularly K^+)

Stitch

A 'stitch', also known as exercise-related transient abdominal pain (ETAP), is a localised, sharp pain in the side. It is commonly brought on during running and can become a temporary mechanism of fatigue. Most individuals, however, can quickly overcome a stitch and continue with exercise. A stitch is thought to occur due to the up-and-down nature of running or jogging, as stitches are less common in non-running based activities such as cycling, kayaking or rowing. The movement of the internal organs with each stride may cause micro-trauma to the digestive system and result in pain. Alternatively, or additionally, the redistribution of blood away from the digestive tract during exercise may be responsible for the development of a stitch during running. Stitches appear to be more common when exercising shortly after a meal and consequently temporary digestive tract ischemia (lack of blood flow) caused by the re-distribution of blood to the exercising muscles may be the underlying cause. Further possible causes of a stitch include ischemia of the diaphragm, stress of the lower diaphragm ligaments, and irritation of the parietal peritoneum.

Key point

A stitch is:

➤ a transient, localised pain

➤ most common during running-based activities

➤ thought to occur due to movement of the internal organs, or ischemia of the digestive tract or diaphragm

Over-reaching and over-training

If the intensity and duration of training is pushed too hard an athlete can experience over-reaching and over-training, both of which have a negative impact on performance. Over-reaching and over-training can be factors that impact on any athlete, regardless of the duration of their activity. An athlete or his or her coach should attempt to ensure that the periodised training load is balanced such that they do not break down in training. From a theoretical standpoint this is easy to understand. However, at the elite level athletes have to push hard, sometimes existing on a knife-edge between maximal performance gains and over-training. This section is included here because much of the early work carried out in the area of over-training was conducted due to the symptoms reported by endurance athletes. It is important to recognise, however, as mentioned above, that the over-training syndrome can affect any athlete regardless of the duration or intensity of their sport.

Over-reaching describes a short-term expression of over-training. When the stresses of training and everyday life result in a short-term decrement in performance, the athlete is said to have over-reached. If training continues, regardless of the symptoms of over-reaching, longer-term negative effects on performance will be realised. It is essential that an athlete's training load incorporates periods of recovery to allow the body to recover from the stresses encountered. After an instance of over-reaching an athlete normally recovers in a period of 3–14 days, the recovery after over-training often takes several months or longer. The symptoms of over-reaching and the longer-term over-training syndrome are: decrements in performance, persistent feelings of general fatigue, sustained muscle soreness, elevated resting heart rate, mood state issues, loss of competitive drive, insomnia, loss of appetite and weight loss. As well as training overloads, psychological stresses, poor diet and insufficient recovery periods can contribute to the occurrence of over-reaching or over-training. A thoroughly planned periodised training programme with clear goals for the year ahead, along with an on-going dialogue between the athlete and their coach, are the best measures to avoid the incidence of either over-reaching or over-training. A periodised training programme should include: variety for an athlete (to avoid staleness), pre-planned recovery periods and regular nutritional reviews to ensure a healthy diet is maintained.

Key points

Over-reaching and over-training:

➤ Intensity of training too great, recovery insufficient, inadequate diet – or combination of all three

➤ Over-reaching
  • Short-term effects
  • Recover within 3–14 days

➤ Over-training
  • Occurs if training continues despite symptoms of over-reaching
  • Long-term effects
  • Recovery takes several months or longer

➤ Over-reaching and over-training symptoms
  • Impaired performance, general fatigue, sustained muscle soreness, elevated resting HR, mood state issues, insomnia, loss of competitive drive, loss of appetite, loss of weight

A periodised training programme and communication with their coach can help athletes avoid the problems associated with over-training

Knowledge integration question

As a coach, or PE teacher, how would you identify an athlete at risk of over-training and how might you help them prevent its occurrence?

14.2 Longer-term health issues, exercise and exercise physiology

McArdle disease

An interesting health issue, from an exercise physiological perspective that relates to glycolysis as was covered in Chapter 10, is the occurrence of McArdle disease. McArdle disease was first reported in 1951 by a London doctor, Dr Brian McArdle, after he assessed the symptoms of a patient and diagnosed a problem relating to glycogen breakdown. His tests also revealed that his patient did not accumulate lactate during anaerobic exercise. The disease, also known as glycogen storage disease type V, is thought to affect around 1 in 100,000 people although only about one-third are diagnosed. It was later discovered that the problem with glycogen breakdown related to an enzyme deficiency, specifically, glycogen phosphorylase. As can be seen from

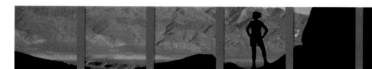

CASE STUDY

Extract from a blog written by a 52-year-old with McArdle disease

I was diagnosed with McArdle disease in 1991 at the age of 32, though I had been suffering from the classic symptoms of McArdle disease from the age of 10.

Years ago when I was about 15 and before I was diagnosed with McArdle disease I tried my legs at running, but it was a hopeless effort

because my muscles wouldn't work the way they should have, I even tried running with a local running club, . . . but basically I was just tagging along. Even when I was doing my Duke of Edinburgh Award the physical activity was an ordeal on its own because it involved running which I hopelessly struggled with. Going up . . . mountains was an even bigger test for my muscles as anyone knows McArdle disease and mountains have an ardent dislike of each other.

Today some friends of mine whom I've met on the internet through Facebook and who suffer with McArdle disease are doing something that I would love to do, they are walking the route of the **London Marathon,** which is done over two days . . . Two of them have already, with others last year, done the 'Walk over Wales' and later this year will walk Snowdonia.'

Figure 10.3 (in Chapter 10), glycogen phosphorylase, also known as myophosphorylase, catalyses and regulates the breakdown of glycogen to glycogen-1-phosphate-2. Patients have symptoms from childhood but it is common for the disease not to be correctly diagnosed until adulthood. This was the case for the person who wrote the following blog extract.

The symptoms of the disease include early fatigue onset, muscle pain (myalgia), cramps, and muscle weakness. People with McArdle disease have great difficulty at the start of activity or exercise, but experience a 'second wind' phenomenon whereby symptoms ease somewhat after approximately 5–10 minutes when the fatty acid metabolism can more readily meet the demands of exercise. A history of painful cramps that occur within a few minutes of initiating exercise and which subside rapidly with rest, in conjunction with a raised serum creative kinase (CK) (see Chapter 9) is highly suggestive of McArdle disease.

The disease can be diagnosed through DNA analysis or through muscle biopsy and the assessment of myophosphorlyase levels and glycogen concentration. An absence of this enzyme can be used to confirm a diagnosis of McArdle disease. It is also possible to perform an ischemic (lack of blood flow) or non-ischemic forearm exercise test to indicate the possibility of McArdle disease. In the ischemic version, a sphygmomanometer cuff (blood pressure cuff) is applied to the exercising arm prior to starting the test and then inflated to 250 mmHg. In this way blood flow is cut-off to the forearm during exercise. However, this test may produce a fixed contracture of the muscle and it is possible to complete the test

without the use of a sphygmomanometer, but still obtaining a similar result. The test involves exercising (repeat contractions) for one minute using a hand-grip dynamometer. For a person with McArdle disease, his or her lactate level would not rise above resting level despite the anaerobic exercise.

For people with McArdle disease, the absence of lactate accumulation during exercise is often associated with a rise in ammonia levels. This is the result of a compensatory reliance on the adenylate deaminase reaction which is triggered by the build up of ADP during high-intensity exercise. Due to the inhibition of glycogenolysis in a McArdle patient when attempting high-intensity exercise, there is an increased reliance on the phosphagen and aerobic energy systems.

It is also interesting to note from an exercise physiological standpoint that individuals with McArdle disease, due to their absence of lactate accumulation during exercise, were used in a study by Hagberg et al. (1982) to demonstrate the uncoupling of the anaerobic threshold and the lactate threshold. (This aspect of the transition between anaerobic and aerobic metabolism is covered in more detail in Chapter 11.) Briefly, however to recap, Hagberg and colleagues' research revealed that while McArdle patients displayed a normal breakaway ventilation profile, they did not demonstrate a similar breakaway or rise in lactate production. Previously, Davies and colleagues had suggested that the point of lactate and anaerobic threshold were linked and so non-invasive gas analysis could be used to infer the lactate threshold. Through his experiment with McArdle patients, Hagberg and co-workers were able to demonstrate that such a relationship could not be presumed and that the two transitions did not always occur at the same point.

Knowledge integration question

In terms of the transition from aerobic to increasing anaerobic exercise, what important information did exercise physiologists learn from the study of McArdle patients?

Asthma and exercise

Asthma (from the Greek word ásthma, meaning 'panting') is a chronic inflammatory condition of the airways characterised by airway hyper-reactivity (abnormally responsive) resulting in an obstruction to the airflow; this can vary widely from mild to severe. The restriction of airflow by narrowing or obstruction of the airways can occur by contraction of smooth muscle, inflammation of the airway lining, or production of mucus.

The triggers and symptoms of asthma

Asthma is thought to be due to a combination of environmental and genetic factors. It can be triggered by a variety of stimuli, including environmental factors (allergens and pollutants), viral respiratory tract infections, and inhalation of cold, dry air. The symptoms of asthma include wheezing, coughing, chest tightness and dyspnea (shortness of breath), and are more prevalent during early morning or at night. These are usually accompanied by some degree of airflow obstruction which may improve spontaneously or require inhalation of a bronchodilator (β_2-agonist), to relax and widen the airways. Individuals experience different symptoms and levels of severity in response to a variety of triggers. As each person's response differs, interventions for the control of asthma must be tailored to the individual. In severe cases asthma can be deadly with 11 deaths every day from asthma in the USA alone, many of which would be avoidable with the correct treatment and care.

Asthma affects millions of people worldwide

The high incidence and economic cost of asthma is a major public health concern. As of 2010, around 300 million people worldwide suffer from the disease. The majority of developed countries have a prevalence of asthma around 6%; however, Australia and New Zealand currently have the worst rates. Data from 2007–8 indicate 10% of

Australians suffer from asthma, while New Zealand has one of the highest rates of asthma, with ~17% of adults and 25% of children suffering from the disease. The reason for this much higher rate remains unclear, although it is likely due to environmental factors. The prevalence of asthma is higher in children than adults with more boys suffering from the condition than girls (children under 15 years of age). In contrast, more adult women are asthmatic than men. The total annual cost of asthma within the USA is estimated to be nearly $18 billion per year.

Key points

Asthma is a chronic inflammatory condition of the airways affecting around 300 million people worldwide.

It is characterised by an obstruction to the airflow, resulting from:

➤ contraction of airway smooth muscle

➤ inflammation of airway lining

➤ Production of mucus

Triggers of asthma are:

➤ genetic factors

➤ environmental factors (allergents, pollutants)

➤ viral respiratory tract infections

➤ inhalation of cold, dry air

Symptoms of asthma are:

➤ wheezing

➤ coughing

➤ chest tightness

➤ dyspnea (shortness of breath)

Exercise-induced bronchospasm

Regular physical activity improves the function of the respiratory system and is especially important in asthmatic individuals. It reduces the responsiveness of the airway helping to lower the incidence of asthmatic episodes. Many individuals (80–90% of asthmatics), however, experience symptoms of asthma during or following exercise, known as exercise-induced bronchospasm (EIB). This condition is also commonly referred to as exercise-induced asthma (EIA). The restriction to airflow in EIB is primarily the result of smooth muscle in the walls of the airways contracting. Inflammation and its associated swelling plays a minimal role (Andersen & Kippelen, 2008). For this reason, the bronchospasm normally reverses itself within 30 minutes of stopping exercise. The two most important triggers for EIB are the increased ventilation and drying of the airways associated with exercise.

The occurrence of EIB can often result in an individual withdrawing from exercise rather than getting medical advice for the appropriate management of the condition. When properly controlled, asthma should not affect your involvement in sport and exercise, with many elite athletes, such as Paula Radcliffe (British long-distance runner), Jackie Joyner-Kersee (USA heptathlete), Ian Botham (England cricketer), Paul Scholes (England soccer player), Danyon Loader (NZ swimmer), and Adrian Moorhouse (British swimmer), suffering from asthma during their sporting careers. This is summed up nicely by Paula Radcliffe who said 'If you learn to manage your asthma and take the correct medication there is no reason why you should not be the best'.

> ## Key points
>
> Exercise-induced bronchospasm (EIB) is experienced by 80–90% of asthmatics.
>
> Primary triggers for EIB are increased ventilation and drying of the airways.
>
> EIB should not affect your involvement in sport and exercise.

Diagnosis of asthma

Asthma is generally diagnosed with the use of pulmonary function tests. The magnitude of airflow obstruction associated with asthma varies greatly between individuals but, in the majority of cases, it is reversible spontaneously or with β_2-agonist inhalation. In the general population, asthma is diagnosed when airflow obstruction decreases the forced expiratory volume in one second (FEV_1) (measured with a peak flow meter) by $\geq$ 20%, which is then increased again by $\geq$ 12% (or a 200 mL increase) following the use of a short-acting inhaled β_2-agonist.

The diagnosis of EIB in elite athletes showing recurrent symptoms of bronchial obstruction can be verified with a variety of tests. As mentioned previously, athletes hoping to compete in the Olympic Games must provide documented evidence of EIB to obtain approval for the use of inhaled β_2-agonists or corticosteroids. This must include a history of symptoms and a clinical examination focusing on the signs of bronchial obstruction. Following a positive response to the clinical examination, a further positive test is required. This may involve the demonstration of EIB with an exercise challenge, reversibility of symptoms to inhaled β_2-agonists as measured by lung function tests

(as discussed above), or the demonstration of bronchial hyper-responsiveness to direct (methacholine or histamine) or indirect (inhalation of cold or dry air) stimuli.

The American Thoracic Society has recommended exercise testing for the diagnosis of EIB to involve a 6–8 min treadmill run at 80–90% of the calculated maximum load in an ambient temperature and humidity of 20–5°C and <50%, respectively. Following the test, a reduction in FEV_1 of $\geq$10% from baseline is indicative of EIB. Direct bronchial responsiveness can be measured by breathing nebulised methacholine, which is a bronchoconstrictor. The use of spirometry can verify the existence of EIB, with asthmatics reacting to lower levels of methacholine. Eucapnic voluntary ventilation is the easiest test to perform, and has been shown to correlate well with EIB in both summer and winter sport athletes. The test, conducted with the participant is stationary (not exercising), involves breathing dry gas at room temperature with a normal carbon dioxide concentration (4.9%) at 85% of maximal voluntary ventilation for 6 min. The FEV_1 response to the challenge is monitored with a $\geq$10% reduction being a positive test for EIB.

Treatment

Treatment of asthma is dependent upon the severity of the patient's condition.

Asthma is characterised by a reduction of airflow to the lungs which is caused by a narrowing of the airways, inflammation and the production of mucus. Several medications are available to reduce symptoms:

a. **Bronchodilators** act by relaxing smooth muscle within the respiratory tree (trachea, bronchi, bronchioles etc.). Drugs known as β_2-agonists are effective
   i. Salbutamol and terbutaline, if taken by inhalation: either of these compounds acts rapidly giving relief within 1–2 minutes. They are therefore useful to treat acute attacks, but their action is short-lived (~4h)
   ii. Formoterol and Salmeterol are slower-acting compounds but they have a much longer effect. Because of the delayed action they should be used in combination with inhaled steroids.

b. **Histamine reducers:** the release of histamine within the respiratory tree causes smooth muscle to contract so narrowing the airway.
   i. Sodium cromoglycate is of value in controlling exercise-induced asthma, if it is inhaled half-an-hour beforehand. It acts by stabilising the plasma membrane of histamine-containing cells preventing or minimising its release.

c. **Corticosteroids:** these are effective in the treatment of asthma since they reduce bronchial mucosal inflammation, which reduces oedema and secretion of mucus into the airways. A common example is beclomethasone dipropionate. Leukotriene-receptor antagonists, such as Montelukast, can augment the effect of corticosteroids in mild and moderate asthma.

Intermittent asthma may only require the occasional use of an inhaled β_2-agonist for its control. Persistent asthma, however, requires the use of an anti-inflammatory drug (e.g. inhaled corticosteroid) in combination with a long-acting β_2-agonist if the severity is moderate or severe. In all instances a short-acting β_2-agonist is used as required. It is essential that each patient is provided with an individualised programme for their asthma control, as a wide variation exists in the severity of symptoms and the triggers responsible for their induction.

Key point

Bronchodilators (β_2-agonists) and anti-inflammatory drugs (corticosteroids) are most commonly used in the treatment of asthma.

Elite sport and asthma

There is no doubt that asthma has the potential to have a negative effect on performance. It is important, therefore, for athletes to properly control and manage their asthma for optimisation of performance. In 2002, the International Olympic Committee (IOC) was concerned about the increasing use of β_2-agonists by athletes, due to their bronchodilator function having a potential ergogenic effect for healthy elite athletes. As a result β_2-agonists joined the WADA prohibited list, and athletes suffering from asthma must now follow strict criteria, including the submission of a Therapeutic Use Exemption, to obtain permission for the use of both corticosteroids and β_2-agonists. Recent research, found the inhalation of β_2-agonists by non-asthmatic athletes to have no performance-enhancing effect suggesting there is no basis for restriction of their use (Kindermann, 2007).

The prevalence of asthma in elite athletes has increased over the last couple of decades, as indicated by an elevated incidence in American Olympians from 11% in 1984 to >20% in 1996 (Weiler et al., 1986, 1998). The prevalence of asthma is higher in elite athletes than both recreational athletes and the general population. The condition is most prevalent within endurance athletes, particularly swimmers, cross-country skiers, long-distance runners and cyclists, compared with all other athletes. Indeed, the incidence of asthma in long-distance runners (17%) has been found to be greater than that of power and speed athletes (8%) (Helenius et al., 1997). The risk of asthma has been found to be about six times higher in elite endurance athletes and around 3.5 times greater in power sport athletes than control subjects (Helenius et al., 1998). A further difference in the incidence of asthma is that between winter sport athletes (22%) and summer endurance athletes (5–17%). Classically, an early onset of asthma occurs within childhood whereas athletes appear to be a unique population with a late onset of symptoms often emerging during a sports career and disappearing upon retirement from sport. This is supported by the finding that of all potential Finnish Olympic athletes with symptoms of asthma, 20% had a history of asthma from childhood while the majority developed symptoms during their sports career. These findings raise some interesting questions. Why should training and competition for an elite sport increase the risk of asthma, and what mechanisms are involved?

The increased demand by the muscles for oxygen during exercise is met by elevated ventilation, increasing the amount of oxygen transported from the atmosphere to the alveoli where it diffuses into the blood for transport to the exercising muscles. In elite sport, large volumes and high intensities of training are encountered on a regular basis resulting in long periods of increased ventilation which may reach values up to 280 L·min^{-1}. This imposes a great stress on the respiratory tract which is an important stimulus for the onset of EIB in athletes. The greater stress experienced by the airways of elite athletes appears to be responsible for their greater risk of asthma than the general population. The repeated exposure of the airway wall to hyperventilation results in heat and water loss, the combined effect of which is drying and cooling of the airway, which initiates a neural response stimulating bronchoconstriction. The effects of increased ventilation on the airways are exacerbated in cold environments, hence increasing the risk of bronchoconstriction and the development of asthma symptoms in winter sports like cross-country skiing compared with summer sports. Longer periods of high ventilation, and the resultant increased exposure to pollutants and allergens (common triggers of asthma), are encountered by endurance athletes compared with power sport athletes perhaps explaining the difference in asthma incidence between these sport categories. Indeed, bronchoconstriction and symptoms of asthma may occur as a result of hyperventilation and exposure to allergens and pollutants (both indoors and outdoors) even in those with no clinical asthma.

Key points

Asthma in elite athletes:

➤ Corticosteroids and β$_2$-agonists are on the WADA prohibited list, asthmatic athletes must request an exemption for their use in competition.

➤ Prevalence is highest in elite athletes, particularly those involved in endurance sports, and winter sports.

➤ Prolonged exposure to elevated ventilation and resultant cooling of the airways triggers EIB.

Swimming and asthma – a unique situation

Similar to all endurance sports, large increases in ventilation can be experienced for long durations in swimmers. The swimming environment, however, differs from the outdoor or indoor environment of most sports. While swimming, the warm, humid layer of air just above the water surface is what you breathe between strokes. This air contains both water droplets and chemicals, due to the disinfection of swimming pools with chlorine. Symptoms of asthma, the obstruction of airflow and an increased bronchial responsiveness can all be induced by inhalation of chlorine derivatives (Drobnic et al., 1996). Swimmers, therefore, have a high incidence of EIB due to the repeated exposure to chlorinated swimming pools which is ameliorated upon completion of their sporting career.

The female athlete triad

The female athlete triad (Triad) involves the interrelationship between three conditions that exist on a continuum of severity, from a healthy state to one of seriously impaired health. The three components of the Triad are:

• Low energy availability/disordered eating
• Menstrual irregularity/amenorrhea
• Bone loss/osteoporosis

The observation of these symptoms in athletes resulted in the recognition of the Triad in 1992. The female athlete triad and the continuum of severity is illustrated in Figure 14.1. One end of the continuum demonstrates health: high energy availability, healthy menstrual functioning and a healthy BMD. At the opposite end we find the clinical conditions of low energy availability (with or without eating disorder), amenorrhea and osteoporosis. Moving along the continuum from health to disease, there is a gradual change in each of the components. In many situations, therefore, an athlete will present with intermediate, or subclinical, symptoms of the three components. It may be, therefore, that an athlete involved in a sport requiring leanness may show signs of restricted eating but does not meet the criteria for an eating disorder. Menstrual irregularities, such as **anovulation** or **oligomenorrhea**, may be present but the situation of amenorrhea has not yet been reached. Likewise, BMD may be falling, but is still within the normal range, hence osteoporosis is not diagnosed. An important point to make is that the three components can move along the continuum of severity at differing

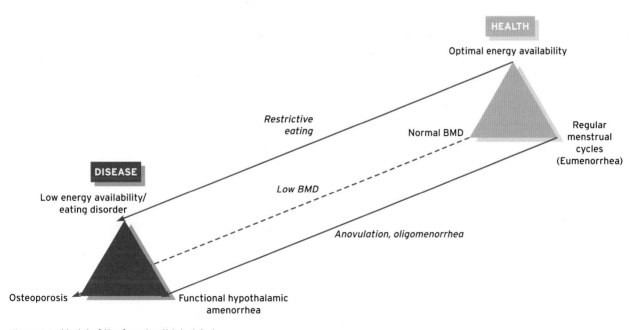

Figure 14.1 Model of the female athlete triad.

rates. However, due to the clear associations between the components, it is likely that an athlete suffering from one of the components is also suffering from the other two.

Energy availability

Energy availability refers to the difference between energy intake and that expended during exercise, hence relating to the energy available for cellular maintenance, thermoregulation, growth and reproduction. When energy availability is low, physiological mechanisms lower the energy use for the above functions, which, despite the restoration of energy balance, impairs health. Low energy availability may result from one of two situations. Firstly, the increase in an athlete's training load may not be accompanied by an increase in caloric intake inadvertently resulting in a negative energy balance. In this situation the energy deficit occurs in the absence of an eating disorder, it is simply that there appears to be no biological mechanism to balance energy intake with exercise-induced expenditure. This highlights the role of nutritional guidance for elite athletes. A research study found that restricting caloric intake by the omission of a meal increased hunger. However, when the same energy deficit was induced through exercise there was no appetite response to promote the athlete to eat (Hubert et al., 1998).

Secondly, an energy deficit may result from a restricted caloric intake with the potential development of an eating disorder such as *anorexia nervosa* (restrictive eating) or *bulimia nervosa* (binge-eating and purging). There are several reasons why an athlete may slip into a disordered eating pattern. In particular elite female athletes involved in sports that emphasise a lean build or small body size are most at risk. The scenario in which an athlete is told she must lose weight, the words used to tell her, and the availability of weight loss guidance, may influence the route taken (consciously or subconsciously), to meet the required weight or body shape for her particular sport. Irrespective of the process involved, low energy availability (<30 kcal·kg^{-1}LBM·day^{-1}) appears to be the primary factor impairing both reproductive and skeletal health. Energy availability can change rapidly due to altered dietary or exercise behaviours. The effect of an energy deficit on menstrual function, however, will not become apparent for up to a month, while a decline in BMD may not be detectable for a year or more.

Menstrual function

There is a common misconception that the absence of regular menstrual cycles is a normal consequence of training and competing at the elite level. This, however, should not be sustained and amenorrhea, brought on by low energy availability, forms one of the points of the Triad triangle (Figure 14.1). If menstrual cycles have been absent for three or more months the condition is termed *secondary amenorrhea*, whereas *primary amenorrhea* relates to a delayed age of menarche. In the Triad, menstrual disorders result from the impaired secretion of luteinising hormone from the pituitary gland and, this type of amenorrhea is referred to as *functional hypothalamic amenorrhea*. The relationship between amenorrhea and sports training appears to remain unclear, although one study found ballet dancers to experience menarche at a later age, albeit at the same height and weight as in non-dancers (Warren, 1980).

Bone health

The reduction of bone mineral density is directly influenced by low energy availability through the suppression of hormones involved in bone formation. Additionally, an indirect effect occurs through the development of amenorrhea with the resulting fall in oestrogen leading to increased bone reabsorption. Combined, these effects during childhood and adolescence result in the sub-optimal accumulation of bone mineral and can result in the development of osteoporosis, increasing bone fragility and the risk of stress fractures. An athlete presenting with a stress fracture, therefore, may be indicative of poor bone health and, particularly if combined with menstrual or eating irregularities, the individual should be screened for the Triad.

The onset of amenorrhea does not immediately cause osteoporosis but a gradual decline in the mineralisation of bone begins. The resumption of regular menses results in a gradual improvement of BMD. However, depending on the duration of amenorrhea and resultant effects on bone health, it may not be possible to fully restore BMD levels (Keen & Drinkwater, 1997; Warren et al., 2002).

Key points

The female athlete triad involves the interrelationship between three conditions:

1. Low energy availability/disordered eating
2. Menstrual irregularity/amenorrhea
3. Bone loss/osteoporosis

These components exist on a continuum of severity from health to disease.

Low energy availability impairs reproductive and bone health.

Amenorrhea, through the reduction of oestrogen, lowers BMD.

Health consequences of the Triad

As discussed above, sustained low energy availability can impair health through a variety of physiological changes. In some instances it manifests as a clinical eating disorder, and whether or not this is the case, menstrual function is disrupted and BMD falls, increasing the risk of bone fracture. It appears that, upon the improvement of energy availability and return of regular menses, the decline in bone health may never fully recover. It has been found that 83% of athletes with an eating disorder partially recover, with a sustained recovery of weight, menstrual function and eating behaviour occurring in only 33% (Herzog et al., 1999). Education of athletes, coaches, parents and health professionals should therefore focus on healthy methods of weight manipulation with emphasis on the prevention of eating disorders, explaining why this is important. In addition to these physiological responses, psychological health may be impaired in instances where an eating disorder develops as these are related to low self-esteem, anxiety and depression. Indeed, 5.4% of athletes with an eating disorder have been reported to have attempted suicide, reflecting the seriousness of this condition (Sundgot-Borgen, 1994).

Prevalence

The female athlete triad is composed of three separate components: eating disorder, amenorrhea and osteoporosis. The prevalence of all three conditions in athletes is largely unknown. Recently, however, it has been suggested that the prevalence is low, with 1.2% of high school athletes and 1.9% of Malaysian athletes reported as being a victim of the female athlete triad (Quah et al., 2009; Thein-Nissenbaum & Carr, 2011). Female athletes of all ages and all levels of competition are at risk of the Triad. Although athletes of all sports could potentially develop the Triad, those involved in sports in which leanness or small body size is important appear to be at greatest risk.

> ### Key points
>
> The prevalence of the full Triad appears to be low. However, **individual** components are more common in athletes than the general population.
> The Triad is most commonly found in sports emphasising leanness or small body size.

The prevalence of the Triad appears to be low. However, the presence of the individual components is high compared to the general population. The incidence of eating disorders in elite female athletes of leanness sports is 31%

compared to 5.5% in controls. One in four (25%) females involved in elite endurance sports, aesthetic sports and weight-class sports has an eating disorder while this figure is much lower (9%) in the general population. In gymnastics, a sport well known for the pressures on young females to maintain a small and lean physique, a very high prevalence (62%) of eating disorders has been reported.

Elite participation in sport from a young age can result in primary amenorrhea. The general population has a prevalence of primary amenorrhea less than 1% compared to over 22% in elite female athletes of sports such as diving, cheerleading and gymnastics. Secondary amenorrhea in elite athletes is dependent on several factors including age, training volume and body weight, hence its occurrence varies widely between sports. The influence of these factors was clearly demonstrated in a study by Sanborn and colleagues (1982) which found the prevalence of secondary amenorrhea in distance runners to rise from 3% to 60% when training mileage was increased from <13 to >113 km$\cdot$wk^{-1}, and body weight fell from >60 to <50 kg. Some of the highest incidences have been reported in dancers (69%) and long-distance runners (65%) compared with a low (2–5%) occurrence within the general population.

Disordered eating can negatively influence BMD in the presence or absence of amenorrhea. Amenorrheic athletes, however, have a lower BMD than eumenorrheic (normal menstruation) athletes. Compared with the prevalence of disordered eating and amenorrhea within elite female athletes, a low BMD has been reported in far fewer (0–13%). In general, however, this incidence is greater than that expected in the general population (2.3%). In Chapter 7 the importance of childhood physical activity, particularly that of a high-impact nature, in the development of healthy bone was discussed. Although elite athletes in a wide range of sports subject their bones to repeated high stresses, if an energy deficit exists, potentially combined with the negative effects of amenorrhea, conditions will be sub-optimal for the healthy growth or required remodelling of the bones.

Screening and diagnosis

The physiological and psychological health consequences of the Triad are not readily apparent to a coach or a health professional. The identification of an eating disorder or amenorrhea is often dependent upon information provided by the athlete in response to questionnaires or discussion. Low BMD in an athlete may only be detected following the development of a stress fracture if other symptoms of the Triad also become apparent. The screening for, and diagnosis of, the Triad is therefore challenging.

Elite female athletes should be screened for the Triad during their pre-participation physical or annual health check. If an athlete approaches a health professional with one or more problems related to the Triad, such as amenorrhea, stress fractures, recurrent illness or injury, they should also be screened at that time. Diagnosis is highly dependent on acquiring an accurate patient history with regard to energy intake, weight fluctuations, eating behaviours, menstrual functioning, training volumes and injuries. If an athlete's history is suggestive of one or more of the Triad components, further testing is required. A physical examination and blood analyses should be undertaken to help identify an eating disorder. Symptoms such as fatigue, anaemia, electrolyte abnormalities or depression are associated with dieting and may alert a health professional to the diagnosis of the Triad.

The risk of bone loss increases with the duration of amenorrhea, hence short-term amenorrhea is an early indicator for the Triad. There are no tests for the diagnosis of functional hypothalamic amenorrhea, hence tests to exclude other treatable causes of amenorrhea are required. A history of amenorrhea or disordered eating for six months or more, or a history of stress fractures, indicates bone health may be poor and BMD should be assessed by DXA (as described in Chapter 7). To aid prevention and allow early intervention, the education of athletes, coaches, health professionals, parents, and other family members, regarding the causes and signs of the Triad, is very important. This will help to prevent a serious decline in the health and performance of the athlete.

Treatment

The treatment of the Triad should involve a multidisciplinary team involving a combination of the following: physician, dietician, coach, exercise physiologist and parents. In addition, if an eating disorder is present, a mental health practitioner should be involved. The treatment of the Triad can involve a combination of factors; lifestyle changes (diet), hormone replacement therapy, and family involvement.

The initial aim of treatment is to increase the energy available as this is the main root of the problem. A dietician will educate and monitor the patient for adequate nutrition, with an expected weight gain of $0.23–0.45$ kg·wk^{-1} until the goal weight is reached. Athletes with a low calcium intake are at a higher risk of a stress fracture, hence adequate dietary calcium must be ensured. In addition, a daily supplementation of vitamin D may help to facilitate calcium absorption. Although the intensity of exercise should be decreased by 10–20% during the initial few months, there is no need to stop exercising completely.

The effectiveness of hormone replacement therapy on bone mineral loss in female athletes suffering from the Triad is unclear, with most evidence supporting its use in post-menopausal women. As three years of amenorrhea can result in irreversible bone loss, consideration of HRT after six months of amenorrhea may be appropriate. The use of oral contraceptives and cyclic oestrogen/progesterone have been used in the treatment of functional hypothalamic amenorrhea. It should be remembered, however, that the main goal is to regain regular menses through proper nutrition, reduced training and ultimately, body weight maintenance.

The involvement of family members may be crucial to the success of treatment. With appropriate education, family members can support the athlete and encourage them throughout the treatment process. Family support is especially important for adolescent athletes.

> ### Key point
>
> Treatment of the Triad should involve a multidisciplinary team.
>
> The main aim is to increase energy availability through proper nutrition, to regain regular menses and prevent or limit bone mineral loss.

Physical activity and the ageing process

A common issue in health promotion is the education of older individuals on the benefits of physical activity and initiating the engagement of these individuals in regular exercise. The benefits of physical activity in the ageing population are numerous, both from a physiological and psychological perspective. The current overall annual health care cost of the elderly ($\geq$65 year old) in Japan has been estimated at Japanese ¥339,366 (US \$4,437) per person (Aoyagi & Shephard, 2011). These costs could be eased substantially by an increase in physical activity levels of the older population due to the positive roles of physical activity in the promoting health and preventing disease. In addition to physical health, the psychological health of adults in the developed world countries is poor, with depression indicated as becoming the leading cause of death or disability this century (World Health Organization). Involvement in activity is associated with more positive psychological attributes and lower depressive symptoms, hence its role in enhancing psychological health is an important one. The influence of exercise on depression is discussed in the following section, with the main focus in the current section being on the physiological effects of ageing and the positive role which physical activity can play.

Physiological changes with ageing and the role of physical activity

Ageing is associated with the impairment of many physiological parameters, some of which can be modified through the participation in regular physical activity. The changes in body composition with ageing can negatively affect the musculoskeletal and cardiovascular systems, and metabolic function. These natural ageing processes are discussed in the following paragraphs, alongside the interpretation of any physical activity benefits.

Body composition changes and resultant musculoskeletal function

Body fat changes with ageing

During ageing the composition of the body changes with relation to both fat mass and lean body mass. There is an increase in total body fat, with a particular accumulation in the visceral (abdominal) region – a risk factor for cardiovascular disease and type II diabetes (discussed in more detail later in this chapter). Regular participation in aerobic and/or resistance activities decreases the accumulation of total body fat, with even small decreases being associated with a substantial reduction in visceral fat. This is important in the prevention or management of many common chronic conditions, including cardiovascular disease, type II diabetes, hypertension, osteoarthritis, depression and impaired mobility.

Osteoporosis – a major health concern

Lean body mass falls with ageing due to a reduction in both bone and muscle mass. The health of bone is dependent on the application of forces through both muscular contractions and ground reactions. In youth, weight-bearing and high-impact activities are emphasised to optimise the development of healthy bone, while a shift toward resistance training and balance exercises occurs with ageing. An improved balance in the elderly will give them more confidence on their feet and may reduce the risk of falling. The reduction in bone mass with ageing is gradual and is associated with a reduced density and quality of bone which increases the risk of fractures. This condition is known as **osteoporosis**, literally meaning '*porous bone*'. In women, an accelerated bone loss and a rapid fall in BMD occurs at the menopause due to a decline in the sex hormone oestrogen. Within 3–5 years of the menopause the rate of bone loss is restabilised at a new higher rate than that prior to menopause. The lowered oestrogen level results in an increased rate of bone reabsorption. Evidence suggests that oestrogen deficiency stimulates the formation of osteoclasts (cells responsible for bone reabsorption) by increasing the production of osteoclastogenic cell signalling molecules (cytokines) and increasing the number of osteoclast precursors (D'Amelio et al., 2008). When the formation of bone is less than the volume of bone reabsorbed there is a loss of bone mass and increased bone fragility.

Osteoporosis is a major public health concern, primarily affecting post-menopausal women and elderly men. Due, in part, to the biological changes during the menopause, more women suffer from osteoporosis than men, with a greater proportion of women sustaining an osteoporotic fracture. Estimated to affect 200 million women worldwide, with an estimation of 9 million osteoporotic fractures at the turn of the century, the economic cost of osteoporosis is vast, with the yearly direct cost in the USA alone exceeding $19.1 billion as a result of over 2.1 million fractures. As may be expected, the incidence of osteoporosis and rates of fractures vary between countries, as illustrated in Tables 14.1 and 14.2, respectively. As the current bone health in the USA, and indeed around the world, is very poor and of great concern, the American Orthopaedic Association launched an initiative called 'Own the Bone' in 2009 (Bunta, 2011). It aims to limit the predicted increase in osteoporosis and associated fractures by lowering the

Table 14.1 The incidence of osteoporosis (%) for women and men over 50 years of age.

Country	Women (%)	Men (%)
Canada	25	>12.5
China	50.1	22.5
Denmark	41	18

Table 14.2 The risk of osteoporotic fracture (%) for women and men over 50 years of age. US data is based on the white ethnic population.

Country	Women (%)	Men (%)
Australia	51	42
UK	50	20
USA	40	13

risk of a future fracture in older patients (50 years and older) through education and behavioural change.

In the older population, exposure to regular physical activity including organised sports, unstructured activity, and household and occupational tasks, can attenuate the loss of bone mass and density associated with ageing. In addition, an *increase* in bone mass has been found to result from resistance training or weight-bearing aerobic exercise in both pre- and post-menopausal women. Regular exercise has also been estimated to improve bone mineral density by 1–2% per year compared with sedentary individuals. For the future bone health of the next generation, participation in sport and exercise during childhood should be actively encouraged as this has been suggested to be crucial for the prevention of osteoporosis in later life.

Sarcopenia – loss of muscle mass and strength with ageing

Increasing age is associated with a fall in muscle mass (**sarcopenia**) resulting in a reduction in muscular strength. Due to muscle inactivity there is a gradual loss in fibre number and size, resulting in a reduced muscle cross-sectional area of 25–30% and a 30–40% reduction in strength by the age of 70 years (Porter et al., 1995). As the muscle atrophy occurs primarily in type II fibres, muscle characteristics transition towards those of type I fibres, reducing the force-producing capabilities of the muscle along with the rate of contraction. The consequences of sarcopenia are varied, from an increased risk of falls and fractures, to impaired metabolic rate and thermoregulatory ability, resulting in an overall loss in functional capacity and ability to perform everyday tasks. Thankfully, these life-changing age-related effects of sarcopenia are reversible and significant increases in muscle mass and muscle strength can be stimulated in the older individual through resistance training and the resultant hypertrophy of muscle. These adaptations function to improve the individual's functional capacity enabling an independent lifestyle for an increased number of years.

Key points

Ageing results in several physiological changes:

➤ Increased total body fat, especially visceral fat

➤ Osteoporosis

➤ Sarcopenia

Regular physical activity can attenuate these processes of ageing.

Exercise capacity

The process of ageing markedly reduces exercise capacity, including a fall in aerobic power and HR_{max}. Participation in regular physical activity can attenuate some of these detrimental changes, although the decline in peak HR and hence aerobic power cannot be prevented with training. The cardiovascular and musculoskeletal adaptations to regular physical activity, however, allow for improvements in sub-maximal exercise. Adaptations to training include a lowered cardiorespiratory response to sub-maximal exercise, in terms of HR and blood pressure, and the maintenance of a higher workload with a delayed onset of fatigue. The reduction in sarcopenia with regular physical activity allows for greater strength, power and endurance, also contributing to the attenuation of exercise capacity decline.

Mortality and chronic disease

Physical activity level is inversely related to all-cause mortality and chronic disease risk. The promotion of an active lifestyle with ageing is, therefore, vital for optimal health and the prevention or management of chronic diseases. Regular aerobic exercise influences many factors which are related to cardiovascular disease. The level of a cardio-protective factor, HDL-cholesterol, is increased. Carbohydrate metabolism is improved as shown by an improved glucose tolerance and elevated insulin sensitivity, both resulting in a reduced risk of coronary heart disease. The increase in arterial blood pressure with ageing, a risk factor for several cardiovascular disorders, is attenuated through regular physical activity. Physical activity may influence the prevalence of chronic disease through its influence on physiological capacity, psychological health or risk factors for cardiometabolic disease. There are many examples of chronic conditions that can be prevented by, benefit from or be managed by, regular physical activity. These include conditions which are experienced by many, with the likelihood that you know of someone suffering from one of them; cardiovascular disease, stroke, type II diabetes, obesity, hypertension, depression, anxiety, osteoarthritis and osteoporosis. The incorporation of physical activity into the everyday life of older individuals can substantially improve their physiological functioning and psychological health with a reduction in the risk of developing a chronic disease. This improved health and functional capacity will allow the ageing population to perform everyday tasks and increase the duration of their independent lifestyle.

Exercise and depression

A significant number of people experience depression, pervasive feelings of low mood and lethargy, at some point in their lives. Depression is thought to affect around 10% of the population in developed countries, and interestingly, it appears to be almost twice as prevalent for females than for males. Depression is associated with negative feelings of sadness, worthlessness, guilt, restlessness, irritability and hopelessness. Recent research suggests that the hippocampus is an important centre associated with the development of depression and many anti-depression medications appear to take their effect on that area of the brain. A number of different factors have been implicated as possible triggers for depression and these include differences in brain structure, chemical and hormonal imbalances, personality differences, social isolation, and psychological trauma earlier in life.

Exercise and physical activity appear to be closely connected with depression. Research indicates that regular physical activity can help to alleviate symptoms as well as serving a preventative role. Former New Zealand rugby player John Kirwan, who is featured in the case study below, is a strong advocate for physical activity as a treatment for depression. It appears that a balance must be maintained however, for research has also highlighted the increased risk of depression in cases of overtraining.

Regular physical activity appears to have beneficial effects for people with depression, with exercise interventions improving their mood, confidence and ability to concentrate on tasks. It is thought the benefits relate to one, or a combination of, the following factors:

- Alterations in hormonal functioning, including dopamine, serotonin and noradrenaline, all of which act as neurotransmitters within the body.
- Improved self-esteem associated with increased fitness and skill development through participation in sport.
- Increased metabolism and body temperature associated with exercise may alter physiological functioning and brain neurotransmission.
- Taking part in physical activity may provide an alternative focus, taking a person's mind off their illness, even if only for a relatively short time period.

Research suggests that as little as 30 minutes of exercise, 1 or 2 days per week is sufficient to alleviate the symptoms of depression. The optimal levels of exercise needed to treat and prevent depression require further research. Similarly, the types and intensities of exercise required to alleviate depression need further investigation. Nevertheless, physical activity does appear to provide both a treatment and a preventative measure for people suffering with depression.

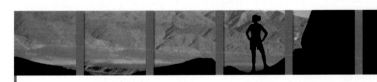

CASE STUDY

Former All-Black (NZ rugby player) John Kirwan is currently leading a campaign to help those people in New Zealand who have depression. As a former elite sportsperson who suffered from depression himself, Kirwan places an importance on regular physical activity as a treatment for the illness. Kirwan has stated 'looking back when I first experienced depression staying active was probably one of the best things I could have done. I didn't realise it at the time, but these days I know that if I don't work out at least 3 or 4 times a week I just don't feel good. Now it's not the physical buzz that makes me feel good, it's the mental buzz, its that little feeling of self-reward or goodness that comes from moving around that helps me feel better mentally.'

Obesity

Research indicates that there are close links between obesity, physical inactivity, the development and progression of cardiovascular disease (CVD) and the onset of Type II diabetes mellitus. As a result we review these important aspects of health in the sections below. In Chapter 2, we examined recent government recommendations for average daily calorie intake and fat intake, the role of cholesterol within the body and components of a healthy diet, all of which are linked to the aspects of health considered in this section.

The rapidly increasing levels of obesity occurring in a number of developed countries in recent years, has implications for the incidence of CVD and Type II diabetes in those countries, and is closely linked to increasing physical inactivity. The increasing incidence of obesity is, however, a much more complex issue for health than a simple balance between food intake and the level of physical activity (energy intake versus energy expenditure). Research indicates that the rising incidence of obesity relates to a far more complex interaction of genetic, medical, sociological, psychological, physiological, employment and historical factors, the interaction of which differ between countries and indeed individuals. In this section we provide an overview of a complex subject that is now the focus of a number of textbooks in the field. Suggestions for further reading are included in the reference list at the end of this textbook.

Obesity refers to an excess of body fat. A comparison between 2002 and 2010 World Health Organization (WHO) figures for the top 20 countries in the world regarding obesity is provided in Table 2.7 (Chapter 2). Importantly, for us as physical education teachers, exercise scientists and coaches, in many of these countries the incidence of obesity is rising in children as well as in adults. This makes obesity a lifelong illness and a progressive process that has links to a wide number of co-morbidities (associated conditions). Table 14.3 provides an overview of these co-morbidities, which, in addition to leading to premature death can also severely impair the quality of life and functional mobility in the intervening years. The complex nature of obesity can be highlighted by the example of depression. Research and clinical studies clearly show that people suffering from depression can put on weight as a result of the illness. Equally however, obesity and the societal stigmas associated with the illness can trigger a bout of depression. This can cause a downward spiral for an increasingly obese person who is also prone to depression. As a consequence, obesity as an illness can be complex to treat and requires a significant desire to change and make

Table 14.3 Co-morbidities associated with obesity.

Co-morbidity
Cardiovascular disease
Hypertension
Type II diabetes
Stroke
Cancer
Renal disease
Hepatic disease
Reproductive disorders
Musculoskeletal injury
Arthritis
Depression
Sleep disturbance and snoring

alterations in lifestyle to bring about a positive shift in body mass and composition. Obesity is clearly linked with body composition, one of the components of fitness listed in Table 8.2 (Chapter 8). As such we will consider body composition within this section prior to examining the classification of severity of obesity.

Key points

➤ Obesity, an excess of body fat, is closely linked with:
  • Physical inactivity
  • Cardiovascular disease
  • Type II diabetes mellitus

➤ Obesity can impair quality of life and lead to premature death

➤ There are rapidly increasing levels of obesity in both adults and children in many developed countries

Body composition and its analysis

Body composition refers to the physical make-up of the body. In its broadest sense, this refers to the size and shape of an individual. In the past, this was commonly assessed using somatotyping, which provided a score (1–7) for each of three classifiers, endomorphy (the roundness, fatness aspect), mesomorphy (the muscularity, low-fat aspect) and ectomorphy (the long thin, low-fat aspect). Using somatotyping a pure ectomorph would score 1–1–7, a mesomorph

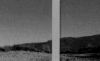

CALCULATION

Body Mass Index example

For a participant with a mass of 63 kg and height of 1.67 m:

$$\text{BMI (kg} \cdot \text{m}^{-2}) = 63 \div (1.67 \times 1.67)$$

$$\text{BMI (kg} \cdot \text{m}^{-2}) = 63 \div 2.7889$$

$$\text{BMI} \qquad = 22.6 \text{ kg} \cdot \text{m}^{-2}$$

would score 1–7–1 and an endomorph would score 7–1–1. Developed in the 1940s this system is seldom used by physiologists who now use more modern techniques, such as bioelectrical impedance analysis (BIA) and dual-energy X-ray absorptiometry (DXA), which provide more detailed analysis of body composition. In a health context, the body mass index (BMI) is often calculated to estimate body composition. However, there are a number of problems associated with the use of this measure. The calculation and use of BMI are covered in the following section. For physiologists, body composition most commonly refers to the relationship between two components; fat mass (FM) and lean body mass (LBM) (or fat free mass – FFM).

Research regarding the body composition of elite athletes suggest that mean body fat percentages are typically between 5–10% for males and 10–20% for females. The lowest recorded values are typically found for distance runners, triathletes and cross country skiers. Body composition has health implications for all athletes, but for weight-categorised sports such as judo, boxing, weightlifting and taekwondo, the way in which body weight is maintained (in and out of competition) is also important for current and future health . For all athletes, and those wanting to improve their health, an increased training volume with no change in dietary energy intake will normally lead to a positive shift in body composition (i.e. a decrease in fat percentage in relation to lean body mass).

Methods of body composition assessment

Body Mass Index (BMI)

There is a wide variety of instruments and calculations that can be used to assess body composition. One of the most straightforward estimations of body composition, often

used in a health context, is the body mass index (BMI). This is calculated using a participant's height and mass (bodyweight). The equation for BMI is:

$$\text{BMI} = \frac{\text{Mass (kg)}}{\text{Height (m)}^2}$$

The advantage of using BMI as a measure of body composition is that the components can be measured simply and the index calculated quickly. The disadvantage of BMI is that the mass component of the equation does not take into account the ratio of fat mass to lean body mass. This would mean that two participants of the same height and mass, but completely different body fat percentages would be given the same BMI score. It is for this reason that a number of methods and calculations have been developed to provide a more detailed analysis of an individual's body composition.

Skinfolds and Bioelectrical Impedance Analysis (BIA)

Figure 14.2 provides an illustration of two instruments that are commonly used to assess body composition: skinfold calipers and a bioelectrical impedance analyser. Traditionally, exercise physiologists used skinfold calipers to measure a participant's body fat percentage. Using this method, a fold of skin is measured between the calipers at a number of anatomical sites around the body. The skinfolds (measured in mm) at the selected sites are entered into a prediction equation to provide an estimation of body fat percentage. To ensure accuracy of results there must be a high degree of intratester (test-retest) and intertester (agreement between all testers) reliability. Bioelectrical impedance analysis (BIA) is increasingly being used by physiologists as a faster, and often equally accurate, method for assessing body composition. This method

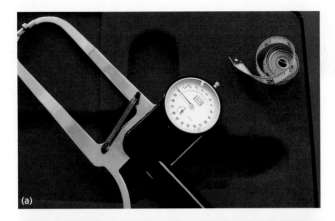

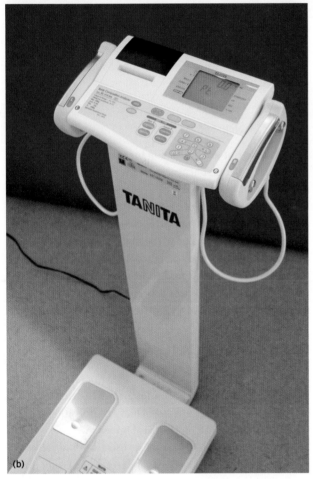

Figure 14.2 Methods of body composition analysis, (a) skinfold calipers and (b) bioelectrical impedance analysis. (*Source*: Nicky Norris)

involves a participant standing still on the analyser with bare feet and, in some analyser models, holding two handholds with arms not touching the body. An undetectable, low level electrical current is passed through the body. Prior to standing on the analyser, the participant should empty their pockets and remove any jewellery, to avoid

disturbance of the electrical current. Body water is high in electrolytes and so is an excellent electrical conductor. Lean body mass has a relatively high water content compared to fat mass and, as a consequence, the differences in impedance to conductivity can be used to assess body fat percentage. Bioelectrical impedance analysers provide an estimate (using prediction equations based on bioelectrical impedance results) of total fat mass, lean body mass and often the fat mass for each limb and the trunk. As the calculation of the results is based on body water content and the resultant electrical conductivity, the hydration status of an individual will directly affect the results. When a participant last ate, drank or exercised before a test will impact on the results and therefore needs to be controlled to maintain the integrity of the analysis.

Two key concerns with the assessment of body composition relate to the reliability of measurements and the way in which results are used. Increasingly, athletes and those involved in an exercise programme to improve their health are concerned about their body composition. Such concerns are fuelled by the widely portrayed images of the perfect body in the media and by the increasing levels of obesity in many western countries. As a consequence, teachers, coaches and health professionals need to handle discussion of body composition results in a sensitive manner. Even when dealing with professional athletes who, when compared with the majority of society, have healthy body compositions, results of a body composition analysis can cause distress. Given the potential sensitivity of the data and the possible sources of measurement error, the measurement and communication of body composition data should be handled with care.

Key points

Obesity is clearly linked with body composition, the relationship between fat mass and lean body mass

Techniques commonly used to assess body composition include:

➤ Bioelectrical impedance analysis (BIA)

➤ Dual-energy X-ray absorptiometry (DXA)

➤ Body mass index (BMI) (mass (kg)/height (m)^2)

➤ Skinfold thicknesses

Classification, development and treatment of obesity

Obesity is typically classified by BMI and by waist circumference. Table 14.4 provides a comparative table based on

Table 14.4 Classification of overweight and obesity, and risk of disease relating to body mass index and waist circumference.

Waist circumference	Underweight BMI <18.5 kg·m^{-2}	Normal BMI 18.5−24.9 kg·m^{-2}	Overweight BMI 25−29.9 kg·m^{-2}	Class I obesity BMI 30−34.9 kg·m^{-2}	Class II obesity BMI 35−39.9 kg·m^{-2}	Class III obesity BMI ≥40 kg·m^{-2}
≤102 cm (males) ≤88 cm (females)	Least risk	Lower risk	Increased risk	High risk	Very high risk	Extremely high risk
>102 cm (males) >88 cm (females)	Lower risk	Increased risk	High risk	Very high risk	Very high risk	Extremely high risk

Note: BMI = body mass index.

For BMI categories – WHO: http://apps.who.int/bmi/index.jsp?introPage=intro_3.html. NHLBI Obesity Education Initiative. *The practical guide: Identification, evaluation and treatment of overweight and obesity in adults*. National Institutes of Health (NIH Publication Number 00-4084), 2000.

these two measurements and indicates the degree of disease risk associated with a particular BMI classification or waist circumference. It is clear that the higher the BMI and the higher the waist circumference, the greater is the risk to an individual of developing a disease.

Fat mass within the body increases through two mechanisms. Most commonly, a gain in fat mass is through an increase in the *size* of the specialist fat cells, the adipocytes. In other words, fat cell hypertrophy through increased fat storage in each fat cell. In cases of extreme obesity, however, adipocytes can reach their maximal storage capacity (around 1.0 µg fat per cell) and this can lead to hyperplasia, an increase in the total number of fat cells.

As a result of the complicated interaction of genetic, medical, sociological, psychological, physiological, employment and historical factors associated with obesity, treatment for the illness is made more complex. Treatments include: diet modification, physical activity (described in more detail below), surgery (including gastric bypass and liposuction) and behavioural interventions (such as psychotherapy, support groups, weight loss camps, hypnosis). As physical educators and coaches, a real concern regarding this illness is around childhood obesity. Research clearly indicates obese children can and currently do go on to be obese (and often more obese) adults. To combat this trend, which is an aim for many governments worldwide, a multi-agency approach may be required. If current trends continue, physical education teachers will work with increasing numbers of overweight and obese students. It is possible for physical educators to play an integral role in the development of whole-school and community approaches to the treatment of obesity. A community-based approach, in which physical educators and exercise

scientists work alongside other professionals and the local community is perhaps the most likely method through which to halt and reverse the advance of obesity. The pervasiveness of this disease, the rate of its increase and its complicated aetiology make this a challenging illness for individuals to face alone.

Key points

➤ Obesity is typically classified as BMI ≥ 30 kg·m^{-2}

➤ Elevated BMI and waist circumference are associated with a greater degree of disease risk

➤ Treatment for obesity is complex, it may include:
  • Diet modification
  • Physical activity
  • Surgery
  • Behavioural interventions
  • A community based approach may be most likely to halt and reverse the advance of obesity

Knowledge integration question

Obesity is a worldwide epidemic. With consideration to its causes and methods of treatment, how could you, as a PE teacher or sports coach, help lower the incidence of childhood and adulthood obesity?

Cardiovascular disease

Diseases affecting the heart and the vascular system are collectively known as cardiovascular diseases (CVDs). These include, but are in no means limited to, coronary

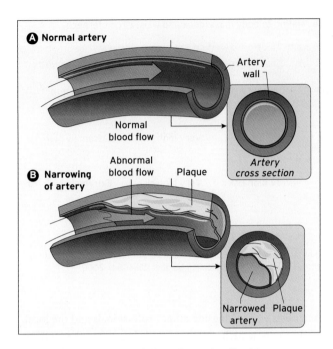

A Normal artery

Artery wall

Normal blood flow

Artery cross section

B Narrowing of artery

Abnormal blood flow   Plaque

Narrowed   Plaque
artery

Figure 14.3 Illustration depicting atherosclerotic plaque development.

heart disease (CHD) (also called coronary artery disease (CAD)), stroke, hypertension, and chronic heart failure. The underlying cause of CVD lies in the health of the arteries. Coronary heart disease involves the narrowing of the coronary arteries, those that supply oxygen-rich blood to the heart, through the deposition of fats, cholesterol and other substances to form hard plaques. The formation of arterial plaques, illustrated in Figure 14.3, results in the hardening (arteriosclerosis) and narrowing (atherosclerosis) of the arteries over a period of many years. This serves to reduce the supply of oxygenated blood to the heart muscle and increase blood pressure, a condition known as hypertension (systolic BP > 140 mmHg or diastolic BP > 90 mmHg). Eventually, the arterial plaque may crack or rupture, with the resultant formation of a blood clot on the plaque surface. This blood clot, or indeed a dislodged piece of plaque, may restrict or completely block the flow of blood along the coronary artery to the heart. If a section of the heart becomes ischaemic, due to a sudden blockage of blood flow, the heart muscle will become damaged or die and a heart attack or myocardial infarction will ensue. Over time, myocardial ischaemia and hypertension can lead to chronic heart failure, the inability of the heart to supply the oxygen needs of the body. Similar to a heart attack, a stroke involves an ischaemic insult but in this instance the tissue involved is the brain. For this reason, a stroke is sometimes referred to as a 'brain attack'.

The prevalence of cardiovascular disease

A recent report by the World Health Organization (WHO), entitled 'Global atlas on cardiovascular disease prevention and control', includes disturbing statistics relating to CVD. Cardiovascular diseases are the leading causes of death and disability in the world, with 17.3 million people estimated to have died from a CVD in 2008. This represented 30% of all global deaths, with coronary heart disease (7.3 million) and stroke (6.2 million) responsible for the majority. Of these CVD deaths in 2008, 80% occurred in low- and middle-income countries, with no difference in the incidence between men and women.

Although a fall in the number of deaths from CVD has occurred in several countries, due to the implementation of national action plans such as 'Our healthier nation' in the UK (1999), CVD, and in particular coronary heart disease, remains the biggest killer. A disheartening finding is that 80% of the deaths caused by CVD in 2008 were preventable, through behavioural and lifestyle changes. This is promising, however, as there is great potential for lowering the incidence of CVDs in the future, as has already been instigated in several countries, including the UK, the USA and Australia.

Symptoms of cardiovascular disease

The narrowing and hardening of the arteries, due to the gradual build-up of plaque over many years, is often asymptomatic. As the health of the arteries plays a major role in CVD, the occurrence of a myocardial infarction or a stroke may, therefore, be the first indication of a diseased cardiovascular system. This highlights the importance of having regular blood pressure, blood glucose and blood lipid checks, in an attempt to detect any potential problems before they manifest in a serious clinical condition.

Incomplete perfusion of the heart muscle is associated with symptoms of *angina pectoris*, such as pains or pressure in the central chest that spreads to the shoulders, neck or arms. The complete blockage of blood flow to part of the heart results in a heart attack, during which a wide range of symptoms can develop: angina; elbow, jaw or back pain; a shortness of breath or difficulty in breathing; feeling nauseous or vomiting; feeling light-headed or faint; breaking into a cold sweat; or becoming pale. In contrast, an ischaemic insult to the brain results in a stroke, the greatest cause of disability in older individuals, which involves neurological disturbances. For this reason, symptoms of a stroke differ substantially from those of a heart attack. They include a sudden weakness or numbness of the face, arm and leg, most often on one side of the body, visual disturbances, speech difficulties and confusion, struggling to walk, dizziness, loss of balance or coordination, severe headache, fainting or unconsciousness. Awareness of symptoms of a heart attack or stroke can greatly improve the prognosis through acquiring immediate medical attention.

Cardiovascular disease risk factors

It is clear that CVD is a leading cause of death, and its diagnosis may not be made until following a serious event. What, therefore, can we do to reduce the risk of CVD? There are many risk factors, some of which are outwith our control, such as age, sex and family history. The modifiable risk factors, however, are the ones that we can target in our attempt to lower the alarming prevalence of these diseases worldwide. An unhealthy diet, sedentary lifestyle and smoking can lead to increases in blood pressure (hypertension), blood glucose concentration, blood lipid level, low-density lipoprotein (LDL) cholesterol and the development of Type II diabetes and obesity, all of which are risk factors for the development of a CVD. An increase in physical activity, consumption of a healthy diet and the cessation of smoking, therefore, are all lifestyle changes that can significantly reduce the risk of CVD. These three factors are discussed below.

Physical inactivity

Earlier sections in the book have clearly illustrated the benefits of physical activity for a variety of conditions, including depression, obesity, osteoporosis and sarcopenia. A physically inactive lifestyle is associated with twice the risk of developing coronary artery disease, once again highlighting the importance of exercise for health. Cardiorespiratory fitness (CRF), associated with physical activity level, is a strong predictor of CVD mortality. An enhanced CRF through regular physical activity serves to improve insulin sensitivity, blood lipid profile, body composition, inflammation and blood pressure (Lee et al., 2010), thereby greatly reducing the risk of CVD.

It has been suggested that the total duration of exercise, rather than the intensity of exercise, is the most important factor for improving lipid profile and insulin sensitivity, although lower durations of exercise remain beneficial compared to a sedentary lifestyle (Houmard et al., 2004; Kraus et al., 2002). High-density lipoprotein (HDL) concentration, referred to as 'good cholesterol' (refer to Chapter 2,

'Lipoproteins' section), is elevated with regular endurance exercise. As part of the lipid profile, this increase in HDL cholesterol lowers the risk of CVD in physically active individuals compared with those leading a sedentary lifestyle. An interesting current discussion amongst the experts regards the individual roles of cardiorespiratory fitness and body fatness on CVD risk. The most recent reviews indicate that, even in the absence of body weight loss, an improved cardiorespiratory fitness through regular physical activity will lower the risk of cardiovascular mortality (Fogelholm, 2010; Gaesser et al., 2011).

Diet

The consumption of a healthy diet, as outlined in Chapter 2, is crucial for lowering the risk of CVD. Diet is directly linked to the development of atherosclerosis, the underlying cause of CVD. Additionally, diet can play a role in the development of obesity and hypertension. The modification of diet for the prevention or treatment of obesity, also reduces the incidence of diabetes which is an independent risk factor for CVD. It has long been known that consuming a healthy diet contributes toward lowering the risk of CVD.

The risk of CVD can be lowered through several simple dietary changes. A reduction in dietary fat, especially saturated and trans-fats, can help reduce blood LDL cholesterol levels which are involved in the build up of arterial plaque, the underlying cause of CVD. The inclusion of more dietary fruit and vegetables, wholegrains and soluble fibre, are also good for the heart, potentially through moderation of LDL cholesterol levels and effects. A reduction in salt intake can lower the risk of CVD through the lowering of blood pressure.

Smoking

Cigarette smoking is thought to be the single most preventable cause of heart disease. It is associated with a two- to three-fold increase in coronary artery disease and stroke. The longer an individual has smoked, and the greater the number of cigarettes smoked per day, the greater the increased risk of CVD. Chemicals in the smoke are thought to stimulate the constriction of vascular smooth muscle, contributing to hypertension and subsequent injury of the vascular wall. The injury site then becomes the site of plaque formation as fats and cholesterol start to build up. As mentioned previously, this development of atherosclerosis is the underlying cause for CVD.

Blood oxygen levels are compromised in smokers. Carbon monoxide in cigarette smoke binds to haemoglobin, reducing the oxygen-carrying capacity of the blood and subsequent delivery to the tissues. In addition, lung diseases associated with cigarette smoking result in lowered blood oxygen content, hence the heart must work harder to supply the tissues with oxygen. This fall in blood oxygen content, combined with the smoking-related hypertension and atherosclerosis, may lead to heart failure. Quitting smoking will therefore reduce the risk of developing CVD. After one year of being smoke-free the risk of heart disease is halved.

Exercise rehabilitation for heart attack patients

Previously, strict bed rest was recommended following cardiovascular surgery or a heart attack. Due to the resultant loss of strength and aerobic capacity with enforced inactivity, however, rehabilitation was slow and difficult. As a result, cardiac rehabilitation programmes now commence within a few days of the event, allowing for minimal bed rest. During hospitalisation, stable patients should be encouraged to spend time in a seated or upright position, to provide an orthostatic stress; this increases the heart rate and blood pressure, stimulating an increased oxygen uptake by the myocardium. Following 2–3 days, the patient should progress to walking a few steps, building up to several hundred feet 2–4 times per day. Following discharge from hospital, participation of heart attack patients in an exercise-based rehabilitation programme lowers death rate by 20–5%.

Exercise training for cardiac rehabilitation may be best conducted in a monitored group-based session, especially for individuals at higher risk of further cardiovascular problems. Due to the cost and travel involved in these group sessions, however, medically directed home-based exercise rehabilitation may be just as beneficial for stable heart disease patients. The exercise prescribed should involve a combination of aerobic and resistance training with the goals of improving aerobic endurance, muscular endurance and strength to reduce the risk of a secondary event and lower mortality risk. Cardiovascular training typically focuses on walking-based activities; however, other forms of aerobic exercise may be included. Exercise should be conducted at least three times per week for 30–60 continuous or accumulated minutes (e.g. three bouts of 10 minutes), for at least 12 weeks' duration at a moderate intensity. This should be supplemented by an increase in everyday activities, such as gardening, using the stairs instead of taking the lift, going for a walk during a work break, parking further from destination and walking. Strenuous activities and sudden start-stop activities place a greater strain on the heart, especially in previously sedentary individuals, hence the recommendation of moderate intensity exercise for cardiac patients. The American Heart Association has indicated that maximum benefits are gained from 5–6 hours activity per week, which could include a combination of structured exercise and increased daily activities, for the prevention of heart attack and death in those with CHD. Practical methods for guiding exercise intensity include an increase in heart rate of no more than 20–30 beats·min^{-1}, the use of the RPE (rating of perceived exertion) scale (score of 9–11) or the 'talk test' (can talk comfortably during exercise). These intensities equate to 70–85% of maximal heart rate. As rehabilitation progresses, the intensity and duration of exercise should be developed. Resistance training, for the development of muscular strength and endurance, is recommended to involve the completion of one set of 8–10 exercises (that involve the major muscle groups) 2–3 times per week. The load applied should result in moderate fatigue upon completion of 10–15 repetitions.

Although physical activity is strongly encouraged during cardiac rehabilitation, each patient will differ with regards to optimal exercise intensity and duration. It is important that the increase in exercise volume is gradual and timed for each individual. There are four symptoms that cardiac patients should be made aware of, that indicate a worsening of their cardiac condition. These are as follows:

1. New onset or recurring angina pain
2. Unaccustomed shortness of breath
3. Dizziness or light-headedness
4. Heart arrhythmia (abnormal heart rhythm)

If any of these symptoms are experienced, the individual should discontinue exercise and obtain medical advice.

Despite the clear physiological and metabolic benefits of regular physical activity, only 11–20% of heart disease patients participate in medically supervised rehabilitation programmes. If this statistic wasn't disturbing enough, cardiac exercise programmes typically have a high (50%) dropout rate after 3–6 months. This highlights the importance of educating cardiac patients on the benefits of physical activity, whilst also providing them with dietary advice, information on smoking cessation and, very importantly, providing them with strategies to help with behavioural change.

Key points

Cardiovascular disease:

➤ Narrowed arteries (atherosclerosis) is underlying cause

➤ Is the biggest killer, accounting for 30% of all global deaths in 2008

➤ 80% of these CVD deaths were preventable (2008 data)

➤ The most common CVDs are coronary heart disease and stroke

➤ Symptoms of CVD

- Occurrence of heart attack or stroke may be first indication of CVD
- Heart attack symptoms – angina, shortness of breath, nausea or vomiting, feeling faint, cold sweats, becoming pale
- Stroke symptoms – numbness, visual disturbances, speech difficulties, dizziness, loss of balance, headache, fainting or unconsciousness

➤ Main modifiable risk factors include

- Smoking
- Physical inactivity
- Unhealthy diet

➤ Physical activity is important in CVD rehabilitation

Diabetes mellitus

The development of diabetes mellitus is closely associated with the hormone insulin and its role in glucose regulation (refer to the endocrine system in Chapter 4). There are two main forms of diabetes, Type I, also known as insulin-dependent diabetes mellitus (IDDM) or juvenile onset diabetes, and Type II, non-insulin-dependent diabetes mellitus (NIDDM) which is also known as adult onset diabetes. The common signs and symptoms of diabetes include, excessive thirst, frequent urination, the presence of glucose in the urine (glycosuria), unexplained weight loss, increased hunger, fatigue, irritability, blurred vision, wounds being slow to heal and an increased frequency of infection.

Type I diabetes

Insulin-dependent diabetes mellitus (Type I), is the least common of the main forms of diabetes, usually with <10% of the diabetic population having this form of the disease. Although sometimes referred to as juvenile onset, because most cases are diagnosed in individuals under the age of 20 years, this form of diabetes can occur later and sometimes, though rarely, when people are in their 40s. As

described in Chapter 4, insulin is produced by the β cells of the pancreas and, as the name of the disease suggests, this form of diabetes is caused by a reduction or failure of the β cells to produce insulin. Usually, in contrast to Type II diabetes, the onset of Type I diabetes is often sudden and can lead to ketoacidotic coma. Ketoacidosis, which can be fatal, results from increased lipid metabolism which is triggered by impaired glucose metabolism. The relative increase in lipid metabolism, which results in the production of acidic ketone bodies, arises because the lack of insulin production, and hence impaired cellular glucose uptake, necessitates a favouring of lipid metabolism. Additionally, the presence of insulin inhibits lipid metabolism, hence in the absence of insulin the rate of lipid metabolism rises thereby increasing ketoacidosis. This failure of the β cells to produce insulin most likely results from an autoimmune response which causes the destruction of the β cells or leads to their impaired functioning. As a consequence, those with Type I diabetes must either inject or infuse (with a pump) rapid-acting and slow-acting insulin to regulate glucose metabolism. The presence of too much insulin via injection or infusion can lead to very low blood glucose levels, known as hypoglycaemia. In contrast, if an individual takes insufficient insulin, blood glucose will rise to high levels (hyperglycaemia). When carefully managed, it is possible for a person with Type I diabetes to lead an otherwise completely normal life and compete at the highest levels in sport. Soccer player Gary Mabbutt has Type I diabetes, but played over 600 professional games for England, Tottenham Hotspur and Bristol Rovers while managing his diabetes on a daily basis. Other athletes who managed diabetes and played sport at the highest level include cricketer Wasim Akram, tennis player Arthur Ashe, the boxer Smokin' Joe Frasier, and multiple Olympic Gold medallist rower Sir Steve Redgrave.

Type II diabetes

Type II diabetes used to be known as adult onset diabetes as most cases were diagnosed in individuals over the age of 40 years. This form of diabetes, however, is increasingly being diagnosed in adolescents. As a consequence, Type II diabetes may become a paediatric illness of which physical education teachers and coaches may need to become more aware. This form of diabetes is not caused by a lack of insulin production, but by a resistance to insulin (decreased sensitivity) particularly in the skeletal muscles. The resultant reduction in glucose uptake by the muscles leads to blood glucose levels remaining elevated above normal. The onset of Type II diabetes, in contrast to Type I, is normally slower and progressive. If left untreated it can lead to blindness, the need for lower-limb amputation due to poor circulation, increased CVD risk and renal failure.

Type II diabetes is very closely related to obesity, with over 80 % of people with this form of diabetes being overweight or obese. This relationship is due to the fact that obesity reduces insulin receptor sensitivity. The causes of the disease are complex, but are thought to relate to diet and lack of physical exercise. More recently there has been speculation that there is also a genetic component to the development of the disease. Until recently it has been thought that there is no cure for Type II diabetes, and so the only option for an individual was to manage their diabetes by careful consideration of the diet, through physical activity, and where necessary, medication. A recent (2011) study in the UK, however, has reported the first cases of a reversal in Type II diabetes brought about through a dietary intervention.

The role of regular physical activity

Regular physical activity can benefit both Type I and Type II diabetics. Before commencing a physical activity programme, however, diabetics should undergo a medical examination to identify any underlying complications, such as cardiovascular, eye, kidney, feet or nervous system problems. There are several considerations required for diabetics during exercise. Foot care is essential. It is important for diabetics to wear appropriate footwear, possibly with additional accessories, to prevent blisters, to keep the feet dry and to minimise trauma. Maintaining hydration before and during exercise is also important due to the adverse effects of dehydration on blood glucose levels and heart function.

Prior to exercise, it is important for Type I diabetics to have their diabetes under good control to prevent the occurrence of hyper- or hypoglycaemia. An improved insulin sensitivity in the active Type I diabetic means they may require a lower level of insulin replacement. Although several research studies have failed to show an independent effect of physical activity on glycaemic control, there is no doubt that regular exercise is an important behavioural change with multiple health benefits.

Regular physical activity improves several risk factors of CVD, such as obesity, atherosclerosis, hypertension and increased LDL-cholesterol, all of which are associated with Type II diabetes. In addition to the benefits of these changes for those with established Type II diabetes, regular physical activity also plays an important role in the prevention of this disease. Although physical activity is closely

related with obesity, and as such may be beneficial, it can also independently reduce the severity of Type II diabetes. Linked with the etiology of the disease, an improved sensitivity to insulin with regular exercise is clearly beneficial in reducing the severity of Type II diabetes. This response to exercise, however, is acute in nature, emphasising the importance of regular exercise in the treatment of diabetes.

Similar to CVD rehabilitation, a recommended exercise programme for diabetics includes 30–60 minutes of moderate intensity aerobic exercise on 4–6 days per week. Intense exercise is also beneficial for decreasing insulin requirements in diabetics, although care should be taken in those at high risk of CVD. Moderate intensity resistance training can also be included in an exercise programme for the majority of diabetics, so long as it is in combination with more prolonged aerobic activities. High intensity training may also be conducted by young diabetics. However, it is not recommended for older individuals or those with long-standing diabetes.

Key points

Diabetes mellitus develops due to the absence of insulin production (Type I) or an increased resistance to insulin (Type II) – both lead to impaired glucose regulation.

➤ Type I diabetes – absence of insulin production:
  - Early onset – most cases diagnosed under the age of 20 years
  - Onset is often sudden and can lead to a coma
  - Treatment: injection or infusion of insulin, regular physical activity
  - Able to lead a normal life and compete in elite sport

➤ Type II diabetes:
  - Adult onset – most cases diagnosed in individuals over 40 years of age – but becoming more prevalent in adolescents
  - Onset is slower and progressive
  - Closely associated with obesity
  - Treatment: managed through dietary manipulation and regular physical activity

Metabolic syndrome

Obesity, CVD and diabetes, as well as being health risks factors individually, are also associated with a more recently identified multifactorial health concern – the metabolic syndrome. In the 1980s researchers identified a number of factors that increase the risk of developing coronary heart disease, Type II diabetes and stroke. Other factors associated with a diagnosis of metabolic syndrome include insulin resistance, abnormal lipid metabolism and hypertension. Some researchers believe that poor diet and lack of physical activity are also key factors in the development of metabolic syndrome.

Knowledge integration question

What is the role of regular physical activity in health, with special consideration to obesity, cardiovascular disease and diabetes mellitus risk?

14.3 Physical activity for health and well-being

Physical activity at its most basic level is any muscular movement that causes an increase in energy expenditure. As exercise scientists, physical education teachers and sports coaches, we tend to intrinsically believe that exercise is good for us, but is this really true? How does physical activity improve our health and well-being? The simple way to address this question is to turn it around and ask, what are the detrimental effects of a sedentary lifestyle? Research clearly demonstrates that physical inactivity is associated with decreases in health and well-being. The risks of obesity, of developing cardiovascular disease and diabetes are all increased through leading a sedentary lifestyle.

Benefits of regular physical activity

Physiological

An increase in sedentary behaviour occurs with increasing age. Research findings indicate that regular exercise can help to offset the effects of ageing (see section, above, on physical activity and ageing for full details), as well as helping to maintain health and well-being. An overview of the benefits of regular physical activity is provided in Table 14.5. For example, weight-bearing and strength training exercise has been demonstrated to be beneficial in protecting against and decreasing the effects of osteoporosis. Furthermore, whereas it had previously been thought that aerobic power declines with age, more recent research has demonstrated that an individual's aerobic power does not have to follow a classic pattern of decline with age. Indeed, regular physical activity and training can help to facilitate a plateau in aerobic power until much

Table 14.5 Benefits of physical activity.

Reduced risk factors	Improved functioning factors
Mortality rate	Quality of life
Cardiovascular disease	Cardiovascular functioning
Obesity	Endocrine functioning
Type II diabetes	Metabolic functioning
Cancer risk (colon and breast cancer)	Sleep patterns
Osteoporosis	Self-esteem
Depression	Self-confidence
Anxiety	Health choices and behaviours
Incidences of falling	Locus of control
	Mood and attitude to life
	Coordination and functional movement

later in life. The reduction in muscular strength, power and endurance with ageing can be attenuated through regular physical activity. This, combined with the maintenance of balance and coordination, can reduce the risk of falling.

Psychological

As well as the physiological benefits of physical activity, the alterations in endocrine functioning can improve psychological well-being. The release of hormones such as endorphins resulting from involvement in endurance exercise can stimulate improvements in self-esteem, self-confidence, locus of control and feelings of well-being. In addition, physical activity carried out in a social environment can help people to make social connections and form friendships which also contribute to enhanced mental health. Sufferers of mental illnesses such as depression (described above), can benefit greatly from physical activity through a particularly important mechanism for improving feelings of well-being and locus of control.

Key points

Benefits of regular physical activity:

➤ Physiological and psychological improvements lead to improved quality of life

Table 14.6 Some examples of current (2011) governmental recommendations for physical activity.

Age group	USA (Centre for Disease Control and Prevention)	UK (Department of Health, Chief Medical Officer)	Australia (Department for Health and Ageing)	New Zealand (Department for Health)
Children (5 or 6-17 yrs)	60 min physical activity every day. 3 days per week vigorous **and** muscle strengthening 3 days per week (as part of 60 mins) **and** bone strengthening 3 days per week (as part of 60 mins).	60 min moderate physical activity each day including 2 days a week which involve activities to improve bone health, muscle strength and flexibility.	5-12 yrs 60 min moderate and vigorous activities a day. 12-18 yrs 60 min of physical activity a day (moderate and vigorous) <2 hr day TV or computer or game use.	60 min moderate physical activity each day to vigorous exercise Active play as well <2 hr day TV or computer or game use.
Adults (18-64 yrs)	2 hr 30 min per week (Avg. 30 min per day × 5 days) moderate activity **and** muscle strengthening 2 days a week **or** 1 hr 15 min per week vigorous activity **and** muscle strengthening 2 days a week **or** a mix of moderate and vigorous **and** muscle strengthening 2 days a week.	Total of at least 30 min a day (in one session or shorter ones of 10 min) on 5 or more days a week.	Total of at least 30 min a day (in one session or shorter ones of 10-15 min) on most, but preferably all days.	30 min moderate physical activity most if not all days and vigorous exercise if possible.
Older adults (>65 yrs)	Recommendation same as for adults.	Recommendation same as for adults.	Recommendation same as for adults.	Not stated separately, so as for adults.

How much physical activity is enough?

The evidence about the benefits of physical activity leads to another important question. Given that physical activity is good for you, how much should an individual engage in to maintain his or her health and well-being? As can be seen from Table 14.6, governmental recommendations are similar between countries, 60 minutes per day for children and young people (under 18 years of age) and 30 minutes per day for adults most, if not all, days of the week. Interestingly, the US Government recommendations now specifically mention bone and muscle strengthening exercise and the Chief Medical Officer in the UK now recommends flexibility exercise as well as bone and muscle strengthening in addition to the guidelines for aerobic exercise.

Key points

Physical activity to maintain health and well-being:

➤ Children and adolescents (< 18 years of age) – 60 minutes per day

➤ Adults – 30 minutes per day on most/all days

➤ Activity should include aerobic exercise, bone and muscle strengthening exercises and flexibility exercises

Training programme development for health

In the USA moderate exercise is defined as exercise that, on a subjective scale from 0–10 pts (0 being stationary – 10 being maximal exercise), is an intensity of 5–6 pts, whereas vigorous exercise would be 7–8 pts of an individual's personal maximal capacity. By way of example, they include walking briskly (5 km·hr^{-1}), water aerobics and tennis doubles as moderate intensity physical activity, and lap swimming, race walking, skipping (jump rope), singles tennis and aerobic dance as vigorous exercise. Typically, moderate exercise relates to an intensity that is 40–60% of HR$_{max}$ (3–6 METS), while vigorous exercise is around 70–85% of HR$_{max}$ (> 6 METS).

With regard to developing a training programme for someone wishing to improve their health, beyond the frequency, intensity and duration recommendations in Table 14.6, the guidelines for exercise prescription in Chapter 8 would also be usefully applied. The general principles of training such as overload, progression and specificity, equally apply to a training programme developed for health reasons as for one developed to improve athletic performance. As indicated in Table 14.6, consideration should also be given to strength training, bone health (weight-bearing) and flexibility exercises to promote health and well-being. Exercise prescription for strength training was considered in Chapter 9 and the basis of such training could be applied to a health programme, as could the flexibility exercises described in Chapter 8.

> **Key point**
>
> The general principles of training should be applied during the development of a training programme for health benefits

Increasing physical inactivity

Despite the benefits and the relatively short time required to engage in physical activity, studies indicate that physical activity levels are decreasing in many countries. The reasons behind this trend and the implications for health are multifactorial, complex and relate heavily to societal changes in recent years.

One of the reasons behind the trend towards increased physical inactivity relates to change in employment. Research indicates that many forms of modern employment require less physical activity than was required in jobs for previous generations.

In schools, the selling-off of playing fields or closing of swimming pools (to save costs) has been accompanied by increases in health and safety regulations in some countries which may be contributing to a reduction of physical activity for children. In addition, the pressure on schools to improve academic results has led to a trend in many countries to reduce physical education time for each student. At a time when governments are developing guidelines to increase physical activity levels, the time available for physical education is being reduced. In this context, physical education teachers might need to lobby hard at a school, regional and national level to facilitate an improvement in time for physical education. Such a trend is not helped by the direction countries such as the UK, have taken with regard to elite sport. In recent years the development of elite sport has led to a changed focus in schools, away from participation and lifelong exercise and towards talent identification. Such a change might be beneficial for elite sport; however it may prove detrimental for the health of a nation.

Perhaps national physical education organizations such as the American Alliance for Health, Physical Education,

Recreation and Dance (AAHPERD), Physical Education New Zealand (PENZ), the Association for Physical Education in the UK (afPE), Australian Council for Health, Physical Education and Recreation (ACHPER) and those in other countries around the world need to lobby both on a national and an international level about the role of physical education in schools. The decline in hours for physical education classes in the school curriculum combined with the increased time devoted to examination physical education, increases in physical inactivity and rising levels of obesity have important implications for all physical educators and physical education associations. It may also be time, given the fairly traditional physical education curricula in many countries to examine what is taught in schools. There is, perhaps, an increasing divergence between the curricula taught in schools and the leisure trends of adolescents outside school.

While the decline in physical education in schools might provide one possible reason for the decline in physical activity in some countries, there are many other factors that perhaps also influence the trend towards increasing physical inactivity. Certainly, leisure trends for many people appear to be moving towards less physically active choices, such as computer gaming and social networking. When interviewed, people who are physically inactive cite lack of time, motivation and facilities as key factors behind their sedentary lifestyle choices. In the next section we examine the role of high-intensity interval training as a time-efficient form of physical activity that helps to improve physical activity levels and health.

> **Key points**
>
> Increasing physical inactivity is a major health problem and may be the result of several factors:
>
> ➤ Employment is less physically active
>
> ➤ Closure of school sports facilities and reduction in the time for physical education
>
> ➤ Leisure activities less physically active, e.g. television, computer gaming, social networking
>
> ➤ Lack of time, motivation and facilities

Firstly in this section we consider an alternative, intermittent exercise intervention for improving health for previously sedentary or obese individuals or those at risk of developing.

High-intensity interval training

Traditionally, sedentary individuals who want to lose weight, who want to improve their fitness or who are at risk of developing (or who have) diabetes or CVD, have been prescribed various forms of moderate intensity endurance exercise as a way to improve their health status. The health risks associated with obesity, diabetes and CVD were above, along with examples of lower-intensity training and methods for conducting such programmes. Research, however, has shown in many studies that sedentary people often describe 'lack of time' as an important reason behind their physical inactivity, explaining to researchers that if they had more time they would exercise more regularly. This finding was partly responsible for more recent research aimed at finding a strategy which was less time-consuming and yet beneficial in improving health and fitness. High-intensity interval training (HIIT) of shorter duration was adopted which might prove to be equally successful in decreasing the risks of diabetes and CVD. (See 'Classic research summary' on p. 463.)

Risk factor reduction through HIIT

In 2005 Warburton and colleagues, working in British Columbia, Canada, conducted a study with coronary artery disease (CAD) patients, presenting some interesting and hopeful findings regarding the possibilities of HIIT as an alternative exercise prescription. In this study 14 males (mean age 56 yrs, height 1.73 m, body mass 82 kg) who had undergone recent (within the last six months) coronary artery bypass surgery completed a 16-week training programme where they were assigned to either traditional or interval training. The traditional exercise programme consisted of a 10-minute warm-up before completing 30 minutes of continuous exercise at 65% of $HR/\dot{V}O_2$ reserve, followed by a standardised weight training programme and finally a 10-minute cool-down. The HIIT group completed the same warm-up, weight training programme and cool-down. However, for their 30 min exercise programme participants completed 2 minutes of high-intensity exercise (90% of $HR/\dot{V}O_2$ reserve) followed by a 2 min recovery phase at 40% of $HR/\dot{V}O_2$ reserve. In this way, participants completed 7×2 min high-intensity repetitions in each 30 min training session. Both groups completed five days of training each week, with the continuous training group completing five continuous sessions, while the HIIT group completed three continuous and two HIIT sessions.

Prior to starting the training programme, and at the end of the study, participants completed a range of laboratory tests over two days which included a $\dot{V}O_{2peak}$ test using the Bruce protocol (described in Chapter 12) and an exercise to exhaustion test the following day. Results indicated that both groups had similar, statistically significant, improvements in $\dot{V}O_{2peak}$. However, the time to exhaustion was significantly longer for the HIIT group when compared with the traditional training group. Results indicated that interval training could match, and even better, improvements in fitness for CAD patients, supportive of the findings of Rognmo et al., (2004). But what of other at-risk groups?

Studies by a combined Norwegian and UK research group have provided further information regarding the potential benefits of interval training for other at-risk groups. A study led by Wisløff and colleagues (2007) investigated the effects of interval training at 95% HR_{peak} and continuous moderate training (70% HR_{peak}) on 27 heart failure patients. Those patients in the HIIT group improved their $\dot{V}O_{2peak}$ (46% versus 14%) and left ventricular function to a greater extent following a 12-week programme (3 sessions per week), than the traditional training group. In a study with 32 metabolic syndrome patients, by the same research group but this time led by Tjønna (2008), the participants followed a 16-week (3 sessions per week) exercise training programme, following either an interval training (90% HR_{peak}) or continuous training (90% HR_{peak}) protocol for the duration of the study. Again increased gains were made by the HIIT group when compared with the continuous training group. The HIIT group had a larger improvement in $\dot{V}O_{2max}$ (35% versus 16%) and a more substantial decrease in the risk factors associated with metabolic syndrome. Results indicated that interval training could match, and even better, improvements in fitness for CAD and heart failure patients as well as those with metabolic syndrome, but what of time-saving? Research findings regarding the time-saving benefits of HIIT were to follow from other research groups.

Time-saving and HIIT

In 2006 Gibala and colleagues, working in Ontario, Canada, published results for a sprint training programme that was conducted with 16 active healthy males and provided an important step forward into a possible time-saving effect of HIIT. The participants (mean age 21.5 years, height 1.83 m, body mass 80 kg) were assigned to an endurance training (ET) or a sprint interval training (SIT) group. The SIT group completed 4–6 30-second sprints, with 4-minute recoveries for each training session, while the ET group completed 90–120 min continuous exercise. The training and testing for both groups was completed on a cycle ergometer. During the two weeks of training participants completed a total of six training sessions, one on each Monday, Wednesday and Friday. As a result of the difference in training regimes, the SIT group completed around 2.5 hours of training while the ET group completed 10.5 hours during the two weeks of the study, which represented a significant time saving for the SIT group.

Prior to starting the training programmes the participants completed a 50 kJ and a 750 kJ ride, during which participants were required to cycle until they had expended the required kJ for each test. In addition, participants had a muscle biopsy taken from their vastus lateralis muscle. The same testing procedure was repeated at the end of the study. Results indicated that the time taken for the 750 kJ ride decreased by 10.1% for the SIT group and 7.5% for the ET group. The differences in the 50 kJ tests were smaller, with the SIT group 4.1% and the ET group 3.5% quicker to complete the test. The muscle biopsy findings indicated that participants in both groups significantly improved their muscle oxidative capacity, but despite the differences in training volumes, there were no statistical differences between the improvements for the SIT and ET groups. Similarly, muscle buffering capacity and glycogen content improved more for the SIT group than the ET group, but there were no statistical differences between the groups. The key conclusions from this study were that (a) fitness and metabolic markers improved when the total training volume was structured to enable time-saving and (b) that SIT provided an alternative form of training to traditional ET producing similar improvements in exercise performance, muscle oxidative capacity and buffering. Given these findings it appeared that HIIT

training, in this case in the form of SIT, could provide a time-efficient training method for improving exercise performance for young active males.

This research group, working this time in association with a researcher in Australia, and led by Burgomaster (2008), then examined the potential benefits of a longer-duration training intervention. The active untrained male participants completed SIT (4–6 × 30-second sprints with 4.5-minute recovery) and ET (40–60 minute at 65% $\dot{V}O_{2peak}$) three times and five times a week (respectively). These exercise protocols resulted in the SIT group completing 1.5 hours each week versus 4.5 hours completed by the ET group. Despite the difference in training volume both training programmes produced similar changes in $\dot{V}O_{2peak}$, HR response to sub-maximal exercise (cycling), mitochondrial function and lipid oxidation. The authors concluded that HIIT again produced a time-saving exercise strategy that was equal to ET with regard to metabolic and exercise performance improvements. But what of the rest of the population, could similar findings be replicated for female as well as male participants and for older and less active people?

In 2012 a study led by Draper, Lunt and colleagues in New Zealand addressed these questions. In addition, the researchers set the exercise protocols in a real-world rather than laboratory setting with participants completing the exercise sessions at the local park. The 49 participants (aged 35–60 years) were randomly assigned to one of three exercise groups ET, HIIT and SIT and followed the protocols shown in Figure 14.4.

Pre- and post-training, participants completed an adapted version of the modified Bruce protocol to assess their aerobic capacity ($\dot{V}O_{2max}$), along with various anthropometric and clinical measures. Results of the study indicated that both SIT and HIIT resulted in similar

Figure 14.4 Exercise protocols for study led by Draper and Lunt (2012). Participants completed three exercise sessions per week for 12 weeks. ET = endurance training, HIIT = high-intensity interval training, SIT = sprint interval training, WU = warm up, CD = cool down.

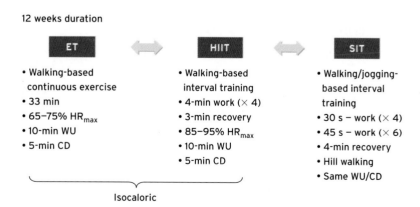

12 weeks duration

ET	HIIT	SIT
• Walking-based continuous exercise	• Walking-based interval training	• Walking/jogging-based interval training
• 33 min	• 4-min work (× 4)	• 30 s – work (× 4)
• 65–75% HR_max	• 3-min recovery	• 45 s – work (× 6)
• 10-min WU	• 85–95% HR_max	• 4-min recovery
• 5-min CD	• 10-min WU	• Hill walking
	• 5-min CD	• Same WU/CD

Isocaloric

aerobic capacity gains to traditional ET exercise prescription, but with a significant time saving for the SIT group. There were also significant improvements in sub-maximal exercise response ($\dot{V}O_2$ and HR), resting blood pressure and waist circumferences, again with no statistical differences between the groups. These results indicated that (a) HIIT and SIT can provide similar reductions in health risk factors and improvements in aerobic endurance ability compared to ET in a real-world setting and (b) SIT can provide a time-efficient method of exercise for improving health and fitness. The results of the study also indicated that the increased intensity for the SIT group, along with the increased loading on the body associated with ascending and descending a slope, resulted in an increased injury incidence when compared with HIIT and ET. Consequently, researchers and health professionals involved in exercise prescription should consider the use of reduced or non-weight bearing exercise for a SIT intervention to decrease the potential risk of injury. Results from each of the studies, however, support the notion that HIIT training has the potential to provide a useful, time-saving alternative for improving health and fitness to traditional endurance training.

Knowledge integration question

What is the physiological justification of prescribing high-intensity interval training for health benefits?

Check your recall
Fill in the missing words.

➤ Delayed onset muscle soreness may occur _____ to _____ days following exercise, particularly if _____ contractions have been involved in the activity.

➤ The mechanisms responsible for DOMS are thought to be micro-trauma to the muscle fibres and _____.

➤ The most common treatments of muscular cramp are _____ and the replacement of fluid and _____.

➤ The risks of developing obesity, diabetes mellitus and cardiovascular disease can be reduced through the participation in regular _____ _____.

➤ Many sedentary individuals cite '_____ _____ _____' as a reason for their physical inactivity

➤ _____ _____ _____ _____ (HIIT) provides a time-efficient method for improving aerobic fitness in CAD, heart failure, and metabolic syndrome patients

Review questions

1. What is DOMS? Explain why DOMS occurs and its significance for physical activity and training.

2. Discuss the possible mechanisms responsible for muscular cramps and strategies successful in its treatment.

3. What is the likely cause of the runner's stitch?

4. Through experimentation of what disease did Brooks and colleagues demonstrate that the lactate and ventilatory thresholds do not always occur at the same time point? Why was this the case in these patients?

5. What is the biggest killer worldwide and how is physical activity related to its prevention and treatment?

6. What are the health benefits of high-intensity interval training?

7. What are the likely causes and treatment for asthma?

8. Name the three groups of medication that can be prescribed in the treatment of asthma?

9. Explain the difference between overtraining and overreaching.

10. How does exercise serve to benefit people suffering from depression?

Teach it!
In groups of three, choose one topic and teach it to the rest of the study group.

1. Discuss the ways in which physical activity can benefit health.

2. Outline the key physiological changes occurring through the aging process.

3. Explain the female triad.

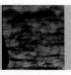

CLASSIC RESEARCH SUMMARY

High-intensity interval training and coronary artery disease patients by Warburton et al. (2005)

Exercise is commonly used in the rehabilitation of coronary artery disease (CAD) patients, resulting in an increased cardiorespiratory fitness and an overall improvement of their health. Continuous aerobic exercise training and low-intensity interval training have been shown to benefit health, including lowering the cardiac mortality rates. The aim of this classic paper by Warburton and colleagues, therefore, was to determine the health benefits of high-intensity interval training (HIIT) in CAD patients.

In this study 14 males (mean age 56 years, height 1.73 m, body mass 82 kg), who had undergone recent (within the last six months) coronary artery bypass surgery, completed a 16-week training programme where they were assigned to either traditional or interval training. The traditional exercise programme consisted of a 10-minute warm-up before completing 30 min of continuous exercise at 65% of $HR/\dot{V}O_2$ reserve, followed by a standardised weight training programme and finally a 10 min cool-down. The HIIT group completed the same warm-up, weight-training programme and cool-down. However, for their 30 min exercise programme participants completed 2 minute of high-intensity exercise (90% of $HR/\dot{V}O_2$ reserve) followed by a 2-minute recovery phase (40% of $HR/\dot{V}O_2$ reserve). In this way, participants completed 7×2 minutes high-intensity repetitions in each 30 min training session. Both groups completed 5 days of training each week, with the continuous training group completing five continuous sessions, while the HIIT group completed three continuous and two HIIT sessions.

Prior to starting the training programme, and at the end of the study, participants completed a range of laboratory tests over two days which included a $\dot{V}O_{2peak}$ test using the Bruce protocol (described in Chapter 12) and an exercise to exhaustion test the following day. Results indicated that both groups had similar, statistically significant, improvements in $\dot{V}O_{2peak}$. However, the time to exhaustion was significantly longer for the HIIT group when compared with the traditional training group. These results indicate that HIIT can match, or even better, improvements in fitness for CAD patients. The findings of Warburton and colleagues have subsequently been extended to show that heart failure and metabolic syndrome patients also experience greater benefits from HIIT, and that this protocol of exercise training can be used to save time for those with a busy lifestyle.

Reference: Warburton, D.E.R., McKenzie, D.C., Haykowsky, M.J., Taylor, A., Shoemaker, P., Ignaszewski, A.P. and Chan, S.Y. (2005). Effectiveness of high-intensity interval training for the rehabilitation of patients with coronary artery disease. *American Journal of Cardiology*, 95: 1080–4.

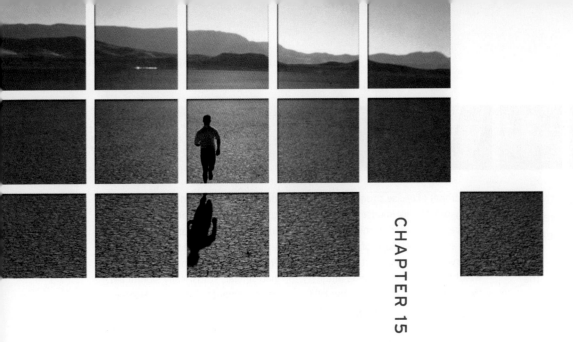

Applied exercise physiology and the environment

Learning objectives

After reading, considering and discussing with a study partner the material in this chapter you should be able to:

➤ **explain human thermoregulation**

➤ **describe the mechanisms of heat transfer**

➤ **discuss the effects of exercise in hot environments**

➤ **summarise the effects of exercising in cold environments**

➤ **teach others about the stages in water immersion and the effects on physiological functioning**

➤ **compare and contrast the physiological effects of hyperbaric and hypobaric environments on the physiological demands of exercise**

In this the final chapter of this textbook we discuss an interesting and important aspect of applied physiology, that of the environment and its effects on physiological functioning. There are a wide number of sports that take place in potentially dangerous environments, outdoor education is a curriculum area within physical education in many countries and many people live near potentially dangerous hazards such as rivers, lakes and oceans. For physical educators who are involved in outdoor education programmes, or athletes and coaches involved in sports

that take place in challenging conditions, an understanding of environmental threats to homeostasis is important to individual and group safety and health. This chapter provides a brief introduction to environmental physiology as it relates to involvement in sports that take place in a variety of environments. It begins with an introduction to thermoregulation as this is an important aspect of homeostasis that can be threatened when exercising in some environments. Following this we consider exercise in hot and cold environments, the effects of water immersion, hypobaria and hyperbaria on physiological functioning.

15.1 Thermoregulation

Humans belong to a group of mammals and birds called homeotherms. Homeotherms, as a part of their homeostatic mechanisms, attempt to maintain a constant core temperature (T_c) (at around 37°C for humans). Exercise in hot or cold environments, including sports which involve, or may involve, water immersion, threatens homeostasis and our immediate health. To preserve normal physiological function, T_c has to be regulated within a narrow range (35–41°C).

Thermoregulation is the control of body temperature within a narrow range and involves a variety of mechanisms to either increase or reduce body temperature. Humans regulate their body temperature to maintain an optimal internal environment for the cells of the body. Research indicates, for example, that when T_c falls below 37°C there is a concomitant slowing in brain cell activity and a decrease in performance. In addition, the enzymes that catalyse metabolic reactions function optimally within a narrow temperature range. The internal thermal balance is maintained by a variety of mechanisms that are initiated by the hypothalamus in response to sensory input from hot and cold receptors located in the skin, muscles, spinal cord and brain. The body's thermoregulatory mechanisms attempt to maintain T_c at, or close to, 37°C.

Measurement of core temperature

Body temperature can be measured by a variety of methods. Commonly, in the home, sub-lingual (under the tongue) or tympanic (ear) temperature is used as an estimate of deep body or core temperature. The results of this type of measurement can be influenced by drinks taken prior to measurement or warming of the ear, such as wearing a hat. In addition, temperature at the body's surface is not always reflective of T_c, for instance, in thermo-neutral conditions the skin temperature is normally around 33°C, 4°C lower than T_c. As a consequence, in a research setting T_c is measured using methods that provide the most accurate information. These include the use of a swallowed radio telemetry pill (T_{in} – intestinal), a rectal probe (T_{re}), or an oesophageal probe (T_{os}). Most commonly in laboratory research T_{re} is used due to the expense of using telemetry pills (around £30–50/US$50–70/AUS$60–75/NZ$80–100 each) and the discomfort felt with T_{os}.

Thermoregulatory zone

Human thermoregulation normally operates within a thermoneutral or thermoregulatory zone. Figure 15.1 provides an illustration of these zones. Within the thermoneutral zone T_c can be maintained by alterations in blood flow alone, keeping skin temperature around 33°C. Beyond the thermoneutral zone, but within the thermoregulatory zone, T_c can be maintained by inducing shivering or sweating. If the naked body is exposed to a temperature outwith the thermoregulatory zone it will not be able to defend T_c and, as a consequence, body temperature will continue to rise (in hot environments) or fall (in cold environments) inducing hyperthermia or hypothermia, respectively. For a naked adult standing in air the thermoneutral zone is 26–30°C. The thermoneutral temperature for humans in water is around 35–35.5°C. The thermoneutral zone is higher and narrower for water than for air, due to the greater conductivity of water compared with air. When the environmental temperature is above or below the thermoneutral temperatures, the body activates behavioural and internal mechanisms to protect core temperature.

Mechanisms of heat transfer

Heat transfer occurs through four mechanisms: radiation, convection, conduction and evaporation. Body temperature can be raised internally through metabolism and externally by conduction, convection and radiation. For example, the sun on a summer day can provide a major source of radiation heat energy. Body heat is lost via conduction, convection, radiation and evaporation.

Conduction

Conduction involves the transfer of heat from one material to another through direct molecular contact. Heat

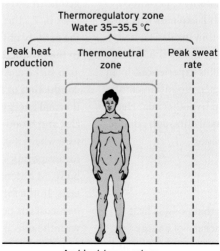

Figure 15.1 Thermoregulation in humans: the thermoneutral and thermoregulatory zones. (*Source:* Adapted from Mekjavic and Bligh (1987))

produced by the muscles during exercise can be conducted to the skin. If you sit on a storage heater to warm up at the end of a day's paddling, heat will be conducted to your body. Sports involving cold water immersion can result in a rapid loss of body heat as it is transferred to the boundary layer of water molecules surrounding the body. It is for this reason that you commonly see triathletes wearing wetsuits during the open water swim element of their race.

Convection

Convection is a specific form of conduction involving the movement of a fluid (gas or liquid) across a warmer surface (solid, liquid or gas). Boundary layer molecules of the fluid are heated by conduction. This is how a wetsuit functions to keep you warm in open water – an initial layer of cold water enters between the skin and the wetsuit which is subsequently warmed by conduction from your body heat. In this situation, the warmed boundary layer acts as insulation. However, in open water, the warmed boundary layer has a reduced density, creating buoyancy, and the warmed fluid begins to rise. Cool fluid replaces the boundary layer and the process of conduction, movement and replacement continues. This process is called convection. Both air and water colder than the skin can transfer heat away from the body by convection and this will result in faster cooling than straightforward conduction.

Water or air molecules heated through contact with the body (conduction) can also be stripped away from the body if there is an air current (wind) or water flow (river current or tidal movement) through the process of *advection* or *forced convection*. The continuous, rapid replacement of the boundary layer during forced convection can result in a faster heat transfer than convection. This effect is often referred to as 'wind chill' and is commonly experienced in a mountain environment. Wind chill explains why on a breezy day it can be warmer to wear thin insulation under a light windproof outer garment rather than a thicker non-windproof garment. If wind chill is experienced in an already cold environment, such as when mountain climbing, great care must be taken to avoid hypothermia. Heat loss during water immersion is primarily through conduction and convection or forced convection.

Radiation

Radiation is emitted from all objects that possess heat energy. Radiation is composed of 'packets' of energy called photons which travel at the speed of light. The sun heats the earth by thermal radiation since these photons are able to travel though the vacuum of space without being affected by it. The main photons responsible for heat transfer belong in the infrared spectrum which is an energy level just below that of visible light. The energy in infrared radiation will heat solid or liquid objects when it comes into contact with them. When we stand facing the sun we can feel its heat as we are absorbing its radiation. Light-coloured surfaces absorb less thermal radiation than dark ones, so during exercise light-coloured clothing in the summer can help keep you cooler. As heat-generating homeotherms, humans also emit radiation and at rest this represents the major heat loss mechanism. During exercise the relative amount of heat loss through radiation decreases and evaporation provides the major pathway for heat dissipation. In water, because we are surrounded by a liquid, heat loss by radiation is greatly decreased (occurring mainly from the head) because infrared radiation through liquid is extremely limited. It is for this reason, along with the thermal conductivity of water, that conduction and convection represent the major heat loss mechanisms during water immersion.

Evaporation

Evaporation, the use of energy to convert a liquid to a gas, forms the major source of heat loss during exercise. At rest the major source of heat loss for humans, around 60%, is through radiation. During exercise in low humidity conditions, evaporation provides the mechanism for about 80% of our heat loss. In humid conditions, when the water vapour content in air is high, evaporation is reduced but still remains the major source for heat loss. In addition to water vapour content, the evaporation of sweat is dependent on air velocity, with still conditions being disadvantageous. In response to exercise or environmentally induced rises in T_c, the hypothalamus stimulates an increase in the activity of the sweat glands. This results in an increase in the production of sweat which is secreted onto the skin surface. At the same time, vasodilation increases the conduction of heat from the body core to the skin. The thermal energy that is transferred from the active muscles and blood to the skin warms the sweat to a temperature where it can evaporate. The heat absorbed by sweat for evaporation results in the removal of heat from the body. Maintenance of T_c is vital for maintaining homeostasis. In the following sections we examine the threats to homeostasis posed by hot and cold environments along with the effects of water immersion on physiological functioning.

15.2 Physiological challenge of thermal stress

Taking part in high-intensity aerobic endurance sports, particularly those of a longer duration, can require an athlete to exercise in environments that expose them to extremes of thermal stress. The combined stresses of exercise and heat or cold create multiple threats to homeostasis for an athlete. This section examines the effects of heat and cold on performance during aerobic endurance sports.

The physiological stress of hot environments

Exercise in the heat provides a dual challenge to the body: thermal stress from the environment and physical stress from the exercise. The primary mechanisms for coping with the thermal stress associated with heat are vasodilation (i.e. increasing blood flow to the skin) and an increased sweat rate. Thermoreceptors, mainly located close to the hypothalamus and sensitive to temperature changes as small as 0.01°C, relay information to the hypothalamus, the body's thermostat. The hypothalamus stimulates blood flow alterations and increases in sweat gland activity. In short-duration sports, such as those that were the focus of Chapters 9 and 10, exposure to a hot environment is minimised and consequently has a minimal impact on performance. For longer-duration sports, such as aerobic endurance sports (the focus of Chapters 11 and 12) or intermittent sports (the focus of Chapter 13), where the exposure to a hot environment is more sustained, heat stress provides a greater threat to homeostasis and a greater challenge to the body's thermoregulatory functioning. The longer the duration and the higher the intensity of exercise, the greater the challenge to thermal balance. The risks of dehydration and hyperthermia, and their deleterious effects on performance, are increased as the environmental temperature rises. The degree of shade from direct sunlight and the amount of reflected solar radiation will also affect the thermal stress placed on an athlete. In addition, the relative humidity and air movement (wind) will affect the degree of heat stress, as mentioned above. Research indicates that the higher an athlete's level of fitness the better they are able to cope with the additional stress of exercise in the heat.

Physiological responses to exercise in the heat

As mentioned, exercise in the heat creates a dual challenge to physiological functioning. Exercise creates an increased demand for oxygen and blood flow to the muscles, while thermal stress diverts blood flow to the skin and stimulates an increase in sweat rate in response to thermal stress. The enhanced activity of the sweat glands increases their demand for oxygen and energy. Exercise in hot environments, therefore, creates a competitive demand for blood flow and results in an increased rate of glycogen usage. Research shows that exercise in the heat results in higher lactate concentrations which are indicative of a shift to increased fast-rate glycolysis. In addition, exercise in hot environments increases ventilation rate and heart rate, and reduces time to glycogen depletion and fatigue. The alterations in blood flow in hotter environments result in a decreased venous return and as a consequence a decrease in stroke volume. To compensate for this and maintain cardiac output, heart rate has to rise during exercise in the heat. This rise in HR, associated with maintenance of cardiac output during exercise, is termed cardiovascular drift and was described in more detail earlier in this chapter.

Sweat rate and composition

The key mechanism for heat loss during exercise, is evaporation. When the exercise intensity and environmental temperature are low the sweat rate is correspondingly low and consequently sodium and chloride ions within sweat are reabsorbed as the sweat makes its journey from the sweat gland to the skin via the sweat duct. Thus the mineral content of sweat during low-intensity exercise in cooler environments is lower than that at higher intensities and temperatures. The reabsorption takes place from the walls of the sweat duct and returns sodium and chloride ions to the bloodstream, reducing electrolyte loss. However, potassium and other minerals such as calcium and magnesium, also lost in sweat, cannot be reabsorbed in this way and must be replaced by dietary intake. At higher intensities of exercise, sweat rate is increased and consequently travels via the sweat ducts to the skin much more quickly. As a result the reabsorption of sodium and chloride is reduced, resulting in an increased rate of electrolyte loss.

When exercising at higher intensity levels fluid loss through sweating can be as high as 2.0 L·hr^{-1}. For the average 70 kg adult performing a 60 min endurance session, this represents a 2.9% drop in body weight through fluid loss, and as was described earlier, research indicates a drop of only 1% has been shown to equate to a 2% drop in performance (speed during running). During the course of an endurance race in the heat, such as a marathon, performers can lose as much as 6–10% of bodyweight through sweat loss. A 2–3% drop in bodyweight through fluid loss is sufficient to decrease plasma volume, contributing to cardiovascular drift, and impairing the sweat response. To offset the negative effects of dehydration, athletes must employ a rehydration strategy during exercise in the heat. The use of electrolyte drinks as part of a rehydration strategy is discussed in Chapter 12. In addition to the negative effect on performance, dehydration incurred during exercise heat stress contributes to the incidence of heat exhaustion and heat stroke which are potentially life-threatening. The use of a fluid rehydration strategy in hot environments can help to reduce the incidence of heat-related illness during participation in aerobic endurance sports.

Knowledge integration question

The evaporation of sweat is vital for thermoregulation during exercise in a hot environment. What are the drawbacks of excessive sweating during a long-duration endurance event in the heat, and what influence do these factors have on performance?

Key points

The body's primary mechanisms for heat loss include vasodilation (enhancing skin blood flow) and increasing sweat rate aiding evaporative cooling.

Evaporative cooling is enhanced by increased air movement and decreased relative humidity.

Increased rates of sweating increase the risks of dehydration. Exercise in the heat can lead to heat exhaustion and heat stroke.

Heat illnesses

At rest, body temperature is normally maintained within 1°C of mean body temperature (37°C). Humans are better able to tolerate a fall in temperature than a rise above normal. A temperature of 42°C can be fatal, whereas a human can survive drops in core temperature to 25–27°C. As a consequence, heat illnesses (heat exhaustion and heat stroke) should be treated seriously. The three causes of hyperthermia (increased body temperature), are high exercise intensity, high environmental temperature and high humidity, which combine to increase the likelihood of heat illness. Children, who are less fit, or are obese, or who are suffering from illness, are at greater risk in the heat.

Heat exhaustion

Heat exhaustion results from hypovolaemia brought about through alterations in blood flow to the skin for cooling, and fluid loss through sweating. The competition for blood supply between the skin and muscles during exercise results in a decrease in blood volume returning to the heart. The subsequent decrease in stroke volume impairs cardiac output and results in a decrease in blood pressure leading to circulatory 'shock'. Signs of heat exhaustion include dizziness, fatigue, moist clammy skin, feeling faint, vomiting, low blood pressure and a weak rapid pulse. A person displaying symptoms of heat exhaustion should be treated as for shock: if possible remove the person from the immediate environment to a cooler place, lay the person down with legs raised to increase venous return, provide an electrolyte drink and seek medical help. If the symptoms are untreated heat exhaustion can progress to heat stroke. (See also 'Classic research summary' on p. 486.)

Heat stroke

Heat stroke results from a failure of the body's thermoregulatory mechanisms to cope with heat exposure. It is a life-threatening illness and requires immediate medical attention. In addition to exposure to hot environmental conditions, heat stroke can also occur during high-intensity endurance exercise in relatively moderate temperatures. The failure of the thermoregulatory system in heat stroke leads to a continuing rise in core temperature which impairs CNS functioning and leads to coma, tissue damage, and if untreated, death. Symptoms of heat stroke include very high body temperature, dry hot skin associated with a cessation of sweating, an increase in blood pressure, confusion and unconsciousness.

Key point

Exercise in the heat can lead to serious heat illnesses, heat exhaustion and heat stroke.

Heat acclimatisation

It is well established that the body can acclimatise to exercise in the heat. If an athlete is going to compete at a venue where the environmental temperature is greater than that in which they normally train and compete, then the adoption of an acclimatisation strategy will result in an improvement in their competition performance. To benefit from a heat acclimatisation strategy an athlete must exercise during the heat of the day; resting exposure is not sufficient. It appears that an acclimatisation period of 5–10 days should be sufficient to alter the thermoregulatory response. During this period the exercise intensity should be reduced to below normal for any given training session and attention should be paid to rehydration both during and following exercise. This type of strategy appears to reduce sodium and chloride loss and increase water retention such that pre-exercise water levels are 10–20% above normal. The hormone aldosterone increases the reabsorption of sodium and water at the kidneys and the sweat glands, and anti-diuretic hormone stimulates the kidneys to conserve water. These alterations increase blood volume (plasma), stroke volume and arterial pressure, along with lowering core temperature. In addition the heart rate is lowered, as is the core temperature at which sweating is initiated; there is less sodium and chloride lost in sweat and feelings of fatigue are reduced.

Knowledge integration question

With the approach of a major competition in a hot environment, what factors relating to performance should be considered?

In some instances, athletes are unable to spend much time at the venue prior to competition, whether due to cost or personal circumstances. In this situation, adaptation to heat stress in artificial conditions (e.g. a heat chamber), is of great benefit for physiological preparation when a competition is to be held in a hotter environment than that to which the athlete is accustomed.

Key point

Heat acclimatisation will improve an athlete's performance in a hot environment through the following physiological adaptations:

➤ Increased blood volume and stroke volume = lower heart rate
➤ Decreased core temperature
➤ Sweating is initiated at a lower core temperature
➤ Sweat sodium concentration is reduced
➤ Feelings of fatigue are lowered

The physiological stress of cold environments

The physiological stresses presented by exercise in cold environments relate to the air temperature, wind strength, relative humidity and the presence of rain. The lower the temperature, the greater the wind strength and the lower the relative humidity (or the presence of rain), the greater the threat to homeostasis. When environmental temperature falls below that of the skin, the body will lose heat through radiation, a loss which is exacerbated by air movement (wind). Dry air creates an increased risk of exercise induced bronchospasm (asthma) which presents a threat to health and the completion of any exercise. The presence of rain has been shown to decrease the insulative properties of clothing and consequently decreases the time to fatigue. To meet the challenge of a cold environment, athletes wear clothing to insulate core temperature and protect the skin from exposure to the environment. The insulative effect of such clothing can result in sweating during exercise in the cold, with sweat rate increasing as the intensity of exercise is raised. Evaporation of sweat on the skin or in clothing is enhanced by air movement. Sweating during exercise, particularly in the presence of wind, increases the cooling effect of the environment and hence the threat to maintaining core temperature. It is for this reason that the adage 'to stay warm in the hills, stay slightly cold' came about.

Physiological responses to exercise in the cold

The body's physiological response to cold air is similar to its response to cold water immersion which is described in more detail in below. In response to sensory stimulation from cold thermoreceptors, found mainly in the skin, the hypothalamus stimulates vasoconstriction and piloerection to preserve heat. To increase heat production in cold air environments the hypothalamus stimulates an increase in muscle tone, shivering and an endocrine-driven increase in metabolism. During cold water immersion, conduction and convection represent the key mechanisms for heat loss. Specialist insulative clothing such as wetsuits and drysuits (ideally with additional insulation worn underneath) can help to protect against the cooling effects. The main heat loss mechanisms during exercise in cold air are radiation and evaporation. Appropriate use of insulative clothing, and the use of changes of clothing (to replace wet or damp clothing resulting from sweat production during exercise), can help to greatly reduce the effects of cooling on core temperature during exercise in cold air environments.

Key points

The degree of physiological stress during exercise in a cold environment depends on the relative humidity, wind strength and the presence of rainfall.

Responses to cold exposure:

➤ vasoconstriction

➤ piloerection

➤ addition of extra clothing layers

➤ increased muscle tone

➤ shivering

Effects of cold environments on performance

Exercise in the cold affects performance in a variety of ways. Insulative clothing, which is often bulky, can inhibit movement and increase frictional drag as clothing rubs leading to a decrease in efficiency and a higher metabolic cost at any given workload. The initiation of increased muscle tone and shivering in cold environments to increase heat production comes at a metabolic cost. Research indicates that exercise in cold environments can result in a higher metabolic response for each workload, when compared to a thermoneutral environment. As with the cold water immersion response (below), vasoconstriction and cooling of the skin can lead to a decrease in the functioning of sensory receptors in the hands, resulting in a loss of manual dexterity. This loss is sometimes, as is described in more detail below, reduced after a short time due to the Hunter's reaction or response. Research indicates that, after an initial period of vasoconstriction of the blood vessels in the hand, there is a subsequent vasodilation that serves to counteract the loss of manual dexterity.

Muscular strength and power have been found to decrease in response to cold stress due to an increase in time for muscular contraction, along with a decrease in the fluid viscosity and enzymatic activity of the muscle fibres. At any given sub-maximal workload, ventilation, oxygen consumption and lactate accumulation are higher in cold when compared with thermoneutral environments.

Cardiovascular endurance decreases in cold environments due to a number of factors. When the blood temperature falls below 37°C it has been shown to reduce oxygen dissociation from haemoglobin resulting in decreased oxygen delivery to the muscles. Blood flow to the limbs is reduced due to vasoconstriction in the cold and this adds to the decreased oxygen delivery to the muscles. The decreases in oxygen transport result in the inhibition of fat metabolism and complete oxidation of food substrates. This leads to an increased reliance on glycogen and anaerobic energy production resulting in rises in blood lactate concentration and an earlier occurrence of fatigue. Through these mechanisms, research has shown that $\dot{V}O_{2max}$ is reduced in cold environments.

Key point

A cold environment can decrease muscular strength and power, and impair cardiovascular endurance.

Cold exposure illness and injury

Exposure to cold environments can lead to hypothermia and frostbite. Hypothermia is most commonly diagnosed at a core temperature of 35°C or below. It can be triggered by a sudden water immersion, such as the result of a kayak or canoe capsize, or a slower onset such as might occur during a mountain marathon, adventure/multisport race. The symptoms of hypothermia include shivering, a change to a greyish colour for those with lighter skin colouring, slurred speech, irritability, clumsiness and drowsiness. When the core temperature drops to 31°C shivering will cease, representing a significant point in hypothermia. At this point, an individual is unable to re-warm themselves without external heating. In cases of mild hypothermia, removing the person from the wind (an emergency shelter is excellent for this purpose), replacing wet clothing, increasing insulation and providing food and drink can help the person to recover quite quickly. As the person begins to recover, decisions can be made about how best to evacuate. In cases of severe hypothermia, the above measures should be completed where possible but medical assistance should be sought as quickly as circumstances allow. A further problem of exercise in cold environments is frostbite which can occur in skin exposed to sub-zero temperatures. In mild cases, limbs can be re-warmed in body temperature (37°C) water, or in the case of a hand, by placing it under the armpit. In severe cases of frostbite, especially if there is a danger of the limb refreezing if warmed, medical assistance should be sought for treatment.

Cold acclimatisation

Research indicates that it may be possible to habituate the body to cold exposure and consequently decrease the effects of exposure on performance. Results of research into cold acclimatisation, however, are less conclusive than for hot environments. A decreased sympathetic response (delayed shivering, increased vasoconstriction, decreases in blood pressure and heart rate) following cold acclimatisation has been suggested. However, other studies have failed to repeat these findings. The incidence of Hunter's response (a periodic vasodilation in the blood vessels of the hands which facilitates manual dexterity in cold conditions) often observed with fishermen, who spend frequent periods with their hands in cold water or in contact with cold objects, has been cited as an example of habituation. Cold water swimmers and marathon runners have been found to have a delayed shivering response and Aborigines, who sleep with very little clothing during very cold desert nights, have been found to tolerate mild hypothermia without a shivering response.

Key points

Cold exposure can lead to hypothermia and frostbite.

Cold acclimatisation may be beneficial for those competing regularly in cold environments.

15.3 Physiological challenge of cold water immersion

Any individual involved in a water-based sport may at some stage have to deal with the additional demands placed on the body by water immersion. In adventure sports such as surfing, diving or freediving, the water immersion, by the nature of the sport, is prolonged and therefore a major issue for

these performers with regard to water-induced hypothermia. In sports like kayaking, canoeing and sailing, hypothermia presents a potential threat to homeostasis, but in addition, a sudden and often unplanned water immersion can lead to cold shock. Gaining understanding of the effects of short-term and long-term water immersion on physiological functioning is essential for those involved in water-based sports, a number of which have been a focus of this chapter. Having an understanding of the threats to homeostasis presented by water immersion is important for teachers or coaches planning a day's river descent, for a group of sea kayakers planning a sea journey, or a sailor dealing with a sudden capsize during a race. Anyone involved in water-based adventure sports, if for no other reason than safety, should have a knowledge of the effects of water immersion.

In the summer months around New Zealand and Britain the mean sea temperature is around 15°C, in the winter months this temperature falls to an average of 5°C. Rivers around the world often have a temperature variation between summer and winter months of over 20°C to just above freezing. Even in summer months there can be a great variation in river temperatures. The Kaituna River in New Zealand benefits from geothermal warming and, to a British paddler, feels like paddling in bath water. In contrast, a summer capsize when paddling glacier-fed alpine rivers, such as the Inn in Austria or many rivers in New Zealand, can result in a sudden change from a high ambient temperature to a low (10°C or less) water immersion temperature. The effects of a capsize and roll (or capsize and swim) create an additional physiological stress, over and above the exercise demands of the activity. The body has a variety of mechanisms through which to attempt to overcome stress induced by water immersion.

Water immersion survival

Weather changes or boat problems during ocean sailing races such as the Sydney to Hobart Race (described by Ben Ainslie in the Sport in Action section in Chapter 12) or the Vendée Globe single-handed, non-stop, round-the-world race can, in an instant, change the focus from racing to survival. An example of this can be seen through the survival of Tony Bullimore during the 1996 Vendée Globe race. Two months into the race (in January 1997) disaster struck for Tony Bullimore, who was 56 years old at that time and an ex-Royal Marine from Bristol. In the middle of 60-knot winds and 15-metre waves, his yacht, the Exide Challenger, lost its keel and capsized. Fortunately for Bullimore, who was below deck at the time of the capsize, the yacht had a series of compartments which trapped sufficient air for his survival.

Nevertheless, he found himself without light and waist-deep in water. Despite these problems Bullimore was able to activate his Emergency Position Indicating Radio Beacon (EPIRB) and construct a hammock (from a cargo net) above the water line which enabled him to stay out of the water. It was five days before he was rescued by HMS Adelaide, an Australian naval ship responding to his EPIRB, by which time he was suffering from hypothermia, frostbite and dehydration. He had sustained himself during his wait for rescue with limited water supplies and chocolate. His experience as a Royal Marine and sailor provided him with the knowledge necessary to survive the effects of his water immersion.

Thermal transfer in water

When immersed in water below body temperature, heat will move from the core and heat a boundary layer of water next to the skin. This boundary layer heating process results in heat loss from the core. When the water is moving or a person swims, the boundary layer will be disturbed and a new cooler boundary layer forms around the body. This movement of water against the skin in the sea (or a river) will enhance conductive cooling. It is partly for this reason that, unless they are close enough to shore or a vessel, people are now advised not to swim as the movement of swimming will increase the rate at which the body cools. The properties of water make it far more effective as a medium through which heat transfer takes place when compared with air, i.e. heat is lost much more quickly in water than in air. Due to its increased density, water has a greater thermal conductivity (about 24–25 times that of air) which results in humans cooling around four times faster in water than in air. In addition, whereas normal clothing creates an insulative barrier to cooling in air, in water the body is almost 100% exposed to cooling as the barrier is lost.

Water immersion misconceptions

A number of common misconceptions have developed regarding the implications of water immersion as a threat to homeostasis. It is only in more recent years that research by physiologists such as Frank Golden, Michael Tipton and colleagues has led to a clearer understanding of the physiological stress associated with water immersion. For instance, in the 1960s and 70s it was regarded as beneficial to undress in water after an accidental immersion to avoid the clothing weighing you down and impeding swimming. Associated with this during an accidental immersion, victims were encouraged to swim around to keep warm. In survival training courses, trainees were encouraged to put their heads in the water as a method of drown-proofing. Research into the

effects of water immersion has shown that, contrary to these beliefs, clothes should be kept on to preserve heat, movement should be kept to a minimum in order to avoid further heat loss and that head immersion for drown-proofing purposes accelerates the onset of hypothermia. The increased depth of understanding regarding the implications of cold water immersion presents an excellent aid for all water sport athletes, teachers, coaches and outdoor educators.

Key points

Certain sports involve planned (e.g. diving) or potentially accidental water immersion (e.g. kayaking).

Knowledge of the effects of water immersion is important for performance and safety.

Physiological responses to water immersion

In early research relating to the consequences of unplanned (cold) water immersion, drowning and hypothermia were alternatively highlighted as the key concerns for survival. In 1981, responding to statistics gathered on fatalities in open water swimming, Golden and Hervey established a series of stages in water immersion that more accurately described its risks. Research in the 1970s indicated that over half the people who died as a result of open-water immersion did so within three metres of safety and two out of three of these individuals were reported as good swimmers. There was clearly an inherent risk in open-water immersion that did not relate to hypothermia as a cause of death, and consequently Golden and Hervey suggested that the risks involved should be classified by the length of time of the immersion. Their risk classification system is shown in Table 15.1 along with a summary of the predominant risk factors during each stage of immersion.

Initial response (cold shock)

The initial response begins immediately on contact with water and peaks at around 30 seconds. Symptoms begin to subside as the immersion duration approaches three minutes. The initial or cold shock response does not occur on entry to warm water and is thought to be a response initiated by cold receptor stimulation. Research indicates that a greater response occurs the colder the water and for those who have had fewer cold water immersions. The cold shock response is thought to be the primary cause of death in incidents when individuals drown within three metres of safety. The cold receptors primarily trigger CNS-driven alterations in breathing and circulation. On entry to cold

Table 15.1 Stages in response to water immersion.

Specific risk	Timing of response	Summary of risks
Initial response	0–3 minutes	**Cold shock:** Immediate vasoconstriction, rise in BP, HR and breathing rate **Associated risks:** Cardiac problems and arrhythmia, gasp response, dizziness, confusion, panic, reduced breath-hold capacity, drowning.
Short-term response	3–30 minutes	**Associated risks:** Loss of manual dexterity, impaired coordination and swimming ability, decreasing strength, drowning.
Long-term response	Over 30 minutes	**Associated risks:** Hypothermia, drowning
Post-immersion response	On and post rescue	**Associated risks:** After-drop in temperature, cardiac problems

Source: Adapted from Golden, F. and Tipton, M. (2002).

water (below 15°C) there is an immediate increase in the respiratory drive. This results in an individual taking an initial large gasp of air (around 2–3 litres) followed by the initiation of hyperventilation, where the rate of breathing is increased without an increase in depth of breathing. The incidence of hyperventilation can cause dizziness and confusion and is consequently thought to add to the panic associated with the immersion. Golden and colleagues believe that the most significant risk involved in the cold shock response relates to a decrease in breath-hold time – reduced from around 60 s on land to around 10 s in the water. The decrease in breath-hold time results in an increased risk of water inhalation and drowning.

Concomitant with the increases in breathing rate are CNS-driven alterations in circulation. Initial entry into cold water creates an immediate rise in blood pressure and heart rate along with triggering vasoconstriction. These responses establish an increase in cardiac output that is thought to present a cardiac or stroke risk for those with cardiovascular disease. In addition, cold water immersion has been associated with the occurrence of cardiac arrhythmias created by a HR conflict between the cold shock HR response (to increase HR) and the dive reflex. The dive reflex, common to many mammals, triggers vasoconstriction, breath-holding and slowing of the heart rate upon entry into water. Cardiac arrhythmia results from the competition between the cold shock response and diving reflex to control HR during cold water immersion. Golden and Tipton have suggested a number of factors that appear to affect the cold shock response and could help during an accidental immersion. Firstly, safety measures should be put in place wherever possible to avoid the risk of accidental water immersion. The use of clothing appropriate to the risk of accidental immersion and the use of a buoyancy aid

or lifejacket, as appropriate to the activity, can alleviate the cold shock response. Knowledge of the effects of initial cold water immersion can help the person to cope better with the effects. Where possible an individual should hold on to something and remember that the symptoms will pass. Research indicates that the cold shock response is blunted in those who have a lower body fat percentage and are aerobically fitter. In addition, the use of habituation strategies, acclimatising an individual to cold water immersions, has been shown to reduce the cold shock response. This has implications for kayakers possibly using one or more habituation rolls in cold water before and during a river descent to lessen the cold shock response in a must-roll situation.

Key points

The four stages of physiological response to cold water immersion:

1. Initial response (cold-shock)
2. Short-term response
3. Long-term response
4. Post-immersion response

Initial, cold shock response

➤ Lasts for 3 min after immersion
➤ Peaks around 30 s after immersion
➤ Physiological responses
  • Increases breathing rate (hyperventilation)
  • Increases HR – but in competition with the diving reflex which decreases HR, can lead to cardiac arrhythmias
➤ Thought to be responsible for many of the deaths which occur within three metres of safety

Short-term response

Beyond three minutes of immersion the short-term responses to water immersion become the predominant concern for an individual. The short-term responses relate to cold-induced decreases in muscular strength, manual dexterity and coordination. Research relating to swimming ability in cold water has shown that performance is impaired as part of a vicious circle of decreasing streamlining. Swimming, even for experienced swimmers, in cold water results in an increased breathing frequency. The increased breathing rate results in a less streamlined swimming position, which in turn leads to an increased oxygen demand, creating a further rise in breathing rate and a worsening in body position in the water (the body becoming more vertical as the individual eventually becomes static in the water and effort becomes focused on breathing and keeping the head above water). In a study with competent fully clothed swimmers in 25°C water all 10 completed a 10-minute swim. In water of 5°C only three managed to complete the 10-minute swim. Increases in breathing rate and stroke rate, and a decrease in swim streamlining, were found to be higher in those that failed to complete the swim as compared with those who succeeded. Golden and colleagues suggested that this knowledge should be made widely available to enable any individual to make an informed decision about swimming for shore in cold water. In addition, where possible, try to complete manual tasks such as life-jacket inflation as early as possible due to the decreasing manual dexterity and strength associated with short-term water immersion. Golden and Tipton recommend keeping swimming to a minimum and avoiding waving to rescuers to retain as much air trapped in clothing as possible.

Key points

Short-term responses to water immersion:

➤ Occurs between 3 and 30 min after water immersion

➤ Impairs muscle strength, manual dexterity and coordination

  • Can impair ability to swim, to self-inflate life jacket, to release flares

Long-term response

After 30 minutes of immersion, the primary concern becomes continued heat loss and hypothermia. Survival time during long-term water immersion is related to the rate of hypothermia and to the type of clothing worn. In response to continued water immersion the body's key mechanism to generate heat and protect core body temperature is shivering. The shivering response is initiated soon after entry into cold water. In the early stages of the onset of hypothermia shivering begins as an intermittent response. As temperature continues to decline shivering becomes continuous until carbohydrate stores are exhausted. After this point muscles go into a spasm pulling the body into a flexed foetal-like position and the individual becomes incapable of assisting in their rescue. At a core body temperature below 34°C brain function is impaired and leads to unconsciousness. Heart failure follows as body temperature reaches around 28°C. To protect against the progressive drop in core temperature during continued water immersion the primary measures include clothing choice when taking part in water-based adventure activities and, in the instance of an accidental cold water immersion, removal from the water (e.g. onto a floating object). Although it may feel colder in the wind, the rate of cooling would be slowed. In light of the loss of strength and manual dexterity that is associated with short-term immersion, removing yourself from the water should be effected as quickly as possible.

Key point

Beyond thirty minutes of water immersion, during the long-term response, the key concern is continued core temperature cooling. Shivering, to protect core temperature, continues until glycogen depletion.

Post-immersion response

A number of risks associated with rescue have been identified and should be considered for individuals who have been involved in cold water immersion. First identified in the 1790s by James Currie, a physician, individuals who survive a water immersion episode often experience an 'afterdrop' in core body temperature following removal from the water. This afterdrop has been linked with post-immersion fatalities. It has been suggested that such deaths are caused by cold blood from the periphery entering central circulation leading to cardiac failure. More recently, Golden and Hervey suggested that post-immersion afterdrop is a consequence of the physics of heat transfer. Even after removal from water an individual will experience a continued movement of heat from the warmer core to the periphery down the thermal gradient until the periphery is re-warmed. In the instance of an afterdrop fatality Golden and Hervey suggested that the continued cooling post-immersion results in the individual's core temperature dropping to an unrecoverable level.

An important theory regarding post-immersion death has been identified from the change in pressure on the body that occurs on removal from the water. As was described earlier in this section, head-out water immersion leads to a hydrostatic squeeze on the body resulting in an increase in venous return. Now that more blood is entering the heart, the cardiac output increases raising the blood pressure. In addition, the vasoconstriction associated with cold water immersion adds to this effect. To adjust to the increase in blood volume detected by blood vessel receptors, plasma is removed from the blood and passed from the body via the kidneys as urine. In this way the blood volume is decreased. When removed from the water survivors are often lifted in a vertical position – either into a boat or at the end of a helicopter strop. It is believed that vertical removal from the water results in the greatest challenge to a survivor's circulation. On removal from the water a survivor faces a drop in blood pressure, blood volume and cardiac output due to the removal of the hydrostatic squeeze. The reduced blood volume (hypovolemia), a cold-induced impairment of baroreceptor response to adjust blood pressure and a drop in cardiac output may be the cause of post-immersion unconsciousness (lack of blood and oxygen to the brain) and cardiac problems. It is for this reason that many air-sea rescues are completed with horizontal recovery of the victim, which has been shown to decrease the post-immersion circulatory stress.

For anyone involved in water-based sports, especially those involved in water-based adventure sports, an understanding of the effects of water immersion is essential if they are to be fully prepared to act appropriately. Recognition of the stages in water immersion could save the life of a member of a group or a stranger encountered during a day sailing or kayaking.

Key points

Post-immersion stage of water immersion

➤ Body initially experiences a continued drop in temperature – the 'afterdrop'

➤ Removal of hydrostatic squeeze

• Drop in blood pressure, blood volume and cardiac output

• Horizontal evacuation from water is safer than vertical rescue

15.4 Physiological challenge of hyperbaric and hypobaric environments

The physiological challenges associated with the ascent of mountain peaks above 1,500 m or underwater exploration, involve entry into hypobaric and hyperbaric environments. Hypobaric environments, encountered at high altitude, have a lower environmental pressure than that at sea level. Free diving and SCUBA (self-contained underwater breathing apparatus) diving, whether for pleasure or for commercial purposes, present a number of physiological challenges, a significant one being the increased atmospheric pressure. Operating at atmospheric or environmental pressures that are higher or lower than sea level presents additional stress to an athlete. This section begins with a review of the physiological challenge of exercise at altitude and then examines the effects of the underwater environment on physiological functioning during diving.

Exercise in a hypobaric environment

The sport of mountaineering involves exercise in an environment that presents a thermal and hypobaric challenge to the athlete. The physiological challenge of the mountain environment has been of great interest to physiologists for many centuries. As a comparative environment, altitude study has provided researchers with an improved understanding of physiological functioning at sea level. Subsequently, research has focused on improving knowledge about the challenge of the hypobaric environment and the physiological response to prolonged stays at altitude. Ascent to altitude provides at least three physiological stressors: exercise, altitude and cold. The general physiological response to exercise has been covered widely throughout this textbook and the thermal challenge of cold environments was described above. This section examines the physiological challenge of exercise at altitude. The challenge of the mountain environment is primarily concerned with the decreasing atmospheric pressure associated with increasing altitude. Altitude is commonly defined as commencing at a height of 1,500 m. Below 1,500 m, increases in height have a minimal effect on performance, while above this level, rises in altitude have an increasing affect on physiological function. *High altitude* refers to heights between 1,500 m and 3,000 m above sea level, *very high altitude* between 3,000 m and 5,500 m and *extreme altitude* from 5,500 m and above. Consequently, Mitre Peak in New Zealand represents a high altitude peak, the summit of Mont Blanc in France is at very high altitude and an ascent of Aconcangua in Chile would represent an extreme altitude expedition. Around 15 million people worldwide are thought to live at an altitude above 3,000 m, with the limit of permanent human habitation being at around 5,300–5,500 m in the Andes Mountains. Humans visit extreme altitude for relatively short periods of time. The main stress associated with exercise at altitude occurs due to the sub-normal partial pressure of oxygen (compared to sea level), known as **hypoxia**.

The effect of altitude on the oxygen cascade

As altitude increases the atmospheric pressure falls. Atmospheric pressure represents the pressure exerted by the weight of the air pressing down on us. A mountain ascent, therefore, is accompanied by an increase in altitude and a fall in atmospheric pressure. Atmospheric pressure is measured with a barometer, developed by Evangelista Torricelli in 1644. The earliest experiment to investigate the effects of altitude on atmospheric pressure was carried out by Blaise Pascal in 1648. In his experiment, Pascal showed that atmospheric pressure was lower at the top of the 1,465 m Puy de Dôme (now the venue for many Tour de France stage finishes) than in the valley below. Subsequent research has shown that atmospheric pressure continues to fall with increasing altitude. At sea level the average atmospheric pressure is 760 mmHg. Table 15.2 provides an illustration of the fall in atmospheric pressure with increasing altitude. There is an initial fall in atmospheric pressure of 86 mmHg from sea level to 1000 m. However, as one continues to ascend, the rate at which pressure falls declines to only a to

36 mmHg drop from 8,000 m to 9,000 m. If the atmospheric pressure had been 760 mmHg at sea level on the day of Blaise Pascal's experiment, then the pressure on the summit of the Puy de Dôme would have been around 635 mmHg, more than sufficient to reveal a clear drop in pressure to Pascal.

It is not, however, the fall in atmospheric pressure itself that creates the physiological stress of altitude, but the fall in the partial pressure of oxygen (PO_2). In Chapter 6 the oxygen cascade was described. As air moves from the atmosphere to the blood, the partial pressure of oxygen (PO_2) falls at each stage (trachea, alveoli, blood). The higher PO_2 in the alveoli compared to the blood is critical for the diffusion of oxygen into the bloodstream, as oxygen diffuses from high to low concentrations. The atmospheric PO_2 and tracheal PO_2 are shown in Table 15.2. A secondary environmental oxygen cascade is clearly evident with increasing altitude. Whereas the atmospheric PO_2 at sea level is 159 mmHg, the summit of Chomolangma (Mount Everest) has a PO_2 of 49–50 mmHg (the summit of Chomolangma is around 8,850 m, hence PO_2 is slightly greater than that illustrated for 9,000 m).

At sea level the oxygen cascade results in a fall in PO_2 from 159 mmHg to 103 mmHg as air moves from the atmosphere to the alveoli. This decrease in PO_2 is shown in more detail in Table 6.2 (Chapter 6). The partial pressure of oxygen in blood arriving at the capillaries surrounding the alveoli is around 40 mmHg which creates a pressure gradient of 63 mmHg (alveolar PO_2 is 103 mmHg minus capillary PO_2 of 40 mmHg = 63 mmHg). The fall in atmospheric pressure with increasing altitude

Table 15.2 Changes in atmospheric pressure and partial pressure of oxygen with altitude ascent.

Altitude (m)	Atmospheric pressure (mmHg)	Atmospheric PO_2 (mmHg)	Tracheal PO_2 (mmHg)	Mountain with similar altitude	1st ascent
Sea level	760	159	149		
1,000	674	141	131	**Yr Wyddfa**, Snowdonia, Wales (1085 m)	Not known
2,000	596	125	115	**Mitre Peak**, South Island, New Zealand (2000 m)	1910
3,000	526	110	100	**Mount Dixon**, South Island, New Zealand (3019 m)	1931
4,000	462	97	87	**Pikes Peak**, Rockies, USA (4300 m)	1806
5,000	405	85	75	**Mount Steele**, Yukon, Canada (5073 m)	1935
6,000	354	74	64	**Kilimanjaro**, Tanzania (5895 m)	1889
7,000	308	64	55	**Aconcagua**, Andes, Chile (6959 m)	1897
8,000	267	56	46	**Shishapangma**, Himalaya (8027 m)	1964
9,000	231	48	38	**Chomolangma** (aka Sagarmatha or Everest) (8848 m)	1953

(Table 15.2) directly affects PO_2 throughout the oxygen cascade and results in decreasing oxyhaemoglobin saturation with increasing altitude. For instance, on the summit of Mount Dixon (3,019 m) the atmospheric PO_2 is around 110 mmHg leading to an alveolar PO_2 of 71 mmHg. This results in a decrease in the pressure gradient for oxygen transfer from 63 mmHg at sea level to 31 mmHg on Mount Dixon (alveolar PO_2 at an altitude of 3,000 m is 71 mmHg – capillary PO_2 40 mmHg = 31 mmHg). It is the combined effect of decreased PO_2 and reduced oxyhaemoglobin saturation that results in cellular hypoxia, presenting a physiological challenge during and following ascent to altitude. This is the reason why exercise intensity during altitude training has to be lower than that at sea level (refer to the previous section on altitude training).

The oxyhaemoglobin dissociation curve

As described above, the oxygen partial-pressure gradient responsible for the diffusion of oxygen from the lungs to the blood differs between sea level and altitude with resultant effects on the oxygen saturation of the blood. Oxygen dissolves and diffuses across the gaseous exchange membrane (between the alveoli and the capillaries) as a direct consequence of this pressure or concentration gradient. At sea level, this results in an almost complete oxygen saturation of haemoglobin (97–98%) (i.e. the extent to which haemoglobin combines with oxygen). Christian Bohr, who was described in more detail in Chapter 1, found that the level of haemoglobin oxygen saturation was determined by the PO_2. He found that, graphically, the oxygen saturation of haemoglobin occurs in a sigmoid (S–shaped) curve. An illustration of the oxyhaemoglobin dissociation curve is shown in Figure 15.2. The Sigmoid curve reveals that up to around 80% saturation, haemoglobin saturation rises rapidly in response to relatively small increases in PO_2. Beyond 80% saturation, the curve flattens as the haemoglobin oxygen saturation moves closer to 100% saturation. At an alveolar PO_2 of 103 mmHg the oxyhaemoglobin saturation is close to 100%.

Factors affecting the oxyhaemoglobin dissociation curve

In addition to PO_2, the oxygen saturation of haemoglobin is affected by blood pH (acidity), blood temperature, and 2,3-diphosphoglycerate (2,3-DPG). A decrease in blood pH (rise in acidity) or an increase in body temperature weakens the bond between oxygen and haemoglobin, hence an increased offloading of oxygen at the tissues occurs. This

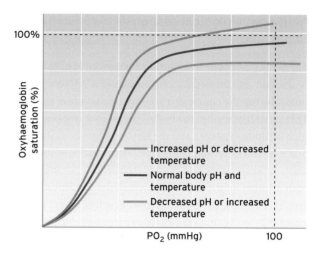

Figure 15.2 The effects of changes in pH and body temperature on the oxyhaemoglobin dissociation curve.

reduction in the affinity of haemoglobin for oxygen is represented by a rightward shift of the oxyhaemoglobin curve and is known as the Bohr effect. During strenuous exercise, pH falls (due to the rise in lactate and associated rise in H^+) and body temperature increases above 37°C (due to muscular heat production). As such, exercise can shift the curve to the right, facilitating the offloading of oxygen to the tissues where it is required, particularly skeletal muscle.

Produced during erythrocyte glycolysis, 2,3-DPG has been shown to be coupled with decreased haemoglobin affinity for oxygen. Similar to increased acidity and temperature, therefore, increased 2,3-DPG shifts the oxyhaemoglobin curve to the right. The effect of exercise on 2,3-DPG levels remains equivocal. However, some well-designed experiments suggest no change, or even a slight decrease, in 2,3-DPG concentration during moderate or severe exercise, or during an incremental test to exhaustion (Mairbaurl et al., 1986 Spodaryk & Zoladz, 1998). It appears, therefore, that 2,3-DPG plays no major role in the enhanced offloading of oxygen to the tissues during exercise. However, as discussed in the following section, it contributes to improving tissue oxygen supply upon exposure to altitude.

Key points

At sea level the oxygen saturation of blood is 97–98%

Increasing altitude = decreased atmospheric pressure and PO_2

The lower the PO_2, the lower the oxygen saturation of the blood – illustrated by the oxyhaemoglobin dissociation curve

The offloading of oxygen to the tissues is increased during exercise due to a fall in pH and an increased body temperature

Acute physiological response to altitude

The body's response to hypoxia experienced at altitude can be divided into immediate responses and adaptations that occur during the course of a stay at any particular altitude. This section examines the body's immediate responses to high-altitude exposure and the next section on acclimatisation examines the adaptations that occur with a sojourn at altitude. Respiratory and cardiovascular functioning are both affected by the lower PO_2 experienced at altitude. On arrival at altitude the body's chemoreceptors detect the lower PO_2 in the thinner air – lower atmospheric pressure air containing fewer oxygen molecules. The chemoreceptors, located in the aorta and common carotid arteries, stimulate the alterations in cardiovascular and respiratory function.

Respiratory response to acute altitude

The respiratory driver, located in the medulla oblongata and the pons (part of the brain stem), interpret the sensory information from the chemoreceptors and increase pulmonary ventilation in response to the lower PO_2 encountered at altitude. Hyperventilation, associated with arrival at altitude, increases the alveolar PO_2 towards the levels in ambient air and facilitates oxygen transfer to the bloodstream. In this way, hyperventilation serves to improve oxygen supply to the muscles and counters the hypoxia experienced at altitude. The increase in pulmonary ventilation, while beneficial to oxygen supply, upsets the acid-base balance of the blood. Hyperventilation increases the PO_2 but at the same time decreases alveolar PCO_2. At high altitude the PCO_2 in the lungs can fall to 20 mmHg compared with a sea level mean value of 39 mmHg (see Table 6.2). With pulmonary capillary PCO_2 remaining at 46 mmHg this increases the pressure gradient from 7 mmHg to 26 mmHg. The rise in partial pressure differential results in an increased unloading of carbon dioxide at the lungs. As was described in the section on gas transport in the blood in Chapter 6, carbon dioxide is most commonly carried in the blood as bicarbonate ions which provide a pH lowering effect to maintain blood pH. With increased pulmonary ventilation and unloading of carbon dioxide the level of carbonic acid in the blood falls (converted to carbon dioxide and water) resulting in a rise in blood alkalinity and upsetting the acid-base balance. This is known as respiratory alkalosis.

Cardiovascular response to acute altitude

In response to the decreased PO_2 at altitude, the cardiovascular system makes a number of alterations in functioning to improve oxygen supply to the muscles. After a few hours at altitude a decrease in blood plasma volume occurs. Plasma volume can be decreased by over 20% when compared with sea level, and this condition is maintained for several weeks after arrival at altitude. As the blood plasma volume decreases the remaining blood has an increased concentration of erythrocytes (red blood cells) and an increased relative oxygen-carrying capacity. This brings about an enhanced oxygen delivery to the tissues.

Within a short time of arrival at altitude, to compensate for the lowered PO_2, cardiac output ($\dot{Q}$) is increased. Cardiac output, as was described in Chapter 6, is the product of stroke volume and heart rate – the volume of blood ejected with each heart beat multiplied by the heart rate (beats·min^{-1}). By increasing the $\dot{Q}$ the body can enhance oxygen transport around the body. The decrease in blood plasma volume initiated after arrival at altitude results in an increased blood viscosity. The rise in blood 'thickness' – ratio of cellular components (red blood cells, white blood cells and platelets) to plasma – leads to a decrease in stroke volume so any rise in $\dot{Q}$ has to be brought about through increases in heart rate.

On arrival at altitude HR rises at rest and in response to any given sub-maximal exercise intensity, when compared with sea level. The increased load on the heart is only sustained for a short period of time (a few days) after which there is an increase in oxygen extraction by the muscles to compensate for the lowered blood PO_2. This enables the heart rate response to fall towards normal. The increased oxygen release to the muscles is brought about through increases in erythrocyte production of 2,3-diphosphoglycerate (2,3-DPG) and the associated reduction in haemoglobin affinity for oxygen. This action results in a greater oxygen release to the tissues of the body and reduces the demands on the heart to increase the circulation of blood. An additional mechanism that is thought to bring about compensation for reduced PO_2 occurs through rises in pulmonary artery blood pressure. The pulmonary arteries are responsible for transport of the blood from the heart's right ventricle to the lungs for gaseous exchange. It appears that on arrival at altitude pulmonary blood pressure rises through vasoconstriction. This rise in blood pressure results in an increase in blood flow to the upper sections of the lungs, enhancing the volume of blood available for gaseous exchange, including oxygen loading.

Key points

The initial exposure to altitude results in changes to:

➤ Respiratory functioning

- Hyperventilation – improves oxygen supply to tissues but disrupts acid-base balance

➤ Cardiovascular functioning

- Decreased plasma volume – increased RBC concentration and relative O_2 carrying capacity
- Increased cardiac output – due to elevated HR
- Increased 2,3-DPG (after a few days) – enhanced O_2 extraction by the muscles (reduces demands on heart)
- Increased pulmonary artery blood pressure – increases volume of blood for gaseous exchange

Altitude illnesses

Despite these compensatory mechanisms, exposure to altitudes above 2,500 m can lead to a number of altitude-related illnesses. The most commonly occurring altitude illness being *acute mountain sickness* (AMS). Many people experience the symptoms of AMS when they arrive at altitude or move to a higher altitude. Symptoms normally occur within 24 hours of arrival, but subside within a week as the individual acclimatises. The symptoms of AMS include headache, mood change, nausea, fatigue, sleep disturbance, loss of appetite and dizziness. It is thought that AMS is triggered by short-term decreases in cerebral oxygen saturation. If symptoms are intolerable, descent to a lower altitude has been shown to induce a fast recovery. Slow rates of ascent, rest days at specific altitudes and climb high-sleep low strategies have been found to reduce the incidence of AMS. *High altitude pulmonary edema/ odema* (HAPE) occurs in only a minority of individuals who travel to altitude. It is thought that HAPE occurs more commonly in response to rapid mountain ascents without sufficient time for acclimatisation and as a result of hard physical exertion at extreme altitude. Symptoms of HAPE include stronger headaches (than experienced with AMS), excessive hyperventilation, disruption of bowel and bladder function and decreases in trunk control. It is thought that pulmonary oedema (an excess build-up of fluid in cells or tissues of the lungs) causes damage to the gaseous exchange barrier. Again, descent to lower altitude initiates recovery for an individual suffering from HAPE, although this process can take several days. *High altitude cerebral edema/odema* (HACE), although rare, is the most serious of altitude-related illnesses and requires immediate medical treatment. It develops from the symptoms of

AMS which can make early diagnosis difficult. Symptoms include coordination and walking problems, severe fatigue, chest pain and impaired mental functioning, lapsing into unconsciousness. It appears that HACE, which leads to increased fluid pressure on the brain, results from cerebral vasodilation leading to increased fluid and protein movement across the blood-brain barrier. To recover from this potentially life-threatening illness descent from altitude and medical attention are essential.

Exercise at altitude

Exercise performance is generally impaired at altitude. Not surprisingly, in response to the decreased PO_2, aerobic capacity as measured through $\dot{V}O_{2max}$ is reduced at altitude. Research indicates that $\dot{V}O_{2max}$ falls by 5–10% for each 1000 m increase in altitude, although the percentage decline increases more rapidly at higher altitudes. At the summit of Aconcagua, at an altitude of around 7000 m, $\dot{V}O_{2max}$ is approximately half that at sea level. On the summit of Chomolangma it is reduced to 10–20% of sea level values. In agreement with these findings, endurance performance declines with increasing altitude resulting in longer times for race completion when compared with sea level. In contrast, performance in anaerobic events, particularly power and power endurance sports, is either not affected by high altitude exposure or is improved as a result of the thinner air.

Key points

Medical problems associated with altitude include:

➤ Acute mountain sickness (AMS)

➤ High altitude pulmonary edema (HAPE)

➤ High altitude cerebral edema (HACE)

Altitude acclimatisation

Adaptation to altitude can be simulated in a laboratory, known as **acclimation**, or brought about by a period spent living at altitude (**acclimatisation**). Full acclimatisation to high altitude appears to take around two weeks, with another week required for each further 600 m increment of ascent. It is brought about by a range of respiratory, cardiovascular and metabolic adaptations to the reduced PO_2. Alkalosis brought about through hyperventilation (which remains elevated even during prolonged stays at altitude) is compensated for by increases in the excretion of bicarbonate (HCO_3^-). The decrease in blood bicarbonate associated with reducing respiratory alkalosis is thought to be partly responsible for the decreased anaerobic performance and reduced lactate concentration experienced during prolonged stays at altitude. The decrease in blood bicarbonate concentration, however, restores the acid-base balance in the blood.

Perhaps the most significant adaptation to altitude comes through the stimulation of red blood cell production brought about through the release of the hormone erythropoietin from the kidneys. Erythropoietin secretion is stimulated in response to the decreased PO_2 experienced at altitude and results in an increase in red blood cell production. Altitude-induced polycythemia (an increase in the number of red blood cells above normal) can realise increases in haematocrit from sea level values of 40–45% to 60–65% at very high altitude (see Chapter 6 for more information on sea level haematocrit). The rise in erythrocyte number, and as a consequence the haemoglobin concentration, enhances the blood's oxygen-carrying capacity. Athletes who perform at sea level have become interested in altitude training primarily as a result of this response to lowered PO_2. On return to sea level after a sojourn at altitude, erythrocyte numbers remain elevated providing an athlete with an increased oxygen-carrying capacity relative to pre-altitude training levels. Consequently, it is thought by many athletes that altitude training has an ergogenic effect on performance.

One impact of acclimatisation to altitude that is commonly reported, is that of weight loss. As a result of a stay at altitude both fat mass and lean body mass (fat-free mass) have been found to decline. The weight loss associated with prolonged exposure to altitude is related to: loss of appetite, increased energy expenditure, impaired nutrient absorption from digestion, increased water loss due to higher rates of evaporation in the cool dry air, increased urination to decrease plasma volume and inadequate drinking to replace fluid loss. During training at altitude athletes should consciously maintain fluid intake as dehydration, which is well known to adversely affect performance, is a common problem associated with a period spent at altitude.

Research into acclimatisation has identified a number of additional effects associated with prolonged exposure. However, some of these findings have been equivocal, most likely due to the different altitudes and methods employed between studies. It is generally agreed that muscle fibres decrease in size at altitude, which is attributed to decreased training and exercise intensities associated with reduced oxygen availability. Some researchers have reported increased capillarisation in response to chronic (continued) altitude exposure, while others have suggested that the increase in capillary density is the result of decreases in muscle fibre size and consequently, capillaries being closer

together. With regard to improvements in aerobic metabolism, researchers have found increases in mitochondrial size and number in response to a sojourn at altitude, along with reported incidences of increased aerobic enzyme activity (succinate dehydrogenase and citrate synthase). These adaptations, along with increases in myoglobin concentration, appear to contribute to improving oxidative mechanisms in response to the decreased PO_2.

Catecholamine (adrenaline and noradrenaline) secretion increases in response to the initial exposure to altitude. As you adapt, however, catecholamine secretion is reduced and this has an important link with an apparent *lactate paradox*. On arrival at altitude blood lactate response is found to increase for a given form of exercise and this is attributed to the decreased PO_2 and increased reliance on fast-rate glycolysis. One might expect lactate response to sub-maximal exercise at altitude to remain higher than at sea level, despite acclimatisation, as a result of the decreased buffering capacity (associated with bicarbonate buffer excretion) and the fact that $\dot{V}O_{2max}$ does not increase with prolonged altitude exposure. The lactate paradox occurs because blood lactate levels at altitude decrease to a similar level as the equivalent exercise intensity at sea level. This paradox is thought to exist due to the decreased adrenaline response associated with acclimatisation. Adrenaline secretion with acute exposure to altitude stimulates increased glycogen catabolism (glycogenolysis) (refer to Chapter 10, Control of the rate of glycolysis) which, when combined with the lower PO_2, results in an increase in fast-rate glucose metabolism and the formation of lactate. It appears that the improved oxidative functioning associated with acclimatisation (e.g. increased red blood cell production) is sufficient to blunt the stimulus for adrenaline secretion which results in a decrease in lactate production. In addition, it has been speculated that after acclimatisation to altitude muscles oxidise more lactate, directly resulting in a decreased release into the blood.

Key points

Acclimatisation to altitude:

➤ Takes around two weeks, subsequent 600 m ascent requires a further week

➤ Physiological adaptations

- Increased excretion of bicarbonate – acid-base balance regained
- Increased secretion of erythropoietin – increased number of RBCs
- Weight loss
- Reduced catecholamine response leads to decreased lactate response

Exercise in a hyperbaric environment

Breath-hold diving represents the earliest form of exploration of the environment below the open water surface. The earth's hyperbaric environment presents a unique physiological challenge to humans. As was described in the section on hypobaria, the average atmospheric pressure at sea level is 760 mmHg. This pressure is created by the air in the atmosphere 'pressing' down on objects at sea level. In diving terms, this is known as one atmosphere or 1 bar. The density of water is 775 times greater than that of air, subsequently, you need only descend below the surface to reach the point at which the pressure exerted on the body is double that encountered at sea level. Figure 15.3 provides an illustration of the effect of underwater depth on pressure, along with its effect on the volume of any gas. As can be seen from this figure, the environmental pressure doubles at a water depth of 10 m. The pressure at this point is referred to as 2 bar and represents that of two atmospheres (one atmosphere for air and one atmosphere for the 10 m of water).

The pressure associated with increasing depth of dive presents one of the main challenges to the diver. As is shown in Figure 15.3, an increase in water depth results in a linear decrease in the volume of any gas. The law that describes the relationship between gas volume and pressure was discovered by Robert Boyle (whose work was described in more detail in Chapter 1). When a gas held at a constant temperature is placed under increasing pressure its volume decreases (the gas molecules are forced closer together into a smaller volume). The effects of increases in pressure on the volume of a gas are shown in Figure 15.3, such that at two atmospheres the gas volume is a half, and at four atmospheres it is a quarter, of its volume at sea level. As well as the pressure associated with underwater exploration, and its effect on the body's gases, the key challenge is the lack of oxygen available underwater. Freedivers overcome this challenge by breath-hold during submersion, whereas SCUBA divers and submariners carry an oxygen supply with them. A third challenge associated with underwater exploration is that of the cold temperatures encountered during water immersion: this aspect of diving has already been covered in the chapter. The following sections examine the physiological challenges of freediving and SCUBA diving.

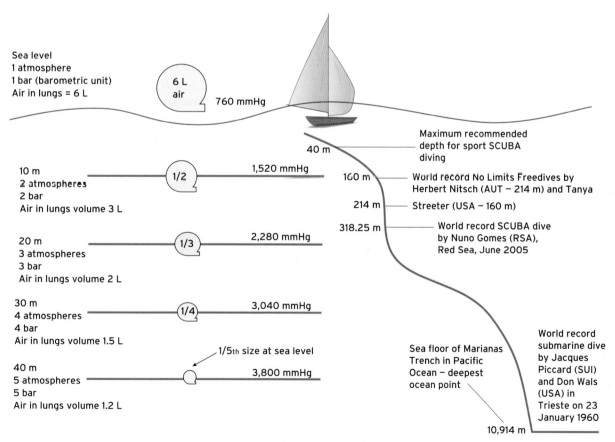

Figure 15.3 Increasing atmospheric pressure with increasing depth and its relationship with gas volume.

Freediving (breath-hold diving)

Breath-hold diving has a recorded history dating back around 5,000 years. Carried out for pleasure, food, salvage and military purposes, perhaps the most famous breath-hold divers are the Japanese women Ama divers. Although there are less than 1,000 Ama divers today, in the 1920s there were as many as 13,000 who worked collecting pearls. The Ama divers descend to a depth of around 20 m, carrying a lead weight on a cord attached to their waists which they use to assist their descent. On return to the surface the Ama divers offload collected shells and ready themselves for another dive, often making 50–100 dives per day. Not surprisingly, a greater incidence of eardrum ruptures and ear infections have been recorded for Ama divers when compared with non-diving females in the towns where they live.

From these origins breath-hold diving has grown into the competitive sport of freediving which is governed by the International Association for the Development of Apnea (absence of breathing) now often referred to as the International Association for the Development of Freediving (AIDA). There are eight different categories of freediving world record, and a world championships is held for the activity every year. In fact, the 8th AIDA World Championship were held in September 2011 in Kalamata, Greece. The world records for men and women in each of the eight AIDA disciplines are shown in Table 15.3.

The *static apnea* record involves breath-holding in a swimming pool or open water with the mouth and nose submerged, without moving. This is the only record where the measurement is of time rather than distance. *Dynamic apnea* (with and without fins) can also be conducted in a swimming pool, although the minimum pool length must be 25 m, and involves swimming underwater for as far as possible. When using fins the record can be attempted using long fins or a monofin. *Constant weight* freediving (with and without fins) is the most basic of the depth descents where the competitor uses their body and any ballast they wish to carry to assist the descent. With a rope to guide the dive, they must return to the surface carrying the same weight with which they descended. *Free immersion* involves the use of a rope, without swimming propulsion, to pull hand-over-hand as far down as possible before using the rope to ascend. In *variable weight* freediving a weight is attached to the diver or a 'sled' is used to enhance their descent. In *no limits* diving a sled is used for descent and ascent is completed using a compressed-air-filled balloon or compartment in the diver's wetsuit that is released on reaching the maximal descent point.

These records are exceptional, when it is considered that average breath-hold in a normal untrained adult is around 1–2 minutes. One of the key aspects that enables such endurance records to be set, and is used by Ama divers, is hyperventilation. As introduced in the section on the hypobaric environment, hyperventilation results in a 'blowing-off' of carbon dioxide and a reduction in the alveolar and blood PCO_2. In breath-hold diving hyperventilation is used to decrease the carbon dioxide levels within the body just prior to submerging. Carbon dioxide concentration is detected by chemoreceptors and provides the key stimulus for increasing breathing rate during exercise. These receptors are found

Table 15.3 Freediving world records.

Discipline	Men's record	Year	Record holder	Women's record	Year	Record holder
Static apnea	20.21 min	2010	R da Gama Bahia (BRA)	18.32 min	2009	Karol Meyer (BRA)
Dynamic apnea (no fins)	265 m	2010	Dave Mullins (NZL)	160 m	2010	Natalia Molchanova (RUS)
Dynamic apnea (fins)	212 m	2010	Dave Mullins (NZL)	225 m	2010	Natalia Molchanova (RUS)
Constant weight (no fins)	101 m	2010	W Trubridge (NZL)	62 m	2009	Natalia Molchanova (RUS)
Constant weight (fins)	124 m	2010	Herbert Nitsch (AUT)	96 m	2009	Sara Campbell (GBR)
Free immersion	120 m	2010	Herbert Nitsch (AUT)	85 m	2008	Natalia Molchanova (RUS)
Variable weight	142 m	2007	Herbert Nitsch (AUT)	126 m	2010	Annelie Pompe (SWE)
No limit	214 m	2007	Herbert Nitsch (AUT)	160 m	2002	Tanya Streeter (USA)

in the common carotid arteries and close to the medulla oblongata and pons (the location of the respiratory driver). By hyperventilating prior to submersion, breath-hold divers are able to reduce carbon dioxide levels in their blood which helps to decrease the respiratory drive and extend dive time. This technique is not, however, without risks and has led to the death of those involved in breath-hold swimming. The decreased carbon dioxide levels brought about through hyperventilation, while delaying the desire to breathe, can lead to fainting before the PCO_2 has increased to a level sufficient to stimulate the desire to take a breath. These blackouts appear to be linked to a fall in PO_2 below a critical level in the alveoli and blood. It appears that hyperventilation increases the risk of oxygen depletion during a dive which can lead to fainting. A further risk, linked with diving in colder waters, is the slowing in heart rate associated with the dive reflex. The dive reflex is described in more detail above in the section on water immersion. In breath-hold diving it is believed that performers can face problems associated with cardiac arrhythmias brought about in response to the diving reflex. Success in freediving has been linked to total lung volume, with those having larger lung volume showing significantly improved breath-hold times.

Key points

Breath-hold diving/freediving

➤ Occurs in a hyperbaric environment

➤ Hyperventilation prior to a dive lowers blood PCO_2 reducing the stimulus to breathe and extending dive time

➤ Risks include:

- Hyperventilation increases risk of oxygen depletion during dive which can lead to fainting and death
- Cold water slows the HR
- May suffer from cardiac arrhythmias

SCUBA diving

In the early days of diving the air supply for breathing was supplied by a tube from the surface of the water. It was not until 1943 that two French divers, Jacques Cousteau and Emile Gagnan, developed a system whereby the air supply was carried with the diver. The development of the SCUBA system enabled divers to explore the underwater environment without the need for a supply line from the surface. Originally developed for commercial purposes, one of the earliest uses of SCUBA involved de-mining at the end of the second world-war. After the excellent underwater films

produced by Jacques Cousteau, SCUBA diving became a popular recreational adventure sport. The SCUBA system is comprised of four components that enable breathing underwater; an air tank, two regulators and a breathing valve. The compressed air for breathing is contained in one or more tanks which are carried on the back. The air tanks are normally compressed to around 200 bar (3,000 psi). This pressure is far too great for breathing purposes and so two regulators are fitted to the tank to reduce the pressure. The first regulator decreases the pressure of the air to about 9.5 bar (140 psi) and the second one, which supplies air on demand, matches the air pressure to the pressure of the water around the diver. Lastly, a one-way mouthpiece enables air to be inhaled from the regulator but then exhaled into the water, rising to the water surface as bubbles. This type of SCUBA is called open-circuit, because the exhaled air is released into the water. For military stealth purposes a second expired air collection tank, normally worn on the chest, has been used to avoid the release of air bubbles into the water. This type is known as a closed-circuit system. A variety of air mixtures is used in diving including, pure oxygen, nitrox (oxygen and nitrogen) and heliox (helium and oxygen) to extend the duration and depth of diving. Using a compressed air system the length of a dive is normally limited by any previous dives that day, the number of air tanks carried, the depth of the dive and the efficiency of movement and air usage. 'Over-breathing', or inefficient use of air during a dive can more than halve the possible submersion time. The pressure encountered in SCUBA diving provides the main potential hazard associated with this type of adventure sport. The complications that can be associated with SCUBA diving include the ear, sinus and mask squeezes, pneumothorax, nitrogen narcosis, and decompression sickness, as discussed below.

Squeezes

A *squeeze* (ear, sinuses and mask) can occur when you descend and pressure increases on air trapped within the body or between your face and the face mask. The pain is caused by the air trying to equalise pressure on either side of a block. Normally as you descend you need to clear your ears at regular intervals by blowing gently with your nose blocked, stretching your jaw muscles or yawning to allow the pressure to equalise between your middle ear and the external pressure. If you have a blockage of the eustachian tube it may not be possible to equalise pressure, causing pain. If you cannot equalise the pressure you should not continue to dive, as it is possible to rupture the eardrum. Normally with eye and nose masks you do not get a mask squeeze with SCUBA diving; however, if you cannot clear your sinuses, not only will it lead to pain but it can also create the potential for a face mask squeeze. To avoid the pain associated with a squeeze you should not dive when you have a cold or other upper respiratory tract infection.

Pneumothorax

When ascending from a dive it is important to continue to breathe normally. While exploring the underwater environment during a dive you are breathing air under pressure equal to that of the water depth you are in. As you rise, the fall in pressure results in an increased volume of air in your lungs (refer to Figure 15.3). If you continue to breathe normally throughout the pressure changes of ascent the air in the lungs will continually re-equalise. During times of stress, however, divers sometimes hold their breath on ascent which can leads to serious lung problems. Breath-holding maintains the same air within your lungs, hence, the fall in pressure upon ascent will increase the volume of air inside your lungs, potentially leading to the bursting of alveoli. This situation results in air entering the pleural space (see section on the structure of the lungs in Chapter 6). As an ascent continues, the air in the pleural space will continue to expand creating pressure on the lung tissue and causing a sudden collapse of the lung known as a **pneumothorax**. A diver can simply avoid this problem by maintaining exhalation on ascent.

Nitrogen narcosis

In deeper and longer-duration dives, nitrogen, an inert gas during respiration, can begin to have an intoxicating and anaesthetic effect on the body. The increase in pressure associated with deeper dives establishes a higher partial pressure of nitrogen (PN_2) leading to more entering the body. Known as **nitrogen narcosis** or *rapture of the deep*, the euphoria associated with this condition can impair judgement and functioning. It has led divers to continue to descend in situations where they have insufficient air for a deeper dive, and on occasions to remove their SCUBA believing they no longer need it. As such, it is a potentially life-threatening risk associated with SCUBA diving; however, the symptoms quickly disappear if the diver ascends.

Knowledge integration question

What are the negative physiological effects of hypobaric and hyperbaric environments? How can a hypobaric environment be used in a positive way for sea-level sports performance?

Decompression sickness (the bends)

Deep and prolonged dives create another potential nitrogen-associated problem for the diver if they ascend too quickly. During a longer dive nitrogen slowly enters the tissues of the body due to the increased PN_2. If you ascend slowly the nitrogen can pass harmlessly from the tissues as you rise. If, however, you rise rapidly by mistake or in an emergency, the nitrogen dissolved in your body does not have time to leave your body harmlessly, forming bubbles in the tissues, fluids and joints of your body. This condition is known as **decompression sickness** or *the bends* after the effect it has on the body. A diver who has surfaced with the bends is often seen to bend over to try to relieve the pain from nitrogen in the joints. Treatment for decompression sickness is essential and requires immediate use of a recompression chamber. In a recompression chamber the pressure can be returned to a level such that the nitrogen bubbles re-dissolve into the tissues and can then leave the body slowly as the pressure in the chamber is gradually reduced. Although more common now, recompression chambers are not normally available to sport divers, hence great attention should be paid to the rate of ascent to avoid an incidence of the bends.

Key points

SCUBA diving:

➤ Physiological challenge relates to the high pressures encountered in the hyperbaric underwater environment.

➤ Problems associated with diving include:
- Squeezes
- Pneumothorax
- Nitrogen narcosis
- Decompression sickness (the bends)

➤ These concerns can normally be avoided by close monitoring of dive time and a planned, slow ascent.

Check your recall
Fill in the missing words.

➤ The control of core temperature within a narrow range is known as _____.

➤ The four mechanisms of heat transfer are: conduction, _____, radiation and evaporation.

➤ During exercise, the major source of heat loss is through _____.

➤ The body's thermostat is located in the _____.

➤ During exercise in the heat, competition exists between the _____ and the _____ for available blood flow.

➤ Health risks during exercise in a hot environment include heat exhaustion and heat _____.

➤ A decreased performance in cold environments results from impaired cardiovascular endurance, muscular _____ and _____.

➤ In situations of high sweat loss, such as exercise in a hot environment, _____ may also be added to a sports drink.

➤ Sodium loss through sweating can be exacerbated by the consumption of plain water, resulting in the condition of _____, which can present a serious problem to endurance athletes.

➤ The development of _____ is a great risk associated with water immersion, as cooling in water happens at a much _____ rate than in the same temperature of air.

➤ The initial response to water immersion is known as _____ _____.

➤ At altitude (>_____ m), low _____ _____ presents an additional physiological stress.

➤ Oxygen transfer into the blood, and _____ saturation, is severely compromised at high altitude.

➤ The immediate response to the lower PO_2 at altitude is _____.

➤ Despite compensatory physiological mechanisms, the following altitude-related illnesses may occur: _____ _____ _____ (AMS), _____ _____ _____ _____ (HACE) and _____ _____ _____ _____ (HAPE).

➤ Exercise performance is generally _____ at altitude.

➤ Acclimatisation to altitude takes about _____ weeks and involves an increased production of _____ _____ cells.

➤ Altitude training is a common strategy utilised by athletes to improve _____ _____ performance.

➤ In contrast to altitude, diving exposes the body to a _____ environment.

➤ A key technique employed before breath holding is that of _____ which reduces CO_2 concentration, inhibiting the respiratory drive and extending dive time.

➤ The main hazard for SCUBA divers arises from the _____ pressure during dives.

➤ Complications involved with SCUBA diving include _____, _____ and _____.

➤ Decompression sickness can be avoided if the diver ascends _____.

Review questions

1. Humans are homeotherms. What does this mean and what are the thermoneutral and thermoregulatory zones?

2. How does sweating increase the rate of heat loss during exercise? Why does sweat contain higher concentrations of minerals during vigorous exercise in hot environments?

3. What are the physiological adaptations to heat acclimatisation and what duration of acclimatisation regimen is suggested to obtain these benefits?

4. Why is oxygen transport to the muscles inhibited in cold environments? What impact does this have on energy production?

5. Describe the effects of cold shock and the diving reflex during initial immersion in cold water? What implication do these responses have on heart rate?

6. Explain the Hunter's response. How does this help people working in cold environments?

7. How does the human body cope with heat loss during prolonged immersion in cold water? Why is swimming in an attempt to reach a watercraft or the shore not recommended unless you are very close to safety?

8. Why is a high level of V O_{2max} advantageous for a high-altitude mountaineer even though activities may take place at a slow walking pace during an ascent? Why is their blood volume likely to decrease at high altitude?

9. Explain what causes decompression sickness in a SCUBA diver who returns to the surface too quickly?

10. Why might a diver feel particularly euphoric during a deep dive?

Teach it!
In groups of three, choose one topic and teach it to the rest of the study group.

1. A major competition is approaching for a triathlete which is to be held in a hot environment. What risks does the triathlete face and how can these be reduced?

2. What physiological responses will occur upon capsize during a kayaking expedition? How can the kayaker minimise the dangers of water immersion?

3. Explain the changes in physiological responses and adaptations to those who stay at altitude for a length of time.

CLASSIC RESEARCH SUMMARY

Exercise in the heat, carbohydrate ingestion and muscle fatigue in cyclists by Abbiss et al. (2008)

The generation of power during prolonged exercise is impaired when exercise is performed in a high ambient temperature (> 27°C) or when carbohydrate stores are depleted. In reality, racing involves a self-selected pace, and it may be that central mechanisms are involved in regulating this pace to avoid reaching a critical core temperature (39.5–40.5°C). Carbohydrate ingestion can delay the onset of fatigue during prolonged exercise, potentially by a combination of the following factors: reduced rate of glycogenolysis, maintained blood glucose levels and reduced central fatigue. In addition, carbohydrate ingestion may be more beneficial in situations of increased heat stress due to the enhanced energy demands. The paper by Abbiss and colleagues investigated the independent and synergistic effects of carbohydrate ingestion and environmental heat stress on muscle fatigue during cycling.

In a temperate environment, participants (10 endurance-trained male cyclists) performed an incremental cycling test for the determination of VO2max and the identification of the second ventilatory threshold (VT$_2$). Within three minutes, a 16.1-km time trial was performed for familiarisation purposes. They then completed four trials, separated by at least four days and conducted at the same time of day (8:00–9:30). The trials, performed in a randomised, crossover approach, involved a 10-min warm-up, 90-min cycling at a constant power output (80% of VT$_2$) followed by (within 3.3 min) a 16.1-km time trial. They were either performed in a temperate (18.1°C) or hot (32.2°C) environment, with ingestion of either a carbohydrate (CHO) or placebo gel during the 90-min cycling phase (i.e. temperate, CHO; temperate, placebo; hot, CHO; hot, placebo). Water was available to drink *ad libitum* during both the 90-min cycling and the 16.1-km time trial.

In the carbohydrate trials, a CHO gel was consumed directly before the warm-up (0.48 g CHO·kg body wt^{-1}) and every 15 min during the 90-min trial (0.24 g CHO·kg body wt^{-1}). The same volume of placebo gel was consumed, at the same time points, in the placebo trials. Measurements made during the 90-min cycling included oxygen uptake, perceived exertion and thermal sensation (recorded with the use of scales). For the 16.1-km time trial participants were instructed to complete the distance as fast as possible. Power output, cycling speed, vastus lateralis muscle activation (by EMG), rectal, skin and environmental temperatures, and perceived exertion and thermal sensation were recorded during the time trial. Venous blood samples were taken pre-exercise and immediately following the 90-min cycle phase and the 16.1-km time trial, from which plasma lactate, glucose and dopamine concentrations, and serum-free fatty acids, serotonin and prolactin were analysed. Prior to the 90-min cycle stage and immediately (within 60 s) following the time trial, participants performed four 5 s maximal isometric contractions of the quadriceps femoris on an isokinetic dynamometer. During the last two contractions, an electrical stimulus was superimposed to allow the differentiation between peripheral and central fatigue.

Abbiss and colleagues found both carbohydrate ingestion and environmental temperature to affect the rate of muscular fatigue during prolonged cycling. Carbohydrate ingestion was more beneficial during cycling in the heat, as reflected in an improved time trial performance due to an increased power output during the final stages. A faster rate of power output decline, however, was found within the first 6 km of the time trial when conducted in the heat, due, at least in part, to central fatigue. From a practical viewpoint, this paper indicates that carbohydrate ingestion and a high environmental temperature may influence the pacing strategies adopted by endurance trained male cyclists.

Reference: Abbiss, C.R., Peiffer, J.J., Peake, J.M., Nosaka, K., Suzuki, K., Martin, D.T. and Laursen, P.B. (2008). Effect of carbohydrate ingestion and ambient temperature on muscle fatigue development in endurance-trained male cyclists. *Journal of Applied Physiology*, 104: 1021–28.

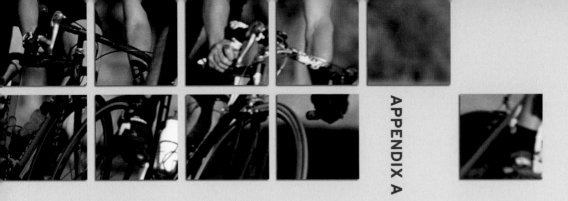

Movement terms

Broad descriptive terms are used to describe movements with reference to the anatomical position

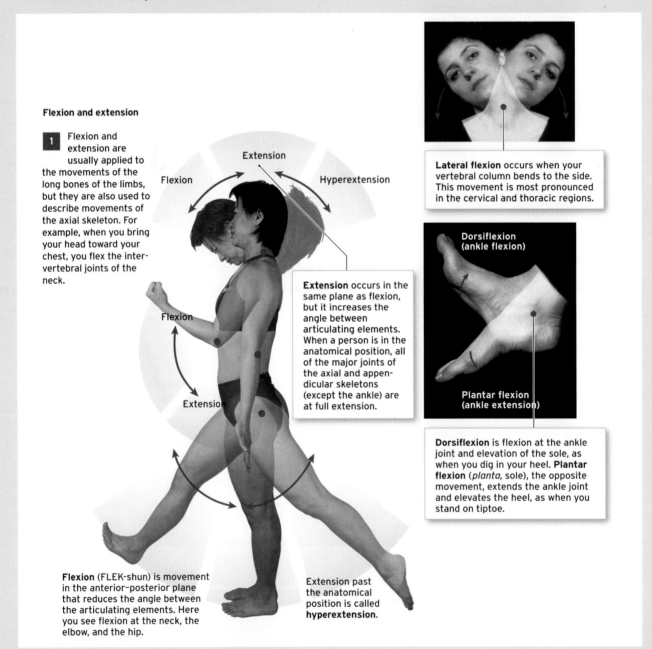

Flexion and extension

1 Flexion and extension are usually applied to the movements of the long bones of the limbs, but they are also used to describe movements of the axial skeleton. For example, when you bring your head toward your chest, you flex the intervertebral joints of the neck.

Extension

Flexion

Hyperextension

Flexion

Extension

Extension occurs in the same plane as flexion, but it increases the angle between articulating elements. When a person is in the anatomical position, all of the major joints of the axial and appendicular skeletons (except the ankle) are at full extension.

Lateral flexion occurs when your vertebral column bends to the side. This movement is most pronounced in the cervical and thoracic regions.

Dorsiflexion (ankle flexion)

Plantar flexion (ankle extension)

Dorsiflexion is flexion at the ankle joint and elevation of the sole, as when you dig in your heel. **Plantar flexion** (*planta*, sole), the opposite movement, extends the ankle joint and elevates the heel, as when you stand on tiptoe.

Flexion (FLEK-shun) is movement in the anterior–posterior plane that reduces the angle between the articulating elements. Here you see flexion at the neck, the elbow, and the hip.

Extension past the anatomical position is called **hyperextension.**

Abduction and adduction

Spreading the fingers or toes apart abducts them, because they move away from a central digit. Bringing them together constitutes adduction. (Fingers move toward or away from the middle finger; toes move toward or away from the second toe.)

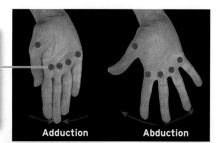

Adduction   Abduction

2 Abduction and adduction always refer to the movements of the appendicular skeleton, not to those of the axial skeleton.

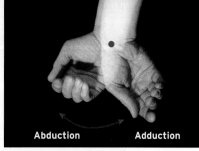

Abduction   Adduction

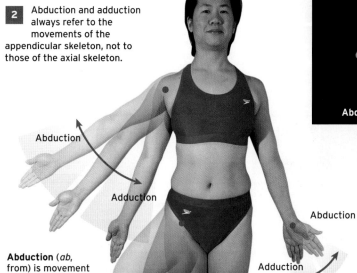

Abduction

Adduction

Abduction

Adduction

Abduction (*ab*, from) is movement away from the longitudinal axis of the body in the frontal plane.

Abduction

Adduction

Adduction (*ad*, to) is movement toward the longitudinal axis of the body in the frontal plane.

Abduction

Adduction

Circumduction

3 Moving your arm as if to draw a big circle on the wall is **circumduction**. In this movement your hand moves in a circle, but your arm does not rotate.

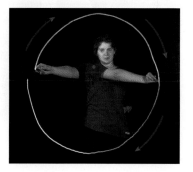

Terms of more limited application describe rotational movements and special movements

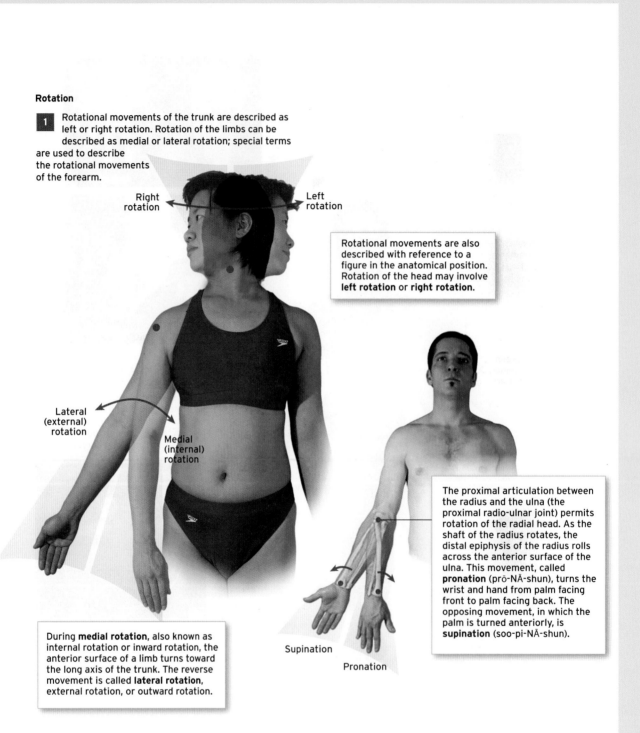

Rotation

1 Rotational movements of the trunk are described as left or right rotation. Rotation of the limbs can be described as medial or lateral rotation; special terms are used to describe the rotational movements of the forearm.

Right rotation

Left rotation

Rotational movements are also described with reference to a figure in the anatomical position. Rotation of the head may involve **left rotation** or **right rotation**.

Lateral (external) rotation

Medial (internal) rotation

The proximal articulation between the radius and the ulna (the proximal radio-ulnar joint) permits rotation of the radial head. As the shaft of the radius rotates, the distal epiphysis of the radius rolls across the anterior surface of the ulna. This movement, called **pronation** (prō-NĀ-shun), turns the wrist and hand from palm facing front to palm facing back. The opposing movement, in which the palm is turned anteriorly, is **supination** (soo-pi-NĀ-shun).

Supination

Pronation

During **medial rotation**, also known as internal rotation or inward rotation, the anterior surface of a limb turns toward the long axis of the trunk. The reverse movement is called **lateral rotation**, external rotation, or outward rotation.

Special movements

2 There are several special terms that apply to specific articulations or unusual types of movement.

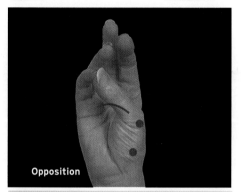

Opposition

Opposition is movement of the thumb toward the surface of the palm or the pads of other fingers. Opposition enables you to grasp and hold objects between your thumb and palm. It involves movement at the first carpo-metacarpal and metacarpophalangeal joints. Flexion at the fifth metacarpophalangeal joint can assist this movement.

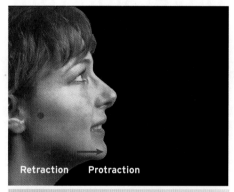

Retraction   Protraction

Protraction entails moving a part of the body anteriorly in the horizontal plane. **Retraction** is the reverse movement. You protract your jaw when you grasp your upper lip with your lower teeth, and you protract your clavicles when you cross your arms.

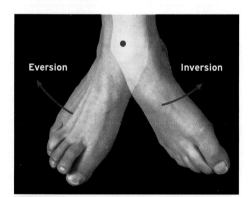

Eversion   Inversion

Inversion (*in*, into + *vertere*, to turn) is a twisting motion of the foot that turns the sole inward, elevating the medial edge of the sole. The opposite movement is called **eversion** (ē-VER-zhun; *e*, out).

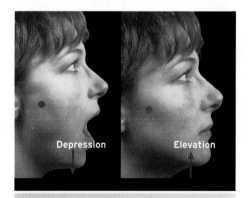

Depression   Elevation

Depression and **elevation** occur when a structure moves in an inferior or a superior direction, respectively.

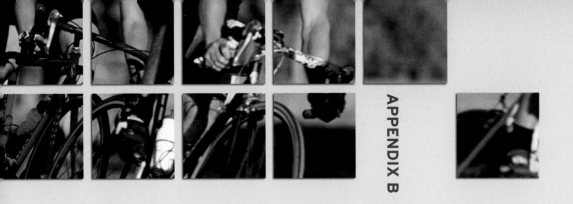

Gas conversion table

Factors (10^{-3}) to reduce moist gas (ATPS) to a dry gas (STPD) at 0 °C and 760 mmHg
From this website: **http://www.sportex.bham.ac.uk/research/hpl/lab8.htm**

Pressure (mmHg)	Temperature °C																	
	15	16	17	18	19	20	21	22	23	24	25	26	27	28	29	30	31	32
700	0.855	851	847	842	838	834	829	825	821	816	812	807	802	797	793	788	783	778
702	857	853	849	845	840	836	832	827	823	818	814	809	805	800	795	790	785	780
704	860	856	852	847	843	839	834	830	825	821	816	812	807	802	797	792	787	783
706	862	858	854	850	845	841	837	832	828	823	819	814	810	804	800	795	790	785
708	865	861	856	852	848	843	839	834	830	825	821	816	812	807	802	797	792	787
710	867	863	859	855	850	846	842	837	833	828	824	819	814	809	804	799	795	790
712	870	866	861	857	853	848	844	839	836	830	826	821	817	812	807	802	797	792
714	872	868	864	859	855	851	846	842	837	833	828	824	819	814	809	804	799	794
716	875	871	866	862	858	853	849	844	840	835	831	826	822	816	812	807	802	797
718	877	873	869	864	860	856	851	847	842	838	833	828	824	819	814	809	804	799
720	880	876	871	867	863	858	854	849	845	840	836	831	826	821	816	812	807	802
722	882	878	874	869	865	861	856	852	847	843	838	833	829	824	819	814	809	804
724	885	880	876	872	867	863	858	854	849	845	840	835	831	826	821	816	811	806
726	887	883	879	874	870	866	861	856	852	847	843	838	833	829	824	818	813	808
728	890	886	881	877	872	868	863	859	854	850	845	840	836	831	826	821	816	811
730	890	888	884	879	875	871	866	861	857	852	847	843	838	833	828	823	818	813
732	895	890	886	882	877	873	868	864	859	854	850	845	840	836	831	825	820	815
734	897	893	889	884	880	875	871	866	862	857	852	847	843	838	833	828	823	818
736	900	895	891	887	882	878	873	869	864	859	855	850	845	840	835	830	825	820
738	902	898	894	889	885	880	876	871	866	862	857	852	848	843	838	833	828	822
740	905	900	896	892	887	883	878	874	869	864	860	855	850	845	840	835	830	825

Pressure (mmHg)	Temperature °C																	
	15	16	17	18	19	20	21	22	23	24	25	26	27	28	29	30	31	32
742	907	903	898	894	890	885	881	876	871	867	862	857	852	847	842	837	832	827
744	910	906	901	897	892	888	883	878	874	869	864	859	855	850	845	840	834	829
746	912	908	903	899	895	890	886	881	876	872	867	862	857	852	847	842	837	832
748	915	910	906	901	897	892	888	883	879	874	869	864	860	854	850	845	839	834
750	917	913	908	904	900	895	890	886	881	876	872	867	862	857	852	847	842	837
752	920	915	911	906	902	897	893	888	883	879	874	869	864	859	854	849	844	839
754	922	918	913	909	904	900	895	891	886	881	876	872	867	862	857	852	846	841
756	925	920	916	911	907	902	898	893	888	883	879	874	869	864	859	854	849	844
758	927	923	918	914	909	905	900	896	891	886	881	876	872	866	861	856	851	846
760	930	925	921	916	912	907	902	898	893	888	883	879	874	869	864	859	854	848
762	932	928	923	919	914	910	905	900	896	891	886	881	876	871	866	861	856	851
764	936	930	926	921	916	912	907	903	898	893	888	884	879	874	869	864	858	853
766	937	933	928	924	919	915	910	905	900	896	891	886	881	876	871	866	861	855
768	940	935	931	926	922	917	912	908	903	898	893	888	883	878	873	868	863	858
770	942	938	933	928	924	919	915	910	905	901	896	891	886	881	876	871	865	860

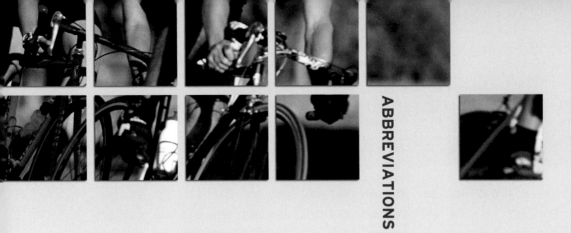

1RM	1 repetition maximum		**BMD**	Bone mineral density
2,3-dpg	2,3-diphosphoglycerate		**BMI**	Body mass index
AAHPERD	American Alliance for Health, Physical Education, Recreation and Dance		**BMR**	Basal metabolic rate
			BP	Blood pressure
AAT	Aerobic-anaerobic transition		**CAD**	Coronary artery disease
ACh	Acetylcholine		**CFS**	Cerebrospinal fluid
ACHPER	Australian Council for Health, Physical Education and Recreation		**CHD**	Coronary heart disease
ADP	Adenosine diphosphate		**CHO**	Carbohydrate
ADR	Adenylate deaminase reaction		**CK**	Creatine kinase
AFL	Australian Football League		**CNS**	Central nervous system
AIDA	International Association for the Development of Freediving		**CoA**	Coenzyme A
			CP	Critical power
AKR	Adenylate kinase reaction		**CRF**	Cardiorespiratory fitness
ALP	Athlete-led protocol		**CVD**	Cardiovascular disease
AMP	Adenosine monophosphate		**DNA**	Deoxyribonucleic acid
AMS	Acute mountain sickness		**DOMS**	Delayed onset muscle soreness
ANS	Autonomic nervous system		**DXA**	Dual-energy X-ray absorptiometry
AnT	Anaerobic threshold		E_a	Energy of activation
AnTT	Anaerobic threshold training		**EDV**	End diastolic volume
ATP	Adenosine triphosphate		**EIA**	Exercise-induced asthma
ATP-PCr	phosphagen system or creatine kinase reaction		**EIB**	Exercise-induced bronchiospasm
			EMD	Electromechanical delay
ATPS	Ambient temperature and pressure saturated		**EPIRB**	Emergency position indicating radio beacon
AWC	Anaerobic work capacity		**EPO**	Erythropoietin
BIA	Bioelectrical impedance analysis		**EPOC**	Excess post-exercise oxygen consumption
BMC	Bone mineral content			

ESV	End systolic volume
ET	Endurance training
ETAP	Exercise-related transient abdominal pain
ETC	Electron transport chain
FAD	Flavin adenine dinucleotide
FCAT	Four corners agility test
F_ECO_2	Fraction of expired carbon dioxide
F_EO_2	Fraction of expired oxygen
FEV_1	Forced expiratory volume in 1 sec
FI	Fatigue index
FIBA	Fédération Internationale de Basketball Amateur
FIFA	Fédération Internationale de Football Association
FIH	Fédération Internationale de Hockey
FIT	Frequency intensity and duration
FM	Fat mass
FMN	Flavin mononucleotide
FR	Fatigue resistance
FVC	Forced vital capacity
FVT	Force-velocity test
G3P	Glyceraldehyde-3-phosphate
GI	Glycemic index
GI tract	Gastro-intestinal tract
GPS	Global positioning system
HACE	High altitude cerebral edema
HAPE	High altitude pulmonary edema
HDL	High-density lipoprotein
HIIT	High-intensity interval training
Hi-lo	Live high train low
HONC	Hydrogen, oxygen, nitrogen and carbon
HR	Heart rate
HR_{max}	Maximal heart rate
HST	High step test
IAnRT	Intermittent anaerobic running test

IDDM	Insulin-dependent diabetes
IFNA	International Federation of Netball Associations
IHIT	Intermittent high-intensity training
IOC	International Olympic Committee
ITA	Intermittent aerobic training
LBM	Lean body mass
LDH	Lactate dehydrogenase
LDL	Low-density lipoprotein
LRT	Lateral reach test
LSD	Long slow distance
LT	Lactate threshold
mCSA	Muscle cross-sectional area
MET	Metabolic equivalent
MLSS	Maximal lactate steady state
MOAD	Maximal accumulated oxygen deficit test
MPO	Mean power output
mRNA	Messenger ribonucleic acid
MSFT	Multi-stage fitness test
MSRT	Multi-stage shuttle run test
MVA	Maximal aerobic velocity
NAD^+	Nicotinamide adenine dinucleotide
NIDDM	Non-insulin-dependent diabetes
NMRS	Nuclear magnetic resonance spectroscopy
NMT	Non-motorised treadmill
OBLA	Onset of blood lactate accumulation
PCO_2	Partial pressure of carbon dioxide
PCr	Phosphocreatine
PDH	Pyruvate dehydrogenase
PENZ	Physical Education New Zealand
PFK	Phosphofructokinase
PHIIRSS	Prolonged high-intensity intermittent running sport simulation
PHV	Peak height velocity
Pi	Phosphate ion or phosphoryl group

PN_2	Partial pressure of nitrogen		SNS	Somatic nervous system
PNS	Peripheral nervous system		SR	Sarcoplasmic reticulum
PO_2	Partial pressure of oxygen		SSC	Stretch-shortening cycle
PPi	Pyrophosphate		SSGT	Squash-specific graded test
PPO	Peak power output		SSIET	Soccer-specific intermittent-exercise test
PWV	Peak weight velocity		Ss_{max}	Steady-state maximum
Q	Cardiac output		STPD	Standard temperature and pressure dry
RAST	Running-based anaerobic sprint test		SV	Stroke volume
RBC	Red blood cell		T_c	Core temperature
RDA	Recommended daily allowance		T_{in}	Intestinal temperature
RER	Respiratory exchange ratio		T_{lim}	Time limit
R_f	Respiratory frequency		TMA	Time and motion analysis
RFU	(English) Rugby Football Union		TMP	Trans-membrane potential
rHuEPO	Recombinant human erythropoietin		T_{os}	Oesophageal temperature
RMR	Resting metabolic rate		T_{re}	Rectal temperature
RNA	Ribonucleic acid		$\dot{V}CO_2$	Volume of carbon dioxide
ROS	Reactive oxygen species		$\dot{V}_E$	Minute ventilation
RPE	Rating of perceived exertion		$\dot{V}O_2$	Volume of oxygen
RQ	Respiratory quotient		$\dot{V}O_{2max}$	Maximal oxygen consumption
RTD	Rate of torque development		$\dot{V}O_{2peak}$	Peak oxygen consumption
SAPT	Swimming anaerobic power test		V_T	Tidal volume
SCUBA	Self-contained underwater breathing apparatus		WADA	World Anti-Doping Agency
SDH	Succinate dehydrogenase		WAnT	Wingate anaerobic test
ShuttleSDT	Shuttle sprint and dribble test		WHO	World Health Organisation
SIT	Sprint interval training		WIST	Water polo intermittent shuttle test
SlalomSDT	Slalom sprint and dribble test		W_{lim}	Work limit

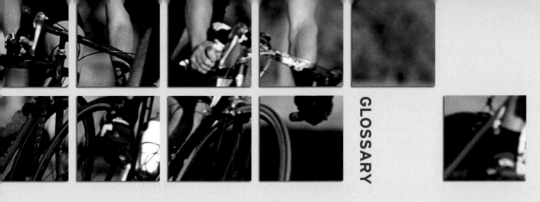

A band the region of a sarcomere containing myosin filaments

Acclimation the physiological adaptation to an artificial environment (e.g. heat chamber, altitude tent) to optimise competition performance

Acclimatisation the physiological adaptation to a natural environment to optimise competition performance

Acetylcholine a neurotransmitter in both the PNS and CNS; the neurotransmitter at the neuromuscular junction

Acetylcholinesterase the enzyme that catalyses the degradation of the neurotransmitter acetylcholine

Acetyl CoA an acetyl group bound to co-enzyme A; formed through the metabolism of carbohydrates and fats for entry to the Krebs cycle

Acid dissociates in solution to release hydrogen ions; increases acidity of solution

Actin the thin myofilament involved in muscle contraction

Action potential a rapid change in the electrical membrane potential of excitable cells

Active flexibility the ability of muscles to move a limb through a range of motion

Adenosine diphosphate adenosine attached to two phosphoryl groups

Adenosine monophosphate adenosine attached to a single phosphoryl group

Adenosine triphosphate adenosine attached to three phosphoryl groups; the energy source for cellular activity

Adenylate deaminase reaction a reaction in which AMP is deaminated to form IMP and NH_3 with the addition of water

Adenylate kinase reaction a reaction supplementary to the phosphagen system which forms ATP and AMP from two molecules of ADP

Adolescent growth spurt a dynamic period of post-natal growth; a milestone of puberty

Aerobic requires oxygen

Aerobic-anaerobic transition the transition from aerobic to increasingly anaerobic metabolism

Aerobic capacity see aerobic power

Aerobic metabolism reactions that require oxygen

Aerobic power the maximal rate of oxygen consumption; also referred to as aerobic capacity

Aerobic system pathways that involve the catabolism of carbohydrates, lipids and proteins to synthesise ATP in the presence of oxygen

Afferent neuron see sensory neuron

Agonist see prime mover

Aldosterone a hormone released from the adrenal cortex which functions to increase sodium reabsorption, water retention and blood pressure.

Allostery/allosteric regulation the fastest-acting regulation of enzyme activity; the effector molecule binds to allosteric site (not the substrate binding site) on enzyme

α(alpha) cells cells of the pancreas that produce glucagon

Altitude an elevation of 1,500 m and above

Alveolar ventilation the exchange of oxygen and carbon dioxide between the alveoli and the bloodstream

Alveoli the terminal structures of the respiratory tract; the sites of gas exchange between the lungs and the blood

Amenorrhea the absence of a menstrual cycle

Amine group NH_2

Amino acids building blocks for proteins

Amphiarthrosis a joint allowing more movement than a synarthrosis but less than a diarthrosis

Anabolism the synthesis of new molecules

Anaerobic does not require oxygen

Anaerobic endurance the ability to maintain high-intensity exercise

Anaerobic threshold the transition between aerobic and anaerobic exercise; also known as the ventilatory threshold

Anion a negatively charged ion

Anovulation a lack of ovulation; the ovaries do not release an oocyte (egg cell) during the menstrual cycle

Antagonist the muscle which opposes the movement of the prime mover

Anti-diuretic hormone a hormone synthesised by the hypothalamus and released by the pituitary gland which functions to conserve water at the kidneys

Aortic valve a valve between the left ventricle and the aorta

Apical surface the surface of a cell oriented to the outside world or central space of an organ or gland

Apnea the suspension of breathing

Aponeurosis a flattened tendinous structure which attaches sheetlike muscles to one or more bones

Appendicular skeleton the 126 bones that make up the upper and lower limbs, the pectoral girdle and the pelvic girdle

Appositional growth growth in diameter, thickness

Arachnoid mater the middle meningeal layer of the CNS, attached to the inner surface of the dura mater

Areal bone mineral density the ratio of bone mineral content to bone cross-sectional area; expressed as $g \cdot cm^{-2}$

Articular capsule a fibrous capsule surrounding the articulating surfaces in a synovial joint

Articular cartilage the hyaline cartilage covering the articulating bone surfaces within synovial joints

Association neuron *see* interneuron

Astrocyte the most abundant CNS neuroglia

Atomic mass the mass of one atom of an isotope, or average atom mass of an element (atomic mass units)

Atomic number the number of protons within the nucleus of an atom

Atrioventricular bundle carries the action potential from the atrioventricular node to the Purkinje fibres; also known as the bundle of His

Atrioventricular node part of the system that coordinates heart rate; a node between the atria and ventricles that conducts the action potential from the atria to the ventricle via the atrioventricular bundle and the Purkinje fibres

Atrioventricular valves valves at the junction of the atria and ventricles that prevent the backflow of blood into the atria

Atrium (pl. atria) a superior collecting chamber of the heart that receives venous blood from the systemic or pulmonary circulation

Autocrines cells which release hormones that take effect at the site of production; the hormones do not enter the bloodstream

Autonomic ganglion a mass of cell bodies of autonomic nerves

Autonomic nervous system part of the peripheral nervous system that acts to control the unconscious functioning of the body

a-v O₂ difference the difference between the oxygen content in a known amount of arterial and venous blood

Axial skeleton the 80 bones that make up the body core (skull, vertebrae and ribs)

Axolemma axon plasma membrane

Axon a specialised filament that generates action potentials and conducts them away from the cell body

Axon collateral a branch of the main axon that leaves the cell body

Axon hillock the site on the neuron cell body from which the axon arises

Axon terminal forms the link with other tissues or neurons

Axoplasm the cytoplasm of an axon

Ball and socket joint the most freely moveable of all synovial joints; allows for movement in two planes, circumduction and rotation

Ballistic stretch motion and momentum are used to induce a stretch

Base accepts hydrogen ions in solution to form hydroxide ions; increases alkalinity of solution

Bends (the) *see* decompression sickness

β (beta) cells cells of the pancreas that produce insulin

β (beta) oxidation the initial pathway for the catabolism of free fatty acids

Bicuspid valve a valve with two cusps between the left atrium and the left ventricle; also referred to as the mitral valve

Bioenergetics the study of energy dynamics in living organisms

Bipolar neuron a neuron with a single dendrite coming to the cell body

Blood-brain barrier surrounds the majority of capillaries in the brain separating the general circulation from the neural tissue of the brain

Blood doping increasing the number of red blood cells by infusion to enhance athletic performance

Body mass index an indication of body composition by expressing body mass relative to height; BMI = body mass (kg) divided by height (m) squared

Bond energy the energy required to break a specific bond between two atoms

Bradycardia a resting heart rate below 60 beats·min⁻¹

Brain-stem the posterior part of the brain providing a link between the brain and the spinal cord

Buffer a compound that removes or adds hydrogen ions to a solution thereby stabilising the pH

Bundle of His *see* atrioventricular bundle

Calorie the amount of heat required to raise the temperature of 1 g of water by 1°C – a common unit of food energy

Canaliculi a microscopic network of canals allowing nutrients and waste products to be transported to and from osteocytes within bone

Carbohydrate loading the manipulation of diet to increase the muscle glycogen stores prior to endurance exercise to optimise performance

Carboxyl group COOH

Cardiac drift *see* cardiovascular drift

Cardiac muscle striated, involuntary muscle found in the walls of the heart; also known as myocardium

Cardiac output the volume of blood ejected from the left ventricle in one minute

Cardiovascular drift a gradual increase in heart rate with no increase in work rate; also known as cardiac drift

Cardiovascular system the body's main transport mechanism; comprised of the heart, the vascular system and the blood

Catabolism the breakdown of a molecule into smaller molecules or its constituent atoms

Catacholamines a family of amine adrenergic neurotransmitters produced and released by the adrenal medulla; includes adrenaline, noradrenaline and dopamine

Cation a positively charged ion

Cell body (neuron) the rounded part of a neuron which contains organelles and nucleus; also known as the soma

Cellular respiration the set of metabolic reactions which results in the formation of ATP

Cellular ventilation the diffusion of oxygen into a cell for use within cellular respiration, and the movement of carbon dioxide from the cell into the blood

Central fatigue a reduced neural drive to working muscles during exercise; increased feelings of fatigue

Central nervous system the brain and the spinal cord

Centriole involved in the organisation of the microtubules of the mitotic spindle during cell division

Centrosome a central organelle from which many of the micro-tubules radiate, contains a pair of centrioles

Cerebellum a posterior portion of the brain which acts as the brain's feedback centre; plays an important role in motor performance

Cerebrum the largest, most superior region of the brain; divided into left and right cerebral hemispheres

Channel protein a transmembrane protein allowing specific ions to enter the cell

Chemical equation a shorthand symbolic form of a chemical reaction

Chemical reaction a process in which a chemical change occurs

Chemoreceptor a sensory receptor which detects changes in the chemical environment

Chondroblast cartilage-forming cell

Chondrocyte cartilage cell

Chyme the semi-fluid substance formed in the stomach when food is mixed with the digestive enzymes

Circular muscle fascicles arranged in a circular fashion around an opening or recess; also known as a sphincter

Cisternae the sac-like structures of endoplasmic reticulum

Coffee-grinding (sailing) the bicycle action used to move cranks on sailing boats

Compact bone one of two types of bone; dense, hard, strong bone arranged in parallel units called osteons; also referred to as cortical bone

Complete tetanus *see* fused tetanus

Complex training training involving the integration of strength and plyometric activities

Compound formed by the bonding of different elements

Concentric contraction a type of muscle contraction where the muscle shortens during force generation

Conduction the transfer of heat from one material to another through direct molecular contact

Conducting zone the section of the respiratory tract which passes air to the alveoli from the nose and mouth to the terminal bronchioles and alveoli

Condyloid joint *see* ellipsoid joint

Continuous conduction the movement of an action potential along an unmyelinated nerve fibre, as a wave of depolarisation

Contraction phase the second phase of a muscle twitch; the time period during which tension develops in the muscle

Convection a specific form of conduction where the movement of a fluid across a warmer surface results in heat transfer

Convergent muscle fascicles spread out like a fan over a broad area with a common attachment site at the apex

Cortex the outer portion of an organ

Cortical thickness the total width of the bone minus the width of the medullary cavity

Covalent bond a chemical link between two atoms by the sharing of electrons between atoms

Covalent modification the activation or inactivation of enzyme activity

Critical power the maximal power attainable for a sustained period of time; represents the upper limit of the heavy intensity exercise zone.

Crossbridge the attachment of a myosin head to a specific binding site on the actin filament

Current the flow of electric charge such as the movement of ions within the body

Cytokine a small signalling protein involved in intercellular communication

Cytoplasm the contents of a cell found between the plasma membrane and the nucleus

Cytoskeleton a cellular protein network within the cytoplasm, consists of microtubules and microfilaments

Cytosol/intracellular fluid gel-like substance which houses and protects the organelles of a cell

Deamination the removal of the amine group from an amino acid

Decompression sickness the formation of nitrogen bubbles within the body following a rapid accent from deep water immersion; also referred to as the bends

Dehydration loss of body water

Dehydrogenase an enzyme that catalyses the removal or addition of hydrogen atoms from or to a substrate

Delayed onset muscle soreness muscle stiffness and soreness that can occur within 1-2 days of intense exercise

Dendrite the sensory process of a neuron

Depolarised the change of a cell's membrane potential to less negative, or more positive, e.g. from −70 mV to around +35 mV during an action potential

Desmin a sarcomere protein which links adjacent Z lines

Desmosome structurally combines cardiac fibres together at intercalated discs

Diaphragm (thoracic) a sheet of skeletal muscle which separates the thoracic cavity from the abdominal cavity; plays a role in respiration

Diaphysis the shaft of a long bone

Diarthrosis *see* synovial joint

Diastolic blood pressure the lowest level of arterial pressure in the vascular system; occurs between contractions of the heart

Diencephalon the posterior region of the forebrain including the epithalamus, thalamus and hypothalamus

Digestion the breakdown of food

Dorsal root an afferent (sensory) root of a spinal nerve

Dorsal root ganglion a mass of cell bodies of afferent (sensory) nerves; also referred to as spinal ganglion

Dorsiflexion the movement which brings the toes toward the shin

Dura mater the outer layer of the CNS meninges found immediately beneath the skull

Dynamic balance the combination of balance, agility and coordination

Eccentric contraction a type of muscle contraction where the muscle lengthens during force generation

Efferent neurons *see* motor neurons

Eicosanoid formed by the oxygenation of one of three 20-C essential fatty acids; control inflammatory and immunity process and act as messengers in the CNS

Elastic cartilage a flexible cartilage due to the presence of elastin

Electrocardiogram the trace of the heart's electrical activity produced by an electrocardiograph

Electrocardiograph equipment used to detect the electrical activity of the heart

Electrolyte a soluble compound whose ions can conduct an electrical current

Electron transport chain (ETC) the site of electron transfer to facilitate the production of ATP by oxidative phosphorylation; occurs within the inner mitochondrial membrane

Ellipsoid joint a synovial joint that allows movement in two planes; also referred to as a condyloid joint

End-diastolic volume the volume of blood in the left ventricle at the end of diastole (relaxation)

Endergonic a reaction in which energy is absorbed; not a spontaneous reaction

Endocrines cells which release hormones that travel some distance within the body to take effect

Endocrine gland secrete material directly into the blood (ductless)

Endocrine system the body's slower, sustained regulation mechanism; consists of the endocrine glands and organs which secrete hormones directly into the blood stream

Endomysium a connective tissue sheath surrounding each individual skeletal muscle fibre; continuous with the tendon or aponeurosis of the muscle

Endoneurium a delicate layer of connective tissue that surrounds individual nerve fibres

Endoplasmic reticulum an organelle that functions in intracellular transport, synthesis, packaging, storage and secretion of a variety of molecules

Endorphin a neurotransmitter released into the blood; blocks feelings of pain and promotes feelings of well-being

Endothermic energy is absorbed, normally in the form of heat

End-systolic volume the volume of blood remaining in the left ventricle at the end of systole (contraction)

Energetics the study of energy transfer

Energy of activation the energy required for a reaction to take place

Enthalpy the change in energy between reactants and products

Entropy the dispersal or disorder of energy

Enzyme a protein within the body that catalyses (speeds up) a specific reaction

Ependymal cell a CNS neuroglia that aids the flow of cerebrospinal fluid

Epimysium a connective tissue sheath surrounding a skeletal muscle; continuous with the tendon or aponeurosis of the muscle

Epineurium an outer layer of dense connective tissue surrounding multiple fascicles of a peripheral nerve

Epiphyseal line replaces the epiphyseal plate upon completion of long bone growth

Epiphyseal plate the cartilage remaining between the primary and secondary ossification centres; the site of long bone growth; also referred to as the growth plate

Epiphyses the heads of a long bone

Epithelia a layer of cells lining the surfaces and hollow organs of the body

Equilibrium (chemical) a state of balance in which the concentrations of reactants and products are constant

Ergogenic aid a substance, technique or technological enhancement that can be used to improve performance

Erythrocyte red blood cell

Erythropoietin a hormone produced primarily by the kidneys which stimulates the production of red blood cells (erythrocytes)

Euhydration a state of water balance, normal water content

Evaporation the use of energy to convert a liquid (e.g. sweat) to a gas resulting in heat loss

Excitable capable of conducting an electrical impulse

Excitation-contraction coupling the process of nervous stimulation leading to muscular contraction

Excess post-exercise oxygen consumption the post-exercise elevation in oxygen consumption; also referred to as oxygen debt

Exercise economy the energy required for a given pace or power output

Exergonic a reaction in which energy is released; a spontaneous reaction

Exocrine glands release secretions into ducts that open on to epithelial surface

Exocytosis the fusion of a vesicle with the plasma membrane to enable release of an intracellular substance to the extracellular space

Exothermic energy is released, normally in the form of heat

Extension a movement that increases the angle between two bones at a joint

External intercostals the primary inspiratory muscles; contraction causes rib cage to rise

Extracellular fluid all fluid outwith cells, includes plasma and interstitial fluid

Exocytosis the process by which a cell removes the contents of a vesicle by fusion with the plasma membrane

Fartlek training continuous training during which the exercise intensity is varied throughout the session

Fascicle a small bundle of skeletal muscle fibres bound together by the perimysium

Fast rate glycolysis pyruvate bond with hydrogen atoms to produce lactate

Fat-free mass see lean body mass

Fat mass the mass of fat within the body

Female athlete triad the interrelationship of under-nutrition, menstrual irregularity and bone loss

Fibrocartilage an intermediate cartilage with a mixture of strength and compression resistance

Flavin adenine dinucleotide a co-enzyme carrier for hydrogen atoms; can exist in a reduced or oxidised state

Flexibility the range of motion at a joint

Flexion a movement that decreases the angle between two bones at a joint

Forced expiratory volume a measure of lung efficiency; normally measured as the volume of air that can be forcefully expired, following maximal inhalation, in one second (FEV_1)

Forced vital capacity a measure of the voluntary capacity of the lungs; the volume of air that can be forcefully expired following maximal inhalation

Free energy the energy available to do work

Free radicals destructive molecules that develop naturally as a part of metabolism

Fused tetanus high frequency of stimulation resulting in maximal muscle tension, no relaxation between stimuli; a smooth, sustained contraction; also referred to as complete tetanus

Ganglia a small mass of neuron cell bodies located outside the CNS

Gap junction a connection that allows action potentials to spread from one cardiac fibre to the next

Glial cells see neuroglia

Gliding joint a synovial joint with minimal movement where the flat surfaces of bones come together

Glucagon a hormone released by the alpha cells of the pancreas, stimulates the breakdown of glycogen to glucose

Gluconeogenesis the formation of glucose from non-carbohydrate molecules

Glucose a simple sugar (monosaccharide) used as a primary energy source

Glucose-alanine cycle the conversion of alanine to glucose in the liver – a mechanism through which amino acids can become a source of energy

Glycemic index a food rating based on its rate of digestion and absorption

Glycogen a long chain of glucose molecules; stored within muscle and the liver as an energy reserve

Glycogenesis the formation of glycogen

Glycogenolysis the breakdown of glycogen to form glucose

Glycolipid a lipid with attached carbohydrate, a component of the plasma membrane involved in cellular recognition

Glycolysis the catabolism of glucose or glycogen to produce pyruvate and ATP

Glycoprotein a protein containing carbohydrate chains, a component of the plasma membrane involved in cell-cell interactions

Golgi apparatus an organelle responsible for the processing and packaging of newly synthesised proteins

Graded muscle response a graded development of muscle tension dependent on the frequency of stimulation

Grey matter areas of the CNS containing neuronal cell bodies and their dendrites

Growth plate see epiphyseal plate

Haematocrit the percentage of whole blood that is composed of cells; also referred to as the 'packed cell volume'

Haldane transformation a transformation used in the calculation of oxygen uptake; makes allowances for the change in volume between inspired and expired gas samples

Haversian system see osteon

Heart rate the number of times the heart beats per minute

Hiking (sailing) sitting on the windward side of the boat to counteract the force of the wind

Hinge joint a synovial joint that allows movement in one plane

Homeostasis the regulation of the internal environment to maintain a stable, constant condition

Hormone a chemical released by a cell or a gland that initiates a change in the function of the target cells for which it is intended

Hormone-sensitive lipase the key enzyme of lipolysis

Hyaline cartilage a strong, tough and smooth cartilage, comprised mainly of collagen; most common cartilage in the human body

Hydrogenation a chemical reaction between hydrogen and another element or compound

Hydrolysis the breakage of a chemical bond through the addition of a water molecule

Hydrophilic water-loving

Hydrophobic water-fearing

Hydroxyapatite crystals mineralised form of bone

Hyperbaric high atmospheric pressure; experienced during water immersion

Hyperglycaemia high blood glucose concentration (> 13.5 $mmol \cdot L^{-1}$; > 243 $mg \cdot dL^{-1}$)

Hyperplasia an increase in cell number

Hyperpnea an increased ventilation to meet the metabolic demands of the body, e.g. during exercise

Hyperthermia high body temperature; heat dissipation is unable to match heat gain

Hypertrophy an increase in cell size

Hypobaric low atmospheric pressure; experienced at altitude

Hypoglycaemia low blood glucose concentration (< 4 mmol·L^{-1})

Hyponatraemia low serum sodium concentration, < 135 mEq/L

Hypothermia low body temperature ($< 35°C$), below that required for normal metabolism

Hypovolaemia low blood volume resulting from reduced plasma volume

Hypoxia low partial pressure of oxygen (compared to sea level)

H zone the region of a sarcomere containing only myosin filaments

I band the region of a sarcomere containing only actin filaments

Incomplete tetanus see unfused tetanus

Intercalated disc the region which connects adjacent cardio-myocytes; supports the synchronised contraction of cardiac muscle

Interleukin-6 (IL-6) a cytokine with both pro-inflammatory and anti-inflammatory roles

Intermediate filament a component of the cytoskeleton which helps to maintain structure and stabilises the position of the organelles

Intermittent exercise exercise involving a variety of intensities placing demands on both anaerobic and aerobic metabolic pathways

Interneuron a specialised neuron that passes information from one neuron to another; also known as an association neuron

Interstitial fluid the fluid that surrounds tissue cells

Intracellular fluid fluid within cells, the cytosol

Ionic bond an electrostatic force between atoms through the donation of one or more electrons from one atom to another

Isokinetic contraction a type of muscle contraction where the muscle contracts at the same speed; requires an isokinetic machine that can vary the load applied to the muscle

Isomerase an enzyme that changes the structure, but not the chemical composition, of the substrate

Isometric contraction a type of muscle contraction where the muscle remains the same length during force generation

Isotonic contraction a type of muscle contraction where the muscle tension remains constant despite a change in muscle length

Isotope different form of the same substance; same number of protons, different number of neutrons

Kilocalorie the amount of heat required to raise the temperature of 1 kg of water by 1°C – a common unit of food energy

Kinase an enzyme that transfers phosphoryl groups to or from a substrate

Krebs cycle the cycle of aerobic reactions that takes place within the mitochondrial matrix; hydrogen molecules are transferred to the electron transport chain for ATP synthesis; also known as the citric acid cycle or tricarboxylic acid cycle

Lactate a salt of lactic acid; produced from pyruvate in anaer-obic conditions

Lactate threshold the exercise intensity at which lactate begins to accumulate in the body

Lactic acid formed from pyruvic acid in anaerobic conditions

Lacunae small spaces between lamellar rings in compact bone within which osteocytes are enclosed

Lamellae concentric rings of bone within an osteon

Latent period the first phase of a muscle twitch; the time period between the stimulation of muscle and the start of muscle contraction

Lean body mass the total body mass minus the fat mass; includes skeletal muscle, water, connective tissue and the body organs; also known as fat-free mass

Leukocyte white blood cell

Lipolysis the catabolism of triglyceride molecules into their component parts for subsequent metabolism

Lumen the central space of a tubular structure, e.g. a duct or a blood vessel

Lysosome an organelle containing enzymes that break down cellular debris

M line the midline of a sarcomere

Macronutrients the compounds that are potential energy sources for the human body: carbohydrate, fat, protein

Matter everything around you that has a mass, is made of atoms and molecules

Maximal lactate steady state the highest exercise intensity that can be sustained for 30 min with no concurrent accumu-lation of blood lactate (< 1 mM change)

Maximal oxygen uptake (VO$_{2max}$) the maximum capacity of the body to utilise oxygen during incremental exercise

Mechanoreceptors a sensory receptor which detects mechan-ical stimuli, such as touch, pressure, distortion or vibration

Medullary cavity the central cavity within the diaphysis of a long bone

Membrane potential the potential difference created by the cell membrane due to the separation of oppositely charged molecules; this is measured in millivolts (mV)

Meninges three protective, connective tissue membranes surrounding the brain and spinal cord

Meniscus (pl. menisci) a fibrocartilage pad between the articu-lating surfaces of a synovial joint

Metabolic equivalent (MET) a system for estimating exercise intensity based on resting metabolic rate; 1 MET = resting $\dot{V}O_2$ of 3.5 mL·kg·min^{-1}

Metabolism the set of chemical reactions that take place within the body to sustain life

Michaelis constant the point at which enzyme velocity reaches half of its maximum

Microfilament a component of the cytoskeleton which anchors it to the plasma membrane

Microglia a CNS neuroglia involved in the repair of neural tissue

Micronutrients nutrients required by the body in very small quantities for physiological functioning, such as vitamins and minerals

Microtubule a component of the cytoskeleton which provides strength and rigidity

Microtubule (neuron-specific) provides a transport structure through which substances pass between the cell body and the axon

Minerals inorganic micronutrients required for healthy physiological functioning

Minute ventilation the volume of air inspired or expired each minute (tidal volume × respiratory frequency)

Mitochondrion (pl. mitochondria) the primary site of energy production within a cell

Mitral valve *see* bicuspid valve

Mole the quantity of a substance containing 6.02×10^{23} atoms, molecules or ions

Molecule the chemical bonding of two atoms of the same element

Monounsaturated contains one carbon double bond

Motor neuron transmits information away from the central nervous system to the rest of the body; also known as an efferent neuron

Motor unit a motor neuron and all the muscle fibres it innervates

Motor unit recruitment the progressive increase in muscle tension with the successive recruitment of contractile (motor) units

Multipolar neuron has many dendrites connecting to the cell body

Muscle cell *see* muscle fibre

Muscle fibre the cellular unit of skeletal muscle also known as a muscle cell

Muscle insertion the point of muscle attachment to the bone that moves when the muscle contracts

Muscle origin the point of muscle attachment to the bone that does not move when the muscle contracts

Muscle-specific tension the force produced per unit area of muscle

Muscle twitch the contraction–relaxation response of a muscle fibre to a single action potential

Muscular endurance the ability of a muscle to perform repeated contractions or to maintain a contraction for a period of time

Muscular pump the mechanism by which venous return is assisted by the contraction of skeletal muscles squeezing blood within the veins

Muscular strength the amount of force that can be generated during a single maximal contraction

Musculoskeletal system a system allowing for movement through the skeletal and muscular systems

Mutase an enzyme that changes the structure, but not the chemical composition, of the substrate

Myelin sheath a protective insulating fatty sheath around axons; increases the speed of action potential transmission

Myocardium *see* cardiac muscle

Myofibril a group of myofilaments that run the length of a skeletal or cardiac muscle fibre

Myofilaments protein filaments within myofibrils; the main proteins are actin (thin filaments) and myosin (thick filaments)

Myokine a substance (cytokine or other peptides) released by skeletal muscle during physical activity

Myoglobin the oxygen-carrying protein of muscle tissue

Myoplasticity the ability of skeletal muscle to adapt both functionally and structurally to repeated stimulations

Myosin the thick myofilament involved in muscle contraction

Negative feedback the output of a system acts as a corrective mechanism to attenuate changes from normal levels

Nerve impulse *see* action potential

Nervous-endocrine control the interaction of the nervous and endocrine systems in the communication within the body

Nervous system the body's fast-response mechanism; includes a network of neurons

Neurilemma the plasma membrane of the cell body and dendrites of a neuron

Neuroendocrine organ an organ which receives neural input which results in the release of hormones into the blood

Neurofibrils protein filaments which help maintain the structure of a neuron cell body

Neurogenesis the process of neuron generation

Neuroglia cells of nervous tissue provide neurons with structural and metabolic support; also known a glial cells

Neuromuscular junction the junction between a motor neuron axon terminal and a muscle fibre

Neuroplasm the cytoplasm of the neuron cell body

Neuron the excitable cell of nervous tissue which transmits information between cells by electrical and chemical signalling; also known as a nerve cell

Nicotinamide adenine dinucleotide a co-enzyme carrier for hydrogen atoms formed from adenine and niacin; can exist in a reduced or oxidised state

Nitrogen narcosis the euphoric effect of a build-up of nitrogen in the body; associated with diving

Nissl body specific to neurons, small rough endoplasmic reticulum structures responsible for protein synthesis

Nociceptor a sensory receptor that detects potentially damaging stimuli

Nucleoside a compound consisting of a nitrogenous base and a five carbon sugar

Nucleotide a nucleoside bonded to one or more phosphoryl groups

Nucleus the control centre of a cell, the cellular organelle that contains the genetic material

Oligodendrocyte a CNS neuroglia; responsible for creating a myelin sheath around the CNS axons

Oligomenorrhea an irregular menstrual cycle with more than 35 days between cycles

Onset of blood lactate accumulation the exercise intensity at which blood lactate accumulation reaches 4 mM

Organelles subunits within a cell which serve a variety of functions

Ossification the replacement of skeletal cartilage by bone

Osteoblast bone-forming cell

Osteoclast bone removal and resorption cell

Osteocyte bone cell

Osteon the functional unit of compact bone; also referred to as a Haversian system

Osteoporosis a reduction in bone mass associated with reduced bone density; meaning 'porous bone'

Over-reaching a short-term expression of over-training

Over-training a syndrome that can affect any athlete if training intensity and duration are excessive; associated with impaired performance

Oxidative phosphorylation the final step of the ETC involving the phosphorylation of ADP to ATP in the presence of oxygen

Oxidised loss of electrons

Oxygen cascade the fall in the partial pressure of oxygen as air moves from the atmosphere to the alveoli

Oxygen debt *see* excess post-exercise oxygen consumption

Oxygen deficit a temporary oxygen shortage in cells due to the delay in the increase in oxygen consumption at the start of exercise

Oxygen uptake kinetics the rate at which oxygen uptake increases to match the energy demands of the muscle with an increase in exercise intensity

Paracrines cells which release hormones that take effect close to the site of production; the hormones do not enter the bloodstream

Parallel muscle fascicles are arranged parallel to the long axis of the muscle

Parasympathetic nervous system the division of the ANS which returns the body to normal functioning, the 'rest and digest' response

Parietal pleura the outer membrane of the pleural sac lining the thoracic wall and diaphragm

Passive flexibility the range of motion through which a muscle can be placed with the aid of other muscles or gravity; i.e. stretching

Pedagogy the education of children and the study of theories of learning associated with education

Pennate muscle fascicles attach obliquely at a common angle to the tendon

Pericardium a double-walled, fluid-filled sac that surrounds the heart

Perikaryon *see* cell body (neuron)

Perimysium a connective tissue sheath surrounding the fascicles of skeletal muscles; continuous with the tendon or aponeurosis of the muscle

Perineurium a connective tissue sheath surrounding the fascicles of the peripheral nervous system

Periodisation a system of programme design which divides training into specific phases to allow peaking for a major event or season while avoiding exhaustion

Periosteum a connective tissue sheath surrounding a bone

Peripheral fatigue impaired functioning at the muscle level

Peripheral nervous system includes all neural tissue outwith the central nervous system

Peristalsis the movement of food by waves of muscular contraction of the digestive tract smooth muscle

Peroxisome an organelle containing enzymes linked with the breakdown of fatty acids and amino acids

Phagocytosis the cellular process of engulfing solid extracellular material, such as bacteria and cell debris, into the cytoplasm

Phosphagen system the fastest pathway for ATP synthesis; utilises energy released from the catabolism of phosphocreatine for the phosphorylation of ADP

Phospholipid a membrane lipid which contains a hydrophobic and hydrophilic region

Phosphofructokinase the major rate-limiting enzyme of glycolysis

Photoreceptor a sensory receptor which detects light

Pia mater the innermost meningeal layer of the CNS, sticks to the surface of the brain

Pivot joint a synovial joint that allows rotation

Placebo effect the body's response to a substance is determined by the individual's expectation of effect rather than by any physiological effect of the substance

Plantar flexion the movement which points the toes; moves the toes away from the shin

Plasma the fluid portion of the blood

Plasma membrane a thin structure which encloses every cell, acts as a barrier between the external environment and the internal contents of the cell

Platelet a blood cell involved in blood clotting; also referred to as a thrombocyte

Pleural cavity the gap between the parietal pleura and the visceral pleura

Pleural fluid a serous fluid in the pleural cavity

Pleural sac a double-layer serous membrane surrounding the lungs

Plyometric contraction a type of muscle contraction where the muscle varies in length; uses an eccentric contraction to produce a more powerful concentric contraction

Pneumothorax a collapsed lung due to the build up of air in the pleural space

Polarised refers to a cell with a difference in electrical charge between the inside and outside of the cell; maintains a resting membrane potential

Polyacrylamide gel electrophoresis (PAGE) a technique used for the separation of protein molecules of differing size

Polyunsaturated contains more than one carbon bond

Post-ganglionic neuron a neuron that conducts a signal from the autonomic ganglion to the effector organ

Post-synaptic neuron a neuron which receives an action potential from a pre-synaptic neuron

Potential difference *see* membrane potential

Potential energy the energy stored within a body or in a system

Power the application of strength at speed

Pre-ganglionic neuron a neuron that conducts a signal from the CNS to an autonomic ganglion

Pre-synaptic neuron the neuron carrying the action potential toward the synapse

Prime mover the muscle responsible for the movement; also referred to as the agonist

Proprioception the awareness of where the body is in space

Proprioceptive neuromuscular facilitation involves an isometric contraction prior to stretching a specific muscle

Puberty a phase of development during adolescence where an individual becomes physiologically capable of sexual reproduction

Pulmonary circulation carries blood to and from the lungs

Pulmonary valve a valve between the right ventricle and the pulmonary arteries

Pulmonary ventilation breathing; the movement of oxygen into the lungs and carbon dioxide out of the lungs

Purkinje fibres propagate the action potential to the ventricular cardiac muscle initiating contraction of the ventricles

Pyruvate the product of glycolysis; a substrate for the Krebs cycle

Radiation a form of heat transfer; the process by which thermal energy is radiated from the surface of an object (e.g. the skin) in the form of electromagnetic waves

Reactive oxygen species highly reactive chemicals containing oxygen, such as oxygen ions and peroxides; formed in a variety of chemical reactions (including normal metabolism)

Receptor protein a transmembrane protein which provides a receptor site for a specific signal molecule

Recognition protein a transmembrane protein which provides the identity of the cell

Red bone marrow the site of red and white blood cell and platelet production

Redox reaction involves the exchange of electrons between reactants – oxidation of one reactant and reduction of another

Reduced gain of electrons

Relaxation phase the final phase of a muscle twitch; the fall in muscle tension back to resting levels

Reliability how similar test scores are when performed on two separate occasions

Repolarised the return of a depolarised membrane to its resting membrane potential, as occurs following an action potential

Respiratory exchange ratio the ratio between the volume of carbon dioxide produced and the volume of oxygen consumed

Respiratory frequency the rate of breathing

Respiratory membrane the membrane across which gaseous exchange takes place; includes the alveolar and capillary cell walls

Respiratory quotient the use of the respiratory exchange ratio (RER) to estimate the predominant fuel for exercise. An RER of 0.7 indicates that fat metabolism would be predominant whereas an RER Of 1.0 would indicate that carbohydrates provide the main source for ATP synthesis

Respiratory zone the section of the respiratory tract involved in gas exchange; involves the respiratory bronchioles, alveolar ducts, alveolar sacs and alveoli

Resting membrane potential the membrane potential of a cell under homeostasis

Ribosome responsible for the translation of MRNA and protein synthesis

Rough endoplasmic reticulum an organelle responsible for protein synthesis; outer membrane is covered with ribosomes

Saddle joint a synovial joint that allows movement in two planes plus circumduction; does not allow rotation

Sail pumping the drawing of a windsurf sail to and from the windsurfer

Saltatory conduction the rapid movement of an action potential between successive nodes of Ranvier on a myelinated nerve fibre

Sarcolemma the plasma membrane of a muscle fibre

Sarcomere the contractile unit of skeletal muscle fibres

Sarcopenia a reduction in muscle mass

Sarcoplasm the cytoplasm of a muscle fibre

Sarcoplasmic reticulum a tubular network surrounding each myofibril; stores and releases calcium

Satellite cell a PNS neuroglia; supplies the PNS neurons with nutrients

Schwann cell a PNS neuroglia; responsible for creating a myelin sheath around the PNS axons

Semilunar valves valves at the junction of the ventricles and arteries that prevent backflow of blood into the ventricles

Sensory neuron detects internal and external signals and relays them to the central nervous system; also known as an afferent neuron

Sinoatrial node the pacemaker for the heart; stimulates autorhythmic contraction of the heart

Skeletal muscle striated, voluntary muscle which functions along with the skeleton to initiate movement

Sliding filament theory the accepted model of muscular contraction

Slower rate glycolysis pyruvate enters the mitochondria where it is catabolised to carbon dioxide and water

Smooth endoplasmic reticulum an organelle responsible for the synthesis and storage of carbohydrates and lipids

Smooth muscle non-striated, involuntary muscle found in the walls of many visceral organs

Sodium-potassium pump expels three Na^+ from, and imports two K^+ into, a cell

Soma see cell body (neuron)

Somatic nervous system part of the peripheral system that controls the skeletal muscles

Speed the movement from one point to another as quickly as possible

Sphincter see circular muscle

Spinal nerve formed by the binding together of the dorsal and ventral roots; carries motor, sensory and autonomic signal between the body and the spinal cord

Spongy bone one of two types of bone; an irregular lattice of bony struts; also known as trabecular or cancellous bone

Squeeze (SCUBA diving) an increased pressure on air trapped within the body, or between face and mask, during water descent

Static stretch involves holding a position to apply a stretch to the soft tissues surrounding a particular joint

Steady-state exercise an exercise intensity where the energy supply for exercise meets the energy demands; heart rate plateaus when steady-state exercise is reached

Strength see muscular strength

Striated striped in appearance

Stroke volume the volume of blood ejected in one contraction of the left ventricle

Summation the temporal or spatial addition of stimuli which results in a greater response compared to that of a single stimulus

Surfactant a lipid component of alveolar fluid which reduces surface tension thus preventing alveolar collapse

Sympathetic nervous system The division of the ANS responsible for speeding up the body systems, the 'fight or flight' response

Synapse the junction between a neuron and another cell

Synaptic cleft the very small gap between a presynaptic membrane and a postsynaptic membrane

Synarthrosis a joint which permits very little or no movement

Synovial joint a freely moveable joint with a fluid-filled cavity; also referred to as a diarthrosis

Systemic circulation supplies blood to the whole body, with the exception of the lungs (pulmonary circuit)

Systolic blood pressure the peak arterial pressure; occurs during ventricular systole

Tachycardia a heart rate above 100 beats·min^{-1} in adults; out with the normal resting range

Temporal summation an increased muscle tension due to an increased frequency of action potential; also referred to as wave summation

Tendon a rope-like collagenous structure attaching skeletal muscle to bone

Terminal cisternae a pair of enlarged regions of the sarcoplasmic reticulum at the A band/I band junctions

Tetanus the progressive development of muscle tension in response to a number of stimuli in quick succession

Thermoreceptor a sensory receptor that detects changes in temperature.

Thermoregulation the control of body temperature within a narrow range

Tidal volume the volume of air moved into or out of the lungs during quiet breathing

Titin an elastic protein which runs the length of a sarcomere, holding the thick myosin filaments in place

Trabeculae the thin bony struts within spongy bone

Transamination the attachment of an amine group to an α-keto acid to form a new amino acid

Transmembrane protein a protein that spans a membrane

Transport protein a transmembrane protein which actively transports ions and large molecules into the cell

Trapezing (sailing) suspension of the body over the side of the boat while attached to the mast via a harness

Tricuspid valve a valve with three cusps between the right atrium and the right ventricle

Triglyceride a glycerol attached to three fatty acids; the long-term energy store of lipid within adipocytes

Tropomyosin a protein wrapped around the length of the actin filament

Troponin a globular protein complex bound to tropomyosin and actin; binds with calcium to uncover the myosin binding sites on the actin filament, allowing for muscular contraction

T tubules a network of tubules that originates from the infolding of the sarcolemma; encircles each myofibril at the A band/I band junction of sarcomeres, contacting the terminal cisternae of the sarcoplasmic reticulum

Unfused tetanus a rate of stimuli which increases muscle fibre tension but still allows for partial relaxation between stimuli ; also referred to as incomplete tetanus

Unipolar neuron a neuron with a joint dendrite axon process connecting with the cell body

Valency (or valence) the number of bonds an atom can form

Validity (of a test) the extent to which a test measures what it is designed to measure

Valsalva manoeuvre exhalation against a closed airway; used in a sporting context to stabilise the thoracic and abdominal cavities

Vasoconstriction the narrowing of blood vessels; a reduction in the lumen diameter

Vasodilation the widening of blood vessels; an increase in the lumen diameter

Ventilatory threshold see anaerobic threshold

Ventral root an efferent (motor) root of a spinal nerve

Ventricle an inferior chamber of the heart that receives blood from an atrium and discharges it into the systemic or pulmonary circulation

Visceral pertaining to the internal organs

Visceral pleura the inner membrane of the pleural sac which covers the lungs

Vitamin an organic compound required as a micronutrient in very small amounts, must be obtained from the diet as cannot be sufficiently synthesised by the body

Voltage the difference in electric potential between two points

Volumetric bone mineral density the ratio of bone mineral content to bone volume; expressed as g·cm^{-3}

Wave of depolarisation the movement of an action potential along an axon or a muscle fibre

Wave summation see temporal summation

White matter areas of the CNS dominated by myelinated axons

Yellow bone marrow a triglyceride store located within the medullary cavity of long bones

Z line a protein structure which forms the border of a sarcomere; a sarcomere is the region between adjacent Z lines

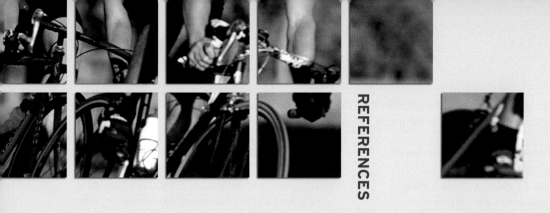

Abbiss, C. R., Peiffer, J. J., Peake, J. M., Nosaka, K., Suzuki, K., Martin, D. T., & Laursen, P. B. (2008). Effect of carbohydrate ingestion and ambient temperature on muscle fatigue development in endurance-trained male cyclists. *Journal of Applied Physiology, 104*(4), 1021-8.

Aherne, W., Ayyar, D. R., Clarke, P. A., & Walton, J. N. (1971). Muscle fibre size in normal infants, children and adolescents: An autopsy study. *Journal of the Neurological Sciences, 14*(2), 171-82.

Ahmad, C. S., Clark, A. M., Heilmann, N., Schoeb, J. S., Gardner, T. R., & Levine, W. N. (2006). Effect of gender and maturity on quadriceps-to-hamstring strength ratio and anterior cruciate ligament laxity. *American Journal of Sports Medicine, 34*(3), 370-4.

Ahmaidi, S., Granier, P., Taoutaou, Z., Mercier, J., Dubouchaud, H., & Prefaut, C. (1996). Effects of active recovery on plasma lactate and anaerobic power following repeated intensive exercise. *Medicine & Science in Sports & Exercise, 28*(4), 450-6.

Ainsworth, B. E., Serfass, R. C., & Leon, A. S. (1993). Effects of recovery duration and blood lactate level on power output during cycling. *Canadian Journal of Applied Physiology, 18*(1), 19-30.

Alberga, A. S., Sigal, R. J., & Kenny, G. P. (2011). A review of resistance exercise training in obese adolescents. *Physician and Sports Medicine, 39*(2), 50-63.

Allen, D. G., Lamb, G. D., & Westerblad, H. (2008). Impaired calcium release during fatigue. *Journal of Applied Physiology, 104*(1), 296-305.

Allison, B. (1978). A practical application of specificity in netball training. *Sports Coach, 2*(2), 9-13.

Almarwaey, O. A., Jones, A. M., & Tolfrey, K. (2004). Maximal lactate steady state in trained adolescent runners. *Journal of Sports Sciences, 22*(2), 215-25.

American Academy of Pediatrics Committee on Sports, Fitness, & Committee on School (2000). Physical fitness and activity in schools. *Pediatrics, 105*(5), 1156-7.

Amtmann, J., & Cotton, A. (2005). Strength and conditioning for judo. *Strength & Conditioning Journal, 27*(2), 26-31.

Andersen, R. E., & Montgomery, D. L. (1988). Physiology of alpine skiing. *Sports Medicine, 6*(4), 210-21.

Anderson, S. D., & Kippelen, P. (2008). Airway injury as a mechanism for exercise-induced bronchoconstriction in elite athletes. *Journal of Allergy and Clinical Immunology, 122*(2), 225-35.

Anderssen, S. A., Cooper, A. R., Riddoch, C., Sardinha, L. B., Harro, M., Brage, S., & Andersen, L. B. (2007). Low cardiorespiratory fitness is a strong predictor for clustering of cardiovascular disease risk factors in children independent of country, age and sex. *Journal of Cardiovascular Risk, 14*(4), 526-31.

Andersson, J., Schagatay, E., Gislén, A., & Holm, B. (2000). Cardiovascular responses to cold-water immersions of the forearm and face, and their relationship to apnoea. *European Journal of Applied Physiology, 83*(6), 566-72.

Andreoli, A., Monteleone, M., Van Loan, M., Promenzio, L., Tarantino, U., & De Lorenzo, A. (2001). Effects of different sports on bone density and muscle mass in highly trained athletes. *Medicine & Science in Sports & Exercise, 33*(4), 507-11.

Anton, M. M., Spirduso, W. W., & Tanaka, H. (2004). Age-related declines in anaerobic muscular performance: weightlifting and powerlifting. *Medicine & Science in Sports & Exercise, 36*(1), 143-7.

Aoyagi, Y., & Shephard, R. J. (2011). A model to estimate the potential for a physical activity-induced reduction in healthcare costs for the elderly, based on pedometer accelerometer data from the Nakanojo study. *Sports Medicine, 41*(9), 695-708.

Araneda, O. F., García, C., Lagos, N., Quiroga, G., Cajigal, J., Salazar, M. P., & Behn, C. (2005). Lung oxidative stress as related to exercise and altitude. Lipid peroxidation evidence in exhaled breath condensate: a possible predictor of acute mountain sickness. *European Journal of Applied Physiology, 95*(5), 383-90.

Argus, C. K., Gill, N. D., Keogh, J. W. L., Hopkins, W. G., & Beaven, C. M. (2009). Changes in strength, power, and steroid hormones during a professional rugby union competition. *Journal of Strength & Conditioning Research, 23*(5), 1583-92.

Ariel, G., & Saville, W. (1972). Anabolic steroids: the physiological effects of placebos. *Medicine & Science in Sports & Exercise, 4*(2), 124-6.

Armstrong, L. E. (2000). *Performing in extreme environments.* Champaign, ILL: Human Kinetics.

Armstrong, L. E., Costill, D. L., & Fink, W. J. (1985). Influence of diuretic-induced dehydration on competitive running performance. *Medicine & Science in Sports & Exercise, 17*(4), 456-61.

Armstrong, N., & Barker, A. (2011). Endurance Training and Elite Young Athletes. *The Elite Young Athlete, 56,* 59-83.

Armstrong, N., & McManus, A. M. (2010). *The Elite Young Athlete* (Vol. 56). Basel, Switzerland: Karger Publishers.

Armstrong, N., Tomkinson, G., & Ekelund, U. (2011). Aerobic fitness and its relationship to sport, exercise training and habitual physical activity during youth. *British Journal of Sports Medicine, 45*(11), 849-58.

Armstrong, N., & Welsman, J. (2001). Peak oxygen uptake in relation to growth and maturation in 11-to 17-year-old humans. *European Journal of Applied Physiology, 85*(6), 546-51.

Armstrong, N., & Welsman, J. (2007). Aerobic fitness: what are we measuring? *Medicine and Sport Science, 50*(R), 5-25.

Armstrong, N., & Welsman, J. R. (1994). Assessment arid interpretation of aerobic fitness in children and adolescents. *Exercise and Sport Sciences Reviews, 22*(1), 435-76.

Armstrong, N., & Welsman, J. R. (2000). Development of aerobic fitness during childhood and Adolescence. *Pediatric Exercise Science, 12*(2), 128-44.

Armstrong, N., Welsman, J. R., & Chia, M. Y. H. (2001). Short term power output in relation to growth and maturation. *British Journal of Sports Medicine, 35*(2), 118-24.

Armstrong, N., Welsman, J. R., Williams, C. A., & Kirby, B. J. (2000). Longitudinal changes in young people's short-term power output. *Medicine & Science in Sports & Exercise, 32*(6), 1140-5.

Ashcroft, F. M. (2001). *Life at the extremes: the science of survival.* London: Flamingo.

Astrand, P., & Rodahl, K. (1986). *Textbook of work physiology: Physiological basis of exercise.* New York: McGraw-Hill.

Åstrand, P. O. (2003). *Textbook of work physiology: physiological bases of exercise.* Champaign, ILL: Human Kinetics.

Atkin, A. J., Gorely, T., Biddle, S. J., Marshall, S. J., & Cameron, N. (2008). Critical hours: physical activity and sedentary behavior of adolescents after school. *Pediatric Exercise Science, 20*(4), 446.

Ayalon, A., Inbar, O., & Bar-Or, O. (1974). Relationships among measurements of explosive strength and anaerobic power. In M. Nelson RC, CA (Ed.), *Biomechanics IV. Int. Series in Sports Sci* (Vol. 1, pp. 572-7).

Baechle, T. R., Earle, R. W. (2000). *Essentials of strength training and conditioning.* Champaign, ILL: Human Kinetics.

Bailey, D. M., & Davies, B. (2001). Acute mountain sickness; prophylactic benefits of antioxidant vitamin supplementation at high altitude. *High Altitude Medicine & Biology, 2*(1), 21-9.

Baker, S., & Atha, J. (1981). Canoeists' disorientation following cold immersion. *British Journal of Sports Medicine, 15*(2), 111-5.

Baldari, C., Videira, M., Madeira, F., Sergio, J., & Guidetti, L. (2005). Blood lactate removal during recovery at various intensities below the individual anaerobic threshold in triathletes. *Journal of Sports Medicine and Physical Fitness, 45*(4), 460-6.

Balsom, P. D., Ekblom, B., Söerlund, K., Sjödln, B., & Hultman, E. (1993). Creatine supplementation and dynamic high-intensity intermittent exercise. *Scandinavian Journal of Medicine & Science in Sports, 3*(3), 143-9.

Baltaci, G., & Ergun, N. (1997). Maximal oxygen uptake in well-trained and untrained 9-11 year-old children. *Developmental Neurorehabilitation, 1*(3), 159-62.

Balyi, I. (1996). Long-term planning of athlete development phase. *British Columbia Coach, 1,* 9-14.

Balyi, I., & Hamilton, A. (1998). Long-term planning can make a difference. *Soccer Journal, 43*(4), 18-23.

Balyi, I., & Way, R. (1995). Long-term planning of athlete development: 'the training to train phase'. *BC Coach,* 1-8.

Bampouras, T. M., & Marrin, K. (2009). Comparison of two anaerobic water polo-specific tests with the Wingate test. *Journal of Strength & Conditioning Research, 23*(1), 336-40.

Bangsbo, J. (2003). 4 Physiology of training. *Science and Soccer,* 47.

Bangsbo, J., Graham, T., Johansen, L., & Saltin, B. (1994). Muscle lactate metabolism in recovery from intense exhaustive exercise: impact of light exercise. *Journal of Applied Physiology, 77*(4), 1890-5.

Bangsbo, J., Iaia, F. M., & Krustrup, P. (2007). Metabolic response and fatigue in soccer. *International Journal of Sports Physiology and Performance, 2*(2), 111-27.

Bangsbo, J., Iaia, F. M., & Krustrup, P. (2008). The Yo-Yo intermittent recovery test: a useful tool for evaluation of physical performance in intermittent sports. *Sports Medicine, 38*(1), 37-51.

Bangsbo, J., Mohr, M., & Krustrup, P. (2006). Physical and metabolic demands of training and match-play in the elite football player. *Journal of Sports Sciences, 24*(07), 665-74.

Baptista, F., Barrigas, C., Vieira, F., Santa-Clara, H., Homens, P., Fragoso, I., Teixeira, P. & Sardinha, L. (2011). The role of lean body mass and physical activity in bone health in children. *Journal of Bone and Mineral Metabolism,* 1-9. doi: 10.1007/s00774-011-0294-4

Bar-Or, O. (1983). *Pediatric sports medicine for the practitioner: from physiologic principles to clinical applications.* Berlin, Germany: Springer Verlag.

Bar-Or, O., & Rowland, T. W. (2004). *Pediatric exercise medicine: from physiologic principles to health care application.* Champaign, ILL: Human Kinetics.

Baron, R. (2001). Aerobic and anaerobic power characteristics of off-road cyclists. *Medicine & Science in Sports & Exercise, 33*(8), 1387-93.

Bartsch, P., Bailey, D. M., Berger, M. M., Knauth, M., & Baumgartner, R. W. (2004). Acute mountain sickness: controversies and advances. *High Altitude Medicine & Biology, 5*(2), 110-24.

Bass, S., Pearce, G., Bradney, M., Hendrich, E., Delmas, P. D., Harding, A., & Seeman, E. (1998). Exercise before puberty may confer residual benefits in bone density in adulthood: studies in active prepubertal and retired female gymnasts. *Journal of Bone and Mineral Research, 13*(3), 500-7.

Bassa, E., Patikas, D., & Kotzaminidis, C. (2005). Activation of antagonist knee muscles during isokinetic efforts in prepubertal and adult males. *Pediatric Exercise Science, 17*(2), 171-81.

Baxter-Jones, A. D. G., Maffulli, N., & Mirwald, R. L. (2003). Does elite competition inhibit growth and delay maturation in some gymnasts? Probably not. *Pediatric Exercise Science, 15*(4), 373-82.

Beaver, W. L., Wasserman, K., & Whipp, B. J. (1985). Improved detection of lactate threshold during exercise using a log-log transformation. *Journal of Applied Physiology, 59*(6), 1936-40.

Beaver, W. L., Wasserman, K., & Whipp, B. J. (1986). A new method for detecting anaerobic threshold by gas exchange. *Journal of Applied Physiology, 60*(6), 2020-7.

Behm, D. G., Faigenbaum, A. D., Falk, B., & Klentrou, P. (2008). Canadian Society for Exercise Physiology position paper: resistance training in children and adolescents. *Applied Physiology, Nutrition and Metabolism, 33*(3), 547-61.

Behringer, M., Vom Heede, A., Matthews, M., & Mester, J. (2011). Effects of strength training on motor performance skills in children and adolescents: a meta-analysis. *Pediatric Exercise Science, 23*(2), 186-206.

Behringer, M., Vom Heede, A., Yue, Z., & Mester, J. (2010). Effects of resistance training in children and adolescents: a meta-analysis. *Pediatrics, 126*(5), e1199-1210.

Belanger, A. Y., & McComas, A. J. (1989). Contractile properties of human skeletal muscle in childhood and adolescence. *European Journal of Applied Physiology and Occupational Physiology, 58*(6), 563-7.

Belcastro, A. N., & Bonen, A. (1975). Lactic acid removal rates during controlled and uncontrolled recovery exercise. *Journal of Applied Physiology, 39*(6), 932-6.

Bellomo, R. (2002). Bench-to-bedside review: lactate and the kidney. *Critical Care, 6*(4), 322-6.

Benefice, E., Mercier, J., Guerin, M. J., & Prefaut, C. (1990). Differences in aerobic and antropometric characteristics between peripubertal swimmer and no swimmers. *International Journal of Sports Medicine, 11*(6), 456-60.

Bencke J., Damsgaard R., Saekmose A., Jørgensen P., Jørgensen K., Klausen K. (2002). Anaerobic power and muscle strength characteristics of 11 years old elite and non-elite boys and girls from gymnastics, team handball, tennis and swimming.

Scandinavian Journal of Medicine in Science and Sports, 12(3), 171-8.

Beneke, R. (1995). Anaerobic threshold, individual anaerobic threshold, and maximal lactate steady state in rowing. *Medicine & Science in Sports & Exercise, 27*(6), 863.

Beneke, R., Heck, H., Hebestreit, H., & Leithäuser, R. M. (2009). Predicting maximal lactate steady state in children and adults. *Pediatric Exercise Science, 21*(4), 493-505.

Berg, A., & Keul, J. (1988). Biochemical changes during exercise in children. *Young Athletes: A Biological, Psychological and Educational Perspective.* Champaign, ILL: Human Kinetics, 61-7.

Berg, J. M., Tymoczko, J. L., & Stryer, L. (2010). *Biochemistry.* New York: W. H. Freeman.

Bergh, U., & United States Ski, T. (1982). *Physiology of cross-country ski racing.* Champaign, IL: Human Kinetics.

Bergh, U. L. F. (1987). The influence of body mass in cross-country skiing. *Medicine & Science in Sports & Exercise, 19*(4), 324-31.

Bergman, B. C., Wolfel, E. E., Butterfield, G. E., Lopaschuk, G. D., Casazza, G. A., Horning, M. A., & Brooks, G. A. (1999). Active muscle and whole body lactate kinetics after endurance training in men. *Journal of Applied Physiology, 87*(5), 1684-96.

Bergström, J., Hermansen, L., Hultman, E., & Saltin, B. (1967). Diet, muscle glycogen and physical performance. *Acta Physiologica Scandinavica, 71*(2-3), 140-50.

Bergström, J., & Hultman, E. (1966). Muscle glycogen synthesis after exercise: an enhancing factor localized to the muscle cells in man. *Nature, 210*(5033), 309-10.

Berntsen, S., Wisløff, T., Nafstad, P., & Nystad, W. (2008). Lung function increases with increasing level of physical activity in school children. *Pediatric Exercise Science, 20*(4), 402-10.

Bhasin S., Woodhouse L., and Storer T. W. (2001). Proof of the effect of testosterone on skeletal muscle. *Journal of Endocrinology, 170*(1), 27-38. Review.

Billat, V., Palleja, P., Charlaix, T., Rizzardo, P., & Janel, N. (1995). Energy specificity of rock climbing and aerobic capacity in competitive sport rock climbers. *Journal of Sports Medicine and Physical Fitness, 35*(1), 20-24.

Billaut, F., & Bishop, D. (2009). Muscle fatigue in males and females during multiple-sprint exercise. *Sports Medicine, 39*(4), 257-78.

Bird, S., George, M., Balmer, J., & Davison, R. C. R. (2003). Heart rate responses of women aged 23-67 years during competitive orienteering. *British Journal of Sports Medicine, 37*(3), 254-7.

Bisciotti, N. G., Sagnol, J. M., & Filaire, E. (2000). Aspetti bioenergetici della corsa frazionata nel calcio. *Scuola Dello Sport 50*, 21-7.

Bishop, D. (2000). Physiological predictors of flat-water kayak performance in women. *European Journal of Applied Physiology, 82*(1), 91-7.

Bishop, D. (2003a). Warm up I: potential mechanisms and the effects of passive warm up on exercise performance. *Sports Medicine, 33*(6), 439-54.

Bishop, D. (2003b). Warm up II: performance changes following active warm up and how to structure the warm up. *Sports Medicine, 33*(7), 483-98.

Bishop, D. (2004). The validity of physiological variables to assess training intensity in kayak athletes. *International Journal of Sports Medicine, 25*(1), 68-72.

Bishop, D., Bonetti, D., & Dawson, B. (2001). The effect of three different warm-up intensities on kayak ergometer performance. *Medicine & Science in Sports & Exercise, 33*(6), 1026-32.

Bishop, D., & Claudius, B. (2005). Effects of induced metabolic alkalosis on prolonged intermittent-sprint performance. *Medicine & Science in Sports & Exercise, 37*(5), 759-67.

Bishop, D., Ruch, N., & Paun, V. (2007). Effects of active versus passive recovery on thermoregulatory strain and performance in intermittent-sprint exercise. *Medicine & Science in Sports & Exercise, 39*(5), 872-9.

Bishop, D. C., Smith, R. J., Smith, M. F., & Rigby, H. E. (2009). Effect of plyometric training on swimming block start performance in adolescents. *Journal of Strength & Conditioning Research, 23*(7), 2137-43.

Bishop, P., Smith, J., Kime, J., Mayo, J., & Tin, Y. (1992). Comparison of a manual and an automated enzymatic technique for determining blood lactate concentrations. *International Journal of Sports Medicine 13*(1), 36-9.

Blimkie, C. J. (1992). Resistance training during pre-and early puberty: efficacy, trainability, mechanisms, and persistence. *Canadian Journal of Sport Sciences / Journal canadien des sciences du sport, 17*(4), 264-79.

Blimkie, C. J. (1993). Resistance training during preadolescence. Issues and controversies. *Sports Medicine, 15*(6), 389-407.

Blimkie, C. J. R. (1989). Age-and sex-associated variation in strength during childhood: anthropometric, morphologic, neurologic, biomechanical, endocrinologic, genetic, and physical activity correlates. *Perspectives in Exercise Science and Sports Medicine, 2*, 99-163.

Blimkie, C. J. R., Roache, P., Hay, J. T., & Bar-Or, O. (1988). Anaerobic power of arms in teenage boys and girls: relationship to lean tissue. *European Journal of Applied Physiology and Occupational Physiology, 57*(6), 677-83.

Bloomfield, J., Fricker, P. A., & Fitch, K. D. (eds.) (1995). *Science and medicine in sport.* Chichester, UK: Blackwell.

Bogdanis, G. C., Nevill, M. E., Lakomy, H. K. A., Graham, C. M., & Louis, G. (1996). Effects of active recovery on power output during repeated maximal sprint cycling. *European Journal of Applied Physiology and Occupational Physiology, 74*(5), 461-9.

Bonini, S., & Craig, T. (2008). The elite athlete: Yes, with allergy we can. *Journal of Allergy and Clinical Immunology, 122*(2), 249-50.

Boot, A. M., de Ridder, M. A. J., Pols, H. A. P., Krenning, E. P., & de Muinck Keizer-Schrama, S. M. P. F. (1997). Bone mineral density in children and adolescents: relation to puberty, calcium intake, and physical activity. *Journal of Clinical Endocrinology & Metabolism, 82*(1), 57-62. doi: 10.1210/jc.82.1.57

Booth, J., Marino, F., Hill, C., & Gwinn, T. (1999). Energy cost of sport rock climbing in elite performers. *British Journal of Sports Medicine, 33*(1), 14-18.

Borer, K. T. (2003). *Exercise endocrinology.* Champaign, ILL: Human Kinetics.

Bosquet, L., Léger, L., & Legros, P. (2002). Methods to determine aerobic endurance. *Sports Medicine, 32*(11), 675-700.

Bouchard, C., Lesage, R., Lortie, G., Simoneau, J. A., Hamel, P., Boulay, M. R., Perusse, L., Theriault, G., & Leblanc, C. (1986). Aerobic performance in brothers, dizygotic and monozygotic twins. *Medicine & Science in Sports & Exercise, 18*(6), 639-46.

Bouchard, C., Malina, R. M., Hollmann, W., & Leblanc, C. (1977). Submaximal working capacity, heart size and body size in boys 8-18 years. *European Journal of Applied Physiology and Occupational Physiology, 36*(2), 115-26.

Bouchard, C., & Rankinen, T. (2001). Individual differences in response to regular physical activity. *Medicine & Science in Sports & Exercise, 33*(6), S446-S451.

Bouhlel, E., Chelly, M. S., Tabka, Z., & Shephard, R. (2007). Relationships between maximal anaerobic power of the arms and legs and javelin performance. *Journal of Sports Medicine and Physical Fitness, 47*(2), 141-46.

Boutcher, S. H. (2011). High-Intensity intermittent exercise and fat loss. *Journal of Obesity, 2011.*

Bowden, D. H., & Goyer, R. A. (1960). The size of muscle fibers in infants and children. *Archives of Pathology, 69*, 188-9.

Boyle, R., & Hall, M. B. (1965). *Robert Boyle on natural philosophy: an essay, with selections from his writings.* Indiana University Press.

Bradley, P. S., Mohr, M., Bendiksen, M., Randers, M. B., Flindt, M., Barnes, C., Hood, P., Gomez, A., Andersen, J. L., & Di Mascio, M. (2011). Sub-maximal and maximal Yo-Yo intermittent endurance test level 2: heart rate response, reproducibility and application to elite soccer. *European Journal of Applied Physiology*, 1-10.

Bradwell, A. R., & Coote, J. H. (1987). The BMRES 1984 Medical Research Expedition to the Himalayas. *Postgraduate Medical Journal, 63*(737), 165-7.

Brannan, J. D., & Turton, J. A. (2010). The inflammatory basis of exercise-induced bronchoconstriction. *Physician and Sportsmedicine, 38*(4), 67-73.

Bray, J. J. (1999). *Lecture notes on human physiology.* Chichester, UK: Wiley-Blackwell.

Bredeweg, S. (2003). The elite volleyball athlete. *Handbook of Sports Medicine and Science: Volleyball*, 183-91.

Brewer, J., & Davis, J. (1995). Applied physiology of rugby league. *Sports Medicine, 20*(3), 129-35.

Brickley, G., Doust, J., & Williams, C. (2002). Physiological responses during exercise to exhaustion at critical power. *European Journal of Applied Physiology, 88*(1), 146-51.

Briner, W. W. (1996). Tympanic membrane vs rectal temperature measurement in marathon runners. *JAMA: the journal of the American Medical Association, 276*(3), 194.

Brolinson, P. G., & Elliott, D. (2007). Exercise and the immune system. *Clinics in Sports Medicine, 26*(3), 311-9.

Brooks, G. A. (1985). Anaerobic threshold: review of the concept and directions for future research. *Medicine & Science in Sports & Exercise, 17*(1), 22-34.

Brooks, G. A., Dubouchaud, H., Brown, M., Sicurello, J. P., & Butz, C. E. (1999). Role of mitochondrial lactate dehydrogenase and lactate oxidation in the intracellular lactate shuttle. *Proceedings of the National Academy of Sciences, 96*(3), 1129-34.

Brooks, G. A., Fahey, T. D., & Baldwin, K. M. (2005). *Exercise physiology: human bioenergetics and its applications.* New York: McGraw-Hill.

Brooks, G. A., Hittelman, K. J., Faulkner, J. A., Beyer, R. E. (1971) Temperature, liver mitochondrial respiratory functions, and oxygen debt. *Medicine and Science in Sports 3*(2), 72-74.

Bruce-Low, S., & Smith, D. (2007). Explosive exercises in sports training: a critical review. *Journal of Exercise Physiology-online, 10*(1), 21-33.

Buchheit, M. (2008). The 30-15 intermittent fitness test: accuracy for individualizing interval training of young intermittent sport players. *Journal of Strength & Conditioning Research, 22*(2), 365-74.

Buchheit, M., Al Haddad, H., Chivot, A., Leprêtre, P. M., Ahmaidi, S., & Laursen, P. B. (2010). Effect of in-versus out-of-water recovery on repeated swimming sprint performance. *European Journal of Applied Physiology, 108*(2), 321-7.

Bull, A. J., Housh, T. J., Johnson, G. O., & Rana, S. R. (2008). Physiological responses at five estimates of critical velocity. *European Journal of Applied Physiology, 102*(6), 711-20.

Bunc, V., & Heller, J. (1994). Ventilatory threshold and work efficiency during exercise on cycle and paddling ergometers in young female kayakists. *European Journal of Applied Physiology and Occupational Physiology, 68*(1), 25-9.

Bunta, A. D. (2011). It is time for everyone to own the bone. *Osteoporosis International, 22*, 477-82.

Bunting, C. J., Tolson, H., Kuhn, C., Suarez, E., & Williams, R. B. (2000). Physiological stress response of the neuroendocrine system during outdoor adventure tasks. *Journal of Leisure Research, 32*(2), 191-207.

Burgomaster K. A., Howarth K. R., Phillips S. M., Rakobowchuk M., Macdonald M. J., McGee S. L., Gibala M. J. (2008). Similar metabolic adaptations during exercise after low volume sprint interval and traditional endurance training in humans. *Journal of Physiology, 586*(1), 151-60.

Burke, D. G., MacNeil, S. A., Holt, L. E., Mackinnon, N. C., & Rasmussen, R. O. Y. L. (2000). The effect of hot or cold water immersion on isometric strength training. *Journal of Strength & Conditioning Research, 14*(1), 21-5.

Burnley, M., Doust, J. H., & Jones, A. M. (2005). Effects of prior warm-up regime on severe-intensity cycling performance. *Medicine & Science in Sports & Exercise, 37*(5), 838-45.

Burr, J. F., Jamnik, R. K., Baker, J., Macpherson, A., Gledhill, N., & McGuire, E. J. (2008). Relationship of physical fitness test results and hockey playing potential in elite-level ice hockey players. *Journal of Strength & Conditioning Research, 22*(5), 1535-43.

Butterfield, S. A., Lehnhard, R. A., Loovis, E. M., Coladarci, T., & Saucier, D. (2009). Grip strength performances by 5-to 19-year-olds. *Perceptual and Motor Skills, 109*(2), 362-70.

Butterfield, S. A., Lehnhard, R. A., Mason, C. A., & McCormick, R. (2008). Aerobic performance by children in grades 4 to 8: a repeated-measures study. *Perceptual and Motor Skills, 107*(3), 775-90.

Byrne, A. P. H. N. M. (2010). An overview of physical growth and maturation. *Cytokines, Growth Mediators and Physical Activity in Children During Puberty, 55*, 1-13.

Byrnes, W. C., & Kearney, J. T. (1997). Aerobic and anaerobic contributions during simulated canoe/kayak sprint events 1256. *Medicine & Science in Sports & Exercise, 29*(5), 220.

Cabello Manrique, D., & González-Badillo, J. J. (2003). Analysis of the characteristics of competitive badminton. *British Journal of Sports Medicine, 37*(1), 62.

Caine, D., Lewis, R., O'Connor, P., Howe, W., & Bass, S. (2001). Does gymnastics training inhibit growth of females? *Clinical Journal of Sport Medicine, 11*(4), 260-70.

Calbet, J. A. L., Dorado, C., Diaz-Herrera, P., & Rodriguez-Rodriguez, L. P. (2001). High femoral bone mineral content and density in male football (soccer) players. *Medicine & Science in Sports & Exercise, 33*(10), 1682-7.

Campbell, B., Roberts, M., Kerksick, C., Wilborn, C., Marcello, B., Taylor, L., Nassar, E., Leutholtz, B., Bowden, R., & Rasmussen, C. (2006). Pharmacokinetics, safety, and effects on exercise performance of l-arginine [alpha]-ketoglutarate in trained adult men. *Nutrition, 22*(9), 872-81.

Carling, C., Le Gall, F., Reilly, T., & Williams, A. M. (2009). Do anthropometric and fitness characteristics vary according to birth date distribution in elite youth academy soccer players? *Scandinavian Journal of Medicine & Science in Sports, 19*(1), 3-9.

Carlsen, K. H., & Kowalski, M. L. (2008). Asthma, allergy, the athlete and the Olympics. *Allergy, 63*(4), 383-6.

Carranza-García, L. E., George, K., Serrano-Ostáriz, E., Casado-Arroyo, R., Caballero-Navarro, A. L., & Legaz-Arrese, A. (2011). Cardiac biomarker response to intermittent exercise bouts. *International Journal of Sports Medicine, 32*(5), 327-31.

Casajus, J. A. (2001). Seasonal variation in fitness variables in professional soccer players. *Journal of Sports Medicine and Physical Fitness, 41*(4), 463-9.

Casas, A. (2008). Physiology and methodology of intermittent resistance training for acyclic sports. *Journal of Human Sport and Exercise, 3*(1), 23-52.

Casey, A., Constantin-Teodosiu, D., Howell, S., Hultman, E., & Greenhaff, P. L. (1996). Creatine ingestion favorably affects performance and muscle metabolism during maximal exercise in humans. *American Journal of Physiology-Endocrinology And Metabolism, 271*(1), E31-E37.

Castagna O., Brisswalter J. (2007). Assessment of energy demand in Laser sailing: influences of exercise duration and performance level. *European Journal of Applied Physiology, 99*(2), 95-101.

Castagna, C., Impellizzeri, F. M., Rampinini, E., D'Ottavio, S., & Manzi, V. (2008). The Yo-Yo intermittent recovery test in basketball players. *Journal of Science and Medicine in Sport, 11*(2), 202-8.

Cavanagh, P. R., & Komi, P. V. (1979). Electromechanical delay in human skeletal muscle under concentric and eccentric contractions. *European Journal of Applied Physiology and Occupational Physiology, 42*(3), 159-63.

Cè, E., Margonato, V., Casasco, M., & Veicsteinas, A. (2008). Effects of stretching on maximal anaerobic power: the roles of active and passive warm-ups. *Journal of Strength & Conditioning Research, 22*(3), 794-800.

Cerny, F. J., & Burton, H. (2001). *Exercise physiology for health care professionals.* Champaign, ILL: Human Kinetics.

Chamari, K., Chaouachi, A., Hambli, M., Kaouech, F., Wisløff, U., & Castagna, C. (2008). The five-jump test for distance as a field test to assess lower limb explosive power in soccer players. *Journal of Strength & Conditioning Research, 22*(3), 944-50.

Chaouachi, A., Manzi, V., Wong, D. P., Chaalali, A., Laurencelle, L., Chamari, K., & Castagna, C. (2010). Intermittent endurance and repeated sprint ability in soccer players. *Journal of Strength & Conditioning Research, 24*(10), 2663-9.

Chatagnon, M., Pouilly, J. P., Thomas, V., & Busso, T. (2005). Comparison between maximal power in the power-endurance relationship and maximal instantaneous power. *European Journal of Applied Physiology, 94*(5), 711-7.

Chatterjee, P., Banerjee, A. K., & Majumdar, P. (2006). Energy expenditure in women boxing. *Kathmandu University Medical Journal (KUMJ), 4*(3), 319-23.

Chelly, M. S., Hermassi, S., & Shephard, R. J. (2010). Relationships between Power and Strength of the Upper and Lower Limb Muscles and Throwing Velocity in Male Handball Players. *Journal of Strength & Conditioning Research, 24*(6), 1480-7.

Cheng, B., Kuipers, H., Snyder, A. C., Keizer, H. A., Jeukendrup, A., & Hesselink, M. (1992). A new approach for the determination of ventilatory and lactate thresholds. *International Journal of Sports Medicine, 13*, 518-22.

Chin, M. K., Steininger, K., So, R. C., Clark, C. R., & Wong, A. S. (1995). Physiological profiles and sport specific fitness of Asian elite squash players. *British Journal of Sports Medicine, 29*(3), 158-164.

Chin, M. K., Wong, A. S., So, R. C., Siu, O. T., Steininger, K., & Lo, D. T. (1995). Sport specific fitness testing of elite badminton players. *British Journal of Sports Medicine, 29*(3), 153-7.

Church, J. B., Wiggins, M. S., Moode, F. M., & Crist, R. (2001). Effect of warm-up and flexibility treatments on vertical jump performance. *Journal of Strength and Conditioning Research, 15*(3), 332-6.

Clayton, P. (2001). *Health Defence.* Aylesbury, UK: Accelerated Learning Systems.

Close, G. L., Kayani, A., Vasilaki, A., & McArdle, A. (2005). Skeletal muscle damage with exercise and aging. *Sports Medicine, 35*(5), 413-27.

Cohen, R. C. R., Mitchell, C. M. C., Dotan, R. D. R., Gabriel, D. G. D., Klentrou, P. K. P., & Falk, B. F. B. (2010). Do neuromuscular adaptations occur in endurance-trained boys and men? *Applied Physiology, Nutrition, and Metabolism, 35*(4), 471-9.

Cole, J., Kanaley, J., & Gero, N. (2005). Increased bone accrual in premenarcheal gymnasts: a longitudinal study. *Pediatric Exercise Science, 17*(2), 149-60.

Collet, C., Guillot, A., Lebon, F., MacIntyre, T., & Moran, A. (2011). Measuring motor imagery using psychometric, behavioral, and psychophysiological tools. *Exercise and Sport Sciences Reviews, 39*(2), 85-92.

Colling-Saltin, A. S. (1980). Skeletal muscle development in the human fetus and during childhood. *Children and Exercise, 9*, 193-207.

Connolly, D. A. J. (2002). The energy expenditure of snow-shoeing in packed vs. unpacked snow at low-level walking speeds. *Journal of Strength & Conditioning Research, 16*(4), 606-10.

Connolly, D. A. J., Brennan, K. M., & Lauzon, C. D. (2003). Effects of active versus passive recovery on power output during repeated bouts of short term, high intensity exercise. *Journal of Sports Science and Medicine, 2*(2), 47-51.

Connolly, D. A. J., Sayers, S. P., & McHugh, M. P. (2003). Treatment and prevention of delayed onset muscle soreness. *Journal of Strength and Conditioning Research, 17*(1), 197-208.

Cook, P., Jones, T. A., & Webb, B. (1977). *The Complete Book of Sailing.* New York: Doubleday.

Corbin, C. B., & Noble, L. (1980). Flexibility: a major component of physical fitness. *Journal of Physical Education and Recreation, 51*(6), 23-60.

Corder, K. P., Potteiger, J. A., Nau, K. L., Figoni, S. E., & Hershberger, S. L. (2000). Effects of active and passive recovery conditions on blood lactate, rating of perceived exertion, and performance during resistance exercise. *Journal of Strength & Conditioning Research, 14*(2), 151-6.

Cormack, S. J., Newton, R. U., McGuigan, M. R., & Cormie, P. (2008). Neuromuscular and endocrine responses of elite players during an Australian rules football season. *International Journal of Sports Physiology and Performance, 3*(4), 439-53.

Cormie, P., McBride, J. M., & McCaulley, G. O. (2008). Power-time, force-time, and velocity-time curve analysis during the jump squat: impact of load. *Journal of Applied Biomechanics, 24*(2), 112-20.

Cormie, P., McCaulley, G. O., & McBride, J. M. (2007). Power versus strength-power jump squat training: influence on the load-power relationship. *Medicine & Science in Sports & Exercise, 39*(6), 996-1003.

Cormie, P., McGuigan, M. R., & Newton, R. U. (2011a). Developing Maximal Neuromuscular Power: Part 1 Biological Basis of Maximal Power Production. *Sports Medicine, 41*(1), 17-38.

Cormie, P., McGuigan, M. R., & Newton, R. U. (2011b). Developing maximal neuromuscular power: Part 2 Training considerations for improving maximal power production. *Sports Medicine, 41*(2), 125-46.

Costill, D. L., Dalsky, G. P., & Fink, W. J. (1978). Effects of caffeine ingestion on metabolism and exercise performance. *Medicine & Science in Sports & Exercise, 10*(3), 155-58.

Costill, D. L., Verstappen, F., Kuipers, H., Janssen, E., & Fink, W. (1984). Acid-base balance during repeated bouts of exercise: influence of HCO_3. *International Journal of Sports Medicine, 5*(5), 228-31.

Couillard, C., Despres, J. P., Lamarche, B., Bergeron, J., Gagnon, J., Leon, A. S., Rao, D. C., Skinner, J. S., Wilmore, J. H., & Bouchard, C. (2001). Effects of endurance exercise training on plasma HDL cholesterol levels depend on levels of triglycerides: evidence from men of the Health, Risk Factors, Exercise Training and Genetics (HERITAGE) Family Study. *Arteriosclerosis, Thrombosis, and Vascular Biology, 21*(7), 1226-32.

Courteix, D., Lespessailles, E., Jaffre, C., Obert, P., & Benhamou, C. L. (1999). Bone mineral acquisition and somatic development in highly trained girl gymnasts. *Acta Paediatrica, 88*(8), 803-8.

Creagh, U., & Reilly, T. (1997). Physiological and biomechanical aspects of orienteering. *Sports Medicine, 24*(6), 409-18.

Crewther, B., Cronin, J., & Keogh, J. (2005). Possible stimuli for strength and power adaptation: acute mechanical responses. *Sports Medicine, 35*(11), 967-89.

Crewther, B., Cronin, J., & Keogh, J. (2006). Possible stimuli for strength and power adaptation: acute metabolic responses. *Sports Medicine, 36*(1), 65-78.

Crewther, B., Keogh, J., Cronin, J., & Cook, C. (2006). Possible stimuli for strength and power adaptation: acute hormonal responses. *Sports Medicine, 36*(3), 215-38.

Croix, M. B. A. D. S., Croix, M. B. D. S., Deighan, M. A. D. M. A., Ratel, S. R. S., & Armstrong, N. A. N. (2009). Age-and sex-associated differences in isokinetic knee muscle endurance between young children and adults. *Applied Physiology, Nutrition, and Metabolism, 34*(4), 725-31.

Cronin, J., & Sleivert, G. (2005). Challenges in understanding the influence of maximal power training on improving athletic performance. *Sports Medicine, 35*(3), 213-34.

Cronin, J. B., & Owen, G. J. (2004). Upper-body strength and power assessment in women using a chest pass. *Journal of Strength & Conditioning Research, 18*(3), 401-4.

Cular, D., Krstulovic, S., & janovic, M. T. (2011). The differences between medalists and non-medalists at the 2008 Olympic Games Taekwondo tournament. *Human Movement, 12*(2), 165-70.

Cunningham, P. (2004), The physiological demands of elite single-handed dinghy sailing. Unpublished Ph.D. thesis, University of Chichester.

Cutts, A., & Bollen, S. R. (1993). Grip strength and endurance in rock climbers. *ARCHIVE: Proceedings of the Institution of Mechanical Engineers, Part H. Journal of Engineering in Medicine 1989-1996 (vols 203-210), 207*(28), 87-92.

D'Amelio, P., Grimaldi, A., Di Bella, S., Brianza, S. Z. M., Cristofaro, M. A., Tamone, C., Giribaldi, G., Ulliers, D., Pescarmona, G. P., & Isaia, G. (2008). Estrogen deficiency increases osteoclastogenesis up-regulating T cells activity: a key mechanism in osteoporosis. *Bone, 43*(1), 92-100.

Daanen, H. A. M. (2003). Finger cold-induced vasodilation: a review. *European Journal of Applied Physiology, 89*(5), 411-26.

Danis, A., Kyriazis, Y., & Klissouras, V. (2003). The effect of training in male prepubertal and pubertal monozygotic twins. *European Journal of Applied Physiology, 89*(3), 309-18.

Darling, J. L., Linderman, J. K., & Laubach, L. L. (2005). Energy expenditure of continuous and intermittent exercise in college-aged males. *Journal of Exercise Physiology-online, 8*(4), 1-8.

Dassonville, J., Beillot, J., Lessard, Y., Jan, J., André, A. M., Le Pourcelet, C., Rochcongar, P. & Carré, F. (1998). Blood lactate concentrations during exercise: effect of sampling site and exercise mode. *Journal of Sports Medicine and Physical Fitness, 38*(1), 39-46.

Davies, C. T. M., & Young, K. (1984). Effects of external loading on short term power output in children and young male adults. *European Journal of Applied Physiology and Occupational Physiology, 52*(3), 351-4.

Davis, J. A. (1985). Anaerobic threshold: review of the concept and directions for future research. *Medicine and Science in Sports and Exercise, 17*(1), 6-21.

Davis, J. K., & Green, J. M. (2009). Caffeine and anaerobic performance: ergogenic value and mechanisms of action. *Sports Medicine, 39*(10), 813-32.

Davison, R. R., Van Someren, K. A., & Jones, A. M. (2009). Physiological monitoring of the Olympic athlete. *Journal of Sports Sciences, 27*(13), 1433-42.

Dawson, E. A., Shave, R., George, K., Whyte, G., Ball, D., Gaze, D., & Collinson, P. (2005). Cardiac drift during prolonged exercise with echocardiographic evidence of reduced diastolic function of the heart. *European Journal of Applied Physiology, 94*(3), 305-9.

De Schepper, J., De Boeck, H., & Louis, O. (1996). Measurement of radial bone mineral density and cortical thickness in children by peripheral quantitative computed tomography. *Paediatric Osteology - New Developments in Diagnostics and Therapy. Amsterdam, Elsevier*, 135-40.

De Ste Croix, M., Deighan, M. A., & Armstrong, N. (2003). Assessment and interpretation of isokinetic muscle strength during growth and maturation. *Sports Medicine, 33*(10), 727-43.

De Ste Croix M. B., Deighan M. A., Ratel S, Armstrong N. (2009). Age- and sex-associated differences in isokinetic knee muscle endurance between young children and adults. *Applied Physiology, Nutrition and Metabolism, 34*(4), 725-31.

de Villarreal, S. S., Gonzalez-Badillo, J., & Izquierdo, M. (2007). Optimal warm-up stimuli of muscle activation to enhance short and long-term acute jumping performance. *European Journal of Applied Physiology, 100*(4), 393-401.

Degoutte, F., Jouanel, P., & Filaire, E. (2003). Energy demands during a judo match and recovery. *British Journal of Sports Medicine, 37*(3), 245-9.

Dehnert, C., Hutler, M., Liu, Y., Menold, E., Netzer, C., Schick, R., Kubanek, B., Lehmann, M., Boning, D. & Steinacker, J. M. (2002). Erythropoiesis and performance after two weeks of living high and training low in well trained triathletes. *International Journal of Sports Medicine, 23*(8), 561-6.

Deighan, M., & De Ste, C. (2006). Measurement of maximal muscle cross-sectional area of the elbow extensors and flexors in children, teenagers and adults. *Journal of Sports Sciences, 24*(5), 543-6.

Dekerle, J., Baron, B., Dupont, L., Vanvelcenaher, J., & Pelayo, P. (2003). Maximal lactate steady state, respiratory compensation threshold and critical power. *European Journal of Applied Physiology, 89*(3), 281-8.

Dekerle, J., Brickley, G., Hammond, A. J. P., Pringle, J. S. M., & Carter, H. (2006). Validity of the two-parameter model in estimating the anaerobic work capacity. *European Journal of Applied Physiology, 96*(3), 257-64.

Dekerle, J., Brickley, G., Sidney, M., & Pelayo, P. (2006). Application of the critical power concept in swimming. *Portuguese Journal of Sport Sciences, 6*(2), 121-4.

Dekerle, J., Vanhatalo, A., & Burnley, M. (2008). Determination of critical power from a single test. *Science & Sports, 23*(5), 231-8.

Dekerle, J., Williams, C., McGawley, K., & Carter, H. (2009). Critical power is not attained at the end of an isokinetic 90-second all-out test in children. *Journal of Sports Sciences, 27*(4), 379-85.

Delextrat, A., & Cohen, D. (2008). Physiological testing of basketball players: Toward a standard evaluation of anaerobic fitness. *Journal of Strength & Conditioning Research, 22*(4), 1066-72.

Dellal, A., Keller, D., Carling, C., Chaouachi, A., Wong, D. P., & Chamari, K. (2010). Physiologic effects of directional changes in intermittent exercise in soccer players. *Journal of Strength & Conditioning Research, 24*(12), 3219-26.

Dencker, M., Thorsson, O., Karlsson, M. K., Lindén, C., Eiberg, S., Wollmer, P., & Andersen, L. B. (2007). Gender differences and determinants of aerobic fitness in children aged 8-11 years. *European Journal of Applied Physiology, 99*(1), 19-26.

Dencker, M., Thorsson, O., Karlsson, M. K., Lindén, C., Svensson, J., Wollmer, P., & Andersen, L. B. (2006). Daily physical activity and its relation to aerobic fitness in children aged 8-11 years. *European Journal of Applied Physiology, 96*(5), 587-92.

Department of Health of Great Britain (1991). *Dietary reference values for food energy and nutrients for the United Kingdom: report of the Panel on Dietary Reference Values of the Committee on Medical Aspects of Food Policy.* London: HMSO.

De Ste Croix M. B., Deighan M. A., Ratel S, Armstrong N. (2009). Age- and sex-associated differences in isokinetic knee muscle endurance between young children and adults. *Applied Physiology, Nutrition and Metabolism, 34*(4), 725-31.

Devienne M. F. & Guezennec, C. Y. (2000). Energy expenditure of sailing. *European Journal of Applied Physiology, 82,* 499-503.

Di Prampero, P. E. (1986). The energy cost of human locomotion on land and in water. *International Journal of Sports Medicine, 7*(2), 55-72.

Diallo, O., Dore, E., Duche, P., & Van Praagh, E. (2001). Effects of plyometric training followed by a reduced training programme on physical performance in prepubescent soccer players. *Journal of Sports Medicine and Physical Fitness, 41*(3), 342-8.

Dipla, K., Tsirini, T., Zafeiridis, A., Manou, V., Dalamitros, A., Kellis, E., & Kellis, S. (2009). Fatigue resistance during high-intensity intermittent exercise from childhood to adulthood in males and females. *European journal of applied physiology, 106*(5), 645-53.

Doherty, M., Smith, P. M., & Schroder, K. (2000). Reproducibility of the maximum accumulated oxygen deficit and run time to exhaustion during short-distance running. *Journal of Sports Sciences, 18*(5), 331-8.

Dollman, J., Olds, T. S., Esterman, A., & Kupke, T. (2010). Pedometer step guidelines in relation to weight status among 5- to 16-year-old Australians. *Pediatric Exercise Science, 22*(2), 288-300.

Doré, E., Bedu, M., & Van Praagh, E. (2008). Squat Jump Performance During Growth in Both Sexes: Comparison With Cycling Power. *Research Quarterly for Exercise and Sport, 79*(4), 517-24.

Doré, E., Martin, R., Ratel, S., Duche, P., Bedu, M., & Van Praagh, E. (2005). Gender differences in peak muscle performance during growth. *International Journal of Sports Medicine, 26*(4), 274-80.

Douris, P., McKenna, R., Madigan, K., Cesarski, B., Costiera, R., & Lu, M. (2003). Recovery of maximal isometric grip strength following cold immersion. *Journal of Strength & Conditioning Research, 17*(3), 509-13.

Doyon, K. H., Perrey, S., Abe, D., & Hughson, R. L. (2001). Field testing of VO2peak in cross-country skiers with portable breath-by-breath system. *Canadian Journal of Applied Physiology, 26*(1), 1-11.

Draper, H. H. (1977). The aboriginal Eskimo diet in modern perspective. *American Anthropologist, 79*(2), 309-16.

Draper, N., Bird, E. L., Coleman, I., & Hodgson, C. (2006). Effects of active recovery on lactate concentration, heart rate and

RPE in climbing. *Journal of Sports Science and Medicine, 5,* 97-105.

Draper, N., & Hodgson, C. (2008). *Adventure Sport Physiology.* Chichester, UK: Wiley-Blackwell.

Drobnic, F., Freixa, A., Casan, P., Sanchis, J., & Guardino, X. (1996). Assessment of chlorine exposure in swimmers during training. *Medicine & Science in Sports & Exercise, 28*(2), 271-4.

Duché, P., Falgairette, G., Bedu, M., Fellmann, N., Lac, G., Robert, A., & Coudert, J. (1992). Longitudinal approach of bio-energetic profile in boys before and during puberty. In Condert, E. and Van Praagh E. (eds.). *Pediatric work physiology methodological physiological and practical aspects. Paris: Masson,* 43-5.

Duncan, C. S., Blimkie Jr, C., Cowell, C. T., Burke, S. T., Briody, J. N., & Howman-Giles, R. (2002). Bone mineral density in adolescent female athletes: relationship to exercise type and muscle strength. *Medicine & Science in Sports & Exercise, 34*(2), 286-94.

Dupont G., Blondel N., & Berthoin S. (2003). Performance for short intermittent runs: active recovery vs. passive recovery. *European Journal of Applied Physiology, 89*(6), 548-54.

Dupont, G., & Berthoin, S. (2004). Time spent at a high percentage of VO2max for short intermittent runs: Active versus passive recovery. *Canadian Journal of Applied Physiology, 29,* S3-S16.

Dupont, G., Moalla, W., Guinhouya, C., Ahmaidi, S., & Berthoin, S. (2004). Passive versus active recovery during high-intensity intermittent exercises. *Medicine & Science in Sports & Exercise, 36*(2), 302-8.

Duthie, G., Pyne, D., & Hooper, S. (2003). Applied physiology and game analysis of rugby union. *Sports Medicine, 33*(13), 973-91.

Duthie, G., Pyne, D., & Hooper, S. (2005). Time-motion analysis of 2001 and 2002 super 12 rugby. *Journal of Sports Sciences, 23*(5), 523-30.

Duthie, G. M. (2006). A framework for the physical development of elite rugby union players. *International Journal of Sports Physiology and Performance, 1*(1), 2-13.

Eberle, S. G. (2000). *Endurance sports nutrition* (Vol. 10). Champaign, IL: Human Kinetics.

Edwards, A. M., Clark, N., & Macfadyen, A. M. (2003). Lactate and ventilatory thresholds reflect the training status of professional soccer players where maximum aerobic power is unchanged. *J Sports Sci Med, 2,* 23-9.

Edwards, R. H. T., Ekelund, L. G., Harris, R. C., Hesser, C. M., Hultman, E., Melcher, A., & Wigertz, O. (1973). Cardiorespiratory and metabolic costs of continuous and intermittent exercise in man. *Journal of Physiology, 234*(2), 481-97.

Eglin, C. M., & Tipton, M. J. (2005). Repeated cold showers as a method of habituating humans to the initial responses to cold water immersion. *European Journal of Applied Physiology, 93*(5), 624-9.

Ehrman, J. K. (2009). *Clinical Exercise Physiology.* Champaign, IL: Human Kinetics.

Eiberg, S., Froberg, K., & Hasselstrom, H. (2005). Physical Fitness as a Predictor of Cardiovascular Disease Risk Factors in 6- to 7-Year-Old Danish Children: The Copenhagen School Child Intervention Study. *Pediatric Exercise Science, 17*(2), 161-70.

Eisenman, P. A., & Golding, L. A. (1975). Comparison of effects of training on VO2 max in girls and young women. *Medicine & Science in Sports, 7*(2), 136-8.

Eisenmann, J. C., Katzmarzyk, P. T., Perusse, L., Tremblay, A., Despres, J. P., & Bouchard, C. (2005). Aerobic fitness, body mass index, and CVD risk factors among adolescents: the Quebec family study. *International Journal of Obesity, 29*(9), 1077-83.

Ekelund, U., Poortvliet, E., Nilsson, A., Yngve, A., Holmberg, A., & Sjöström, M. (2001). Physical activity in relation to aerobic fitness and body fat in 14- to 15-year-old boys and girls. *European Journal of Applied Physiology, 85*(3), 195-201.

Elferink-Gemser, M. T., Visscher, C., Van Duijn, M. A. J., & Lemmink, K. (2006). Development of the interval endurance capacity in elite and sub-elite youth field hockey players. *British Journal of Sports Medicine, 40*(4), 340-5.

Elliott, B., & Mester, J. (1998). *Training in sport: applying sport science.* Chichester, UK: J. Wiley & Sons.

English, B. (1984). *Total Telemarking.* New York: East River Publishing Company.

Eriksson, A., Forsberg, A., Nilsson, J., & Karlsson, J. (1978). Muscle strength, EMG activity, and oxygen uptake during downhill skiing. *Biomechanics IV-A. University Park Press, Baltimore,* 54-61.

Eriksson, B. O., Gollnick, P. D., & Saltin, B. (1973). Muscle metabolism and enzyme activities after training in boys 11-13 years old. *Acta Physiologica Scandinavica, 87*(4), 485-97.

Essén, B., Hagenfeldt, L., & Kaijser, L. (1977). Utilization of blood-borne and intramuscular substrates during continuous and intermittent exercise in man. *Journal of physiology, 265*(2), 489-506.

Evans, W. J., & Cannon, J. G. (1991). The metabolic effects of exercise-induced muscle damage. *Exercise and Sport Sciences Reviews, 19,* 99-125.

Faigenbaum, A., Zaichkowsky, L., Westcott, W., L, M., & Fehlandt, A. (1993). The Effects of a Twice-a-Week Strength Training Program on Children. *Pediatric Exercise Science, 5*(4), 339-446.

Faigenbaum, A. D. (2007). State of the art reviews: resistance training for children and adolescents. Are there health outcomes? *American Journal of Lifestyle Medicine, 1*(3), 190-200.

Faigenbaum, A. D., Kraemer, W. J., Blimkie, C. J., Jeffreys, I., Micheli, L. J., Nitka, M., & Rowland, T. W. (2009). Youth resistance training: updated position statement paper from the national strength and conditioning association. *Journal of Strength and Conditioning Research, 23*(5 Suppl), S60-79.

Faigenbaum, A. D., & Micheli, L. J. (1988). Youth strength training. Current Comment from the American College of Sports Medicine. *Sports Medicine Bulletin, 32*(2), 28.

Faigenbaum, A. D., & Myer, G. D. (2010a). Pediatric resistance training: benefits, concerns, and program design considerations. *Current Sports Medicine Reports, 9*(3), 161-8.

Faigenbaum, A. D., & Myer, G. D. (2010b). Resistance training among young athletes: safety, efficacy and injury prevention effects. *British Journal of Sports Medicine, 44*(1), 56-63.

Faigenbaum, A. D., Westcott, W. L., Loud, R. L., & Long, C. (1999). The effects of different resistance training protocols on muscular strength and endurance development in children. *Pediatrics, 104*(1), e5.

Falgairette, G., Bedu, M., Fellmann, N., Van-Praagh, E., & Coudert, J. (1991). Bio-energetic profile in 144 boys aged from 6 to 15 years with special reference to sexual maturation. *European Journal of Applied Physiology and Occupational Physiology, 62*(3), 151-6.

Falk, B., Braid, S., Moore, M., Yao, M., Sullivan, P., & Klentrou, N. (2010). Bone properties in child and adolescent male hockey and soccer players. *Journal of Science and Medicine in Sport, 13*(4), 387-91.

Falk, B., Brunton, L., Dotan, R., Usselman, C., Klentrou, P., & Gabriel, D. (2009). Muscle strength and contractile kinetics of isometric elbow flexion in girls and women. *Pediatric Exercise Science, 21*(3), 354-64.

Falk, B., & Dotan, R. (2006). Child-adult differences in the recovery from high-intensity exercise. *Exercise and Sport Sciences Reviews, 34*(3), 107-12.

Falk, B., & Eliakim, A. (2003). Resistance training, skeletal muscle and growth. *Pediatric Endocrinology Reviews: PER, 1*(2), 120-7.

Falk, B., Galili, Y., Zigel, L., Constantini, N., & Eliakim, A. (2007). A cumulative effect of physical training on bone strength in males. *International Journal of Sports Medicine, 28*(6), 449-455.

Falk B., and Tenenbaum G. (1996). The effectiveness of resistance training in children. A meta-analysis. *Sports Medicine, 22*(3):176-86.

Falk, B. F. B., Usselman, C. U. C., Dotan, R. D. R., Brunton, L. B. L., Klentrou, P. K. P., Shaw, J. S. J., & Gabriel, D. G. D. (2009). Child-adult differences in muscle strength and activation pattern during isometric elbow flexion and extension. *Applied Physiology, Nutrition, and Metabolism, 34*(4), 609-15.

Farrow, D., Young, W., & Bruce, L. (2005). The development of a test of reactive agility for netball: a new methodology. *Journal of Science and Medicine in Sport, 8*(1), 52-60.

Faude, O., Kerper, O., Multhaupt, M., Winter, C., Beziel, K., Junge, A., & Meyer, T. (2010). Football to tackle overweight in children. *Scandinavian Journal of Medicine and Science in Sports, 20 Suppl 1*, 103-10.

Faude, O., Meyer, T., Rosenberger, F., Fries, M., Huber, G., & Kindermann, W. (2007). Physiological characteristics of badminton match play. *European Journal of Applied Physiology, 100*(4), 479-85.

Febbraio, M. A., & Pedersen, B. K. (2005). Contraction-induced myokine production and release: is skeletal muscle an endocrine organ? *Exercise and Sport Sciences Reviews, 33*(3), 114-19.

Felici, F., Rosponi, A., Sbriccoli, P., Scarcia, M., Bazzucchi, I., & Iannattone, M. (2001). Effect of human exposure to altitude on muscle endurance during isometric contractions. *European Journal of Applied Physiology, 85*(6), 507-12.

Feliu, J., Ventura, J. L., Segura, R., Rodas, G., Riera, J., Estruch, A., Zamora, A. & Capdevila, L. (1999). Differences between lactate concentration of samples from ear lobe and the finger tip. *Journal of Physiology and Biochemistry, 55*(4), 333-9.

Ferrero, F. (2002). *The British Canoe Union Canoe and Kayak handbook*. Pesda Press.

Ferrero, F. (2006). *British Canoe Union Coaching Handbook*. Pesda Press: Caernarvon, UK.

Fiore, D. C., & Houston, J. D. (2001). Injuries in whitewater kayaking. *British Journal of Sports Medicine, 35*(4), 235-41.

Fitts, R. H. (2008). The cross-bridge cycle and skeletal muscle fatigue. *Journal of Applied Physiology, 104*(2), 551-8.

Flodgren, G., Hedelin, R., & Henriksson-Larsen, K. (1999). Bone mineral density in flatwater sprint kayakers. *Calcified Tissue International, 64*(5), 374-9.

Fogelholm, M. (2010). Physical activity, fitness and fatness: relations to mortality, morbidity and disease risk factors. A systematic review. *Obesity Reviews, 11*(3), 202-21.

Fonseca, H., Matos, M. G., Guerra, A., & Gomes Pedro, J. (2011). How much does overweight impact the adolescent developmental process? *Child: Care, Health and Development, 37*(1), 135-42.

Fonseca, R. M., De França, N. M., & Van Praagh, E. (2008). Relationship between indicators of fitness and bone density in adolescent Brazilian children. *Pediatric Exercise Science, 20*(1), 40-49.

Forsyth, J. J., & Farrally, M. R. (2000). A comparison of lactate concentration in plasma collected from the toe, ear, and fingertip after a simulated rowing exercise. *British Journal of Sports Medicine, 34*(1), 35-8.

Foskett, A., Williams, C., Boobis, L., & Tsintzas, K. (2008). Carbohydrate availability and muscle energy metabolism during intermittent running. *Medicine & Science in Sports & Exercise, 40*(1), 96-103.

Foster, M. (1970). *Lectures on the history of physiology during the sixteenth, seventeenth, and eighteenth centuries*. Mineola, NY: Dover Publications.

Fox, S. M., Naughton, J. P., & Haskell, W. L. (1971). Physical activity and the prevention of coronary heart disease. *Annals of Clinical Research, 3*(6), 404.

Fox, N. (1981). Risks in field hockey. In Reilly, T. (ed.), *Sports Fitness and Sports Injuries*. London: Faber and Faber, 112-17.

Fradkin, A. J., Zazryn, T. R., & Smoliga, J. M. (2010). Effects of warming-up on physical performance: a systematic review with meta-analysis. *Journal of Strength & Conditioning Research, 24*(1), 140–48.

Francescato, M. P., Talon, T., & Di Prampero, P. E. (1995). Energy cost and energy sources in karate. *European Journal of Applied Physiology and Occupational Physiology, 71*(4), 355–61.

Franchini, E., Nunes, A. V., Moraes, J. M., & Del Vecchio, F. B. (2007). Physical fitness and anthropometrical profile of the Brazilian male judo team. *Journal of Physiological Anthropology, 26*(2), 59–67.

Franchini, E., Vecchio, F. B. D., Matsushigue, K. A., & Artioli, G. G. (2011). Physiological profiles of elite judo athletes. *Sports Medicine, 41*(2), 147–66.

Froberg, K., & Andersen, L. B. (2005). Mini review: physical activity and fitness and its relations to cardiovascular disease risk factors in children. *International Journal of Obesity, 29*, S34–S39.

Frost, G., Dowling, J., Dyson, K., & Bar-Or, O. (1997). Cocontraction in three age groups of children during treadmill locomotion. *Journal of Electromyography and Kinesiology, 7*(3), 179–86.

Fry, R. W., & Morton, A. R. (1991). Physiological and kinanthropometric attributes of elite flatwater kayakists. *Medicine and Science in Sports and Exercise, 23*(11), 1297–301.

Fuemmeler, B. F., Pendzich, M. K., & Tercyak, K. P. (2009). Weight, dietary behavior, and physical activity in childhood and adolescence: implications for adult cancer risk. *Obesity Facts, 2*(3), 179–86.

Fukuba, Y., Miura, A., Endo, M., Kan, A., Yanagawa, K., & Whipp, B. J. (2003). The curvature constant parameter of the power-duration curve for varied-power exercise. *Medicine & Science in Sports & Exercise, 35*(8), 1413–18.

Fulbrook, P. (1993). Core temperature measurement in adults: a literature review. *Journal of Advanced Nursing, 18*(9), 1451–60.

Gabbett, T. J. (2000). Physiological and anthropometric characteristics of amateur rugby league players. *British Journal of Sports Medicine, 34*(4), 303–7.

Gabbett, T. J. (2005). Science of rugby league football: a review. *Journal of Sports Sciences, 23*(9), 961–76.

Gabbett, T. J. (2010). GPS analysis of elite women's field hockey training and competition. *Journal of Strength & Conditioning Research, 24*(5), 1321–4.

Gabbett, T. J., Jenkins, D. G., & Abernethy, B. (2010). Physiological and skill demands of 'on-side'and 'off-side' games. *Journal of Strength & Conditioning Research, 24*(11), 2979–83.

Gabbett, T. J., Kelly, J. N., & Sheppard, J. M. (2008). Speed, change of direction speed, and reactive agility of rugby league players. *Journal of Strength & Conditioning Research, 22*(1), 174–81.

Gaesser, G. A., & Angadi, S. S. (2011). High-intensity interval training for health and fitness: can less be more? *Journal of Applied Physiology*.

Gaesser, G. A., Angadi, S. S., & Sawyer, B. J. (2011). Exercise and diet, independent of weight loss, improve cardiometabolic risk profile in overweight and obese individuals. *Physician and Sports Medicine, 39*(2), 87–97.

Gaitanos, G. C., Williams, C., Boobis, L. H., & Brooks, S. (1993). Human muscle metabolism during intermittent maximal exercise. *Journal of Applied Physiology, 75*(2), 712–19.

Garber, C. E., Blissmer, B., Deschenes, M. R., Franklin, B. A., Lamonte, M. J., Lee, I., . . . Swain, D. P. (2011). American College of Sports Medicine position stand. Quantity and quality of exercise for developing and maintaining cardiorespiratory, musculoskeletal, and neuromotor fitness in apparently healthy adults: guidance for prescribing exercise. *Medicine & Science in Sports & Exercise, 43*(7), 1334–59.

García-Artero, E., Ortega, F. B., Ruiz, J. R., Mesa, J. L., Delgado, M., González-Gross, M., García-Fuentes, M., Vicente-Rodríguez, G., Gutierrez, A. & Castillo, M. J.(2007). Lipid and metabolic profiles in adolescents are affected more by physical fitness than physical activity (AVENA study). *Revista Español de Cardiología, 60*(6), 581–8.

Garrett, W. E., & Kirkendall, D. T. (2000). *Exercise and Sport Science*. Riverwoods, IL: Lippincott, Williams & Wilkins.

Genovely, H., & Stamford, B. (1982). Effects of prolonged warm-up exercise above and below anaerobic threshold on maximal performance. *European Journal of Applied Physiology and Occupational Physiology, 48*(3), 323–30. doi: 10.1007/bf00430222

Gerbert, W., & Werner, I. (2000). Blood lactate response to competitive climbing. *The Science of Climbing and Mountaineering*, 25–6.

Gero N., Cole J.,l Kanaley, J., van der Meulen, M., and Scerpella, T. (2005). Increased Bone Accrual in Premenarcheal Gymnasts: A Longitudinal Study. *Pediatric Exercise Science, 17*(2), 43–5.

Gibala, M. J., & McGee, S. L. (2008). Metabolic adaptations to short-term high-intensity interval training: a little pain for a lot of gain? *Exercise and Sport Sciences Reviews, 36*(2), 58–63.

Gibbs, J., Harrison, L. M., & Stephens, J. A. (1997). Cross-correlation analysis of motor unit activity recorded from two separate thumb muscles during development in man. *Journal of Physiology, 499*(Pt 1), 255–66.

Girard, O., Chevalier, R., Habrard, M., Sciberras, P., Hot, P., & Millet, G. P. (2007). Game analysis and energy requirements of elite squash. *Journal of Strength and Conditioning Research, 21*(3), 909–14.

Girard, O., Sciberras, P., Habrard, M., Hot, P., Chevalier, R., & Millet, G. P. (2005). Specific incremental test in elite squash players. *British Journal of Sports Medicine, 39*(12), 921–6.

Glaister, M. (2005). Multiple sprint work: physiological responses, mechanisms of fatigue and the influence of aerobic fitness. *Sports Medicine, 35*(9), 757–77.

Glenmark, B., Hedberg, G., Kaijser, L., & Jansson, E. (1994). Muscle strength from aldolescence to adulthood–relationship to muscle fibre types. *European Journal of Applied Physiology and Occupational Physiology, 68*(1), 9-19.

Goddard, D., & Neumann, U. (1994). *Performance rock climbing.* Mechanicsburg, PA: Stackpole Books.

Gökbel, H., Gül, I., Belviranl, M., & Okudan, N. (2010). The effects of coenzyme Q10 supplementation on performance during repeated bouts of supramaximal exercise in sedentary men. *Journal of Strength & Conditioning Research, 24*(1), 97-102.

Golden, F., & Tipton, M. (2002). *Essentials of sea survival.* Champaign, ILL: Human Kinetics.

Gomez-Gallego, F., Santiago, C., Gonzalez-Freire, M., Yvert, T., Muniesa, C. A., Serratosa, L., Altmae, S., Ruiz, J. R. & Lucia, A. (2009). The C allele of the AGT Met235Thr polymorphism is associated with power sports performance. *Applied Physiology, Nutrition, and Metabolism, 34*(6), 1108-11.

Gonyea, W. J. (1980). Role of exercise in inducing increases in skeletal muscle fiber number. *Journal of Applied Physiology, 48*(3), 421-6.

Gonyea, W. J., Sale, D. G., Gonyea, F. B., & Mikesky, A. (1986). Exercise induced increases in muscle fiber number. *European Journal of Applied Physiology and Occupational Physiology, 55*(2), 137-41.

Goosey-Tolfrey, V., Castle, P., & Webborn, N. (2006). Aerobic capacity and peak power output of elite quadriplegic games players. *British Journal of Sports Medicine, 40*(8), 684-87.

Gordon, B. A., Knapman, L. M., & Lubitz, L. (2010). Graduated exercise training and progressive resistance training in adolescents with chronic fatigue syndrome: a randomized controlled pilot study. *Clinical Rehabilitation, 24*(12), 1072-79.

Gore, C. J., & Australian Sports, C. (2000). *Physiological tests for elite athletes.* Champaign, ILL: Human Kinetics.

Goto, S. G. S., Naito, H. N. H., Kaneko, T. K. T., Chung, H. Y. C. H. Y., & Radák, Z. R. Z. (2007). Hormetic effects of regular exercise in aging: correlation with oxidative stress. *Applied Physiology, Nutrition, and Metabolism, 32*(5), 948-53.

Gozal, D., & Kheirandish-Gozal, L. (2009). Obesity and excessive daytime sleepiness in prepubertal children with obstructive sleep apnea. *Pediatrics, 123*(1), 13-18.

Graham, J. E., Boatwright, J. D., Hunskor, M. J., & Howell, D. A. N. C. (2003). Effect of active vs. passive recovery on repeat suicide run time. *Journal of Strength & Conditioning Research, 17*(2), 338-41.

Grant, S., Hasler, T., Davies, C., Aitchison, T. C., Wilson, J., & Whittaker, A. (2001). A comparison of the anthropometric, strength, endurance and flexibility characteristics of female elite and recreational climbers and non-climbers. *Journal of Sports Sciences, 19*(7), 499-505.

Grant, S., Hynes, V., Whittaker, A., & Aitchison, T. (1996). Anthropometric, strength, endurance and flexibility characteristics of elite and recreational climbers. *Journal of Sports Sciences, 14*(4), 301-9.

Grant, S., Shields, C., Fitzpatrick, V., Ming, L. O. H., Whitaker, A., Watt, I., & Kay, J. W. (2003). Climbing-specific finger

endurance: a comparative study of intermediate rock climbers, rowers and aerobically trained individuals. *Journal of Sports Sciences, 21*(8), 621-30.

Gray, S., & Nimmo, M. (2001). Effects of active, passive or no warm-up on metabolism and performance during high-intensity exercise. *Journal of Sports Sciences, 19*(9), 693-700.

Green, H. J., Roy, B., Grant, S., Hughson, R., Burnett, M., Otto, C., Pipe, A., Mckenzie, D. & Johnson, M. (2000). Increases in submaximal cycling efficiency mediated by altitude acclimatization. *Journal of Applied Physiology, 89*(3), 1189-97.

Green, S. (1994). A definition and systems view of anaerobic capacity. *European Journal of Applied Physiology and Occupational Physiology, 69*(2), 168-73.

Greenhaff, P. L., Casey, A., Short, A. H., Harris, R., Soderlund, K., & Hultman, E. (1993). Influence of oral creatine supplementation of muscle torque during repeated bouts of maximal voluntary exercise in man. *Clinical Science, 84*(5), 565-71.

Grodjinovsky, A., Inbar, O., Dotan, R., & Bar-Or, O. (1980). Training effect on the anaerobic performance of children as measured by the Wingate anaerobic test. *Children and Exercise IX*, 139-45.

Grosset, J. F., Mora, I., Lambertz, D., & Pérot, C. (2008). Voluntary activation of the triceps surae in prepubertal children. *Journal of Electromyography and Kinesiology, 18*(3), 455-65.

Guidetti, L., Emerenziani, G. P., Gallotta, M. C., & Baldari, C. (2007). Effect of warm up on energy cost and energy sources of a ballet dance exercise. *European Journal of Applied Physiology, 99*(3), 275-81.

Guidetti, L., Musulin, A., & Baldari, C. (2002). Physiological factors in middleweight boxing performance. *Journal of sports medicine and physical fitness, 42*(3), 309-14.

Gupta, S. (2011). Effect of strength and balance training in children with Down's syndrome: a randomized controlled trial. *Clinical Rehabilitation, 25*(5), 425-32.

Gutin, B., Stallmann-Jorgensen, I., Le, A., Johnson, M., & Dong, Y. (2011). Relations of diet and physical activity to bone mass and height in black and white adolescents. *Pediatric Reports, 3*(1), e10.

Haahtela, T., Malmberg, P., & Moreira, A. (2008). Mechanisms of asthma in Olympic athletes - practical implications. *Allergy, 63*(6), 685-94.

Haake, S. J. (2009). The impact of technology on sporting performance in Olympic sports. *Journal of Sports Sciences, 27*(13), 1421-31.

Haff, G. G., Jackson, J. R., Kawamori, N., Carlock, J. M., Hartman, M. J., Kilgore, J. L., Morris, R. T., Ramsey, M. W., Sands, W. A. & Stone, M. H. (2008). Force-time curve characteristics and hormonal alterations during an eleven-week training period in elite women weightlifters. *Journal of Strength & Conditioning Research, 22*(2), 433-46.

Hagberg, J. M., Coyle, E. F., Carroll, J. E., Miller, J. M., Martin, W. H., & Brooke, M. H. (1982). Exercise hyperventilation in patients with McArdle's disease. *Journal of Applied Physiology, 52*(4), 991-4.

Hague, D., & Hunter, D. (2006). *The self-coached climber: the guide to movement, training, performance*. Mechanicsburg, PA: Stackpole Books.

Hahn, A. G., Pang, P. M., Tumilty, D. M., & Telford, R. D. (1988). General and specific aerobic power of elite marathon kayakers and canoeists. *Excel, 5,* 14-19.

Haj-Sassi, R., Dardouri, W., Gharbi, Z., Chaouachi, A., Mansour, H., Rabhi, A., & Mahfoudhi, M. E. (2011). Reliability and Validity of a New Repeated Agility Test as a Measure of Anaerobic and Explosive Power. *Journal of Strength & Conditioning Research, 25*(2), 472-80.

Hakkinen, K., & Komi, P. V. (1985). Effect of explosive type strength training on electromyographic and force production characteristics of leg extensor muscles during concentric and various stretch-shortening cycle exercises. *Scandenarian Journal of Sports Science, 7*(2), 65-76.

Hale, T. (2003). *Exercise physiology: a thematic approach*. John Wiley and Sons.

Halin, R., Germain, P., Bercier, S., Kapitaniak, B., & Buttelli, O. (2003). Neuromuscular response of young boys versus men during sustained maximal contraction. *Medicine & Science in Sports & Exercise, 35*(6), 1042-48.

Hall, T. S. (1975). *History of general physiology: 600 B.C. to A.D. 1900. Vol. 1: From pre-Socratic times to the enlightenment*. University of Chicago Press.

Hansman, C. F. (1962). Appearance and fusion of ossification centers in the human skeleton. *The American journal of roentgenology, radium therapy, and nuclear medicine, 88,* 476-82.

Hargreaves, M., McKenna, M. J., Jenkins, D. G., Warmington, S. A., Li, J. L., Snow, R. J., & Febbraio, M. A. (1998). Muscle metabolites and performance during high-intensity, intermittent exercise. *Journal of Applied Physiology, 84*(5), 1687-91.

Hargreaves, M., & Spriet, L. L. (2006). *Exercise metabolism*. Champaign, ILL: Human Kinetics.

Harris, L. J. (2010). In fencing, what gives left-handers the edge? Views from the present and the distant past. *Laterality: Asymmetries of Body, Brain, and Cognition, 15, 1*(2), 15-55.

Harris, N. K., Cronin, J. B., Hopkins, W. G., & Hansen, K. T. (2008). Squat jump training at maximal power loads vs. heavy loads: Effect on sprint ability. *Journal of Strength & Conditioning Research, 22*(6), 1742-9.

Harris, R. C., Söderlund, K., & Hultman, E. (1992). Elevation of creatine in resting and exercised muscle of normal subjects by creatine supplementation. *Clinical Science, 83*(3), 367-74.

Harris, R. C., Tallon, M. J., Dunnett, M., Boobis, L., Coakley, J., Kim, H. J., Fallowfield, J. L., Hill, C. A., Sale, C. & Wise, J. A. (2006). The absorption of orally supplied β-alanine and its effect on muscle carnosine synthesis in human vastus lateralis. *Amino Acids, 30*(3), 279-89.

Hart, P. (1988). *Improve your windsurfing*. London: Willow Books.

Harvey, N. C., Cole, Z. A., Crozier, S. R., Kim, M., Ntani, G., Goodfellow, L., . . . Dennison, E. M. (2011). Physical activity, calcium intake and childhood bone mineral: a population-based cross-sectional study. *Osteoporosis International,* 1-10.

Hastie, P., Sinelnikov, O., & Wadsworth, D. (2010). Aerobic fitness status and out-of-school lifestyle of rural children in America and Russia. *Journal of physical activity & health, 7*(2), 150-5.

Haydar, B., Al Haddad, H., Ahmaidi, S., & Buchheit, M. (2011). Assessing inter-effort recovery and change of direction ability with the 30-15 Intermittent Fitness Test. *Journal of Sports Science and Medicine, 10,* 346-54.

Hayes, P. A., & Cohen, J. B. (1987). Further development of a mathematical model for the specification of immersion clothing insulation. RAF, UK: Institute of Aviation Medicine.

Hayward, J. S., Collis, M. L., & Lisson, P. A. (1978). *Survival suits for accidental immersion in cold water: design-concepts and their thermal protection performance*. Victoria, B.C.: University of Victoria. Dept. of Biology.

Heck, H., Mader, A., Hess, G., Mücke, S., & Hollmann, W. (1985). Justification of the 4-mmol/l lactate threshold. *International Journal of Sports Medicine, 6*(3), 117-30.

Hedman, R. (1957). The available glycogen in man and the connection between rate of oxygen intake and carbohydrate usage. *Acta Physiologica Scandinavica, 40*(4), 305-21.

Heelan, K. A., Donnelly, J. E., Jacobsen, D. J., Mayo, M. S., Washburn, R., & Greene, L. (2005). Active commuting to and from school and BMI in elementary school children-preliminary data. *Child: Care, Health and Development, 31*(3), 341-9.

Heigenhauser, N. M., Wiseman, R. W., Bishop, R. A. M., Crampin, E. J., Tabata, I., & George, J. F. (2011). Comments on Point: Counterpoint: Muscle lactate and H$^+$ production do/do'not have a 1:1 association in skeletal muscle. *Journal of Applied Physiology, 110,* 1493-6.

Heinonen, A., McKay, H. A., Whittall, K. P., Forster, B. B., & Khan, K. M. (2001). Muscle cross-sectional area is associated with specific site of bone in prepubertal girls: a quantitative magnetic resonance imaging study. *Bone, 29*(4), 388-92.

Helenius, I. J., Tikkanen, H. O., & Haahtela, T. (1997). Association between type of training and risk of asthma in elite athletes. *Thorax, 52*(2), 157-60.

Helenius, I. J., Tikkanen, H. O., Sarna, S., & Haahtela, T. (1998). Asthma and increased bronchial responsiveness in elite athletes: atopy and sport event as risk factors. *Journal of allergy and Clinical Immunology, 101*(5), 646-52.

Hellemans, J. (2000). *The training intensity handbook for endurance sport*. Napier, NZ: KinEli Publishing.

Heller, J., Bily, M., Pultera, J., & Sadilova, M. (1994). Functional and energy demands on elite female kayak slalom: a comparison of training and competition performances. *Acta Universitatis Carolinae: Kinanthropologica, 30*(1), 59-74.

Heller, J., Bunc, V., & Novotny, J. (1991). Effect of site of capillary blood sampling on lactate concentrations during exercise and recovery. *Acta Universitatis Carolinae: Gymnica, 27*(2), 29-38.

Hermansen, L., & Stensvold, I. (1972). Production and removal of lactate during exercise in man. *Acta Physiologica Scandinavica, 86*(2), 191-201.

Herzog, D. B., Dorer, D. J., Keel, P. K., Selwyn, S. E., Ekeblad, E. R., Flores, A. T., Greenwood, D. N., Burwell, R. A. & Keller, M. B. (1999). Recovery and relapse in anorexia and bulimia nervosa: a 7.5-year follow-up study. *Journal of the American Academy of Child & Adolescent Psychiatry, 38*(7), 829-37.

Hespel, P., Maughan, R. J., & Greenhaff, P. L. (2006). Dietary supplements for football. *Journal of Sports Sciences, 24*(7), 749-61.

Hetzler, R. K., Stickley, C. D., & Kimura, I. F. (2011). Allometric scaling of wingate anaerobic power test scores in women. *Research Quarterly for Exercise and Sport, 82*(1), 70-8.

Hetzler, R. K., Vogelpohl, R. E., Stickley, C. D., Kuramoto, A. N., DeLaura, M. R., & Kimura, I. F. (2010). Development of a Modified Margaria-Kalamen Anaerobic Power Test for American Football Athletes. *Journal of Strength & Conditioning Research, 24*(4), 978-84.

Heyward, V. H. (2010). *Advanced fitness assessment and exercise prescription*. Champaign, IL: Human Kinetics Publishers.

Hibbert, M., Lannigan, A., Raven, J., Landau, L., & Phelan, P. (1995). Gender differences in lung growth. *Pediatric Pulmonology, 19*(2), 129-34.

Hill, D. W. (1993). The critical power concept. A review. *Sports Medicine, 16*(4), 237-54.

Hill, D. W., Borden, D. O., Darnaby, K. M., & Hendricks, D. N. (1994). Aerobic and anaerobic contributions to exhaustive high-intensity exercise after sleep deprivation. *Journal of Sports Sciences, 12*(5), 455-61.

Hill, D. W., & Ferguson, C. S. (1999). A physiological description of critical velocity. *European Journal of Applied Physiology and Occupational Physiology, 79*(3), 290-3.

Hills, A. P. & Byme N. M. (2010) In Jurimae, J, Hills A. P. & Jurimae, T. *Cytokines, Growth Mediators and Physical Activity in Children during Puberty*. Basel, Switzerland: Karger.

Hinckson, E. A., & Hopkins, W. G. (2005). Reliability of time to exhaustion analyzed with critical-power and log-log modeling. *Medicine & Science in Sports & Exercise, 37*(4), 696-701.

Hinrichs T, Franke J, Voss S, Bloch W, Schänzer W, and Platen P. (2010). Total hemoglobin mass, iron status, and endurance capacity in elite field hockey players. *Journal of Strength and Conditioning Research, 24*(3), 629-38.

Hobart, J. A., & Smucker, D. R. (2000). The female athlete triad. *American Family Physician, 61*(11), 3357-64.

Hoch, A. Z., Pajewski, N. M., Moraski, L. A., Carrera, G. F., Wilson, C. R., Hoffmann, R. G., Schimke, J. E. & Gutterman, D. D. (2009). Prevalence of the female athlete triad in high school athletes and sedentary students. *Clinical Journal of Sport Medicine: Official Journal of the Canadian Academy of Sport Medicine, 19*(5), 421-8.

Hoff, J. (2005). Training and testing physical capacities for elite soccer players. *Journal of Sports Sciences, 23*(6), 573-82.

Hoff, J., Wisløff, U., Engen, L. C., Kemi, O. J., & Helgerud, J. (2002). Soccer specific aerobic endurance training. *British Journal of Sports Medicine, 36*(3), 218-21.

Hoffman, J. (2002a). *Physiological aspects of sport training and performance*. Champaign, ILL: Human Kinetics.

Hoffman, J. (2002b). Resistance and training and injury prevention. *American College of Sports Medicine. Current Comment*.

Hoffman, J., Ratamess, N., Kang, J., Rashti, S., & Faigenbaum, A. (2009). Effect of betaine supplementation on power performance and fatigue. *Journal of the International Society of Sports Nutrition, 6*(1).

Hoffman, J. R. (2008). The applied physiology of American football. *International Journal of Sports Physiology and Performance, 3*(3), 387-92.

Hoffman, J. R., Maresh, C. M., Newton, R. U., Rubin, M. R., French, D. N., Volek, J. S., Sutherland, J., Robertson, M., Gomez, A. L. & Ratamess, N. A. (2002). Performance, biochemical, and endocrine changes during a competitive football game. *Medicine & Science in Sports & Exercise, 34*(11), 1845-53.

Hohlrieder, M., Mair, P., Wuertl, W., & Brugger, H. (2005). The impact of avalanche transceivers on mortality from avalanche accidents. *High Altitude Medicine & Biology, 6*(1), 72-7.

Holum, J. R. (1998). *Fundamentals of general, organic, and biological chemistry*. Chichester, UK: Wiley Blackwell.

Hori, N., Newton, R. U., Andrews, W. A., Kawamori, N., McGuigan, M. R., & Nosaka, K. (2008). Does performance of hang power clean differentiate performance of jumping, sprinting, and changing of direction? *Journal of Strength & Conditioning Research, 22*(2), 412-18.

Hörst, E. J. (1994). *How to Climb: Flash Training*. Nashville, TN: Falcon Press.

Hörst, E. J. (2002). *Training for Climbing: The Definitive Guide to Improving Your Climbing Performance*. Nashville, TN: Falcon Press.

Hörst, E. J. (2003). *How to Climb 5.12*. Nashville, TN: Falcon Press.

Hörst, E. J. (2008). *Training for Climbing: The Definitive Guide to Improving Your Performance*. Nashville, TN: Falcon Press.

Horswill, C. A. (1992). Applied physiology of amateur wrestling. *Sports Medicine, 14*(2), 114.

Houmard, J. A., Tanner, C. J., Slentz, C. A., Duscha, B. D., McCartney, J. S., & Kraus, W. E. (2004). Effect of the volume and intensity of exercise training on insulin sensitivity. *Journal of Applied Physiology, 96*(1), 101-6.

Houston, M. E. (2006). *Biochemistry primer for exercise science*. Champaign, ILL: Human Kinetics.

Hubert, P., King, N. A., & Blundell, J. E. (1998). Uncoupling the effects of energy expenditure and energy intake: appetite response to short-term energy deficit induced by meal omission and physical activity. *Appetite, 31*(1), 9-19.

Hugh Morton, R. (2010). Why peak power is higher at the end of steeper ramps: An explanation based on the 'critical power' concept. *Journal of Sports Sciences, 29*(3), 307-9.

Hughes, M. (1988). Computerized notation analysis in field games. *Ergonomics, 31*(11), 1585-1592.

Hultman, E., Soderlund, K., Timmons, J. A., Cederblad, G., & Greenhaff, P. L. (1996). Muscle creatine loading in men. *Journal of Applied Physiology, 81*(1), 232-7.

Hurn, M., & Ingle, P. (1988). *Climbing fit*. Seattle, WA: Cloudcap.

Hurni, M. (2002). *Coaching Climbing: A complete program for coaching youth climbing for high performance and safety*. Nashville, TN: Falcon Press.

Hutchinson, D. C. (1994). *The complete book of sea kayaking*. London: A & C Black.

Iaia, F. M., & Bangsbo, J. (2010). Speed endurance training is a powerful stimulus for physiological adaptations and performance improvements of athletes. *Scandinavian Journal of Medicine & Science in Sports, 20*, 11-23.

Imamura, H., Yoshimura, Y., Nishimura, S., Nakazawa, A. T., Teshima, K., Nishimura, C., & Miyamoto, N. (2002). Physiological responses during and following karate training in women. *Journal of Sports Medicine and Physical Fitness, 42*(4), 431-7.

Imamura, H., Yoshimura, Y., Nishimura, S., Nishimura, C., & Sakamoto, K. (2003). Oxygen uptake, heart rate, and blood lactate responses during 1,000 punches and 1,000 kicks in female collegiate karate practitioners. *Journal of Physiological Anthropology and Applied Human Science, 22*(2), 111-14.

Imamura, H., Yoshimura, Y., Uchida, K., Nishimura, S., & Nakazawa, A. T. (1998). Maximal oxygen uptake, body composition and strength of highly competitive and novice karate practitioners. *Applied Human Science, 17*(5), 215-18.

Impellizzeri, F., Sassi, A., Rodriguez-Alonso, M., Mognoni, P., & Marcora, S. (2002). Exercise intensity during off-road cycling competitions. *Medicine & Science in Sports & Exercise, 34*(11), 1808-13.

Inbar, O., & Chia, M. (2008). Development of maximal anaerobic performance: an old issue revisited.

Ingjer, F., & Strømme, S. (1979). Effects of active, passive or no warm-up on the physiological response to heavy exercise. *European Journal of Applied Physiology and Occupational Physiology, 40*(4), 273-282. doi: 10.1007/bf00421519

Ingle, L., Sleap, M., & Tolfrey, K. (2006). The effect of a complex training and detraining programme on selected strength and power variables in early pubertal boys. *Journal of Sports Sciences, 24*(9), 987-97.

Isacco, L., Lazaar, N., Ratel, S., Thivel, D., Aucouturier, J., Doré, E., Meyer, M. & Duché, P. (2010). The impact of eating habits on anthropometric characteristics in French primary school children. *Child: Care, Health and Development, 36*(6), 835-42.

Janot, J. M., Steffen, J. P., Porcari, J. P., & Maher, M. A. (2000). Heart rate responses and perceived exertion for beginner and recreational sport climbers during indoor climbing. *Journal of Exercise Physiology, 3*(1).

Janz, K. F., Dawson, J. D., & Mahoney, L. T. (2000). Predicting heart growth during puberty: the Muscatine Study. *Pediatrics, 105*(5), e63.

Janz, K. F., Dawson, J. D., & Mahoney, L. T. (2002). Increases in physical fitness during childhood improve cardiovascular health during adolescence: the Muscatine Study. *International journal of sports medicine, 23*(1), 15-21.

Janz, K. F., & Mahoney, L. T. (1997). Three-year follow-up of changes in aerobic fitness during puberty: the Muscatine Study. *Research Quarterly for Exercise and Sport, 68*(1), 1-9.

Jemni, M., Sands, W. A., Friemel, F., & Delamarche, P. (2003). Effect of active and passive recovery on blood lactate and performance during simulated competition in high level gymnasts. *Canadian Journal of Applied Physiology, 28*(2), 240-56.

Jenkins, D. G., & Quigley, B. M. (1990). Blood lactate in trained cyclists during cycle ergometry at critical power. *European Journal of Applied Physiology and Occupational Physiology, 61*(3), 278-83.

Jensen, K., & Karkkainen, L. J. O. P. (1999). Economy in track runners and orienteers during path and terrain running. *Journal of Sports Sciences, 17*(12), 945-50.

Jette, M., Thoden, J. S., & Spence, J. (1976). The energy expenditure of a 5 km cross-country ski run. *The Journal of Sports Medicine and Physical Fitness, 16*(2), 134-7.

Jeukendrup, A. E., & Gleeson, M. (2004). *Sport nutrition: an introduction to energy production and performance*. Champaign, ILL: Human Kinetics.

Joanny, P., Steinberg, J., Robach, P., Richalet, J. P., Gortan, C., Gardette, B., & Jammes, Y. (2001). Operation Everest III (Comex'97): the effect of simulated severe hypobaric hypoxia on lipid peroxidation and antioxidant defence systems in human blood at rest and after maximal exercise. *Resuscitation, 49*(3), 307-14.

Johnston, T., Sproule, J., McMorris, T., & Maile, A. (2004). Time-motion analysis and heart rate response during elite male field hockey: Competition versus training. *Journal of Human Movement Studies, 46*, 189-204.

Jones, A. M., & Doust, J. H. (1998). The validity of the lactate minimum test for determination of the maximal lactate steady state. *Medicine & Science in Sports & Exercise, 30*(8), 1304-13.

Jones, A. M., & Poole, D. C. (2005). *Oxygen uptake kinetics in sport, exercise and medicine*: London: Routledge.

Jones, A. M., Vanhatalo, A., Burnley, M., Morton, R., & Poole, D. C. (2010). Critical Power: Implications for Determination of VO_{2max} and Exercise Tolerance. *Medicine & Science in Sports & Exercise, 42*(10), 1876-90.

Jones, L. C., Cleary, M. A., Lopez, R. M., Zuri, R. E., & Lopez, R. (2008). Active dehydration impairs upper and lower body anaerobic muscular power. *Journal of Strength & Conditioning Research, 22*(2), 455-63.

Jordan, A. N., Jurca, R., Abraham, E. H., Salikhova, A., Mann, J. K., Morss, G. M., Church, T. S., Lucia, A. & Earnest, C. P. (2004).

Effects of oral ATP supplementation on anaerobic power and muscular strength. *Medicine & Science in Sports & Exercise, 36*(6), 983-90.

Joyce, B. R., Weil, M., & Calhoun, E. (2000). *Models of teaching.* Boston, MA: Allyn and Bacon.

Judelson, D. A., Maresh, C. M., Anderson, J. M., Armstrong, L. E., Casa, D. J., Kraemer, W. J., & Volek, J. S. (2007). Hydration and muscular performance: does fluid balance affect strength, power and high-intensity endurance? *Sports Medicine, 37*(10), 907-21.

Judge, L. W., Bellar, D., & Judge, M. (2010). Efficacy of potentiation of performance through overweight implement throws on male and female high-school weight throwers. *Journal of Strength & Conditioning Research, 24*(7), 1804-1809.

Judge, L. W., Bellar, D., Judge, M., & Gilreath, E. (2011). Efficacy of potentiation of performance through overweight implement throws on high school weight throwers. *Journal of Strength & Conditioning Research, 25*, S16.

Kale, M., Asçi, A., Bayrak, C., & Açikada, C. (2009). Relationships among jumping performances and sprint parameters during maximum speed phase in sprinters. *Journal of Strength & Conditioning Research, 23*(8), 2272-9.

Kanehisa, H., Ikegawa, S., Tsunoda, N., & Fukunaga, T. (1995). Strength and cross-sectional areas of reciprocal muscle groups in the upper arm and thigh during adolescence. *International Journal of Sports Medicine, 16*(1), 54-60.

Kanehisa, H., Yata, H., Ikegawa, S., & Fukunaga, T. (1995). A cross-sectional study of the size and strength of the lower leg muscles during growth. *European Journal of Applied Physiology and Occupational Physiology, 72*(1), 150-6.

Karlsson, J. (1978). *The physiology of alpine skiing.* US Ski Coaches Association.

Karlsson, J. (1984). Profiles of cross-country and alpine skiers. *Clinics in Sports Medicine, 3*(1), 245-71.

Kascenska, J. R., Dewitt, J., & Roberts, T. (1992). Fitness guidelines for rock climbing students. *Journal of Physical Education, Recreation & Dance, 63*(3), 73-9.

Kazemi, M., Perri, G., & Soave, D. (2010). A profile of 2008 Olympic Taekwondo competitors. *Journal of the Canadian Chiropractic Association, 54*(4), 243-9.

Keast, D., Cameron, K., & Morton, A. R. (1988). Exercise and the immune response. *Sports Medicine, 5*(4), 248-67.

Keen, A. D., & Drinkwater, B. L. (1997). Irreversible bone loss in former amenorrheic athletes. *Osteoporosis International, 7*(4), 311-15.

Kelley, G. A., & Kelley, K. S. (2007). Aerobic exercise and lipids and lipoproteins in children and adolescents: a meta-analysis of randomized controlled trials. *Atherosclerosis, 191*(2), 447-53.

Kellis, E., & Unnithan, V. B. (1999). Co-activation of vastus lateralis and biceps femoris muscles in pubertal children and adults. *European Journal of Applied Physiology and Occupational Physiology, 79*(6), 504-11.

Kemi, O. J., Hoff, J., Engen, L. C., Helgerud, J., & Wisløff, U. (2003). Soccer specific testing of maximal oxygen uptake. *Journal of Sports Medicine and Physical Fitness, 43*(2), 139-44.

Kemper, H. C. G. (2000). Skeletal development during childhood and adolescence and the effects of physical activity. *Pediatric Exercise Science, 12*(2), 198-216.

Kendall, K. L., Smith, A. E., Graef, J. L., Fukuda, D. H., Moon, J. R., Beck, T. W., Cramer, J. T. & Stout, J. R. (2009). Effects of four weeks of high-intensity interval training and creatine supplementation on critical power and anaerobic working capacity in college-aged men. *Journal of Strength & Conditioning Research, 23*(6), 1663-9.

Khanna, G. L., & Manna, I. (2006). Study of physiological profile of Indian boxers. *Journal of Sports Science and Medicine, 5*, 90-8.

Kim, C. H., Cho, J. Y., Jeon, J. Y., Koh, Y. G., Kim, Y. M., Kim, H. J., Park, M., Um, H. S. & Kim, C. (2010). ACE DD genotype is unfavorable to Korean short-term muscle power athletes. *International Journal of Sports Medicine, 31*(1), 65-71.

Kindermann, W. (2007). Do inhaled 2-agonists have an ergogenic potential in non-asthmatic competitive athletes? *Sports Medicine, 37*(2), 95-102.

Kindermann, W., Simon, G., & Keul, J. (1979). The significance of the aerobic-anaerobic transition for the determination of work load intensities during endurance training. *European Journal of Applied Physiology and Occupational Physiology, 42*(1), 25-34.

Kippelen, P., Caillaud, C., Coste, O., Godard, P., & Prefaut, C. (2004). Asthma and exercise-induced bronchoconstriction in amateur endurance-trained athletes. *International Journal of Sports Medicine, 25*(2), 130-2.

Kirchner, E. M., Lewis, R. D., & O'Connor, P. J. (1996). Effect of past gymnastics participation on adult bone mass. *Journal of Applied Physiology, 80*(1), 226-32.

Klassen, G. A., Andrew, G. M., & Becklake, M. R. (1970). Effect of training on total and regional blood flow and metabolism in paddlers. *Journal of Applied Physiology, 28*(4), 397-406.

Klasson-Heggebø, L., Andersen, L. B., Wennlöf, A. H., Sardinha, L. B., Harro, M., Froberg, K., & Anderssen, S. A. (2006). Graded associations between cardiorespiratory fitness, fatness, and blood pressure in children and adolescents. *British Journal of Sports Medicine, 40*(1), 25-9.

Kodama, S., Saito, K., Tanaka, S., Maki, M., Yachi, Y., Asumi, M., Sugawara, A., Totsuka, K., Shimano, H., Ohashi, Y., Yamada, N. & Sone, H. (2009). Cardiorespiratory fitness as a quantitative predictor of all-cause mortality and cardiovascular events in healthy men and women: a meta-analysis. *Journal of American Medical Association, 301*(19), 2024-35.

Kohl Iii, H. W. (2001). Physical activity and cardiovascular disease: evidence for a dose response. *Medicine & Science in Sports & Exercise, 33*(6), S472-S483.

Kollias, I., Panoutsakopoulos, V., & Papaiakovou, G. (2004). Comparing jumping ability among athletes of various sports:

vertical drop jumping from 60 centimeters. *Journal of Strength & Conditioning Research, 18*(3), 546-50.

König, D., Huonker, M., Schmid, A., Halle, M., Berg, A., & Keul, J. (2001). Cardiovascular, metabolic, and hormonal parameters in professional tennis players. *Medicine & Science in Sports & Exercise, 33*(4), 654.

Kostka, T., Drygas, W., Jegier, A., & Zaniewicz, D. (2009). Aerobic and anaerobic power in relation to age and physical activity in 354 men aged 20-88 years. *International Journal of Sports Medicine, 30*(3), 225-30.

Kotzamanidou, M., Michailidis, I., Hatzikotoulas, K., Hasani, A., Bassa, E., & Kotzamanidis, C. (2005). Differences in recovery process between adult and prepubertal males after a maximal isokinetic fatigue task. *Isokinetics and Exercise Science, 13*(4), 261-6.

Kotzaminidis, C., Patikas, D., & Bassa, E. (2005). Activation of antagonist knee muscles during isokinetic efforts in prepubertal and adult males. *Pediatric Exercise Science, 17*(2), 171-81.

Koukoubis, T. D., Cooper, L. W., Glisson, R. R., Seaber, A. V., & Feagin, J. A. (1995). An electromyographic study of arm muscles during climbing. *Knee Surgery, Sports Traumatology, Arthroscopy, 3*(2), 121-4.

Koutedakis, Y., Ridgeon, A., Sharp, N. C., & Boreham, C. (1993). Seasonal variation of selected performance parameters in épée fencers. *British Journal of Sports Medicine, 27*(3), 171-4.

Kraemer, W. J., Fry, A. C., Rubin, M. R., Triplett-McBride, T., Gordon, S. E., Perry Koziris, L., Lynch, J. M., Volek, J. S., Meuffels, D. E. & Newton, R. U. (2001). Physiological and performance responses to tournament wrestling. *Medicine & Science in Sports & Exercise, 33*(8), 1367-78.

Kraemer, W. J., Vescovi, J. D., & Dixon, P. (2004). The physiological basis of wrestling: Implications for conditioning programs. *Strength & Conditioning Journal, 26*(2), 10-15.

Krahenbuhl, G. S., Skinner, J. S., & Kohrt, W. M. (1985). Developmental aspects of maximal aerobic power in children. *Exercise and Sport Sciences Reviews, 13*(1), 503.

Kraus, W. E., Houmard, J. A., Duscha, B. D., Knetzger, K. J., Wharton, M. B., McCartney, J. S., Bales, C. W., Henes, S., Samsa, G. P. & Otvos, J. D. (2002). Effects of the amount and intensity of exercise on plasma lipoproteins. *New England Journal of Medicine, 347*(19), 1483-92.

Kreider, M. E., Stumvoll, M., Meyer, C., Overkamp, D., Welle, S., & Gerich, J. (1997). Steady-state and non-steady-state measurements of plasma glutamine turnover in humans. *American Journal of Physiology-Endocrinology and Metabolism, 272*(4), E621-E627.

Kreider, R. B., Fry, A. C., & O'Toole, M. L. E. (1998). *Overtraining in sport.* Champaign, ILL: Human Kinetics.

Kriemler, S., Zahner, L., Puder, J. J., Braun-Fahrländer, C., Schindler, C., Farpour-Lambert, N. J., Kränzlin, M. & Rizzoli, R. (2008). Weight-bearing bones are more sensitive to physical exercise in boys than in girls during pre-and early puberty:

a cross-sectional study. *Osteoporosis International, 19*(12), 1749-58.

Kruseman, M., Bucher, S., Bovard, M., Kayser, B., & Bovier, P. A. (2005). Nutrient intake and performance during a mountain marathon: an observational study. *European Journal of Applied Physiology, 94*(1), 151-7.

Krustrup, P., & Bangsbo, J. (2001). Physiological demands of top-class soccer refereeing in relation to physical capacity: effect of intense intermittent exercise training. *Journal of Sports Sciences, 19*(11), 881-91.

Krustrup, P., Mohr, M., Ellingsgaard, H., & Bangsbo, J. (2005). Physical demands during an elite female soccer game: importance of training status. *Medicine & Science in Sports & Exercise, 37*(7), 1242-8.

Krustrup, P., Mohr, M., Steensberg, A., Bencke, J., Kjær, M., & Bangsbo, J. (2006). Muscle and blood metabolites during a soccer game: implications for sprint performance. *Medicine & Science in Sports & Exercise, 38*(6), 1165-74.

Kudlac, J., Nichols, D. L., Sanborn, C. F., & DiMarco, N. M. (2004). Impact of detraining on bone loss in former collegiate female gymnasts. *Calcified Tissue International, 75*(6), 482-487. doi: 10.1007/s00223-004-0228-4

Kuno, S., Takahashi, H., Fujimoto, K., Akima, H., Miyamura, M., Nemoto, I., Itai, Y. & Katsuta, S. (1995). Muscle metabolism during exercise using phosphorus-31 nuclear magnetic resonance spectroscopy in adolescents. *European Journal of Applied Physiology and Occupational Physiology, 70*(4), 301-4.

Kuphal, K. E., Potteiger, J. A., Frey, B. B., & Hise, M. P. (2004). Validation of a single-day maximal lactate steady state assessment protocol. *Journal of Sports Medicine and Physical Fitness, 44*(2), 132-40.

Kyrolainen, H., Santtila, M., Nindl, B. C., & Vasankari, T. (2010). Physical fitness profiles of young men: associations between physical fitness, obesity and health. *Sports Medicine, 40*(11), 907-20.

Laing, E. M., Massoni, J. A., Nickols-Richardson, S. M., Modlesky, C. M., O'Connor, P. J., & Lewis, R. D. (2002). A prospective study of bone mass and body composition in female adolescent gymnasts. *Journal of Pediatrics, 141*(2), 211-16.

Lambertz, D., Mora, I., Grosset, J. F., & Pérot, C. (2003). Evaluation of musculotendinous stiffness in prepubertal children and adults, taking into account muscle activity. *Journal of Applied Physiology, 95*(1), 64-72.

Laplaud, D., Guinot, M., Favre-Juvin, A., & Flore, P. (2006). Maximal lactate steady state determination with a single incremental test exercise. *European Journal of Applied Physiology, 96*(4), 446-52.

Larsson, P., Burlin, L., Jakobsson, E., & Henriksson-Larsen, K. (2002). Analysis of performance in orienteering with treadmill tests and physiological field tests using a differential global positioning system. *Journal of Sports Sciences, 20*(7), 529-35.

Lazaar, N., Aucouturier, J., Ratel, S., Rance, M., Meyer, M., & Duché, P. (2007). Effect of physical activity intervention on body composition in young children: influence of body mass index status and gender. *Acta Paediatrica, 96*(9), 1321-25.

Leatt P., Reilly T., & Troup J. G. (1986). Spinal loading during circuit weight-training and running. *British Journal of Sports Medicine, 20*(3), 119-24.

Lee, D., & Artero, E. G. (2010). Review: Mortality trends in the general population: the importance of cardiorespiratory fitness. *Journal of Psychopharmacology, 24*(4 suppl), 27-35.

Lee, S. M. C., Williams, W. J., & Fortney Schneider, S. M. (2000). Core temperature measurement during supine exercise: esophageal, rectal, and intestinal temperatures. *Aviation, Space, and Environmental Medicine, 71*(9), 939-45.

Leenders, N. M., Lamb, D. R., & Nelson, T. E. (1999). Creatine supplementation and swimming performance. *International Journal of Sport Nutrition, 9*(3), 251-62.

Lees, A. (2003). Science and the major racket sports: a review. *Journal of Sports Sciences, 21*(9), 707-32.

Léger, L. A., & Lambert, J. (1982). A maximal multistage 20-m shuttle run test to predict O 2 max. *European Journal of Applied Physiology and Occupational Physiology, 49*(1), 1-12.

Léger, L. A., Mercier, D., Gadoury, C., & Lambert, J. (1988). The multistage 20 metre shuttle run test for aerobic fitness. *Journal of Sports Sciences, 6*(2), 93-101.

Lemmink, K. A. P. M., Visscher, C., Lambert, M. I., & Lamberts, R. P. (2004). The interval shuttle run test for intermittent sport players: evaluation of reliability. *Journal of Strength & Conditioning Research, 18*(4), 821-7.

Leverve, X. M., & Mustafa, I. (2002). Lactate: a key metabolite in the intercellular metabolic interplay. *Critical Care, 6*(4), 284-5.

Levine, B. D., & Stray-Gundersen, J. (1997). 'Living high-training low': effect of moderate-altitude acclimatization with low-altitude training on performance. *Journal of Applied Physiology, 83*(1), 102-12.

Lewis, T. (1930). Observations upon the reactions of the vessels of the human skin to cold. *Heart, 15*(2), 177-208.

Lexell, J. (1995). Human aging, muscle mass, and fiber type composition. *Journals of Gerontology. Series A, Biological Sciences and Medical Sciences, 50*, 11-16.

Lexell, J., Sjöström, M., Nordlund, A. S., & Taylor, C. C. (1992). Growth and development of human muscle: a quantitative morphological study of whole vastus lateralis from childhood to adult age. *Muscle & Nerve, 15*(3), 404-9.

Lillegard W. A., Brown E. W., Wilson D. J., Henderson R., and Lewis E. (1997). Efficacy of strength training in prepubescent to early postpubescent males and females: effects of gender and maturity. *Pediatric Rehabilitation. 1*(3), 147-57.

Lima, F., De Falco, V., Baima, J., & Gilberto Carazzato, J. (2001). Effect of impact load and active load on bone metabolism and body composition of adolescent athletes. *Medicine & Science in Sports & Exercise, 33*(8), 1318-23.

Livingstone, S. D., Grayson, J., Frim, J., Allen, C. L., & Limmer, R. E. (1983). Effect of cold exposure on various sites of core temperature measurements. *Journal of Applied Physiology, 54*(4), 1025-31.

Locke, S., Colquhoun, D., Briner, M., Ellis, L., O'Brien, M., Wollstein, J., & Allen, G. (1997). Squash racquets. A review of physiology and Medicine. *Sports Medicine, 23*(2), 130-8.

Lohman, T. G., & Going, S. B. (2006). Body composition assessment for development of an international growth standard for preadolescent and adolescent children. *Food and Nutrition Bulletin - United Nations University, 27*(4), S314-S325.

Lopes, B., & McCormack, L. (2005). *Mastering mountain bike skills*. Champaign, ILL: Human Kinetics.

Lothian, F., & Farrally, M. (1992). Estimating the energy cost of women's hockey using heart rate and video analysis. *Journal of Human Movement Studies, 23*, 215-31.

Lothian, F., & Farrally, M. (1994). A time-motion analysis of women's hockey. *Journal of Human Movement Studies, 26*(6), 255-66.

Lowdon, B. J. (1980). The somatotype of international surfboard riders. *Australian Journal of Sports Medicine, 12*, 34-9.

Lowdon, B. J., & Pateman, N. A. (1980). Physiological parameters of international surfers. *Australian Journal of Sports Medicine, 12*(2), 30-33.

Lowdon, B. J., Pateman, N. A., & Pitman, A. J. (1983). Surfboard-riding injuries. *The Medical Journal of Australia, 2*(12), 613.

Lowe, J. (1996). *Ice world: techniques and experiences of modern ice climbing*. Seattle, WA: The Mountaineers Books.

Lu, P. W., Cowell, C. T., Lloyd-Jones, S. A., Briody, J. N., & Howman-Giles, R. (1996). Volumetric bone mineral density in normal subjects, aged 5-27 years. *Journal of Clinical Endocrinology & Metabolism, 81*(4), 1586-90.

Lubans, D. R., Morgan, P. J., Cliff, D. P., Barnett, L. M., & Okely, A. D. (2010). Fundamental movement skills in children and adolescents: review of associated health benefits. *Sports Medicine, 40*(12), 1019-35.

Lythe, J., & Kilding, A. E. (2011). Physical demands and physiological responses during elite field hockey. *International Journal of Sports Medicine, 32*(07), 523-8.

Macdonald, M. J., Green, H. J., Naylor, H. L., Otto, C., & Hughson, R. L. (2001). Reduced oxygen uptake during steady state exercise after 21-day mountain climbing expedition to 6,194 m. *Canadian Journal of Applied Physiology, 26*(2), 143-56.

MacDougall, J. D., Wenger, H. A., Green, H. J., & Canadian Association of Sports, S. (1991). *Physiological testing of the high-performance athlete*. Champaign, ILL: Human Kinetics.

MacRae, H. S. H., Hise, K. J., & Allen, P. J. (2000). Effects of front and dual suspension mountain bike systems on uphill cycling performance. *Medicine & Science in Sports & Exercise, 32*(7), 1276-80.

Maddison, R., Jiang, Y., Vander Hoorn, S., Exeter, D., Mhurchu, C. N., & Dorey, E. (2010). Describing patterns of physical activity in adolescents using global positioning systems and accelerometry. *Pediatric Exercise Science, 22*(3), 392–407.

Magalhães, J., Rebelo, A., Oliveira, E., Silva, J. R., Marques, F., & Ascensão, A. (2010). Impact of Loughborough Intermittent Shuttle Test versus soccer match on physiological, biochemical and neuromuscular parameters. *European Journal of Applied Physiology, 108*(1), 39–48.

Magel, J. R., Foglia, G. F., McArdle, W. D., Gutin, B., Pechar, G. S., & Katch, F. I. (1975). Specificity of swim training on maximum oxygen uptake. *Journal of Applied Physiology, 38*(1), 151–5.

Magnusson, H., Linden, C., Karlsson, C., Obrant, K. J., & Karlsson, M. K. (2001). Exercise may induce reversible low bone mass in unloaded and high bone mass in weight-loaded skeletal regions. *Osteoporosis International, 12*(11), 950–55.

Majumdar, P., Khanna, G. L., Malik, V., Sachdeva, S., Arif, M., & Mandal, M. (1997). Physiological analysis to quantify training load in badminton. *British Journal of Sports Medicine, 31*(4), 342–5.

Malina, R. M., & Bouchard, C. (1991). *Growth, maturation, and physical activity*. Champaign, ILL: Human Kinetics.

Malina, R. M., Bouchard, C., & Bar-Or, O. (2004). *Growth, maturation, and physical activity*. Champaign, ILL: Human Kinetics.

Mandengue, S. H., Seck, D., Bishop, D., Cisse, F., Tsala-Mbala, P., & Ahmaidi, S. (2005). Are athletes able to self-select their optimal warm up? *Journal of Science and Medicine in Sport, 8*(1), 26–34.

Margaria, R., Aghemo, P., & Rovelli, E. (1966). Measurement of muscular power (anaerobic) in man. *Journal of Applied Physiology, 21*(5), 1662–4.

Markovic, G., & Mikulic, P. (2010). Neuro-Musculoskeletal and Performance Adaptations to Lower-Extremity Plyometric Training. *Sports Medicine, 40*(10), 859–95.

Markovic, G., Misigoj-Durakovic, M., & Trninic, S. (2005). Fitness profile of elite Croatian female taekwondo athletes. *Collegium Antropologicum, 29*(1), 93–9.

Marieb, E. M. & Hoehn, K. (2011) *Anatomy and physiology* (4th edn). San Francisco, CA: Benjamin Cummings.

Martin, R. J. F., Dore, E., Twisk, J. O. S., Van Praagh, E., Hautier, C. A., & Bedu, M. (2004). Longitudinal changes of maximal short-term peak power in girls and boys during growth. *Medicine & Science in Sports & Exercise, 36*(3), 498–503.

Martini, F. H. & Nath, J. L. (2009) *Fundamentals of anatomy and physiology*. (8th edn). San Francisco, CA: Benjamin Cummings.

Martini, F. H., Nath, J. L., & Bartholomew, E. F. (2012) *Fundamentals of anatomy and physiology* (9th edn). San Francisco, CA: Benjamin Cummings.

Martini, F., Ober, W. C., & Nath, J. E. (2011). *Visual Anatomy & Physiology*. San Francisco, CA: Benjamin Cummings.

Mathiowetz, V., Wiemer, D. M., & Federman, S. M. (1986). Grip and pinch strength: norms for 6-to 19-year-olds. *The American Journal of Occupational Therapy: Official Publication of the American Occupational Therapy Association, 40*(10), 705–11.

Matveyev, L. P. (1966). *Periodization of sports training*. Moscow, Russia: Fiscultura I Sport.

Maughan R. J., Fenn C. E., Leiper J. B. (1989). Effects of fluid, electrolyte and substrate ingestion on endurance capacity. *European Journal of Applied Physiology and Occupational Physiology, 58*(5), 481–6.

Maughan, R. J., & Gleeson, M. (2004). *The biochemical basis of sports performance*. Oxford: Oxford University Press.

Maulder, P. S., Bradshaw, E. J., & Keogh, J. (2006). Jump kinetic determinants of sprint acceleration performance from starting blocks in male sprinters. *Journal of Sports Science and Medicine, 5*, 359–66.

Maynard, L. M., Guo, S. S., Chumlea, W. C., Roche, A. F., Wisemandle, W. A., Zeller, C. M., Towne, B. & Siervogel, R. M. (1998). Total-body and regional bone mineral content and areal bone mineral density in children aged 8–18 y: the Fels Longitudinal Study. *American Journal of Clinical Nutrition, 68*(5), 1111–17.

Maynard, L. M., Wisemandle, W., Roche, A. F., & Chumlea, W. (2001). Childhood body composition in relation to body mass index. *Pediatrics, 107*(2), 344–50.

Mazess, R. B. (1974). *International conference on bone mineral measurement: a conference held in Chicago, Ill., Oct. 12-13, 1973*: U.S. Department of Health, Education, and Welfare, Public Health Service, National Institutes of Health, National Institute of Arthritis, Metabolism and Digestive Disease.

Mazzeo, R. S., & Tanaka, H. (2001). Exercise prescription for the elderly: current recommendations. *Sports Medicine, 31*(11), 809–18.

Mazzeo, R. S., Wolfel, E. E., Butterfield, G. E., & Reeves, J. T. (1994). Sympathetic response during 21 days at high altitude (4,300 m) as determined by urinary and arterial catecholamines. *Metabolism, 43*(10), 1226–32.

Mbads, C., Deighan, M. A., & Armstrong, N. (2003). Assessment and interpretation of isokinetic muscle strength during growth and maturation. *Sports Medicine, 33*(10), 727–43.

McArdle, W. D., Katch, F. L., & Katch, V. L. (2010). *Exercise Physiology: Nutrition, Energy, and Human Performance*. Riverwoods, IL: Lippincott, Williams & Wilkins.

McBride, J. M., Blow, D., Kirby, T. J., Haines, T. L., Dayne, A. M., & Triplett, N. T. (2009). Relationship between maximal squat strength and five, ten, and forty yard sprint times. *Journal of Strength & Conditioning Research, 23*(6), 1633–6.

McCambridge, T. M., & Stricker, P. R. (2008). Strength training by children and adolescents. *Pediatrics, 121*(4), 835–40.

McGregor, S. J., Nicholas, C. W., Lakomy, H. K. A., & Williams, C. (1999). The influence of intermittent high-intensity shuttle running and fluid ingestion on the performance of a soccer skill. *Journal of Sports Sciences, 17*(11), 895–903.

McGuigan, M. R., Tatasciore, M., Newton, R. U., & Pettigrew, S. (2009). Eight weeks of resistance training can significantly alter body composition in children who are overweight or obese. *Journal of Strength & Conditioning Research, 23*(1), 80–85.

McManus, A. M., Armstrong, N., & Williams, C. A. (1997). Effect of training on the aerobic power and anaerobic performance of prepubertal girls. *Acta Paediatrica, 86*(5), 456-9.

McMillan, C. S., & Erdmann, L. D. (2010). Tracking adiposity and health-related physical fitness test performances from early childhood through elementary school. *Pediatric Exercise Science, 22*(2), 231-44.

McMillian, D. J., Moore, J. H., Hatler, B. S., & Taylor, C. (2006). Dynamic vs. static-stretching warm up: the effect on power and agility performance. *Journal of Strength and Conditioning Research, 20*(3), 492-9.

McNarry, M. A., Welsman, J. R., & Jones, A. M. (2011). The influence of training and maturity status on girls' responses to short-term, high-intensity upper-and lower-body exercise. *Applied Physiology, Nutrition, and Metabolism, 36*(3), 344-52.

Medbo, J. I., Mamen, A., Olsen, O. H., & Evertsen, F. (2000). Examination of four different instruments for measuring blood lactate concentration. *Scandinavian Journal of Clinical and Laboratory Investigation, 60*(5), 367-80.

Meeusen, R., Piacentini, M. F., Busschaert, B., Buyse, L., Schutter, G. D., & Stray-Gundersen, J. (2004). Hormonal responses in athletes: the use of a two bout exercise protocol to detect subtle differences in (over) training status. *European Journal of Applied Physiology, 91*(2), 140-46.

Mekjavic, I., & Bligh, J. (1987). The pathophysiology of hypothermia. *International Reviews on Ergonomics, 1*, 201-18.

Melchiorri, G., Castagna, C., Sorge, R., & Bonifazi, M. (2010). Game Activity and Blood Lactate in Men's Elite Water-Polo Players. *Journal of Strength & Conditioning Research, 24*(10), 2647-51.

Melhim, A. F. (2001). Aerobic and anaerobic power responses to the practice of taekwon-do. *British Journal of Sports Medicine, 35*(4), 231-4.

Melo, X., Santa-Clara, H., Almeida, J. P., Carnero, E. A., Sardinha, L. B., Bruno, P. M., & Fernhall, B. (2011). Comparing several equations that predict peak VO 2 using the 20-m multistage-shuttle run-test in 8-10-year-old children. *European Journal of Applied Physiology, 1-11.*

Mendez-Villanueva, A., Hamer, P., & Bishop, D. (2008). Fatigue in repeated-sprint exercise is related to muscle power factors and reduced neuromuscular activity. *European Journal of Applied Physiology, 103*(4), 411-19.

Mendez-Villanueva J. A. & Bishop D. (2005) Physiological aspects of surfboard riding performance. *Sports Medicine. 35*(1), 55-70

Mendez-Villanueva, J., Bishop, D., & Hamer, P. (2003). Activity patterns of elite surfing competition. (Abstract). *Journal of Science & Medicine in Sport, 6*(Supplement), 11.

Mercier B, Mercier J, Granier P, Le Gallais D, Préfaut C. (1992). Maximal anaerobic power: relationship to anthropometric characteristics during growth. *International Journal of Sports Medicine. 13*(1), 21-6.

Mermier, C. M., Janot, J. M., Parker, D. L., & Swan, J. G. (2000). Physiological and anthropometric determinants of sport climbing performance. *British Journal of Sports Medicine, 34*(5), 359-65.

Mermier, C. M., Robergs, R. A., McMinn, S. M., & Heyward, V. H. (1997). Energy expenditure and physiological responses during indoor rock climbing. *British Journal of Sports Medicine, 31*(3), 224-28.

Meyerhof, O., & Junowicz-Kocholaty, R. (1943). The equilibria of isomerase and aldolase, and the problem of the phosphorylation of glyceraldehyde phosphate. *Journal of Biological Chemistry, 149*(1), 71-92.

Meylan, C., & Malatesta, D. (2009). Effects of in-season plyometric training within soccer practice on explosive actions of young players. *Journal of Strength & Conditioning Research, 23*(9), 2605-13.

Miller, T. D., Balady, G. J., & Fletcher, G. F. (1997). Exercise and its role in the prevention and rehabilitation of cardiovascular disease. *Annals of Behavioral Medicine, 19*(3), 220-29.

Minahan, C., Chia, M., & Inbar, O. (2007). Does power indicate capacity? 30-s Wingate anaerobic test vs. maximal accumulated O2 deficit. *International Journal of Sports Medicine, 28*(10), 836-43.

Minett, G., Duffield, R., & Bird, S. P. (2010). Effects of acute multinutrient supplementation on rugby union game performance and recovery. *International journal of Sports Physiology and Performance, 5*(1), 27-41.

Minkler, S., & Patterson, P. (1994). The Validity of the Modified Sit-and-Reach Test in College-Age Students. *Research Quarterly for Exercise and Sport, 65*(2), 189-92.

Mohr, M., Krustrup, P., Nybo, L., Nielsen, J. J., & Bangsbo, J. (2004). Muscle temperature and sprint performance during soccer matches - beneficial effect of re-warm-up at half-time. *Scandinavian Journal of Medicine & Science in Sports, 14*(3), 156-62.

Molenaar, H. M. T., Selles, R. W., Zuidam, J. M., Willemsen, S. P., Stam, H. J., & Hovius, S. E. R. (2010). Growth diagrams for grip strength in children. *Clinical Orthopaedics and Related Research, 468*(1), 217-23.

Moliner-Urdiales, D., Ortega, F. B., Vicente-Rodriguez, G., Rey-Lopez, J. P., Gracia-Marco, L., Widhalm, K., Sjöström, M., Moreno, L. A., Castillo, M. J. & Ruiz, J. R. (2010). Association of physical activity with muscular strength and fat-free mass in adolescents: the HELENA study. *European Journal of Applied Physiology, 109*(6), 1119-27.

Mønness, E., & Sjølie, A. N. (2009). An alternative design for small scale school health experiments: does daily walking produce benefits in physical performance of school children? *Child: Care, Health and Development, 35*(6), 858-67.

Monod, H., & Scherrer, J. (1965). The work capacity of a synergic muscular group. *Ergonomics, 8*(3), 329-38.

Moore, A., & Murphy, A. (2003). Development of an anaerobic capacity test for field sport athletes. *Journal of Science and Medicine in Sport, 6*(3), 275-84.

Mooren, F., & Völker, K. (2005). *Molecular and Cellular Exercise Physiology*. Champaign, ILL: Human Kinetics.

Moritani, T., Nagata, A., Herrfrt, A. D., & Muro, M. (1981). Critical power as a measure of physical work capacity and anaerobic threshold. *Ergonomics, 24*(5), 339-50.

Morse, C. I., Tolfrey, K., Thom, J. M., Vassilopoulos, V., Maganaris, C. N., & Narici, M. V. (2008). Gastrocnemius muscle specific force in boys and men. *Journal of Applied Physiology, 104*(2), 469-74.

Morton, R. H. (1996). A 3-parameter critical power model. *Ergonomics, 39*(4), 611-619.

Morton, R. H., & Billat, L. V. (2004). The critical power model for intermittent exercise. *European Journal of Applied Physiology, 91*(2), 303-7.

Mosston, M. & Ashworth, S. (2002). *Teaching physical education.* San Francisco, CA: Benjamin Cummings.

Mota, J., Guerra, S., Leandro, C., Pinto, A., Ribeiro, J. É. C., & Duarte, J. É. A. (2002). Association of maturation, sex, and body fat in cardiorespiratory fitness. *American Journal of Human Biology, 14*(6), 707-12.

Mota, J., Ribeiro, J. C., Carvalho, J., Santos, M. P., & Martins, J. (2010). Television viewing and changes in body mass index and cardiorespiratory fitness over a two-year period in schoolchildren. *Pediatric Exercise Science, 22*(2), 245-53.

Mottram, D. R. (2011). *Drugs in Sport.* New York: Taylor & Francis.

Mougios, V. (2006). *Exercise biochemistry.* Champaign, ILL: Human Kinetics.

Mujika, I., Chatard, J. C., Lacoste, L., Barale, F., & Geyssant, A. (1996). Creatine supplementation does not improve sprint performance in competitive swimmers. *Medicine & Science in Sports & Exercise, 28*(11), 1435-41.

Myer, G. D., Faigenbaum, A. D., Chu, D. A., Falkel, J., Ford, K. R., Best, T. M., & Hewett, T. E. (2011). Integrative training for children and adolescents: techniques and practices for reducing sports-related injuries and enhancing athletic performance. *Physician and Sports Medicine 39*(1), 74-84.

Myers, J., & Ashley, E. (1997). Dangerous curves. *Chest, 111*(3), 787-95.

Mygind, E., Andersen, L. B., & Rasmussen, B. (1994). Blood lactate and respiratory variables in elite cross-country skiing at racing speeds. *Scandinavian Journal of Medicine & Science in Sports, 4*(4), 243-51.

Nattiv, A., Loucks, A. B., Manore, M. M., Sanborn, C. F., Sundgot-Borgen, J., & Warren, M. P. (2007). American College of Sports Medicine position stand. The female athlete triad. *Medicine and Science in Sports and Exercise, 39*(10), 1867-82.

Nedeljkovic, A., Mirkov, D. M., Pazin, N., & Jaric, S. (2007). Evaluation of Margaria staircase test: the effect of body size. *European Journal of Applied Physiology, 100*(1), 115-20.

Nettle, H., & Sprogis, E. (2011). Pediatric exercise: truth and/or consequences. *Sports Medicine and Arthroscopy Review, 19*(1), 75-80.

Nichols, J. F., Rauh, M. J., Lawson, M. J., Ji, M., & Barkai, H. S. (2006). Prevalence of the female athlete triad syndrome among high school athletes. *Archives of Pediatrics and Adolescent Medicine, 160*(2), 137-42.

Nickols-Richardson, S. M., Modlesky, C. M., O'Connor, P. J., & Lewis, R. D. (2000). Premenarcheal gymnasts possess higher bone mineral density than controls. *Medicine & Science in Sports & Exercise, 32*(1), 63-9.

Nielens, H., & Lejeune, T. M. (2001). Energy cost of riding bicycles with shock absorption systems on a flat surface. *International Journal of Sports Medicine, 22*(6), 400-404.

Nielsen, S., Moller-Madsen, S., Isager, T., Jorgensen, J., Pagsberg, K., & Theander, S. (1998). Standardized mortality in eating disorders - a quantitative summary of previously published and new evidence. *Journal of Psychosomatic Research, 44*(3-4), 413-34.

Nieman, D. C. (1997). Exercise immunology: practical applications. *International Journal of Sports Medicine, 18*(1), S91-100.

Nieman, D. C., & Pedersen, B. K. (1999). Exercise and immune function: recent developments. *Sports Medicine, 27*(2), 73-80.

Nimmo, M. (2004). Exercise in the cold. *Journal of Sports Sciences, 22*(10), 898-916.

Nishii, T., Umemura, Y., & Kitagawa, K. (2004). Full suspension mountain bike improves off-road cycling performance. *Journal of Sports Medicine and Physical Fitness, 44*(4), 356-360.

Noakes, T. D., & Durandt, J. J. (2000). Physiological requirements of cricket. *Journal of Sports Sciences, 18*(12), 919-29.

Noé, F. (2006). Modifications of anticipatory postural adjustments in a rock climbing task: The effect of supporting wall inclination. *Journal of Electromyography and Kinesiology, 16*(4), 336-41.

Noonan, B. C. (2010). Intragame blood-lactate values during ice hockey and their relationships to commonly used hockey testing protocols. *Journal of Strength & Conditioning Research, 24*(9), 2290-5.

Noordhof, D. A., de Koning, J. J., & Foster, C. (2010). The maximal accumulated oxygen deficit method: a valid and reliable measure of anaerobic capacity? *Sports Medicine, 40*(4), 285-302.

Norton, K. I., Craig, N. P., & Olds, T. S. (1999). The evolution of Australian football. *Journal of Science and Medicine in Sport, 2*(4), 389-404.

Nottin, S., Vinet, A., Stecken, F., N'Guyen, L. D., Ounissi, F., Lecoq, A. M., & Obert, P. (2002). Central and peripheral cardiovascular adaptations to exercise in endurance-trained children. *Acta Physiologica Scandinavica, 175*(2), 85-92.

Nunan, D. (2006). Development of a sports specific aerobic capacity test for karate - a pilot study. *Journal of Sports Science and Medicine, Bursa, v. CSSI*, 47-53.

Nurmi-Lawton, J. A., Baxter-Jones, A. D., Mirwald, R. L., Bishop, J. A., Taylor, P., Cooper, C., & New, S. A. (2004). Evidence of sustained skeletal benefits from impact-loading exercise in young females: a 3-year longitudinal study. *Journal of Bone and Mineral Research, 19*(2), 314-22. doi: 10.1359/jbmr.0301222

O'Connor, T., Dubowitz, G., & Bickler, P. E. (2004). Pulse oximetry in the diagnosis of acute mountain sickness. *High Altitude Medicine & Biology, 5*(3), 341-8.

O'Brien, T. D., Reeves, N. D., Baltzopoulos, V., Jones, D. A., & Maganaris, C. N. (2009). The effects of agonist and antagonist muscle activation on the knee extension moment-angle relationship in adults and children. *European Journal of Applied Physiology, 106*(6), 849-56.

O'Brien, T. D., Reeves, N. D., Baltzopoulos, V., Jones, D. A., & Maganaris, C. N. (2010). In vivo measurements of muscle specific tension in adults and children. *Experimental Physiology, 95*(1), 202-10.

Obert, P., Mandigouts, S., Nottin, S., Vinet, A., N'Guyen, L. D., & Lecoq, A. M. (2003). Cardiovascular responses to endurance training in children: effect of gender. *European Journal of Clinical Investigation, 33*(3), 199-208.

Oertel, G. (1988). Morphometric analysis of normal skeletal muscles in infancy, childhood and adolescence: An autopsy study. *Journal of the Neurological Sciences, 88*(1-3), 303-13.

Ogden, C. L., Carroll, M. D., Curtin, L. R., McDowell, M. A., Tabak, C. J., & Flegal, K. M. (2006). Prevalence of overweight and obesity in the United States, 1999-2004. *Journal of the American Medical Association, 295*(13), 1549-55.

Ojanen, T., Rauhala, T., & Häkkinen, K. (2007). Strength and power profiles of the lower and upper extremities in master throwers at different ages. *Journal of Strength & Conditioning Research, 21*(1), 216-22.

Okudan, N., & Gökbel, H. (2006). The ventilatory anaerobic threshold is related to, but is lower than, the critical power, but does not explain exercise tolerance at this workrate. *Journal of Sports Medicine and Physical fitness, 46*(1), 15-19.

Oliver, J. L., Armstrong, N., & Williams, C. A. (2007). Reliability and validity of a soccer-specific test of prolonged repeated-sprint ability. *International Journal of Sports Physiology and Performance, 2*(2), 137-49.

Olsen, J. (1996). Bicycle suspension systems *in* Burke, E. R (ed.) *Hi-Tech Cycling.* Champaign, ILL: Human Kinetics.

Ooi, C. H., Tan, A., Ahmad, A., Kwong, K. W., Sompong, R., Mohd Ghazali, K., Liew, S. L., Chai, W. J. & Thompson, M. W. (2009). Physiological characteristics of elite and sub-elite badminton players. *Journal of Sports Sciences, 27*(14), 1591-9.

Orr, G. W., Green, H. J., Hughson, R. L., & Bennett, G. W. (1982). A computer linear regression model to determine ventilatory anaerobic threshold. *Journal of Applied Physiology, 52*(5), 1349-52.

Orvanova, E. (1987). Physical structure of winter sports athletes. *Journal of Sports Sciences, 5*(3), 197-248.

Ostojic S. M., Markovic G., Calleja-Gonzalez J., Jakovljevic D. G., Vucetic V. & Stojanovic M. (2010). Ultra short-term heart rate recovery after maximal exercise in continuous versus intermittent endurance athletes. *European Journal of Applied Physiology. 108*(5), 1055-9.

Ostojic, S. M., Mazic, S., & Dikic, N. (2006). Profiling in basketball: Physical and physiological characteristics of elite players. *Journal of Strength and Conditioning Research, 20*(4), 740-4.

Otago, L. (1983). A game analysis of the activity patterns of netball players. *Sports Coach, 7*(1), 24-8.

Otago, L. (2004). Kinetic analysis of landings in netball: is a footwork rule change required to decrease ACL injuries? *Journal of Science and Medicine in Sport, 7*(1), 85-95.

Ozmun, J. C., Mikesky, A. E., & Surburg, P. R. (1994). Neuromuscular adaptations following prepubescent strength training. *Medicine & Science in Sports & Exercise, 26*(4), 510-14.

Payne, V. G., & Isaacs, L. D. (2008). *Human Motor Development: A Lifespan Approach.* New York: McGraw-Hill Education.

Pedersen, B. K. (2009). Edward F. Adolph distinguished lecture: muscle as an endocrine organ: IL-6 and other myokines. *Journal of Applied Physiology, 107*(4), 1006-14.

Pedersen, B. K. (2011). Muscles and their myokines. *Journal of Experimental Biology, 214*(2), 337-46.

Pedersen, B. K., Åkerström, T. C. A., Nielsen, A. R., & Fischer, C. P. (2007). Role of myokines in exercise and metabolism. *Journal of Applied Physiology, 103*(3), 1093-8.

Pedersen, B. K., & Febbraio, M. A. (2008). Muscle as an endocrine organ: focus on muscle-derived interleukin-6. *Physiological Reviews, 88*(4), 1379-1406.

Pedersen, B. K., & Hoffman-Goetz, L. (2000). Exercise and the immune system: regulation, integration, and adaptation. *Physiological Reviews, 80*(3), 1055-81.

Peltonen, J. E., Tikkanen, H. O., & Rusko, H. K. (2001). Cardiorespiratory responses to exercise in acute hypoxia, hyperoxia and normoxia. *European Journal of Applied Physiology, 85*(1), 82-8.

Pendergast, D. R. (1989). Cardiovascular, respiratory, and metabolic responses to upper body exercise. *Medicine & Science in Sports & Exercise, 21*(5), S126-S125.

Pérez-Gomez, J., Rodriguez, G. V., Ara, I., Olmedillas, H., Chavarren, J., González-Henriquez, J. J., Dorado, C. & Calbet, J. A. L. (2008). Role of muscle mass on sprint performance: gender differences? *European Journal of Applied Physiology, 102*(6), 685-94.

Pérez-Landaluce, J., RodríGuez-Alonso, M., Fernandez-Garcia, B., Bustillo-Fernandez, E., & Terrados, N. (1998). Importance of wash riding in kayaking training and competition. *Medicine & Science in Sports & Exercise, 30*(12), 1721-4.

Perriello, G., Nurjhan, N., Stumvoll, M., Bucci, A., Welle, S., Dailey, G., Bier, D. M., Toft, I., Jenssen, T. G. & Gerich, J. E. (1997). Regulation of gluconeogenesis by glutamine in normal postabsorptive humans. *American Journal of Physiology-Endocrinology And Metabolism, 272*(3), E437-E445.

Peters, E. M., Robson, P. J., Kleinveldt, N. C., Naicker, V. L., & Jogessar, V. D. (2004). Hematological recovery in male ultra-marathon runners: the effect of variations in training load and running time. *Journal of Sports Medicine and Physical fitness, 44*(3), 315-21.

Pfeiffer R Francis R. (1986). Effects of strength training on muscle development in prepubescent, pubescent and postpubescent males. *Physician and Sports Medicine 14*(9), 134-43.

Phillips, S. M. (2008). Resistance exercise and strong healthy children: safe when done right! *Appl Physiol Nutr Metab, 33*(3), 545-6.

Pieter, W. (2009). Taekwondo. *Combat Sports Medicine*, 1-24.

Pinheiro, C. H. J., Silveira, L. R., Nachbar, R. T., Vitzel, K. F., & Curi, R. (2010). Regulation of glycolysis and expression of glucose metabolism-related genes by reactive oxygen species in contracting skeletal muscle cells. *Free Radical Biology and Medicine, 48*(7), 953-60.

Polidori, M. C., Mecocci, P., Cherubini, A., & Senin, U. (2000). Physical activity and oxidative stress during aging. *International Journal of Sports Medicine, 21*(3), 154-7.

Popadic Gacesa, J. Z., Barak, O. F., & Grujic, N. G. (2009). Maximal anaerobic power test in athletes of different sport disciplines. *Journal of Strength & Conditioning Research, 23*(3), 751-5.

Porter, M. M., Vandervoort, A. A., & Lexell, J. (1995). Aging of human muscle: structure, function and adaptability. *Scandinavian Journal of Medicine & Science in Sports, 5*(3), 129-42.

Posterino, G. S., & Dunn, S. L. (2008). Comparison of the effects of inorganic phosphate on caffeine-induced Ca2+ release in fast-and slow-twitch mammalian skeletal muscle. *American Journal of Physiology-Cell Physiology, 294*(1), C97-C105.

Potdevin, F. J., Alberty, M. E., Chevutschi, A., Pelayo, P., & Sidney, M. C. (2011). Effects of a 6-week plyometric training program on performances in pubescent swimmers. *Journal of Strength & Conditioning Research, 25*(1), 80-86.

Praagh, E. (1998). *Pediatric anaerobic performance*. Champaign: ILL: Human Kinetics.

Price, M., Moss, P., & Rance, S. (2003). Effects of sodium bicarbonate ingestion on prolonged intermittent exercise. *Medicine & Science in Sports & Exercise, 35*(8), 1303.

Pringle, J. S., & Jones, A. M. (2002). Maximal lactate steady state, critical power and EMG during cycling. *European Journal of Applied Physiology, 88*(3), 214-26.

Pronk, M., Tiemessen, I., Hupperets, M. D. W., Kennedy, B. P., Powell, F. L., Hopkins, S. R., & Wagner, P. D. (2003). Persistence of the lactate paradox over 8 weeks at 3800 m. *High Altitude Medicine & Biology, 4*(4), 431-43.

Psotta R., Blahus P., Cochrane D. J., & Martin A. J. (2005). The assessment of an intermittent high intensity running test. *Journal of Sports Medicine and Physical Fitness. 45*(3), 248-56.

Pyne, D. B., Boston, T., Martin, D. T., & Logan, A. (2000). Evaluation of the Lactate Pro blood lactate analyser. *European Journal of Applied Physiology, 82*(1), 112-16.

Pyne, D. B., Gardner, A. S., Sheehan, K., & Hopkins, W. G. (2005). Fitness testing and career progression in AFL football. *Journal of Science and Medicine in Sport, 8*(3), 321-32.

Quah, Y. V., Poh, B. K., Ng, L. O., & Noor, M. I. (2009). The female athlete triad among elite Malaysian athletes: prevalence and associated factors. *Asia Pacific Journal of Clinical Nutrition, 18*(2), 200-8.

Quaine, F., Vigouroux, L., & Martin, L. (2003). Finger flexors fatigue in trained rock climbers and untrained sedentary subjects. *International Journal of Sports Medicine, 24*(6), 424-7.

Racinais, S., Blonc, S., & Hue, O. (2005). Effects of active warm-up and diurnal increase in temperature on muscular power. *Medicine & Science in Sports & Exercise, 37*(12), 2134-9.

Ramsay, J. A., Blimkie Jr, C., Smith, K., Garner, S., Macdougall, J. D., & Sale, D. G. (1990). Strength training effects in prepubescent boys. *Medicine & Science in Sports & Exercise, 22*(5), 605-14.

Rashad, K. I., Phillips, M. A., Revels, M., & Ujamaa, D. (2010). Contribution of the school environment to physical fitness in children and youth. *Journal of Physical Activity & Health, 7*(3), 333-42.

Ratel, S. (2011). High-intensity and resistance training and elite young athletes. *Medicine and Sport Science, 56*, 84-96.

Ratel, S., Duche, P., Hennegrave, A., Van Praagh, E., & Bedu, M. (2002). Acid-base balance during repeated cycling sprints in boys and men. *Journal of Applied Physiology, 92*(2), 479-85.

Ratel, S., Duché, P., & Williams, C. A. (2006). Muscle fatigue during high-intensity exercise in children. *Sports Medicine, 36*(12), 1031-65.

Ratel, S., Williams, C. A., Oliver, J., & Armstrong, N. (2004). Effects of age and mode of exercise on power output profiles during repeated sprints. *European Journal of Applied Physiology, 92*(1), 204-10.

Rcr, D. (2003). Heart rate responses of male orienteers aged 21-67 years during competition. *Journal of Sports Sciences, 21*(3), 221-8.

Ready, A. E., & van der Merwe, M. (1986). Physiological monitoring of the 1984 Canadian women's Olympic field hockey team. *Australian Journal of Science and Medicine in Sport, 18*, 13-18.

Reeser, J. C. (2003). Introduction: a brief history of the sport of volleyball. *Handbook of Sports Medicine and Science: Volleyball*, 1-7.

Reilly, T., & Ball, D. (1984). The net physiological cost of dribbling a soccer ball. *Research Quarterly for Exercise and Sport, 55*(3), 267-71.

Reilly, T., & Borrie, A. (1992). Physiology applied to field hockey. *Sports Medicine, 14*(1), 10-26.

Reilly, T., & Piercy, M. (1994). The effect of partial sleep deprivation on weight-lifting performance. *Ergonomics, 37*(1), 107-15.

Reilly, T., & Seaton, A. (1990). Physiological strain unique to field hockey. *Journal of sports Medicine and Physical fitness, 30*(2), 142-6.

Richardson, R. S., White, A. T., Seifert, J. D., Porretta, J. M., & Johnson, S. C. (1993). Blood lactate concentrations in elite skiers during a series of on-snow downhill ski runs. *Journal of Strength & Conditioning Research, 7*(3), 168-71.

Rimmer, J. H., & Looney, M. A. (1997). Effects of an Aerobic Activity Program on the Cholesterol Levels of Adolescents. *Research Quarterly for Exercise and Sport, 68*(1), 74-9.

Robergs, R. A., & Landwehr, R. (2002). The surprising history of the 'HRmax= 220-age' equation. *Journal of Exercise Physiology, 5*(2), 1-10.

Roberts, S. P., Stokes, K. A., Weston, L., & Trewartha, G. (2010). The Bath University Rugby Shuttle Test (BURST): a pilot study. *International Journal of Sports Physiology and Performance, 5*(1), 64-74.

Roberts S. P., Trewartha G., Higgitt R. J., El-Abd J. & Stokes K. A. (2008). The physical demands of elite English rugby union. *Journal of Sports Science. 26*(8), 825-33.

Roelands, B., & Meeusen, R. (2010). Alterations in central fatigue by pharmacological manipulations of neurotransmitters in normal and high ambient temperature. *Sports Medicine, 40*(3), 229-46.

Roemmich, J. N., Richmond, E. J., & Rogol, A. D. (2001). Consequences of sport training during puberty. *Journal of Endocrinological Investigation, 24*(9), 708-15.

Rohrbough, J. T., Mudge, M. K., & Schilling, R. C. (2000). Overuse injuries in the elite rock climber. *Medicine & Science in Sports & Exercise, 32*(8), 1369-72.

Rognmo Ø., Hetland E., Helgerud J., Hoff J. & Slørdahl S. A. (2004). High intensity aerobic interval exercise is superior to moderate intensity exercise for increasing aerobic capacity in patients with coronary artery disease. *European Journal of Cardiovascular Prevention and Rehabilitation. 11*(3), 216-22.

Roi, G. S., & Bianchedi, D. (2008). The science of fencing: implications for performance and injury prevention. *Sports Medicine, 38*(6), 465-81.

Roots, H., Ball, G., Talbot-Ponsonby, J., King, M., McBeath, K., & Ranatunga, K. W. (2009). Muscle fatigue examined at different temperatures in experiments on intact mammalian (rat) muscle fibers. *Journal of Applied Physiology, 106*(2), 378-84.

Roth, D. A., & Brooks, G. A. (1990). Lactate transport is mediated by a membrane-bound carrier in rat skeletal muscle sarcolemmal vesicles. *Archives of Biochemistry and Biophysics, 279*(2), 377-85.

Roth, M., & Stamatakis, E. (2010). Linking young people's knowledge of public health guidelines to physical activity levels in England. *Pediatric Exercise Science, 22*(3), 467-76.

Rothschuh, K. E., & Risse, G. B. (1973). *History of physiology.* Malabar, FL: R. E. Krieger Publishing Company.

Rougier, P., & Blanchi, J. P. (1991). Evaluation du niveau d'expertise en escalade par l'analyse de la relation posturocinétique. *Science et Motricité, 14*, 3-12.

Rowland, T., Wehnert, M., & Miller, K. (2000). Cardiac responses to exercise in competitive child cyclists. *Medicine & Science in Sports & Exercise, 32*(4), 747.

Rowland, T. W. (1996). *Developmental exercise physiology.* Champaign, ILL: Human Kinetics.

Rubley, M. D., Haase, A. C., Holcomb, W. R., Girouard, T. J., & Tandy, R. D. (2011). The effect of plyometric training on power

and kicking distance in female adolescent soccer players. *Journal of Strength & Conditioning Research, 25*(1), 129-34.

Ruiz, J., Silva, G., Oliveira, N., Ribeiro, J., Oliveira, J., & Mota, J. (2009). Criterion-related validity of the 20-m shuttle run test in youths aged 13-19 years. *Journal of Sports Sciences, 27*(9), 899-906.

Rundell, K. W. (1995). Treadmill roller ski test predicts biathlon roller ski race results of elite US biathlon women. *Medicine & Science in Sports & Exercise, 27*(12), 1677-85.

Rundell, K. W., & Bacharach, D. W. (1995). Physiological characteristics and performance of top US biathletes. *Medicine & Science in Sports & Exercise, 27*(9), 1302-10.

Rundell, K. W., & Slee, J. B. (2008). Exercise and other indirect challenges to demonstrate asthma or exercise-induced bronchoconstriction in athletes. *Journal of Allergy and Clinical Immunology, 122*(2), 238-46.

Rusko, H., Tikkanen, H., & Peltonen, J. (2004). Altitude and endurance training. *Journal of Sports Sciences, 22*(10), 928-45.

Saavedra, C., LagassÉ, P., Bouchard, C., & Simoneau, J. A. (1991). Maximal anaerobic performance of the knee extensor muscles during growth. *Medicine & Science in Sports & Exercise, 23*(9), 1083-9.

Sagar, H. R. (2001). *Climbing your best: training to maximize your performance.* Mechanicsburg, PA: Stackpole Books.

Sahlin, K., & Harris, R. C. (2011). The creatine kinase reaction: a simple reaction with functional complexity. *Amino Acids,* 1-5.

Sailors, M., & Berg, K. (1987). Comparison of responses to weight training in pubescent boys and men. *Journal of Sports medicine and Physical Fitness, 27*(1), 30-37.

Salo, A. I., Bezodis, I. N., Batterham, A. M., & Kerwin, D. G. (2011). Elite sprinting: are athletes individually step-frequency or step-length reliant? *Medicine and Science in Sports and Exercise 43*(6), 1055-62.

Saltin B. & Essen B. (1971) Muscle glycogen, lactate, ATP, and CP in intermittent exercise. In: Pernow B. and Saltin B. (eds.) *Muscle metabolism during exercise. Advances in experimental medicine and biology,* vol. 11. New York: Plenum Press, 419-24.

Sanborn, C. F., Martin, B. J., & Wagner Jr, W. W. (1982). Is athletic amenorrhea specific to runners? *American Journal of Obstetrics and Gynecology, 143*(8), 859-61.

Santos, P., Guerra, S., Ribeiro, J. C., Duarte, J. A., & Mota, J. (2003). Age and gender-related physical activity: A descriptive study in children using accelerometry. *Journal of Sports Medicine and Physical Fitness, 43*(1), 85-9.

Sardinha, L. B., & Teixeira, P. J. (2005). Measuring adiposity and fat distribution in relation to health. *In* Heymsfied, S, Lohman, T., Wang, Z and Going S., *Human Body Composition,* 2nd edn. Champaign, ILL: Human Kinetics.

Sauka, M., Priedite, I. S., Artjuhova, L., Larins, V., Selga, G., Dahlström, Ö., & Timpka, T. (2011). Physical fitness in northern European youth: Reference values from the Latvian Physical

Health in Youth Study. *Scandinavian Journal of Public Health, 39*(1), 35-43.

Savage, M. P., Petratis, M. M., Thomson, W. H., Berg, K., Smith, J. L., & Sady, S. P. (1986). Exercise training effects on serum lipids of prepubescent boys and adult men. *Medicine and Science in Sports and Exercise, 18*(2), 197-204.

Savourey, G., Garcia, N., Caravel, J. P., Gharib, C., Pouzeratte, N., Martin, S., & Bittel, J. (1997). Pre-adaptation, adaptation and de-adaptation to high altitude in humans: hormonal and biochemical changes at sea level. *European Journal of Applied Physiology and Occupational Physiology, 77*(1), 37-43.

Savourey, G., Launay, J. C., Besnard, Y., Guinet, A., Bourrilhon, C., Cabane, D., Martin, S., Caravel, J. P., Péquignot, J. M. & Cottet-Emard, J. M. (2004). Control of erythropoiesis after high altitude acclimatization. *European Journal of Applied Physiology, 93*(1), 47-56.

Sawka, M. N. (1989). Introduction: upper body exercise: physiology and practical considerations. *Medicine & Science in Sports & Exercise, 21*(5), S121-S125.

Scerpella, T. A., Dowthwaite, J. N., Gero, N. M., Kanaley, J. A., & Ploutz-Snyder, R. J. (2010). Skeletal Benefits of Pre-Menarcheal Gymnastics Are Retained After Activity Cessation. *Pediatric Exercise Science, 22*(1), 21-33.

Scharhag-Rosenberger, F. S. R. F., Carlsohn, A. C. A., Cassel, M. C. M., Mayer, F. M. F., & Scharhag, J. S. J. (2011). How to test maximal oxygen uptake: a study on timing and testing procedure of a supramaximal verification test. *Applied Physiology, Nutrition, and Metabolism, 36*(1), 153-60.

Scherrer J. and Monod H. (1960) Le travail musculaire local et la fatigue chez l'homme. *Journal of Physiology (Paris).* 52:419-501.

Schneiker, K. T., Bishop, D., Dawson, B., & Hackett, L. P. (2006). Effects of caffeine on prolonged intermittent-sprint ability in team-sport athletes. *Medicine & Science in Sports & Exercise, 38*(3), 578-85.

Schöffl, V., Klee, S., & Strecker, W. (2004). Evaluation of physiological standard pressures of the forearm flexor muscles during sport specific ergometry in sport climbers. *British Journal of Sports Medicine, 38*(4), 422-5.

Schöffl, V. R., Möckel, F., Köstermeyer, G., Roloff, I., & Küpper, T. (2006). Development of a performance diagnosis of the anaerobic strength endurance of the forearm flexor muscles in sport climbing. *International Journal of Sports Medicine, 27*(3), 205-11.

Schönau, E. (1998). The development of the skeletal system in children and the influence of muscular strength. *Hormone Research in Paediatrics, 49*(1), 27-31.

Schönau, E. (2006). Bone mass increase in puberty: what makes it happen? *Hormone Research in Paediatrics, 65*(2), 2-10.

Schönau, E., & Fricke, O. (2008). Mechanical influences on bone development in children. *European Journal of Endocrinology, 159*(suppl 1), S27-S31. doi: 10.1530/eje-08-0312

Schönau, E., & Frost, H. M. (2002). The 'muscle-bone unit' in children and adolescents. *Calcified Tissue International, 70*(5), 405-7.

Schönau, E., Neu, C. M., Beck, B., Manz, F., & Rauch, F. (2002). Bone mineral content per muscle cross sectional area as an index of the functional muscle bone unit. *Journal of Bone and Mineral Research, 17*(6), 1095-1101.

Schönau, E., Neu, C. M., Mokov, E., Wassmer, G., & Manz, F. (2000). Influence of puberty on muscle area and cortical bone area of the forearm in boys and girls. *Journal of Clinical Endocrinology & Metabolism, 85*(3), 1095-8.

Schönau, E., Neu, M. C., & Manz, F. (2004). Muscle mass during childhood-Relationship to skeletal development. *Journal of Musculoskeletal and Neuronal Interactions, 4*(1), 105-8.

Schwane, J. A., Johnson, S. R., Vandenakker, C. B., & Armstrong, R. B. (1983). Delayed-onset muscular soreness and plasma CPK and LDH activities after downhill running. *Medicine & Science in Sports & Exercise, 15*(1), 51-6.

Scott, A. C., Roe, N., Coats, A. J. S., & Piepoli, M. F. (2003). Aerobic exercise physiology in a professional rugby union team. *International Journal of Cardiology, 87*(2-3), 173-7.

Scott, K. E., Rozenek, R., Russo, A. C., Crussemeyer, J. A., & Lacourse, M. G. (2003). Effects of delayed onset muscle soreness on selected physiological responses to submaximal running. *Journal of Strength & Conditioning Research, 17*(4), 652-8.

Seeley, R. R., Stephens, T., & Tate, P. (2002). *Essentials of anatomy and physiology.* New York: McGraw-Hill.

Seeley, R. R., Stephens, T. D., & Tate, P. (2000). *Anatomy and physiology.* New York: McGraw-Hill.

Seeman, E. (2001). Clinical review 137: Sexual dimorphism in skeletal size, density, and strength. *Journal of Clinical Endocrinology and Metabolism 86*(10), 4576-84.

Seeman, E. (2008). Structural basis of growth-related gain and age-related loss of bone strength. *Rheumatology (Oxford), 47* Suppl 4, iv, 2-8.

Seger, J. Y., & Thorstensson, A. (2000). Muscle strength and electromyogram in boys and girls followed through puberty. *European journal of applied physiology, 81*(1), 54-61.

Seifert, J. G., Luetkemeier, M. J., Spencer, M. K., Miller, D., & Burke, E. R. (1997). The effects of mountain bike suspension systems on energy expenditure, physical exertion, and time trial performance during mountain bicycling. *International Journal of Sports Medicine, 18*(3), 197-200.

Selye, H. (1956). *The stress of life.* New York: McGraw-Hill.

Semenick, D. (1984). Basketball bioenergetics: Practical applications. *National Strength and Conditioning Association Journal. 6*(6), 44-73.

Shackleton, R., & Christensen, J. (1985). *All about wave skis.* Surfside Press.

Sheel, A. W. (2004). Physiology of sport rock climbing. *British Journal of Sports Medicine, 38*(3), 355-9.

Sheppard J. M., Young W. B., Doyle T. L., Sheppard T. A., & Newton R. U. (2006) An evaluation of a new test of reactive agility and its relationship to sprint speed and change of direction speed. *Journal of Science and Medicine in Sport. 9*(4), 342-9. Epub 2006 J 17.

Shephard, R. J. (1987). Science and medicine of canoeing and kayaking. *Sports Medicine, 4*(1), 19-33.

Sherman, W. M., Costill, D. L., Fink, W. J., & Miller, J. M. (1981). Effect of exercise-diet manipulation on muscle glycogen and its subsequent utilization during performance. *International Journal of Sports Medicine 2*(2), 114-18.

Sherman, W. M., Plyley, M. J., Sharp, R. L., Van Handel, P. J., McAllister, R. M., Fink, W. J., & Costill, D. L. (1982). Muscle glycogen storage and its relationship with water. *International Journal of Sports Medicine, 3*, 22-4.

Sherwood, L. (2008). *Human physiology: from cells to systems.* Brooks/Cole, Salt Lake City, UT: Cengage Learning.

Sidney, K., & Shephard, R. J. (1973). Physiological characteristics and performance of the white-water paddler. *European Journal of Applied Physiology and Occupational Physiology, 32*(1), 55-70.

Simmonds, M. J., Minahan, C. L., & Sabapathy, S. (2010). Caffeine improves supramaximal cycling but not the rate of anaerobic energy release. *European Journal of Applied Physiology, 109*(2), 287-95.

Simpson, R. J., Wilson, M. R., Black, J. R., Ross, J. A., Whyte, G. P., Guy, K., & Florida-James, G. D. (2005). Immune alterations, lipid peroxidation, and muscle damage following a hill race. *Canadian Journal of Applied Physiology, 30*(2), 196-211.

Singh, M. A. F. (2004). Exercise and aging. *Clinics in Geriatric Medicine, 20*(2), 201-22.

Singla, P., Bardoloi, A., & Parkash, A. A. (2010). Metabolic effects of obesity: A review. *World Journal of Diabetes, 1*(3), 76-88.

Sirotic, A. C., & Coutts, A. J. (2007). Physiological and performance test correlates of prolonged, high-intensity, intermittent running performance in moderately trained women team sport athletes. *Journal of Strength and Conditioning Research, 21*(1), 138-44.

Skein, M., Duffield, R., Edge, J., Short, M. J., & Mündel, T. (2011). Intermittent-sprint performance and muscle glycogen after 30 h of sleep deprivation. *Medicine & Science in Sports & Exercise, 43*(7), 1301.

Sklad, M., Krawczyk, B., & Majle, B. (1994). Body build profiles of male and female rowers and kayakers. *Biology of Sport, 11*(4), 249-56.

Slaughter, M. H., Lohman, T. G., Boileau, R. A., Horswill, C. A., Stillman, R. J., Van Loan, M. D., & Bemben, D. A. (1988). Skinfold equations for estimation of body fatness in children and youth. *Human Biology, 60*(5), 709-23.

Sleight, S. (1999). *DK complete sailing manual.* London: Dorling Kindersley.

Smith, D. J., Norris, S. R., & Hogg, J. M. (2002). Performance evaluation of swimmers: scientific tools. *Sports Medicine, 32*(9), 539-54.

Smith, H. K. (1998). Applied physiology of water polo. *Sports Medicine, 26*(5), 317-34.

Smith, M. S. (2006). Physiological profile of senior and junior England international amateur boxers. *Journal of Sports Science and Medicine, 5,* 74-89.

Söderman, K., Bergström, E., Lorentzon, R., & Alfredson, H. (2000). Bone mass and muscle strength in young female soccer players. *Calcified Tissue International, 67*(4), 297-303.

Sparling, P. B., Snow, T. K., & Millard-Stafford, M. L. (1993). Monitoring core temperature during exercise: ingestible sensor vs. rectal thermistor. *Aviation, Space, and Environmental medicine, 64*(8), 760-3.

Sparrow, A. (1997). *The complete caving manual.* Marlborough, UK: The Crowood Press.

Spencer, M., Bishop, D., Dawson, B., & Goodman, C. (2005). Physiological and metabolic responses of repeated-sprint activities. *Sports Medicine, 35*(12), 1025-44.

Spencer, M., Lawrence, S., Rechichi, C., Bishop, D., Dawson, B., & Goodman, C. (2004). Time-motion analysis of elite field hockey, with special reference to repeated-sprint activity. *Journal of Sports Sciences, 22*(9), 843-50.

Spencer, M., Rechichi, C., Lawrence, S., Dawson, B., Bishop, D., & Goodman, C. (2005). Time-motion analysis of elite field hockey during several games in succession: a tournament scenario. *Journal of Science and Medicine in Sport, 8*(4), 382-91.

Spodaryk K., Zoladz J. A. (1998). The 2,3-DPG levels of human red blood cells during an incremental exercise test: relationship to the blood acid-base balance. *Physiological Research, 47*(1), 17-22.

Spurway, N. C. and Burns, R. (1993). Comparison of dynamic and static fitness training programmes. *Medical Science Research, 21*(14), 865-7.

Šrámek, P., Šime ková, M., Janský, L., Šavlíková, J., & Vybiral, S. (2000). Human physiological responses to immersion into water of different temperatures. *European Journal of Applied Physiology, 81*(5), 436-42.

Stamford, B. A., Weltman, A., Moffatt, R., & Sady, S. (1981). Exercise recovery above and below anaerobic threshold following maximal work. *Journal of Applied Physiology, 51*(4), 840.

Stanley, W. C., Gertz, E. W., Wisneski, J. A., Neese, R. A., Morris, D. L., & Brooks, G. A. (1986). Lactate extraction during net lactate release in legs of humans during exercise. *Journal of Applied Physiology, 60*(4), 1116-20.

Starling, E. H., & Visscher, M. B. (1927). The regulation of the energy output of the heart. *Journal of Physiology, 62*(3), 243-61.

Steele, J. R., Australian Sports Commission, All Australia Netball Association, National Sports Research Program (Australia), & University of Wollongong. School of Health Sciences (1987). *The effect of changes to playing surface, footwork rules and throwing technique on ground reaction forces at landing in netball*: School of Health Sciences, University of Wollongong.

Steele, J. R., Chad, K. E. Australian Sports Commission, Applied Sports Research Program (1991). *An analysis of the movement patterns of netball players during match play : implications for designing training programs.* National Sports Research Centre.

Stickley, C. D., Hetzler, R. K., & Kimura, I. F. (2008). Prediction of anaerobic power values from an abbreviated WAnT protocol. *Journal of Strength & Conditioning Research, 22*(3), 958-65.

Stolen, T., Chamari, K., Castagna, C., & Wisloff, U. (2005). Physiology of soccer: an update. *Sports Medicine, 35*(6), 501-36.

Stone, M. H., Sands, W. A., Pierce, K. C., Ramsey, M. W., & Haff, G. G. (2008). Power and power potentiation among strength-power athletes: preliminary study. *International Journal of Sports Physiology and Performance, 3*(1), 55-67.

Stone, N. M., & Kilding, A. E. (2009). Aerobic conditioning for team sport athletes. *Sports Medicine, 39*(8), 615-42.

Stratton, J. R., Levy, W. C., Cerqueira, M. D., Schwartz, R. S., & Abrass, I. B. (1994). Cardiovascular responses to exercise. Effects of aging and exercise training in healthy men. *Circulation, 89*(4), 1648-55.

Strauss, M. B., & Aksenov, I. V. (2004). *Diving science.* Champaign, ILL: Human Kinetics.

Streckis, V., Skurvydas, A., & Ratkevicius, A. (2007). Children are more susceptible to central fatigue than adults. *Muscle & Nerve, 36*(3), 357-63.

Stretch, R. A., Bartlett, R., & Davids, K. (2000). A review of batting in men's cricket. *Journal of Sports Sciences, 18*(12), 931-49.

Stumvoll, M., Meyer, C., Perriello, G., Kreider, M., Welle, S., & Gerich, J. (1998). Human kidney and liver gluconeogenesis: evidence for organ substrate selectivity. *American Journal of Physiology-Endocrinology And Metabolism, 274*(5), E817-E826.

Subudhi, A. W., Davis, S. L., Kipp, R. W., & Askew, E. W. (2001). Antioxidant status and oxidative stress in elite alpine ski racers. *International Journal of Sport Nutrition and Exercise Metabolism, 11*(1), 32-41.

Sunderland, C., Cooke, K., Milne, H., & Nevill, M. E. (2006). The reliability and validity of a field hockey skill test. *International Journal of Sports Medicine, 27*(5), 395-400.

Sundgot-Borgen, J. (1994). Risk and trigger factors for the development of eating disorders in female elite athletes. *Medicine & Science in Sports & Exercise, 26*(4), 414-19.

Sutton, J. R., Coates, G., & Houston, C. S. (1992). *Hypoxia and mountain medicine: proceedings of the 7th International Hypoxia Symposium held at Lake Louise, Canada, February 1991.* New York: Pergamon Press.

Svedahl, K., & MacIntosh, B. R. (2003). Anaerobic threshold: the concept and methods of measurement. *Canadian Journal of Applied Physiology, 28*(2), 299-323.

Svensson, M., & Drust, B. (2005). Testing soccer players. *Journal of Sports Sciences, 23*(6), 601-18.

Symons, J. D., Bell, D. G., Pope, J., VanHelder, T., & Myles, W. S. (1988). Electro-mechanical response times and muscle strength after sleep deprivation. *Canadian Journal of Sport Sciences= Journal canadien des sciences du sport, 13*(4), 225-30.

Sziva, Á., Mészáros, Z., Kiss, K., Mavroudes, M., Ng, N., & Mészáros, J. (2009). Longitudinal differences in running endurance and body mass index – a 25-year comparison. *Acta Physiologica Hungarica, 96*(3), 359-68.

Talag, T. S. (1973). Residual muscular soreness as influenced by concentric, eccentric, and static contractions. *Research Quarterly in Exercise and Sport, 44*(4), 458-69.

Tan, S., Yang, C., & Wang, J. (2010a). Physical training of 9- to 10-year-old children with obesity to lactate threshold intensity. *Pediatric Exercise Science, 22*(3), 477-85.

Tan, S., Yang, C., & Wang, J. (2010b). Physical training of 9- to 10-year-old children with obesity to lactate threshold intensity. *Pediatric Exercise Science, 22*(3), 477-85.

Tanaka, H., Monahan, K. D., & Seals, D. R. (2001). Age-predicted maximal heart rate revisited. *Journal of the American College of Cardiology, 37*(1), 153-6.

Tannheimer, M., Thomas, A., & Gerngross, H. (2002). Oxygen saturation course and altitude symptomatology during an expedition to broad peak (8047 m). *International Journal of Sports Medicine, 23*(5), 329-35.

Tegtbur, U. W. E., Busse, M. W., & Braumann, K. M. (1993). Estimation of an individual equilibrium between lactate production and catabolism during exercise. *Medicine & Science in Sports & Exercise, 25*(5), 620-27.

Tesch, P. A. (1983). Physiological characteristics of elite kayak paddlers. *Canadian Journal of Applied Sport Sciences. Journal canadien des sciences appliquées au sport, 8*(2), 87-91.

Tesch, P. A., & Lindeberg, S. (1984). Blood lactate accumulation during arm exercise in world class kayak paddlers and strength trained athletes. *European Journal of Applied Physiology and Occupational Physiology, 52*(4), 441-45.

Tesch, P. E. R., Piehl, K., Wilson, G., & Karlsson, J. A. N. (1976). Physiological investigations of Swedish elite canoe competitors. *Medicine & Science in Sports & Exercise, 8*(4), 214-18.

Thein-Nissenbaum, J. M., & Carr, K. E. (2011). Female athlete triad syndrome in the high school athlete. *Physical Therapy in Sport, 12*(3), 108-16.

Thomas, J. R., Nelson, J. K., & Church, G. (1991). A developmental analysis of gender differences in health related physical fitness. *Pediatric Exercise Science, 3*, 28-42.

Thomas, K., French, D., & Hayes, P. R. (2009). The effect of two plyometric training techniques on muscular power and agility in youth soccer players. *Journal of Strength & Conditioning Research, 23*(1), 332-5.

Thoreau, H. D. (1980). *Walden, or Life in the Woods* (1854). New York: Signet Classic.

Tikuisis, P., Eyolfson, D., Xu, X., & Giesbrecht, G. (2002). Shivering endurance and fatigue during cold water immersion in humans. *European Journal of Applied Physiology, 87*(1), 50-58.

Tillin, N. A., & Bishop, D. (2009). Factors modulating post-activation potentiation and its effect on performance of subsequent explosive activities. *Sports Medicine, 39*(2), 147-66.

References

Tillin, N. A., Jimenez-Reyes, P., Pain, M. T. G., & Folland, J. P. (2010). Neuromuscular performance of explosive power athletes versus untrained individuals. *Medicine & Science in Sports & Exercise, 42*(4), 781-90.

Tipton, M. J. (1989). The initial responses to cold-water immersion in man. *Clinical Science (London, England: 1979), 77*(6), 581-8.

Tjønna A. E., Lee S. J., Rognmo Ø., Stølen T. O., Bye A., Haram P. M., Loennechen J. P., Al-Share Q. Y., Skogvoll E., Slørdahl S. A., Kemi O. J., Najjar S. M. & Wisløff U. (2008) Aerobic interval training versus continuous moderate exercise as a treatment for the metabolic syndrome: a pilot study. *Circulation, 118*(4), 346-54.

Tkacz, J., Young-Hyman, D., Boyle, C. A., & Davis, C. L. (2008). Aerobic exercise program reduces anger expression among overweight children. *Pediatric Exercise Science, 20*(4), 390-401.

Tolfrey, K., Jones, A. M., & Campbell, I. G. (2000). The effect of aerobic exercise training on the lipid-lipoprotein profile of children and adolescents. *Sports Medicine, 29*(2), 99-112.

Tomlin, D. L., & Wenger, H. A. (2001). The relationship between aerobic fitness and recovery from high intensity intermittent exercise. *Sports Medicine, 31*(1), 1-11.

Tong, T. K., Lu, K., Chung, P. K., & Quach, B. (2008). Load assignment of Wingate test in minor overfat young adults – is counting the fat mass a pitfall? *Journal of Exercise Science & Fitness, 6*(1), 15-20.

Tonson, A., Ratel, S., Fur, Y. L., Cozzone, P., & Bendahan, D. (2008). Effect of maturation on the relationship between muscle size and force production. *Medicine & Science in Sports & Exercise, 40*(5), 918-25.

Tortora, G. J., & Bryan, D. (2006). *Principles of anatomy and physiology*. J. Wiley.

Tortora, G. J., & Derrickson, B. (2008). *Principles of anatomy and physiology*. J. Wiley.

Toubekis, A. G., Douda, H. T., & Tokmakidis, S. P. (2005). Influence of different rest intervals during active or passive recovery on repeated sprint swimming performance. *European Journal of Applied Physiology, 93*(5), 694-700.

Toubekis, A. G., Tsami, A. P., & Tokmakidis, S. P. (2006). Critical velocity and lactate threshold in young swimmers. *International Journal of Sports Medicine, 27*(2), 117-23.

Trivi, T., Drid, P., Obadov, S., & Ostojic, S. (2011). Effect of endurance training on biomarkers of oxidative stress in male wrestlers. *Journal of Martial Arts Anthropology, 11*(2), 6-9.

Trudeau, F., Laurencelle, L., & Shephard, R. J. (2009). Is fitness level in childhood associated with physical activity level as an adult? *Pediatric Exercise Science, 21*(3), 329-38.

Tsaoussoglou, M., Bixler, E. O., Calhoun, S., Chrousos, G. P., Sauder, K., & Vgontzas, A. N. (2010). Sleep-disordered breathing in obese children is associated with prevalent excessive daytime sleepiness, inflammation, and metabolic abnormalities. *Journal of Clinical Endocrinology & Metabolism, 95*(1), 143-50.

Tsolakis, C., Douvis, A., Tsigganos, G., Zacharogiannis, E., & Smirniotou, A. (2010). Acute Effects of Stretching on Flexibility, Power and Sport Specific Performance in Fencers. *Journal of Human Kinetics, 26*(-1), 105-14.

Tsolakis, C., & Vagenas, G. (2010). Anthropometric, physiological and performance characteristics of elite and sub-elite fencers. *Journal of Human Kinetics, 23*(-1), 89-95.

Tumilty, D. (1993). Physiological characteristics of elite soccer players. *Sports Medicine, 16*(2), 80-96.

Turner, A. P., Cathcart, A. J., Parker, M. E., Butterworth, C., Wilson, J., & Ward, S. A. (2006). Oxygen uptake and muscle desaturation kinetics during intermittent cycling. *Medicine & Science in Sports & Exercise, 38*(3), 492-503.

Twight, M., & Martin, J. (1999). *Extreme alpinism: climbing light, fast, & high*. Seattle, WA: The Mountaineers Books.

Urhausen, A., & Kindermann, W. (2002). Diagnosis of overtraining: what tools do we have? *Sports Medicine, 32*(2), 95-102.

Vaccaro, P., Gray, P. R., Clarke, D. H., & Morris, A. F. (1984). Physiological characteristics of world class white-water slalom paddlers. *Research Quarterly in Exercise and Sport, 55*, 206-10.

Van Hall, G., Calbet, J. A. L., Søndergaard, H., & Saltin, B. (2001). The re-establishment of the normal blood lactate response to exercise in humans after prolonged acclimatization to altitude. *Journal of physiology, 536*(3), 963-75.

Van Hall, G., Jensen-Urstad, M., Rosdahl, H., Holmberg, H. C., Saltin, B., & Calbet, J. A. L. (2003). Leg and arm lactate and substrate kinetics during exercise. *American Journal of Physiology-Endocrinology And Metabolism, 284*(1), E193-E205.

Van Praagh, E. (ed.) (1998). *Pediatric anaerobic performance*. Champaign, ILL: Human Kinetics.

Van Praagh, E. (2000). Development of anaerobic function during childhood and adolescence. *Pediatric Exercise Science, 12*(2), 150-73.

Van Praagh, E., & Doré, E. (2002). Short-term muscle power during growth and maturation. *Sports Medicine, 32*(11), 701-28.

Van Praagh, E., Fellmann, N., Bedu, M., Falgairette, G., & Coudert, J. (1990). Gender difference in the relationship of anaerobic power output to body composition in children. *Pediatric Exercise Science, 2*, 336-48.

Van Someren, K. A., & Oliver, J. E. (2002). The efficacy of ergometry determined heart rates for flatwater kayak training. *International Journal of Sports Medicine, 23*(1), 28-32.

Van Someren, K. A., Phillips, G. R., & Palmer, G. S. (2000). Comparison of physiological responses to open water kayaking and kayak ergometry. *International Journal of Sports Medicine, 21*(3), 200-4.

Vandenberghe, K., Goris, M., Van Hecke, P., Van Leemputte, M., Vangerven, L., & Hespel, P. (1997). Long-term creatine intake is beneficial to muscle performance during resistance training. *Journal of Applied Physiology, 83*(6), 2055-63.

Vanhatalo, A., Doust, J. H., & Burnley, M. (2007). Determination of critical power using a 3-min all-out cycling test. *Medicine & Science in Sports & Exercise, 39*(3), 548-55.

Vanhatalo, A., & Jones, A. M. (2009). Influence of prior sprint exercise on the parameters of the 'all out critical power test' in men. *Experimental Physiology, 94*(2), 255-263.

Vanhatalo, A., Jones, A. M., & Burnley, M. (2011). Application of critical power in sport. *International Journal of Sports Physiology and Performance, 6*(1), 128-36.

VanHelder, T., & Radomski, M. W. (1989). Sleep deprivation and the effect on exercise performance. *Sports Medicine, 7*(4), 235-47.

VanPutte, C., Regan, J., & Russo, A. (2009). *Seeley's Essentials of Anatomy & Physiology.* New York: McGraw-Hill.

Vardar, S. A., Tezel, S., Öztürk, L., & Kaya, O. (2007). The relationship between body composition and anaerobic performance of elite young wrestlers. *Journal of Sports Science & Medicine, 6*, 34-8.

Vasankari, T. J., Kujala, U. M., Rusko, H., Sarna, S., & Ahotupa, M. (1997). The effect of endurance exercise at moderate altitude on serum lipid peroxidation and antioxidative functions in humans. *European Journal of Applied Physiology and Occupational Physiology, 75*(5), 396-9.

Vautier, J. F., Vandewalle, H., Arabi, H., & Monod, H. (1995). Critical power as an endurance index. *Applied Ergonomics, 26*(2), 117-21.

Vicente-Rodriguez, G., Ara, I., Perez-Gomez, J., Serrano-Sanchez, J. A., Dorado, C., & Calbet, J. A. L. (2004). High femoral bone mineral density accretion in prepubertal soccer players. *Medicine & Science in Sports & Exercise, 36*(10), 1789-95.

Vigouroux, L., & Quaine, F. (2006). Fingertip force and electromyography of finger flexor muscles during a prolonged intermittent exercise in elite climbers and sedentary individuals. *Journal of Sports Sciences, 24*(2), 181-6.

Voet, D., & Voet, J. G. (2010). *Biochemistry*: J. Wiley.

Vogiatzis, G., De Vito, A., Rodio, A., Madaffari and M. Marchetti. (2002) The physiological demands of sail pumping in Olympic level windsurfers. *European Journal of Applied Physiology 86*, 5, 450-4, DOI: 10.1007/s00421-001-0569-x

Vogiatzis, I., Spurway, N. C., & Wilson, J. (1994). On-water oxygen uptake measurements during dinghy sailing. *Journal of Sports Sciences*, 12, 153-7.

Vrijens, J., Hoekstra, P., Bouckaert, J., & Van Uytvanck, P. (1975). Effects of training on maximal working capacity and haemodynamic response during arm and leg-exercise in a group of paddlers. *European Journal of Applied Physiology and Occupational Physiology, 34*(1), 113-19.

Wakeling, P., & Saddler, S. (1978). Aerobic capacities of some British slalom wild-water racing kayak competitors of international status. *Research Papers in Physical Education, 3*(4), 16-18.

Wall, C. B., Starek, J. E., Fleck, S. J., & Byrnes, W. C. (2004). Prediction of indoor climbing performance in women rock climbers. *Journal of Strength & Conditioning Research, 18*(1), 77-83.

Wallin, D., Ekblom, B., Grahn, R., & Nordenborg, T. (1985). Improvement of muscle flexibility. *The American Journal of Sports Medicine, 13*(4), 263-8.

Walsh, M. L. (2000). Whole body fatigue and critical power: a physiological interpretation. *Sports Medicine, 29*(3), 153-66.

Warburton, D. E. R., McKenzie, D. C., Haykowsky, M. J., Taylor, A., Shoemaker, P., Ignaszewski, A. P., & Chan, S. Y. (2005). Effectiveness of high-intensity interval training for the rehabilitation of patients with coronary artery disease. *American Journal of Cardiology, 95*(9), 1080-4.

Warren, M. P. (1980). The effects of exercise on pubertal progression and reproductive function in girls. *Journal of Clinical Endocrinology & Metabolism, 51*(5), 1150-7.

Warren, M. P. (1999). Health issues for women athletes: exercise-induced amenorrhea. *Journal of Clinical Endocrinology & Metabolism, 84*(6), 1892-6.

Warren, M. P., Brooks-Gunn, J., Fox, R. P., Holderness, C. C., Hyle, E. P., & Hamilton, W. G. (2002). Osteopenia in exercise-associated amenorrhea using ballet dancers as a model: a longitudinal study. *Journal of Clinical Endocrinology & Metabolism, 87*(7), 3162-8.

Wasserman, K. and McIlroy, M. B. (1964) Detecting the threshold of anaerobic metabolism in cardiac patients during exercise. *American Journal of Physiology 14*, 844-52.

Watson R. (1974). Bone growth and physical activity in young males. In Mazess R (ed.) International Conference on Bone Mineral Measurements. Washington, US Government Printing Office, pp. 380-5.

Watts, P., Newbury, V., & Sulentic, J. (1996). Acute changes in handgrip strength, endurance, and blood lactate with sustained sport rock climbing. *Journal of Sports Medicine and Physical Fitness, 36*(4), 255-60.

Watts, P. B. (2004). Physiology of difficult rock climbing. *European Journal of Applied Physiology, 91*(4), 361-72.

Watts, P. B., Daggett, M., Gallagher, P., & Wilkins, B. (2000). Metabolic response during sport rock climbing and the effects of active versus passive recovery. *International Journal of Sports Medicine, 21*(3), 185-90.

Watts, P. B., & Drobish, K. M. (1998). Physiological responses to simulated rock climbing at different angles. *Medicine & Science in Sports & Exercise, 30*(7), 1118-22.

Watts, P. B., Joubert, L. M., Lish, A. K., Mast, J. D., & Wilkins, B. (2003). Anthropometry of young competitive sport rock climbers. *British Journal of Sports Medicine, 37*(5), 420-24.

Watts, P. B., Martin, D. T., & Durtschi, S. (1993). Anthropometric profiles of elite male and female competitive sport rock climbers. *Journal of Sports Sciences, 11*(2), 113-17.

Weber, C. L., Chia, M., & Inbar, O. (2006). Gender differences in anaerobic power of the arms and legs-a scaling issue. *Medicine & Science in Sports & Exercise, 38*(1), 129-37.

Weiler, J. M., Layton, T., & Hunt, M. (1998). Asthma in United States Olympic athletes who participated in the 1996 Summer Games. *Journal of Allergy and Clinical Immunology, 102*(5), 722-6.

Weiler, J. M., Metzger, W. J., Donnelly, A. L., Crowley, E. T., & Sharath, M. D. (1986). Prevalence of bronchial hyperresponsiveness in highly trained athletes. *Chest, 90*(1), 23-8.

Wein, H., & Cadman, J. (1981). *The advanced science of hockey.* London: Pelham Books.

Weinberger, M. (2008). Long-acting β-agonists and exercise. *Journal of Allergy and Clinical Immunology, 122*(2), 251-3.

Wells, C. L., Scrutton, E. W., Archibald, L. D., Cooke, W. P., & De La Mothe, J. W. (1973). Physicial working capacity and maximal oxygen uptake of teenaged athletes. *Medicine & Science in Sports & Exercise, 5*(4), 232-41.

Wells, J. C. K. (2000). A Hattori chart analysis of body mass index in infants and children. *International Journal of Obesity, 24*(3), 325-9.

Welsh, R. S., Mark Davis, J., Burke, J. R., & Williams, H. G. (2002). Carbohydrates and physical/mental performance during intermittent exercise to fatigue. *Medicine & Science in Sports & Exercise, 34*(4), 723-31.

Welsman, J. R., Armstrong, N., Nevill, A. M., Winter, E. M., & Kirby, B. J. (1996). Scaling peak VO2 for differences in body size. *Medicine and Science in Sports and Exercise, 28*(2), 259-65.

Weltman, A., Janney, C., Rians, C. B., Strand, K., Berg, B., Tippitt, S., Wise, J., Cahill, B. R. & Katch, F. I. (1986). The effects of hydraulic resistance strength training in pre-pubertal males. *Medicine and Science in sports and Exercise, 18*(6), 629-38.

Weltman, A., Stamford, B. A., Moffatt, R. J., & Katch, V. L. (1977). Exercise recovery, lactate removal, and subsequent high intensity exercise performance. *Research Quarterly in Exercise and Sport, 48*(4), 786-96.

Werner, I., & Gebert, W. (2000). Blood lactate responses to competitive climbing. In Messenger, N., Patterson, W. and Brook, D. *The Science of Climbing and Mountaineering.* Champaign, ILL: Human Kinetics.

White, C., & Rollitt, P. (2009). Judo. *Combat Sports Medicine,* 1-16.

Wilber, R. L., Zawadzki, K. M., Kearney, J. A. Y. T., Shannon, M. P., & Disalvo, D. (1997). Physiological profiles of elite off-road and road cyclists. *Medicine & Science in Sports & Exercise, 29*(8), 1090-94.

William Sheel, A., Seddon, N., Knight, A., McKenzie, D. C., & R Warburton, D. E. (2003). Physiological responses to indoor rock-climbing and their relationship to maximal cycle ergometry. *Medicine & Science in Sports & Exercise, 35*(7), 1225-31.

Williams, A. D., Cribb, P. J., Cooke, M. B., & Hayes, A. (2008). The effect of ephedra and caffeine on maximal strength and power in resistance-trained athletes. *Journal of Strength & Conditioning Research, 22*(2), 464.

Williams, C. A., Dekerle, J., McGawley, K., Berthoin, S., & Carter, H. (2008). Critical power in adolescent boys and girls-an explor-

atory study. *Applied Physiology, Nutrition, and Metabolism, 33*(6), 1105-11.

Williams, C. A., Doust, J. H., & Hammond, A. (2006). Power output and VO 2 responses during 30 s maximal isokinetic cycle sprints at different cadences in comparison to the Wingate test. *Isokinetics and Exercise Science, 14*(4), 327-33.

Williams, E. S., Taggart, P., & Carruthers, M. (1978). Rock climbing: observations on heart rate and plasma catecholamine concentrations and the influence of oxprenolol. *British Journal of Sports Medicine, 12*(3), 125-8.

Williams, J. R., Armstrong, N., & Kirby, B. J. (1992). The influence of the site of sampling and assay medium upon the measurement and interpretation of blood lactate responses to exercise. *Journal of Sports Sciences, 10*(2), 95-107.

Williams, L. R. T., & Walmsley, A. (2000). Response timing and muscular coordination in fencing: a comparison of elite and novice fencers. *Journal of Science and Medicine in Sport, 3*(4), 460-75.

Williams, M. H. (1998). *The ergogenics edge: pushing the limits of sports performance.* Champaign, ILL: Human Kinetics.

Willoughby, K. L., Dodd, K. J., & Shields, N. (2009). A systematic review of the effectiveness of treadmill training for children with cerebral palsy. *Disability & Rehabilitation, 31*(24), 1971-9.

Wilmore, J. H., & Costill, D. L. (1993). *Training for sport and activity: The physiological basis of the conditioning process.* Champaign, ILL: Human Kinetics.

Wilmore, J. H., & Costill, D. L. (2004). *Physiology of sport and exercise.* Champaign, ILL: Human Kinetics.

Wilmore, J. H., Costill, D. L., & Kenney, W. L. (2008). *Physiology of sport and exercise.* Champaign, ILL: Human Kinetics.

Wilson, G. J., Newton, R. U., Murphy, A. J., & Humphries, B. J. (1993). The optimal training load for the development of dynamic athletic performance. *Medicine and Science in sports and Exercise, 25*(11), 1279-86.

Wilson, K. (1978). *The games climbers play.* Diadem Books Ltd.

Wilson, K., Snydmiller, G., Game, A., Quinney, A., & Bell, G. (2010). The development and reliability of a repeated anaerobic cycling test in female ice hockey players. *Journal of Strength & Conditioning Research, 24*(2), 580-84.

Wisloff, U., Stoylen, A., Loennechen, J. P., Bruvold, M., Rognmo, O., Haram, P. M., Tjonna, A. E., Helgerud, J., Slordahl, S. A. & Lee, S. J. (2007). Superior cardiovascular effect of aerobic interval training versus moderate continuous training in heart failure patients: a randomized study. *Circulation, 115*(24), 3086-94.

Wittekind, A. L., & Beneke, R. (2009). Effect of warm-up on run time to exhaustion. *Journal of Science and Medicine in Sport, 12*(4), 480-84.

Wollstein, J., & Ellis, L. (1995). Applied physiology and fitness training for all squash players. *Australian Squash Coach* (Autumn), 5-7.

Wong, P., Chamari, K., & Wisløff, U. (2010). Effects of 12-week on-field combined strength and power training on physical performance among U-14 young soccer players. *Journal of Strength & Conditioning Research, 24*(3), 644-52.

Wood, L., Dixon, S. J., Grant, C., & Armstrong, N. (2006). Elbow flexor strength, muscle size, and moment arms in prepubertal boys and girls. *Pediatric Exercise Science, 18*(4), 457-69.

Woolford, S., & Angove, M. (1992). Game intensities in elite level netball: position specific trends. *Sports Coach, 15*, 28-32.

Wright, F. V., Boschen, K., & Jutai, J. (2005). Exploring the comparative responsiveness of a core set of outcome measures in a school based conductive education programme. *Child: Care, Health and Development, 31*(3), 291-302.

Yeh, M. P., Gardner, R. M., Adams, T. D., Yanowitz, F. G., & Crapo, R. O. (1983). 'Anaerobic threshold': problems of determination and validation. *Journal of Applied Physiology, 55*(4), 1178-86.

Young, W., Cormack, S., & Crichton, M. (2011). Which jump variables should be used to assess explosive leg muscle function? *International Journal of Sports Physiology and Performance, 6*(1), 51-7.

Zafeiridis, A., Dalamitros, A., Dipla, K., Manou, V., Galanis, N., & Kellis, S. (2005). Recovery during high-intensity intermittent anaerobic exercise in boys, teens, and men. *Medicine & Science in Sports & Exercise, 37*(3), 505-12.

Zafeiridis, A. Z. A., Rizos, S. R. S., Sarivasiliou, H. S. H., Kazias, A. K. A., Dipla, K. D. K., & Vrabas, I. S. V. I. S. (2011). The extent of aerobic system activation during continuous and interval exercise protocols in young adolescents and men. *Applied Physiology, Nutrition, and Metabolism, 36*(1), 128-36.

Zagatto, A. M., Beck, W. R., & Gobatto, C. A. (2009). Validity of the running anaerobic sprint test for assessing anaerobic power and predicting short-distance performances. *Journal of Strength & Conditioning Research, 23*(6), 1820-27.

Zanconato, S., Buchthal, S., Barstow, T. J., & Cooper, D. M. (1993). 31P-magnetic resonance spectroscopy of leg muscle metabolism during exercise in children and adults. *Journal of Applied Physiology, 74*(5), 2214-18.

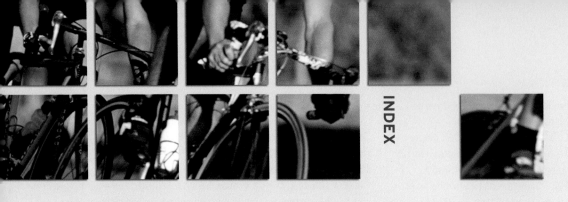